Advanced Researches in Medicine

Advanced Researches in Medicine

Editor: Anthony Clive

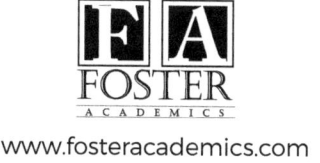

www.fosteracademics.com

www.fosteracademics.com

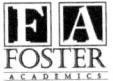
FOSTER
ACADEMICS

Cataloging-in-Publication Data

Advanced researches in medicine / edited by Anthony Clive.
    p. cm.
Includes bibliographical references and index.
ISBN 978-1-63242-518-8
1. Medicine. 2. Medical sciences. I. Clive, Anthony.
R129 .A38 2018
610--dc23

Foster Academics,
118-35 Queens Blvd., Suite 400,
Forest Hills, NY 11375, USA

ISBN 978-1-63242-518-8 (Hardback)

Contents

Preface

This book has been a concerted effort by a group of academicians, researchers and scientists, who have contributed their research works for the realization of the book. This book has materialized in the wake of emerging advancements and innovations in this field. Therefore, the need of the hour was to compile all the required researches and disseminate the knowledge to a broad spectrum of people comprising of students, researchers and specialists of the field.

Medicine as a field of science refers to the diagnosis, treatment, and prevention of varied disorders and diseases. It is a complex study of drugs that are used to treat lethal illnesses like cancer, tumor or non-lethal diseases like common cold, polio, etc. The aim of this text is to present researches that have transformed this discipline and aided its advancement. It will prove helpful to the students by providing information about the various advances and concepts related to the subjects. Different approaches, evaluations, methodologies and advanced studies on medicine have been included in it.

At the end of the preface, I would like to thank the authors for their brilliant chapters and the publisher for guiding us all-through the making of the book till its final stage. Also, I would like to thank my family for providing the support and encouragement throughout my academic career and research projects.

Editor

Comorbid Obsessive-Compulsive Symptoms in Schizophrenia: Insight into Pathomechanisms Facilitates Treatment

Mathias Zink

Central Institute of Mental Health, Department of Psychiatry and Psychotherapy, Medical Faculty Mannheim, Heidelberg University, P.O. Box 12 21 20, 68072 Mannheim, Germany

Correspondence should be addressed to Mathias Zink; mathias.zink@zi-mannheim.de

Academic Editor: Stephen J. Glatt

Insight into the biological pathomechanism of a clinical syndrome facilitates the development of effective interventions. This paper applies this perspective to the important clinical problem of obsessive-compulsive symptoms (OCS) occurring during the lifetime diagnosis of schizophrenia. Up to 25% of schizophrenia patients suffer from OCS and about 12% fulfil the diagnostic criteria of obsessive-compulsive disorder (OCD). This is accompanied by marked subjective burden of disease, high levels of anxiety, depression and suicidality, increased neurocognitive impairment, less favourable levels of social and vocational functioning, and greater service utilization. Comorbid patients can be assigned to heterogeneous subgroups. It is assumed that second generation antipsychotics (SGAs), most importantly clozapine, might aggravate or even induce second-onset OCS. Several epidemiological and pharmacological arguments support this assumption. Specific genetic risk factors seem to dispose patients with schizophrenia to develop OCS and risk-conferring polymorphisms has been defined in *SLC1A1*, *BDNF*, *DLGAP3*, and GRIN2B and in interactions between these individual genes. Further research is needed with detailed characterization of large samples. In particular interactions between genetic risk constellations, pharmacological and psychosocial factors should be analysed. Results will further define homogeneous subgroups, which are in need for differential causative interventions. In clinical practise, schizophrenia patients should be carefully monitored for OCS, starting with at-risk mental states of psychosis and longitudinal follow-ups, hopefully leading to the development of multimodal therapeutic interventions.

1. Introduction

1.1. Insight into Biological Mechanisms of Diseases

1.1.1. Mental Disorders Are a Major Cause of Disability. Clinical research in psychiatry has achieved some important progress both in pathogenetic concepts and in therapeutic interventions over the past decades. However, compared to other medical illnesses and disciplines biological mechanisms of psychiatric disorders are still poorly understood. This leads to a lack of innovative therapeutic interventions in psychiatry compared, for example, to general medicine [1]. Relating to schizophrenia, the market approval of first and second generation antipsychotics (FGA, SGA) has to be acknowledged as the last important and seminal innovation in treatment. Besides pharmacological interventions [2], cognitive behavioral therapy (CBT) is still scarcely implemented in the clinical management, although it is supported by convincing evidence and current treatment guideline recommends its use in schizophrenia [3–8]. As a consequence of missing treatment improvement, problems caused by stigmatization are still apparent today [9].

Differences in the degrees of insight into the biological mechanism of diseases lead to marked differences of effective treatment conditions in general medicine and in psychiatry. Compared to other chronic disorders such as hypertensive heart disease, diabetes mellitus, or even cancer, treatment of schizophrenia is confined to a small number of substances and pharmacological mechanisms. Noteworthy, the effect sizes achieved with core psychopharmacological agents are often in the range of medial and sometimes large improvements [10]. However, the last decades have shown that the time needed for innovative drug development and market approval is much longer in psychiatry [1].

Few examples from general medicine might elucidate how basic research of disease mechanisms facilitated the development of causative treatment: treatment of hypertension gained profit from insight into the regulation of blood pressure by the renin-angiotensin system. As a result of these findings entirely new substances could be developed. In diabetes, several additive mechanisms are currently used for treatment, starting with metformin, sulfonylurea, thiazolidinediones, glucagon-like receptor 1 antagonists, and different formulations of insulin. Finally, the multimodal treatment of cancer implemented antibody-based cytostatic substances based on molecular targets which had been defined in careful basic research.

Of course, in other medical areas, such as several subtypes of cancer, Huntington's disease, and subtypes of dementia the insight into the molecular mechanism did not yet result in causative treatment. In general, further research seems necessary in order to define molecular targets for interventions. This is especially true for major psychiatric conditions such as schizophrenia or obsessive-compulsive disorder (OCD) and even more for their comorbidity.

1.2. Pathogenic Concepts on Schizophrenia and Obsessive-Compulsive Disorder. Schizophrenia [11] is perceived as a common final clinical manifestation of several different and heterogenous neurobiological processes. The interaction of genetic and environmental factors is considered to be of critical importance. Genetic properties alter early neural development and elicit long-lasting effects due to persisting plastic processes of pre- and perinatal development [12–14]. In a neurochemical perspective, alterations of dopaminergic, serotonergic, and amino acid neurotransmission have been defined within the modified dopamine [15] or the glutamate hypothesis of schizophrenia [16, 17]. The final phenotypic manifestation of a psychotic episode occurs rather late in the disease progression of schizophrenia. It has been proposed that therapeutic interventions addressing the early stages of early events in disease progression might be even more effective than curing the late phenotypic stages, namely, the psychotic episode [18, 19]. This paradigmatic change has been propagated by Insel using the term of "rethinking schizophrenia" [20].

Current concepts of OCD localize the critical pathogenic processes within the fronto-striato-thalamocortical circuitry connecting the orbitofrontal cortex (OFC), the anterior cingulate cortex, and the basal ganglia (thalamus and caudate nucleus) [21–24]. Serotonergic neurotransmission seems to play a critical role, because treatment with serotonin-specific reuptake inhibitors (SSRIs) leads to symptomatic improvement and response to cognitive behavioural therapy accompanied by alterations of the brains serotonin system [25–29]. The disease risk is largely determined by genetic factors, but the only linkage finding that has been consistently replicated refers to single nucleotide polymorphism (SNP) in the gene *SLC1A1* on chromosome 9p24, encoding the neuronal glutamate transporter EAAC1 (excitatory amino acid

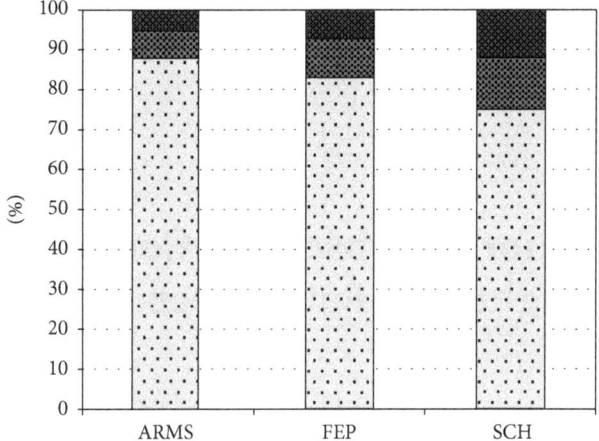

Figure 1: Estimations on prevalence of OCS and OCD according to different samples of patients. (1) Mean prevalence rates in at-risk mental state studies (ARMS). (2) Mean prevalence rates in first episode psychotic patients. (3) Mean prevalence rates in schizophrenia patients.

carrier 1) [30]. This finding supports neurochemical concepts beyond the serotonergic theory of OCD. And indeed, independent lines of evidence support the glutamatergic theory of OCD, most importantly animal models [31–34], human MR spectroscopy [35, 36], treatment approaches addressing the glutamatergic system [37–42], and finally genetic studies [43–45].

1.3. Treatment Resistance. Due to limited insight into the biological mechanisms of both schizophrenia and OCD the modes of treatment are confined to few strategies. Consequently, a large proportion of patients do not sufficiently respond to treatment, even if clinicians follow guidelines for multimodal treatment approaches in schizophrenia [2, 46, 47] or in OCD [25, 48–51]. Faced with treatment resistant patients, pharmacological strategies of polypharmacy are often used in both schizophrenia [47] and OCD [52–54].

Therefore, it is not astonishing that the comorbidity of both syndromes challenges research approaches and treatment options even more. This review has the intention to summarize the current knowledge of the pathogenesis and therapeutic options of obsessive-compulsive symptoms (OCS) in schizophrenia patients and describes necessary future research perspectives.

2. Main Part

2.1. Obsessive-Compulsive Symptoms in Schizophrenia: Epidemiology. Patients with schizophrenia have a high lifetime risk for OCS of about 25% and recent meta-analyses concluded that at least 12% also fulfil the criteria for an OCD (Figure 1) [55–63]. In contrast, in the general population the prevalence rates for OCD are only 1 to 2% [64]. Patients suffering from primary OCD carry a relatively low risk (1.7%) to develop comorbid psychotic symptoms [65].

Schizophrenia patients, who suffer from comorbid OCS, often display pronounced psychotic and sometimes treatment resistant symptoms [66, 67]. In addition, specific neurocognitive deficits have been described [68]. Comorbid patients more often utilize health care services [69] and show heightened levels of anxiety and depression leading to increased risk for suicidality [59]. These pronounced impairments increase the burden of disease; they lead to poorer social and vocational function [70–73] and a less favourable overall prognosis [74].

2.2. Differentiation between OCS and Psychotic Symptoms. Psychotic symptoms and OCS can often be clearly distinguished, but sometimes a marked overlap between dimensions of schizophrenia and the obsessive-compulsive phenotype [75] makes careful differentiation and classification of presented symptoms necessary. The clinical exploration should focus on several aspects that help discriminate delusions or hallucinations from typical OCS to ensure valid and reliable diagnosis [76, 77]. Delusions are defined by the characteristics of certainty, incorrigibility, and impossibility or falsity of their content. The subjects believe in them with absolute conviction, despite compelling counterarguments or proof of the contrary. Thus, delusions describe implausible, bizarre, or patently untrue "facts." Hallucinations are perceived with the character of sensory information originating from an external source. The subject classically attributes this thought content not to his own thinking. In contrast to these psychotic symptoms, obsessions and compulsions are intrusive thoughts/actions that originate from the subjects' own thinking. The patients report insight into the unreasonable nature and try to resist or ignore them. In clinical practice several aspects have to be kept in mind.

The Criterion of Insight. Patients suffering from OCD typically fulfil the abovementioned three symptom characteristics: they attribute the obsessions, impulsive symptoms, and compulsions to their own thinking, declare with insight their unreasonableness, and show some degree of resistance against them. The first characteristics allow a differentiation from hallucinations and delusions. Ruminations or stereotypic egodystonic cognitions with direct relation with the contents of psychotic thinking should not be diagnosed as obsessions.

Stereotypic Behaviour with Relations with the Psychotic Thought Content or Compulsions. Cleaning or checking behaviour should only be diagnosed as compulsions if it is accompanied by typical obsessions and not, if the patient currently suffers from delusions of contamination, intoxication or infection.

Obsessions Presented as Pseudohallucinations. A subgroup of OCS patients experiences their obsessions as extremely aversive and burdening. These patients may try to distance themselves by using expressions such as "voices" or "foreign

thought content," but in most cases these phenomena can be characterized as pseudohallucinations and differ on a phenomenological level from true hallucinations.

Reevaluation of OCS after Remission of Psychotic Symptoms. OCS might manifest for the first time simultaneously with the first psychotic exacerbation. Here, the final decision whether the patient really suffers from a valid comorbid condition should be postponed until the remission of psychotic symptoms.

Differentiation of OCS from Catatonic Symptoms. Particularly catatonic schizophrenia [78] confers several problems to psychopathological assessment in daily clinical practice. Even the established psychometric scales such as the catatonia rating scale [79] and the Yale-Brown-Obsessive-Compulsive Scale [80, 81] share many symptomatic dimensions. Historically, a more precise characterization and differentiation of symptoms was achieved by an undisguised view on the natural long-term course of schizophrenia. The work of Karl Leonhard [82] provided case descriptions that allowed a clear discrimination between OCS and catatonic symptoms most importantly in patients with the so-called "manieristic catatonia."

2.3. Homogeneous Subgroups within the Large Comorbid Sample. The astonishingly large cohort of schizophrenia patients with OCS has been subdivided into several homogeneous subgroups depending on the diverse clinical course and phenotypic presentation. It appears to be necessary to focus on these subgroups with common clinical properties in order to unravel the specific interplay of genetic, psychosocial, and pharmacological factors. The subdivision into such subgroups can be guided by rather simple clinical criteria, such as the time point of first manifestation of comorbid OCS and the clinical course over time.

2.3.1. First Manifestation of OCS. The onset of OCS has been described at different stages during the course of the psychotic disorder:

(1) before psychosis as an independent, coexisting syndrome and diagnosed as OCD;

(2) prior to psychotic manifestation as part of the at-risk mental state (ARMS);

(3) in parallel to the first manifestation of psychosis;

(4) during the course of chronic schizophrenia;

(5) as markedly aggravated or second-onset (*de novo*) OCS after initiation of antipsychotic treatment.

A remarkably large subgroup of patients already suffers from OCS during the ARMS, as recently summarized [83]. The mean prevalence of all reported sample-size weighed rates results in 12.1% (CI: 9.4 to 14.8%) of ARMS patients who report OCS [84–88], whereas 5.2% (CI: 4.1 to 6.3%) fulfil the criteria for OCD [84, 86–92] (Figure 1). In first episode patients slightly higher averaged rates can be found for OCS (17.1%, CI: 14.0 to 20.2) and OCD (7.3%, CI: 5.3

to 9.3%) (Figure 1) [70, 83, 88, 88, 93–95]. Epidemiological data in the referred individual studies largely vary. This might be explained by differences in the ARMS criteria used and differences in the definition and psychometric assessment of OCS or OCD. OCS during the ARMS seems to have an important impact on other clinical variables, but so far findings have been rather heterogeneous. Consistent results have been reported for higher impairment of psychosocial functioning [85, 89, 91, 94] and more severe depressive symptoms [70, 86, 89, 96] in cases with comorbid OCS. In contrast, results investigating the effect of OCS on the transition rates into psychosis [86, 90, 91, 96] have been contradicting. Only preliminary data existed regarding the influence on cognition [85, 96, 97], until the interventional study PREVENT (Secondary Prevention of Schizophrenia: A Randomized Controlled Trial [84]) allowed a multidimensional assessment of a large cohort [83]. Within a sample of 233 ARMS patients 26 patients fulfilled the DSM-IV criteria for concurrent OCD or had a lifetime history of at least subclinical OCS. They were more severely impaired in psychosocial functioning and general psychopathology but not regarding affective symptoms and neurocognitive abilities. Apart from OCS during the ARMS several studies investigated the cooccurrence of OCS during manifest schizophrenia. Whereas some patients experience OCS onset simultaneously with the first episode of psychosis, another and often underestimated subgroup reports OCS development after treatment-start with SGAs. In these cases, a typical order of three events can be observed: first "onset of psychosis," second "start with SGA treatment," and subsequently "*de novo* development of OCS." This sequence suggests the involvement of pharmacodynamic mechanisms in the pathogenesis of OCS in this subgroup of schizophrenia patients (see Figure 2(5) and detailed description in Section 2.6).

2.3.2. Clinical Course of OCS over Time. Not only do the time points of first manifestation of OCS differ between subgroups of comorbid patients, but also the longitudinal course of symptom severity differs (Figure 2). OCS may present as fluctuating symptoms; they may resolve, persist, or even worsen over time. Within patients who reported manifest OCD prior to the psychotic illness, for example, adolescents, OCS most likely persisted or worsened independently of the course of schizophrenia [98]. Only few longitudinal studies investigated quantitative changes of OCS severity within the course of schizophrenia. One large investigation from the Netherlands evaluated participants over a period of 5 years and described a predominantly fluctuating course of OCS severity in over 70% of the comorbid sample: some patients experienced the remission of OCS and others experienced a fluctuating, more or less cyclic course, more or less cyclic course. Smaller groups reported first onset of OCS or persisting symptom severity [70]. A second longitudinal study in a German sample investigated schizophrenia patients during treatment with different modes of antipsychotic monotherapy. Schirmbeck et al. found persisting OCS severity over 12 months in the group treated with clozapine (CLZ) and olanzapine (OLZ) in contrast to low comorbidity rates in the

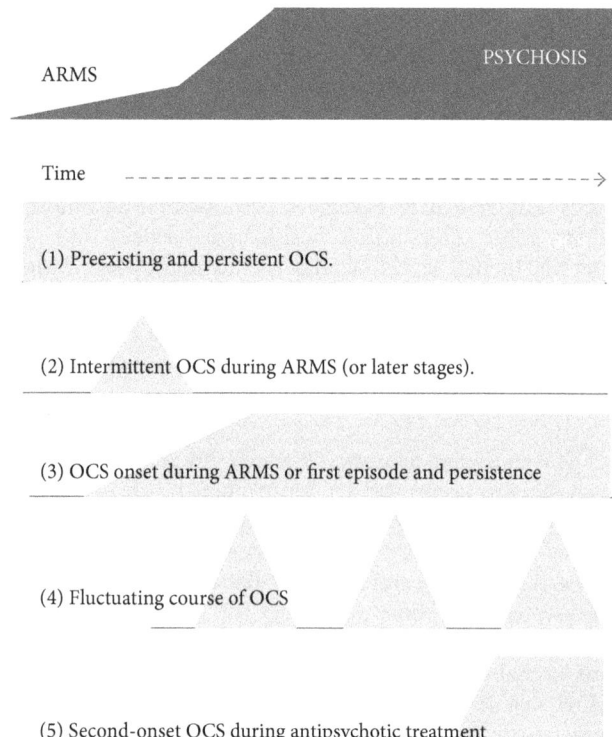

FIGURE 2: Schematic diagram on onset and course of OCS related to stages of schizophrenia. Bright-gray symbols indicate the onset and severity of OCS, dark-gray symbols are related to the at-risk mental state of psychosis (ARMS), the upcoming first episode of schizophrenia or its chronic course. (1) Preexisting and persistent OCS. (2) Intermittent OCS during ARMS or later in the clinical course. (3) OCS onset during ARMS and persistent course, strongly associated with the psychotic symptoms (schizo-obsessive concept). (4) Fluctuating course of OCS. (5) Second-onset OCS during antipsychotic treatment.

group treated with amisulpride (AMS) or aripiprazole (APZ) [68, 99].

In conclusion, the diverse clinical course adds to the heterogeneous clinical presentation and suggests an involvement of different aetiological factors. The influence of environmental factors and/or interactions of psychopathological symptoms on the longitudinal development of comorbid OCS in schizophrenia can be assumed but needs further investigation (see Section 3.1.2).

2.4. Heterogeneous Pathogenic Concepts. On the basis of different time points of first onset and different clinical courses over time, several pathogenetic concepts have been proposed. The proposed theories often overlap in important aspects but sometimes also contradict each other.

The two rather common psychiatric syndromes could of course manifest together by chance, representing a random association. However, based on the abovementioned high prevalence rates and the highly diverse clinical presentations this cannot be the only explanation for OCS in nearly every fourth patient with schizophrenia.

In general, nosological concepts of OCD substantially changed during the history of psychopathology. French and German pioneers of psychiatry published very divergent theories in the 19th and 20th century [100]. The relationship between OCD and the delusional spectrum and the so-called unitary psychosis was a major matter of discussion. Some authors assumed that patients with schizophrenia might develop OCS as an attempt to reduce psychotic symptoms. Thus, the presence of OCS was proposed to have protective effects regarding psychotic disintegration. These explanations were based on single-case analyses or small case series [101, 102]. Quite in line with these statements, Guillem et al., who applied reliable methods of psychopathology and epidemiology, described negative correlations between specific OCS and the severity of psychotic disorganization in thinking and behaviour and proposed compensating mechanisms [103]. In a broader perspective, subsequent research revealed the abovementioned negative impact of comorbid OCS on general severity of illness; for example, a higher severity of psychotic symptoms and more functional impairment of OCS were present [66] (see above).

The cooccurrence of the syndromes might be approached from both the OCD and the schizophrenia spectrum, resulting in different semantic and nosological concepts. In the OCD spectrum perspective, the concept of "schizotypic OCD" has been described [104, 105]. Here authors assume a complex association of primary OCD with schizotypal personality disorder, which meets DSM related criteria. This subgroup of primary OCD patients presents beliefs, which can be classified on a spectrum between obsessions and delusions [100]. They are emphasizing the similarities as being irrational thoughts, the first with insight and the latter lacking insight. Quite similarly, the category of "obsessions without insight" has been integrated into the fourth edition of the Diagnostic and Statistical Manual (DSM IV). It has been hypothesized that OCD patients without insight might represent a subgroup with genetic, phenotypic, and therapeutic vicinity to the schizophrenia-like spectrum [106, 107].

Approaching the cooccurrence from the schizophrenia spectrum, Poyurovsky et al. proposed the so-called "schizo-obsessive" subtype of psychosis, based on careful cross-sectional evaluations [108]. Patients with this subtype are thought to suffer from OCS in addition to positive, negative, and cognitive schizophrenia symptoms [62]. Hwang et al. [109], Bottas et al. [110], and Reznik et al. [111, 112] published similar concepts. So far, the attempts to validate the "schizo-obsessive" subtype on a neurobiological level have been inconsistent. Some but by far not all studies were able to describe specific neurological features [113, 114], cognitive deficits [115, 116], and even structural abnormalities [117].

Finally, the mentioned high prevalence rates of OCS during the ARMS led to the assumption that specific OCS could be a part of the ARMS, in particular the basic symptom cluster in the early course of schizophrenia [118, 119].

The summarized pathogenic concepts reflect the high degree of heterogeneity within the comorbid sample. At present, the number of publications on this topic nearly doubles every year. The main attempt of current research is to elucidate pathogenic mechanisms in order to better understand the diversity in time of onset, clinical course over time, and pathogenic concepts.

2.5. Underlying Neurobiological Mechanisms and Environmental Factors. Whereas the above described explanatory concepts mainly follow a clinical or psychopathological rationale, several investigations focus on a neurobiological perspective. So far, most emphasis has been given to neuropsychology, namely, a multimodal neurocognitive characterization. Preliminary investigations of neurological soft signs [113, 114] and neuroimaging techniques [117, 120] need replication.

2.5.1. Neurocognitive Correlates of OCS in Schizophrenia. In primary OCD specific neurocognitive deficits have consistently been replicated. Especially cognitive shifting abilities, inhibitory control, and the application of effective planning strategies have been described as core cognitive domains [121]. Therefore, the question arose whether OCS in schizophrenia might also be linked to additional cognitive impairment in these OCD-related domains [59]. Several authors tried to differentiate schizophrenia samples with versus without comorbid OCS regarding neuropsychological performance with partially contradicting results. Whereas several authors in some cases small investigations did not find any significant differences [55, 73, 107, 122–126], and others even suggested that OCS may be associated with better cognitive abilities [127, 128], especially in the prodromal states of schizophrenia [83, 85, 96, 97]. Most authors, however, showed more pronounced deficits in the described domains of executive functioning [109, 115, 116, 129], cognitive flexibility [130, 131], and also delayed visual memory [132, 133].

In his recent longitudinal assessment, Lysaker et al. analysed executive functioning and reported that deficits were linked to greater concurrent and prospective self-report of OCS among schizophrenia patients [115]. Our comprehensive and prospective investigation explicitly included OCD-related cognitive domains [121, 134]. Over a period of 12 months we observed that schizophrenia patients with comorbid OCS showed significant pronounced deficits with increasing effect sizes with respect to cognitive flexibility, visuospatial perception, and visual memory. In addition, performance in these domains correlated with OCS severity [68].

These neuropsychological findings have been proposed to reflect possible causal pathways. Here, it has been assumed that pronounced cognitive deficits may reflect an underlying neurobiological risk factor for schizophrenia patients to develop OCS. Within this perspective, at least partially overlapping neurobiological mechanisms with OCD have been assumed. In order to further substantiate this hypothesis neurobiological mechanisms, which might explain the pronounced deficits in the comorbid sample, should be defined. Therefore, pathogenic research should focus on candidate brain regions, which have been described in primary OCD, such as increased activation levels in the orbitofrontal cortex [135, 136] using functional magnetic resonance imaging (fMRI) approaches.

2.5.2. Functional Magnetic Resonance Imaging. Both OCD and schizophrenia patients were thoroughly investigated with different neuroimaging methods, most importantly structural and functional magnetic resonance imaging (fMRI) [135, 137, 138]. Alterations in partly overlapping brain regions were described, but the differences in disease-specific changes are out of the focus of this review. So far, only four neuroimaging studies investigated the neural correlates of OCS in schizophrenia. In a structural approach Aoyama et al. reported a significant volume reduction of the left hippocampus in schizophrenia patients with OCS [139]. Levine et al. found negative associations between OCS and the activation of the left dorsolateral prefrontal cortex during a verbal fluency task [140]. Finally, Bleich-Cohen et al. compared groups in a working memory paradigm. Independently of additional comorbid OCS schizophrenia patients performed worse and showed less activation in dorsolateral prefrontal cortex and right caudate nucleus, when compared to healthy controls [141]. Noteworthy, recruitment in these studies was solely based on the clinical phenotype not accounting for possible underlying pharmacodynamic aspects. Furthermore, no study particularly assessed the fronto-striato-thalamocortical circuitry connecting OFC, anterior cingulate cortex, thalamus, and caudate nucleus, although these regions are thought to play a core role in the pathogenesis of OCD [21, 22, 27].

In our recent investigation of neural correlates of SGA-induced OCS in schizophrenia, we stratified patients according to their antipsychotic monotherapy into two groups ((I) CLZ or OLZ; $n = 21$; (II) AMS or APZ; $n = 19$) and applied a Go/NoGo task assessing inhibitory control and an n-back task measuring working memory.

Patients of group (I) showed significantly more severe OCS and pronounced impairments in specific neurocognitive abilities. Brain activation patterns did not differ during the working memory task, but group (I) patients showed significantly increased activation in the OFC during response inhibition. These alterations in OFC activation were significantly associated with the severity of reported obsessions and impairment in specific neurocognitive tasks [120]. Further longitudinal research seems to be necessary in order to define the neural correlates of an increased risk for OCS, for specific pharmacological side effects (see below) and for specific subtypes of obsessions and compulsions.

2.5.3. Neurotransmitter Systems. Additional neurobiological mechanisms with an impact on OCS have to be acknowledged within the neurochemically defined neurotransmitter systems. Current pathogenic theories of OCD assume a central serotonergic dysfunction in the mentioned network comprising cortical, striatal, and thalamic centres [23]. Therapeutic effects of selective serotonin reuptake inhibitors (SSRIs) and cognitive behavioural therapy (CBT) on serotonergic neurotransmission in this region support this assumption [28, 29]. These findings led to the assumption that the strong serotonergic antagonism of CLZ [142–144] and OLZ [145] might constitute a pathogenic mechanism in the development of second-onset OCS in schizophrenia (for more details see Section 2.6). However, other neurotransmitter systems

also have to be considered. Alterations in dopaminergic activity [146] and in glutamatergic neurotransmission have been related to OCD: support for the involvement of glutamate in the development of OCD [38] comes from animal models [31, 32, 34], human MR spectroscopy [35, 36], treatment approaches addressing the glutamatergic system [37, 39–42], and genetic studies.

2.5.4. Genetic Disposition. While schizophrenia and OCD are common psychiatric disorders with strong heritability [44, 45, 147, 148], the results of family and molecular studies of both disorders do not show much overlap. Regarding OCD genetic association studies on candidate genes of serotonergic and dopaminergic neurotransmission were rather ambiguous. So far, the only linkage finding, which has been consistently replicated, refers to single nucleotide polymorphism (SNP) in the gene *SLC1A1* (solute carrier family) on chromosome 9p24, encoding the neuronal glutamate transporter EAAC1 (excitatory amino acid carrier 1) [30, 149–153]. Recently, Porton et al. reported alternative splicing of SLC1A1 [33]. Three evolutionary conserved and widely expressed isoforms modulate or even inhibit glutamate uptake.

A possible genetic disposition to comorbid OCS in schizophrenia has just recently become a focus of interest (see Section 2.6.3). So far, methodological concerns such as the restriction to mainly cross-sectional evaluations and a lack of power due to small sample sizes added to inconclusive findings. Thus, progress in pathogenic understanding seems most likely if future research focuses on the multimodal characterization of homogeneous subsamples, for example, patients who develop secondary OCS during SGA treatment.

This next section summarizes evidence supporting this hypothesis by reporting epidemiological and pharmacological arguments as well as genetic findings.

2.6. OCS Induced by Second Generation Antipsychotics. Some patients report the mentioned schematic order of first onset or aggravation of OCS after psychotic manifestation and treatment initiation with SGAs. Thus, simple clinical exploration helps identify this homogeneous group of patients. It is important to assess the time points of onset of the first psychotic manifestation, the start of antipsychotic treatment, and the subsequent onset of OCS [99, 154, 155]. During treatment with first generation antipsychotics (FGA) this pattern has rarely been observed. Several authors proposed a pharmacodynamic mechanism and attributed OCS to the important feature of balanced antidopaminergic and antiserotonergic properties of SGAs, in contrast to the low affinity of first generation antipsychotics to serotonergic receptors [156, 157]. In addition, differential effects of FGAs and SGAs on GABAergic and glutamatergic neurotransmission have to be considered [158, 159].

The first reports on OCS as a possible side effect of SGAs [154, 160] were published by Baker et al. [161] and De Haan et al. [162]. Since then several studies showed a clear association between SGA treatment, most importantly CLZ [155], and the *de novo* occurrence of OCS [93, 133, 160, 163]. Causal

TABLE 1: SGAs induce or aggravate OCS.

Clinical observations and epidemiological arguments	
(I)	The prevalence rates of OCS in schizophrenia increased after market approval of SGAs such as clozapine.
(II)	The comorbidity rates in later stages of schizophrenia are higher than during the ARMS or at first manifestation of psychosis.
(III)	In parallel to antipsychotic treatment OCS manifest *de novo* or show a marked aggravation.
(IV)	High prevalence rates of OCS are observed during CLZ treatment.
(V)	Schizophrenia patients with SGA-induced OCS markedly contribute to the entire sample of comorbid patients.
Evidence derived from pharmacological considerations	
(I)	Pharmacodynamic properties modulate the risk for OCS: marked difference between samples treated with first generation antipsychotics or mainly dopaminergic SGAs (such as aripiprazole or amisulpride) compared to CLZ.
(II)	OCS manifest as an unfavourable drug effect *de novo* during treatment with potent antiserotonergic SGAs such as CLZ.
(III)	Indicators of a dose-effect relation: the severity of OCS is positively correlated with duration, dosage, and serum levels of CLZ treatment.
(IV)	OCS severity persists over time in patients under stable CLZ treatment.
(V)	The severity of OCS improves after reduction of CLZ dosage to minimally sufficient levels (due to augmentation or combination).

Summary of epidemiological and pharmacological arguments supporting the induction or at least marked aggravation of OCS by SGA treatment as an unfavourable side effect. CLZ: clozapine, OCS: obsessive-compulsive symptoms, and SGA: second generation antipsychotic agents.

interactions have been proposed resulting in the expression of SGA-induced OCS [154, 160].

Before describing arguments supporting a causal association between CLZ treatment and OCS development, the general significance of CLZ needs to be mentioned. Without a doubt, this SGA must be considered a highly effective and indispensable part of the antipsychotic armament [144, 164–166], especially in cases with otherwise treatment resistant psychoses [167]. Not only the CATIE study [168], but also several other studies have demonstrated its superior antipsychotic efficacy [169–172]. Therefore, CLZ is the antipsychotic of first choice in treatment of resistant schizophrenia. In addition, treatment with CLZ exerts important antisuicidal effects resulting in low mortality rates of CLZ-treated schizophrenia patients [173]. However, important metabolic and haematological side effects have to be kept in mind [169] and related to the topic of this paper the *de novo* occurrence or exacerbation of OCS under antipsychotic treatment has most often been observed with CLZ [154, 155, 163]. In order to formally prove this hypothesis, a randomized controlled trial would be necessary, according to the general criteria suggested by Hill [174]. However, due to legal and ethical restriction such a trial cannot easily be performed. Nevertheless, several epidemiological and pharmacological arguments support this assumption (for summary see Table 1).

2.6.1. Epidemiological Evidence

The Prevalence of OCS Increased after Market Approval of SGAs. The cooccurrence of OCS did not gain much clinical awareness, while treatment with different FGAs was the first-line therapy in schizophrenia. Only few investigations reported comorbidity rates in these samples [69, 71, 175, 176]. The situation markedly changed, when SGAs were formally approved for the treatment of schizophrenia, most importantly CLZ, in the 1970s in Europe and the late 1980s

in the USA [166, 177]. After this paradigmatic change in treatment, the prevalence estimations markedly increased. Of course, a potential publication bias and increased general awareness of this topic over time have to be considered. Nevertheless these data provided a first and indirect hint towards a possible interrelation.

Increased OCS Prevalence in Later Stages of Schizophrenia. Compared to ARMS and first episode samples, the prevalence estimations of OCS and OCD in manifest schizophrenia are significantly higher (12% (OCD) and 25% (OCS); see Figure 1). The higher rates in the later stages of the disease might partly be attributed to antipsychotic treatment with proobsessive SGAs.

Onset of De Novo OCS or Marked Aggravation during Antipsychotic Treatment. In several case reports and cases series, as well as systematic evaluations, the *de novo* emergence of OCS during the treatment with atypical antipsychotics, most importantly CLZ [155], has been described. Although most of these reports are limited to a simple narrative design, the number of independent observations supports the assumption of a causal interrelation.

High Prevalence Rates during CLZ Treatment and Associations Suggesting OCS Induction by SGAs. Impressively high proportions of comorbidity rates have been attributed to the pathogenic process of SGA-induced OCS by several authors. Poyurovski et al. estimated that up to 70% of schizophrenia patients treated with proobsessive SGAs develop secondary OCS [61], while Lykouras et al. reviewed published data and reported *de novo* OCS in 77% of CLZ-treated patients [154]. Further independent studies reported even higher numbers of SGA-induced OCS within their samples of comorbid patients, ranging from 29 of 39 (74%) [178] and 23 of 26 (88%) [179] to 25 of 28 patients (89%) [133]. Furthermore, retrospective assessments of the abovementioned three critical events reveal that most patients experience the onset of OCS after first manifestation of psychosis and the start with SGA treatment [180].

2.6.2. Pharmacological Evidence.
2.6.2. Pharmacological Evidence. Further pharmacological evidence contributes to the assumption of proobsessive SGA effects.

CLZ-Treated Patients Suffer from OCS More Often. When comparing patients according to their mode of antipsychotic treatment, the risk for comorbid OCS markedly differs. As reported, high prevalence rates in CLZ-treated patients [181] contrast with low rates during treatment with FGAs, for instance, haloperidol [67] or other SGAs. These diverging findings might be explained by the mentioned differences in pharmacodynamic properties, in particular regarding inherent serotonergic blockade, monoaminergic reuptake inhibition, or even partial serotonergic agonism [143, 158, 182–184]. In contrast to the high numbers of comorbid OCS during CLZ treatment, APZ, a partial dopaminergic and serotonergic agonist, was associated with an inherent antiobsessive effect in schizophrenia patients with OCS [185–189], quite similar to AMS, a dopamine D3/D2 receptor antagonist [190, 191].

In line with these results we found comorbid OCS in more than 70% of patients treated with CLZ or OLZ, whereas less than 10% of patients treated with AMS or APZ reported OCS [133]. Vice versa, grouping schizophrenia patients according to presence or absence of comorbid OCS revealed that 77% of comorbid patients were treated with CLZ, whereas only 36% of those without OCS received this substance [179]. Although these results clearly suggest an association between CLZ treatment and comorbid OCS, a possible confounding effect due to the selection of specific SGAs for specific subgroups of patients has to be considered.

Associations between Pharmacological Variables and OCS Severity. Recent research indicated a dose-effect relation. The severity of OCS was found to be positively correlated with duration, dosage, and serum levels of CLZ treatment.

Duration of Treatment. Lin et al. [178] compared CLZ-treated patients with and without comorbid OCS and found significantly longer CLZ treatment periods for the comorbid group but no difference in duration of illness. Accordingly, Schirmbeck et al. reported a positive association between OCS severity and duration of CLZ treatment [133] and de Haan et al. reported this association for OLZ [192].

Dosage and Blood Serum Levels. Similar to association with a longer treatment duration, several authors demonstrated positive correlations with dose or serum levels of CLZ [60, 133, 163, 178]. Furthermore, the reduction of daily CLZ dosage, for instance, through the combinations with another SGA, such as APZ, resulted in an alleviation of OCS severity [187, 189, 193]. Noteworthy, this observation might represent both a reduction of the suggested dose-related side effect of CLZ and a consequence of inherent antiobsessive effects of APZ. The latter assumption was supported by a *placebo*

controlled randomized trial, which showed reduced OCS severity after combination with APZ but unchanged CLZ dose during the course of the study [185].

The Longitudinal Course of OCS during Treatment with Different SGAs. A recent longitudinal study revealed differential effects of SGAs on the course of comorbid OCS. Whereas a CLZ/OLZ group showed persistently high OCS severity over a 12-month observational period, AMS/APZ group reported decrease of the initially already low symptom severity. These divergent changes resulted in significant differences between the two pharmacologically diverse groups (completer analysis: $P = 0.006$; full sample analysis: $P = 0.007$) [99].

Noteworthy, contradicting findings regarding the treatment with CLZ have been reported, where the addition of CLZ [194], an increase in CLZ dosage [154], or start with OLZ treatment [108, 195] has been associated with an alleviation of OCS severity. One explanation for these heterogeneous findings relates to the abovementioned diagnostic difficulties to differentiate between OCS and delusional or catatonic symptoms. Patients, who show obsessive ruminations or stereotypic thoughts during acute psychosis or repetitive ritualized behaviour clearly related to the patient's primary psychotic condition might indeed benefit from treatment with CLZ. Furthermore, positive effects of antipsychotics have also been reported in primary OCD, including OLZ, especially in cases with treatment resistance to serotonergic antidepressants [25, 52, 53, 196]. Nevertheless, even in treatment resistant OCD current treatment guidelines do not recommend CLZ as an augmentation strategy. It has been proposed that OCS during CLZ treatment might differ from symptoms in primary OCD [76], but assessments in large samples are missing.

In summary, reported evidence strongly suggests an association between comorbid OCS in schizophrenia and SGA treatment, in particular with CLZ. The published epidemiological and pharmacological evidence hints at causal interactions, suggesting that CLZ's strong inherent antiserotonergic properties [164, 166, 197], most importantly the antagonism at 5-HT1C, 5-HT2A, and 5-HT2C receptors [142, 143, 198], represent an relevant pathogenic mechanism. Low affinities to dopamine receptors result in a very small ratio of dopaminergic/serotonergic receptor blockade, which largely differs from other SGAs such as AMS or APZ [184, 199, 200]. Reciprocal interactions of dopaminergic and serotonergic neurotransmission with glutamatergic and GABAergic functions also need to be considered [158].

Within a broader perspective on SGA-induced OCS, additional questions arise concerning predisposing factors for OCS in schizophrenia. These might comprise external factors such as psychosocial stressors and patient-inherent characteristics (neurocognitive profile, the subtype of psychosis, the stage of the illness, any kind of affective comorbidity, or a family history for anxiety disorders). Not least, the individual genetic disposition seems to be highly important.

2.6.3. Genetic Disposition to Comorbid OCS in Schizophrenia.
2.6.3. Genetic Disposition to Comorbid OCS in Schizophrenia. Based on the replicated associations with the gene *SLC1A1*

in primary OCD patients, a South Korean research group investigated the genetic risk to develop second-onset OCS during treatment with SGAs [160]. Analyses investigating associations between specific SNPs of the candidate gene *SLC1A1* and SGA-induced OCS in this sample showed strong associations with the A/C/G dominant haplotype rs2228622/rs3780413/rs37801412. With an odds ratio of 3.96 the likelihood for patients who carried this A/C/G haplotype was almost 4 times higher to suffer from SGA-induced OCS. A replication approach in 103 schizophrenia patients of European descent could not reproduce these findings either in single marker analyses, or in haplotype analyses. Nonsignificant results and considerably smaller odds rations suggested a lack of power and the necessity that investigations in much larger samples are needed [180].

In a subsequent study, Ryu et al. further described a genetic interaction of the *SLC1A1* polymorphism with variants in the gene *DLGAP3* (disks large associated protein 3) and a link to SGA-induced OCS [201]. Another study of a Chinese sample reported an interaction of SNPs in SLC1A1 and the type 2B subunit of the N-methyl-D-aspartate receptor gene (GRIN2B), as well as significant interactions with OCS severity [202]. Finally, based on associations between the Val66Met polymorphism and OCS in schizophrenia, the brain derived neurotrophic factor (*BDNF*) has recently been proposed as a forth candidate gene [203]. So far, independent replication approaches regarding *BDNF*, *DLGAP3*, and GRIN2B have not been conducted and further studies are needed to untangle the interplay of pharmacological and genetic risk factors for OCS in schizophrenia [180, 204].

The summarized evidence from epidemiological, pharmacological, and genetic studies proves that pharmacotherapy constitutes a relevant environmental factor, which might exert proobsessive effects in schizophrenia patients. Recently, Doyle et al. [205] tried to differentiate CLZ-associated OCS from OCD symptoms in a phenotypic approach. The authors observed in their small samples prevalent "doubting" in CLZ-treated patients, while OCD patients presented predominantly with the behavioural symptom of washing.

3. Discussion of Research Perspectives

3.1. Gene and Environment Interactions. Several frequent and disabling mental disorders manifest as a consequence of both genetic and environmental factors. Schizophrenia, for instance, is commonly perceived as a result of gene and environment interactions (GxEIs), where individual genetic properties dispose to a specific liability and sensitivity for specific stressors. These could include migration to an urban surrounding, other stressful life events, or effects of psychotropic substances [11, 148, 206]. Similar concepts were suggested regarding depression [207], anxiety disorders [208, 209], and obsessive-compulsive disorder [44, 45]. Extending this perspective to common comorbidities it is even more complex and demanding to investigate whether these can also be described on the basis of GxEIs. One example has been illustrated by the described investigation of the risk to develop secondary OCS during treatment with SGAs.

3.1.1. Treatment with Proobsessive SGAs. The above summarized evidence suggests that SGAs increase the risk for secondary OCS via a pharmacodynamic mechanism and thereby represent a relevant environmental factor. Independently, a set of genetic risk constellations, particularly within the gene *SLC1A1*, seem to predispose to OCS. However, the failure to replicate the initial results in the Republic of Korea sample [160, 180] suggests that the general genetic background of a patient (Asian or European) might be of importance when a specific SGA (balance between dopaminergic and serotonergic blockade) is introduced as the treatment of choice. Furthermore, gene-x-gene interactions (SNPs in *SLC1A1*, *BDNF*, DLGAP3, and GRIN2B) also seem to play a role [201, 203] and should be considered in forthcoming studies. It is an important progress in recent neurobiological research to investigate how the interaction of these factors might influence the propensity of schizophrenia patients to suffer from comorbid OCS when being treated with SGAs.

3.1.2. Psychosocial Stressors. In addition, further nonpharmacological environmental factors should be investigated. Such factors might include psychosocial stress induced by critical life events, interpersonal factors, changes of the vocational situation, or the present state of general physical health. Fluctuation of OCS severity in the majority of first episode patients who have been followed up over 5 years [70] strongly suggests that these factors might have an effect on the severity and course of comorbid OCS. In addition, the reciprocal interaction and possible causal directions between OCS and psychotic positive, negative, and cognitive symptoms of schizophrenia must be unravelled and considered.

Detailed follow-up analyses are therefore needed. Patients, who recently reported changes in their OCS, should be investigated by means of an "Experience Sampling Method" (ESM). This approach captures the reactivity to environmental factors and the course of symptoms in detail on a day to day basis, in real life situations. Collected data will help identify the time course of symptom changes and its relation with important contextual triggers of variability.

Within this context it will also be desirable to collect DNA samples in order to analyse predisposing effects of the abovementioned polymorphism and to elucidate an increased risk for the development or aggravation of OCS after being exposed to stressful life events. Thus, combining experience sampling and genetic characterizations might markedly improve our insight into GxEI.

In conclusion, future progress might depend on two aspects. First, well defined homogeneous clinical cohorts should be defined to reduce the number of possible confounding causal factors to a minimum. The investigation of the order of symptom onset, the clinical course, pharmacological treatment, and further environmental factors should be integrated into prospective studies. Second, much larger cohorts have to be recruited in multicenter studies to investigate possible genetic risk constellations. Based on much smaller genetic risk estimations in the European sample [180], power analyses would result in group size calculations of

TABLE 2: Therapeutic interventions addressing OCS in schizophrenia.

	Early recognition and monitoring
(I)	Definition of at-risk constellations
(II)	Detection of subclinical levels of OCS or beginning cognitive impairment using sensitive sets of neurocognitive tests
(III)	Monitoring of apparent OCS
	Add-on of psychotropic agents: polypharmacy
(I)	Augmentation with antidepressants: clomipramine, fluvoxamine, and other SSRIs [level of evidence: RCTs, CS, CR] *Caveat*: additive (anticholinergic) side effects and pharmacokinetic interactions
(II)	Augmentation with mood stabilizers (lamotrigine, valproic acid) aiming at a reduction of SGA-dosage to minimally sufficient levels [level of evidence: CS, CR]
(III)	Combination of proobsessive SGAs with neutral or antiobsessive SGAs (amisulpride, aripiprazole) in order to reduce the clozapine dosage to minimally sufficient levels [level of evidence: RCT, CS, CR]
	Psychotherapy
	Cognitive behavioural therapy including exposure and response prevention [level of evidence: CS, CR]

Summary of therapeutic approaches for schizophrenia patients with comorbid OCS or OCD. The current level of empirical evidence is indicated in square brackets. CR: case report, CS: case series, and RCT: randomized controlled trial.

about five thousand participants, which would be necessary for replication.

3.2. Treatment Approaches of OCS in Schizophrenia. As proposed in the introduction, insight into the biological pathomechanisms and effects of relevant environmental variables on the development and course of OCS in schizophrenia facilitates the development of effective treatment interventions.

3.2.1. Pharmacotherapy. Based on our current knowledge, pharmacological combination and augmentation strategies have been suggested to improve comorbid OCS according to timely reviews [74, 108]. To address possible proobsessive effects of predominantly antiserotonergic SGAs, the add-on of mainly dopaminergic SGAs such as AMS and APZ has been proposed [186–190, 196, 210, 211]. Within augmentation approaches, the treatment with serotonergic antidepressants has been evaluated, for example, with the tricyclic antidepressant clomipramine [175] or with the SSRI fluvoxamine [98, 212, 213]. Results of these trials have been inconsistent with some studies reporting significant reduction of OCS, whereas others failed to observe this intended effect. Noteworthy, additive anticholinergic side effects and pharmacokinetic interactions have to be considered when combining substances. Finally, preliminary findings suggest promising results when augmenting with mood stabilizers such as valproic acid [214, 215] or lamotrigine [41, 216] (see Table 2).

3.2.2. Cognitive Behavioral Therapy. As mentioned in Section 3.1.2, results from ESM studies could provide important information for individualised interventions, including adjusted modules of cognitive behavioural therapy (CBT). However, so far, very limited data exists on the efficacy and safety of CBT for schizophrenia patients with OCS. A recent review of published case reports and case series summarized data of 30 comorbid patients, who were treated with CBT including exposure elements or just exposure and response prevention alone [7]. Results showed favourable outcome measures with significant reduction of OCD severity in 24 patients. Within the included case series by Tundo et al. [217] over 50% of individuals who received CBT were classified as "much or very much" improved. Despite adverse clinical outcomes in 10% and a total dropout rate of 20%, preliminary results suggest meaningful and marked reduction of OCS severity in 80% of participants [74] (see Table 2).

In conclusion, the available evidence is certainly limited by the small case numbers.

Although CBT including exposure and response prevention is considered treatment of first choice for primary OCD with remarkably high effect sizes [48–51], with one exception, currently available CBT manuals for OCD do not provide guidelines for the treatment of OCS in schizophrenia [218–221]. Thus, further controlled clinical trials are certainly needed.

4. Conclusions

The summarized data substantiate the conclusions that OCS is a very frequent and relevant comorbid burden in schizophrenia. The clinical presentation of the cooccurrence is very diverse, suggesting different subgroups with heterogeneous pathogenic mechanisms. First insight into GxEI has been achieved for the subgroup of patients who experienced second-onset OCS during treatment with SGAs. First insight into biological mechanism of the pathogenesis of the comorbid condition has been achieved and creates the bases for the development of innovative therapeutic intervention. Further research should expand to different subgroups of the comorbid sample integrating additional factors which will most likely have an effect on the development and course of OCS. In particular, the effects of environmental stressors and their interaction with genetic properties are incompletely understood. In perspective, a broader set of environmental and genetic variables will have to be analysed in a longitudinal fashion, starting in the ARMS. This will not only improve the characterization of parallel subgroups, but also enhance the risk prediction regarding comorbid OCS. On an individual level risk factors could be assessed aiming at an early recognition and monitoring of emerging symptoms. The definition of an individual framework of predisposing and disease-provoking factors would further have an immediate impact on the application of therapeutic interventions, including both pharmacological and CBT approaches.

Abbreviations

AMS:	Amisulpride
APZ:	Aripiprazole
ARMS:	At-risk mental state
BDNF:	Brain derived neurotrophic factor
CBT:	Cognitive behavioural therapy
CLZ:	Clozapine
CR:	Case report
CS:	Case series
DLGAP3:	Disks large associated protein 3
fMRI:	Functional magnetic resonance imaging
GxEI:	Gene and environment interaction
OCS:	Obsessive-compulsive symptoms
OCD:	Obsessive-compulsive disorder
OFC:	Orbitofrontal cortex
OLZ:	Olanzapine
SGA:	Second generation antipsychotics
SLC1A1:	Solute carrier family gene 1A1
SNP:	Single nucleotide polymorphism
SSRI:	Selective serotonin reuptake inhibitor.

Conflict of Interests

Mathias Zink received unrestricted scientific grants of the European Research Advisory Board (ERAB), German Research Foundation (DFG), Pfizer Pharma GmbH, Servier, and Bristol Myers Squibb Pharmaceuticals; further speaker and travel grants were provided from Astra Zeneca, Lilly, Pfizer Pharma GmbH, Bristol Myers Squibb Pharmaceuticals, Roche, Servier, Otsuka, and Janssen Cilag.

Acknowledgment

Dr. Frederike Schirmbeck contributed valuable comments and careful proofreading to this paper.

References

[1] T. R. Insel and E. M. Scolnick, "Cure therapeutics and strategic prevention: raising the bar for mental health research," *Molecular Psychiatry*, vol. 11, no. 1, pp. 11–17, 2006.

[2] A. Hasan, P. Falkai, T. Wobrock et al., "World Federation of Societies of Biological Psychiatry (WFSBP) Guidelines for Biological Treatment of Schizophrenia, Part 2: update 2012 on the long-term treatment of schizophrenia and management of antipsychotic-induced side effects," *The World Journal of Biological Psychiatry*, vol. 14, no. 1, pp. 2–44, 2013.

[3] W. Gaebel, M. Riesbeck, and T. Wobrock, "Schizophrenia guidelines across the world: a selective review and comparison," *International Review of Psychiatry*, vol. 23, no. 4, pp. 379–387, 2011.

[4] P. M. Grant, G. A. Huh, D. Perivoliotis, N. M. Stolar, and A. T. Beck, "Randomized trial to evaluate the efficacy of cognitive therapy for low-functioning patients with schizophrenia," *Archives of General Psychiatry*, vol. 69, no. 2, pp. 121–127, 2012.

[5] A. F. Lehman, J. A. Lieberman, L. B. Dixon et al., "Practice guideline for the treatment of partients with schizophrenia, second edition," *American Journal of Psychiatry*, vol. 161, no. 2, p. 56, 2004.

[6] F. Sarin, L. Wallin, and B. Widerlöv, "Cognitive behavior therapy for schizophrenia: a meta-analytical review of randomized controlled trials," *Nordic Journal of Psychiatry*, vol. 65, no. 3, pp. 162–174, 2011.

[7] F. Schirmbeck and M. Zink, "Cognitive-behavioural therapy for obsessive-compulsive symptoms in schizophrenia," *The Cognitive Behavioural therapist*, vol. 6, Article ID 175447, 13 pages, 2013.

[8] T. Wykes, C. Steel, B. Everitt, and N. Tarrier, "Cognitive behavior therapy for schizophrenia: effect sizes, clinical models, and methodological rigor," *Schizophrenia Bulletin*, vol. 34, no. 3, pp. 523–537, 2008.

[9] M. C. Angermeyer, H. Matschinger, and G. Schomerus, "Attitudes towards psychiatric treatment and people with mental illness: changes over two decades," *British Journal of Psychiatry*, vol. 203, no. 2, pp. 146–151, 2013.

[10] S. Leucht, S. Hierl, W. Kissling, M. Dold, and J. M. Davis, "Putting the efficacy of psychiatric and general medicine medication into perspective: review of meta-analyses," *British Journal of Psychiatry*, vol. 200, no. 2, pp. 97–106, 2012.

[11] J. van Os and S. Kapur, "Schizophrenia," *The Lancet*, vol. 374, no. 9690, pp. 635–645, 2009.

[12] H. Jakob and H. Beckmann, "Prenatal developmental disturbances in the limbic allocortex in schizophrenics," *Journal of Neural Transmission*, vol. 65, no. 3-4, pp. 303–326, 1986.

[13] H. Jakob and H. Beckmann, "Gross and histological criteria for developmental disorders in brains of schizophrenics," *Journal of the Royal Society of Medicine*, vol. 82, no. 8, pp. 466–469, 1989.

[14] T. J. Raedler, M. B. Knable, and D. R. Weinberger, "Schizophrenia as a developmental disorder of the cerebral cortex," *Current Opinion in Neurobiology*, vol. 8, no. 1, pp. 157–161, 1998.

[15] O. D. Howes, J. Kambeitz, E. Kim et al., "The nature of dopamine dysfunction in schizophrenia and what this means for treatment: meta-analysisof imaging studies," *Archives of General Psychiatry*, vol. 69, no. 8, pp. 776–786, 2012.

[16] A. D. Stan and D. A. Lewis, "Altered cortical GABA neurotransmission in schizophrenia: insights into novel therapeutic strategies," *Current Pharmaceutical Biotechnology*, vol. 13, no. 8, pp. 1557–1562, 2012.

[17] M. Zink, *Plasticity of Brain Development As A Perspective of Basic Science in Psychiatry*, Shaker, 2007.

[18] T. L. Bale, T. Z. Baram, A. S. Brown et al., "Early life programming and neurodevelopmental disorders," *Biological Psychiatry*, vol. 68, no. 4, pp. 314–319, 2010.

[19] A. Schmitt and P. Falkai, "Therapeutic targets in major psychiatric disorders revisited," *European Archives of Psychiatry and Clinical Neuroscience*, vol. 263, no. 8, pp. 619–620, 2013.

[20] T. R. Insel, "Rethinking schizophrenia," *Nature*, vol. 468, no. 7321, pp. 187–193, 2010.

[21] A. M. Graybiel and S. L. Rauch, "Toward a neurobiology of obsessive-compulsive disorder," *Neuron*, vol. 28, no. 2, pp. 343–347, 2000.

[22] S. Karch and O. Pogarell, "Neurobiologie der zwangsstörung," *Der Nervenarzt*, vol. 82, no. 3, pp. 299–307, 2011.

[23] O. Pogarell, C. Hamann, G. Pöpperl et al., "Elevated brain serotonin transporter availability in patients with obsessive-compulsive disorder," *Biological Psychiatry*, vol. 54, no. 12, pp. 1406–1413, 2003.

[24] S. Saxena, A. L. Brody, J. M. Schwartz, and L. R. Baxter, "Neuroimaging and frontal-subcortical circuitry in obsessive-compulsive disorder," *British Journal of Psychiatry*, vol. 173, no. 35, pp. 26–37, 1998.

[25] B. Bandelow, J. Zohar, E. Hollander et al., "World Federation of Societies of Biological Psychiatry (WFSBP) guidelines for the pharmacological treatment of anxiety, obsessive-compulsive and post-traumatic stress disorders—first revision," *World Journal of Biological Psychiatry*, vol. 9, no. 4, pp. 248–312, 2008.

[26] T. Nakao, A. Nakagawa, T. Yoshiura et al., "Brain activation of patients with obsessive-compulsive disorder during neuropsychological and symptom provocation tasks before and after symptom improvement: a functional magnetic resonance imaging study," *Biological Psychiatry*, vol. 57, no. 8, pp. 901–910, 2005.

[27] S. Saxena, A. L. Brody, K. M. Maidment et al., "Localized orbitofrontal and subcortical metabolic changes and predictors of response to paroxetine treatment in obsessive-compulsive disorder," *Neuropsychopharmacology*, vol. 21, no. 6, pp. 683–693, 1999.

[28] D. E. J. Linden, "How psychotherapy changes the brain—the contribution of functional neuroimaging," *Molecular Psychiatry*, vol. 11, no. 6, pp. 528–538, 2006.

[29] S. Saxena, E. Gorbis, J. O'Neill et al., "Rapid effects of brief intensive cognitive-behavioral therapy on brain glucose metabolism in obsessive-compulsive disorder," *Molecular Psychiatry*, vol. 14, no. 2, pp. 197–205, 2009.

[30] J. Veenstra-VanderWeele, S.-J. Kim, D. Gonen, G. L. Hanna, B. L. Leventhal, and E. H. Cook Jr., "Genomic organization of the SLC1A1/EAAC1 gene and mutation screening in early-onset obsessive-compulsive disorder," *Molecular Psychiatry*, vol. 6, no. 2, pp. 160–167, 2001.

[31] N. Albelda, N. Bar-On, and D. Joel, "The role of NMDA receptors in the signal attenuation rat model of obsessive-compulsive disorder," *Psychopharmacology*, vol. 210, no. 1, pp. 13–24, 2010.

[32] D. Joel, "Current animal models of obsessive compulsive disorder: a critical review," *Progress in Neuro-Psychopharmacology and Biological Psychiatry*, vol. 30, no. 3, pp. 374–388, 2006.

[33] B. Porton, B. D. Greenberg, K. Askland et al., "Isoforms of the neuronal glutamate transporter gene, SLC1A1/EAAC1, negatively modulate glutamate uptake: relevance to obsessive-compulsive disorder," *Translational Psychiatry*, vol. 3, article e259, 2013.

[34] X. W. Yang and X.-H. Lu, "Molecular and cellular basis of obsessive-compulsive disorder-like behaviors: emerging view from mouse models," *Current Opinion in Neurology*, vol. 24, no. 2, pp. 114–118, 2011.

[35] G. Starck, M. Ljungberg, M. Nilsson et al., "A ^{1}H magnetic resonance spectroscopy study in adults with obsessive compulsive disorder: relationship between metabolite concentrations and symptom severity," *Journal of Neural Transmission*, vol. 115, no. 7, pp. 1051–1062, 2008.

[36] S. P. Whiteside, J. D. Port, B. J. Deacon, and J. S. Abramowitz, "A magnetic resonance spectroscopy investigation of obsessive-compulsive disorder and anxiety," *Psychiatry Research*, vol. 146, no. 2, pp. 137–147, 2006.

[37] V. Coric, S. Taskiran, C. Pittenger et al., "Riluzole augmentation in treatment-resistant obsessive-compulsive disorder: An open-label trial," *Biological Psychiatry*, vol. 58, no. 5, pp. 424–428, 2005.

[38] M. A. Grados, M. W. Specht, H. M. Sung, and D. Fortune, "Glutamate drugs and pharmacogenetics of OCD: a pathway-based exploratory approach," *Expert Opinion on Drug Discovery*, pp. 1–13, 2013.

[39] D. L. Lafleur, C. Pittenger, B. Kelmendi et al., "N-acetylcysteine augmentation in serotonin reuptake inhibitor refractory obsessive-compulsive disorder," *Psychopharmacology*, vol. 184, no. 2, pp. 254–256, 2006.

[40] C. Pittenger, J. H. Krystal, and V. Coric, "Glutamate-modulating drugs as novel pharmacotherapeutic agents in the treatment of obsessive-compulsive disorder," *NeuroRx*, vol. 3, no. 1, pp. 69–81, 2006.

[41] M. Poyurovsky, I. Glick, and L. M. Koran, "Lamotrigine augmentation in schizophrenia and schizoaffective patients with obsessive-compulsive symptoms," *Journal of Psychopharmacology*, vol. 24, no. 6, pp. 861–866, 2010.

[42] M. Poyurovsky, R. Weizman, A. Weizman, and L. Koran, "Memantine for treatment-resistant OCD," *American Journal of Psychiatry*, vol. 162, no. 11, pp. 2191–2192, 2005.

[43] O. J. Bienvenu, Y. Wang, Y. Y. Shugart et al., "Sapap3 and pathological grooming in humans: results from the OCD collaborative genetics study," *American Journal of Medical Genetics, Part B: Neuropsychiatric Genetics*, vol. 150, no. 5, pp. 710–720, 2009.

[44] H. Nicolini, P. Arnold, G. Nestadt, N. Lanzagorta, and J. L. Kennedy, "Overview of genetics and obsessive-compulsive disorder," *Psychiatry Research*, vol. 170, no. 1, pp. 7–14, 2009.

[45] D. L. Pauls, "The genetics of obsessive-compulsive disorder: a review," *Dialogues in Clinical Neuroscience*, vol. 12, no. 2, pp. 149–163, 2010.

[46] S. Hargreaves, "NICE guidelines address social aspect of schizophrenia," *BMJ*, vol. 326, no. 7391, p. 679, 2003.

[47] M. Zink, S. Englisch, and A. Meyer-Lindenberg, "Polypharmacy in schizophrenia," *Current Opinion in Psychiatry*, vol. 23, no. 2, pp. 103–111, 2010.

[48] I. Gava, C. Barbui, E. Aguglia et al., "Psychological treatments versus treatment as usual for obsessive compulsive disorder (OCD)," *Cochrane Database of Systematic Reviews*, vol. 18, no. 2, 2007.

[49] L. M. Koran, G. L. Hanna, E. Hollander, G. Nestadt, and H. B. Simpson, "Practice guideline for the treatment of patients with obsessive-compulsive disorder work group on obsessive-compulsive disorder," *American Journal of Psychiatry*, vol. 164, no. 7, pp. 1–53, 2007.

[50] A. K. Kuelz and U. Voderholzer, "Psychotherapie der Zwangsstörung," *Der Nervenarzt*, vol. 82, no. 3, pp. 308–318, 2011.

[51] A. I. Rosa-Alcázar, J. Sánchez-Meca, A. Gómez-Conesa, and F. Marín-Martínez, "Psychological treatment of obsessive-compulsive disorder: a meta-analysis," *Clinical Psychology Review*, vol. 28, no. 8, pp. 1310–1325, 2008.

[52] M. H. Bloch, A. Landeros-Weisenberger, B. Kelmendi, V. Coric, M. B. Bracken, and J. F. Leckman, "A systematic

review: antipsychotic augmentation with treatment refractory obsessive-compulsive disorder," *Molecular Psychiatry*, vol. 11, no. 7, pp. 622–632, 2006.

[53] M. Dold, M. Aigner, R. Lanzenberger, and S. Kasper, "Efficacy of antipsychotic augmentation therapy in treatment-resistant obsessive-compulsive disorder a meta-analysis of double-blind, randomised, placebo-controlled trials," *Fortschritte der Neurologie Psychiatrie*, vol. 79, no. 8, pp. 453–466, 2011.

[54] N. A. Fineberg, T. M. Gale, and T. Sivakumaran, "A review of antipsychotics in the treatment of obsessive compulsive disorder," *Journal of Psychopharmacology*, vol. 20, no. 1, pp. 97–103, 2006.

[55] A. M. Achim, M. Maziade, É. Raymond, D. Olivier, C. Mérette, and M.-A. Roy, "How prevalent are anxiety disorders in schizophrenia? a meta-analysis and critical review on a significant association," *Schizophrenia Bulletin*, vol. 37, no. 4, pp. 811–821, 2011.

[56] P. Bosanac, S. Mancuso, and D. Castle, "Anxiety symptoms in psychotic disorders," *Clinical Schizophrenia & Related Psychoses*, vol. 18, pp. 1–22, 2013.

[57] P. F. Buckley, B. J. Miller, D. S. Lehrer, and D. J. Castle, "Psychiatric comorbidities and schizophrenia," *Schizophrenia Bulletin*, vol. 35, no. 2, pp. 383–402, 2009.

[58] E. Hadi, Y. Greenberg, and P. Sirota, "Obsessivecompulsive symptoms in schizophrenia: prevalence, clinical features and treatment. A literature review," *The World Journal of Biological Psychiatry*, vol. 13, no. 1, pp. 2–13, 2012.

[59] P. H. Lysaker and K. A. Whitney, "Obsessive-compulsive symptoms in schizophrenia: prevalence, correlates and treatment," *Expert Review of Neurotherapeutics*, vol. 9, no. 1, pp. 99–107, 2009.

[60] K. Mukhopadhaya, R. Krishnaiah, T. Taye et al., "Obsessive-compulsive disorder in UK clozapine-treated schizophrenia and schizoaffective disorder: a cause for clinical concern," *Journal of Psychopharmacology*, vol. 23, no. 1, pp. 6–13, 2009.

[61] M. Poyurovsky, A. Weizman, and R. Weizman, "Obsessive-compulsive disorder in schizophrenia: clinical characteristics and treatment," *CNS Drugs*, vol. 18, no. 14, pp. 989–1010, 2004.

[62] M. Poyurovsky, J. Zohar, I. Glick et al., "Obsessive-compulsive symptoms in schizophrenia: implications for future psychiatric classifications," *Comprehensive Psychiatry*, vol. 53, no. 5, pp. 480–483, 2012.

[63] M. Swets, J. Dekker, K. van Emmerik-van Oortmerssen et al., "The obsessive compulsive spectrum in schizophrenia, a meta-analysis and meta-regression exploring prevalence rates," *Schizophrenia Research*, vol. 152, no. 2-3, pp. 458–468, 2014.

[64] D. L. Murphy, K. R. Timpano, M. G. Wheaton, B. D. Greenberg, and E. C. Miguel, "Obsessive-compulsive disorder and its related disorders: a reappraisal of obsessive-compulsive spectrum concepts," *Dialogues in Clinical Neuroscience*, vol. 12, no. 2, pp. 131–148, 2010.

[65] L. De Haan, C. Dudek-Hodge, Y. Verhoeven, and D. Denys, "Prevalence of psychotic disorders in patients with obsessive-compulsive disorder," *CNS Spectrums*, vol. 14, no. 8, pp. 415–417, 2009.

[66] R. Cunill, X. Castells, and D. Simeon, "Relationships between obsessive-compulsive symptomatology and severity of psychosis in schizophrenia: a systematic review and meta-analysis," *Journal of Clinical Psychiatry*, vol. 70, no. 1, pp. 70–82, 2009.

[67] A. R. Sa, A. G. Hounie, A. S. Sampaio, J. Arrais, E. C. Miguel, and H. Elkis, "Obsessive-compulsive symptoms and disorder in patients with schizophrenia treated with clozapine or haloperidol," *Comprehensive Psychiatry*, vol. 50, no. 5, pp. 437–442, 2009.

[68] F. Schirmbeck, F. Rausch, S. Englisch et al., "Stable cognitive deficits in schizophrenia patients with comorbid obsessive-compulsive symptoms: a 12-month longitudinal study," *Schizophrenia Bulletin*, vol. 39, no. 6, pp. 1261–1271, 2013.

[69] I. Berman, A. Kalinowski, S. M. Berman, J. Lengua, and A. I. Green, "Obsessive and compulsive symptoms in chronic schizophrenia," *Comprehensive Psychiatry*, vol. 36, no. 1, pp. 6–10, 1995.

[70] L. De Haan, B. Sterk, L. Wouters, and D. H. Linszen, "The 5-year course of obsessive-compulsive symptoms and obsessive-compulsive disorder in first-episode schizophrenia and related disorders," *Schizophrenia Bulletin*, vol. 39, no. 1, pp. 151–160, 2013.

[71] W. S. Fenton and T. H. McGlashan, "The prognostic significance of obsessive-compulsive symptoms in schizophrenia," *American Journal of Psychiatry*, vol. 143, no. 4, pp. 437–441, 1986.

[72] P. H. Lysaker, R. S. Lancaster, M. A. Nees, and L. W. Davis, "Patterns of obsessive-compulsive symptoms and social function in schizophrenia," *Psychiatry Research*, vol. 125, no. 2, pp. 139–146, 2004.

[73] D. Öngür and D. C. Goff, "Obsessive-compulsive symptoms in schizophrenia: associated clinical features, cognitive function and medication status," *Schizophrenia Research*, vol. 75, no. 2-3, pp. 349–362, 2005.

[74] F. Schirmbeck and M. Zink, "Obsessive-compulsive syndromes in schizophrenia: a case for polypharmacy?" in *Polypharmacy In Psychiatric Practice*, M. Ritsner, Ed., ISBN 978-94-007-5798-1, Springer, 2013.

[75] M. Fink and M. A. Taylor, "The many varieties of catatonia," *European Archives of Psychiatry and Clinical Neuroscience*, vol. 251, no. 1, pp. 8–13, 2001.

[76] M. Doyle, A. N. Chorcorain, E. Griffith, T. Trimble, and E. O'Callaghan, "Obsessive compulsive symptoms in patients with Schizophrenia on Clozapine and with Obsessive Compulsive disorder: a comparison study," *Comprehensive Psychiatry*, vol. 55, no. 1, pp. 130–136, 2014.

[77] P. Oulis, G. Konstantakopoulos, L. Lykouras, and P. G. Michalapoulou, "Differential diagnosis of obsessive-compulsive symptoms from delusions in schizophrenia: a phenomenological approach," *World Journal of Psychiatry*, vol. 3, pp. 50–56, 2013.

[78] M. Fink, "Rediscovering catatonia: the biography of a treatable syndrome," *Acta Psychiatrica Scandinavica*, vol. 127, no. 441, pp. 1–47, 2013.

[79] P. Bräunig, S. Krüger, G. Shugar, J. Höffler, and I. Börner, "The catatonia rating scale I—development, reliability, and use," *Comprehensive Psychiatry*, vol. 41, no. 2, pp. 147–158, 2000.

[80] L. de Haan, B. Hoogeboom, N. Beuk, L. Wouters, P. M. A. J. Dingemans, and D. H. Linszen, "Reliability and validity of the Yale-Brown Obsessive-Compulsive Scale in schizophrenia patients," *Psychopharmacology bulletin*, vol. 39, no. 1, pp. 25–30, 2006.

[81] S. R. Woody, G. Steketee, and D. L. Chambless, "Reliability and validity of the Yale-Brown Obsessive-Compulsive Scale," *Behaviour Research and Therapy*, vol. 33, no. 5, pp. 597–605, 1995.

[82] H. Beckmann, A. J. Bartsch, K.-J. Neumarker, B. Pfuhlmann, M. F. Verdaguer, and E. Franzek, "Schizophrenias in the Wernicke-Kleist-Leonhard school," *American Journal of Psychiatry*, vol. 157, no. 6, pp. 1024–1025, 2000.

[83] M. Zink, F. Schirmbeck, F. Rausch et al., "Obsessive-compulsive symptoms in at-risk mental states for psychosis: associations with clinical impairment and cognitive function," *Acta Psychiatrica Scandinavica*.

[84] A. Bechdolf, H. Müller, H. Stützer et al., "Rationale and baseline characteristics of PREVENT: a second-generation intervention trial in subjects at-risk (Prodromal) of developing first-episode psychosis evaluating cognitive behavior therapy, aripiprazole, and placebo for the prevention of psychosis," *Schizophrenia Bulletin*, vol. 37, no. 2, pp. S111–S121, 2011.

[85] J.-W. Hur, N. Y. Shin, J. H. Jang et al., "Clinical and neurocognitive profiles of subjects at high risk for psychosis with and without obsessive-compulsive symptoms," *Australian and New Zealand Journal of Psychiatry*, vol. 46, no. 2, pp. 161–169, 2012.

[86] T. A. Niendam, J. Berzak, T. D. Cannon, and C. E. Bearden, "Obsessive compulsive symptoms in the psychosis prodrome: correlates of clinical and functional outcome," *Schizophrenia Research*, vol. 108, no. 1-3, pp. 170–175, 2009.

[87] T. Shioiri, K. Shinada, H. Kuwabara, and T. Someya, "Early prodromal symptoms and diagnoses before first psychotic episode in 219 inpatients with schizophrenia," *Psychiatry and Clinical Neurosciences*, vol. 61, no. 4, pp. 348–354, 2007.

[88] B. Sterk, K. Lankreijer, D. H. Linszen, and L. De Haan, "Obsessivecompulsive symptoms in first episode psychosis and in subjects at ultra high risk for developing psychosis; onset and relationship to psychotic symptoms," *Australian and New Zealand Journal of Psychiatry*, vol. 45, no. 5, pp. 400–406, 2011.

[89] J. E. DeVylder, A. J. Oh, S. Ben-David, N. Azimov, J. M. Harkavy-Friedman, and C. M. Corcoran, "Obsessive compulsive symptoms in individuals at clinical risk for psychosis: association with depressive symptoms and suicidal ideation," *Schizophrenia Research*, vol. 140, no. 1–3, pp. 110–113, 2012.

[90] L. F. Fontenelle, A. Lin, C. Pantelis, S. J. Wood, B. Nelson, and A. R. Yung, "A longitudinal study of obsessive-compulsive disorder in individuals at ultra-high risk for psychosis," *Journal of Psychiatric Research*, vol. 45, no. 9, pp. 1140–1145, 2011.

[91] P. Fusar-Poli, B. Nelson, L. Valmaggia, A. R. Yung, and P. K. McGuire, "Comorbid depressive and anxiety disorders in 509 individuals with an at-risk mental state: impact on psychopathology and transition to psychosis," *Schizophrenia Bulletin*, vol. 40, no. 1, pp. 120–131, 2014.

[92] I. A. Rubino, E. Frank, R. Croce Nanni, D. Pozzi, T. Lanza Di Scalea, and A. Siracusano, "A comparative study of axis I antecedents before age 18 of unipolar depression, bipolar disorder and schizophrenia," *Psychopathology*, vol. 42, no. 5, pp. 325–332, 2009.

[93] L. De Haan, A. Oekeneva, T. Van Amelsvoort, and D. Linszen, "Obsessive-compulsive disorder and treatment with clozapine in 200 patients with recent-onset schizophrenia or related disorders," *European Psychiatry*, vol. 19, no. 8, p. 524, 2004.

[94] L. de Haan, B. Sterk, and R. van der Valk, "Presence of obsessive compulsive symptoms in first-episode schizophrenia or related disorders is associated with subjective well-being and quality of life," *Early Intervention in Psychiatry*, vol. 7, no. 3, pp. 285–290, 2013.

[95] M. Poyurovsky, C. Fuchs, and A. Weizman, "Obsessive-compulsive disorder in patients with first-episode schizophrenia," *American Journal of Psychiatry*, vol. 156, no. 12, pp. 1998–2000, 1999.

[96] L. F. Fontenelle, A. Lin, C. Pantelis, S. J. Wood, B. Nelson, and A. R. Yung, "Markers of vulnerability to obsessive-compulsive disorder in an ultra-high risk sample of patients who developed psychosis," *Early Intervention in Psychiatry*, vol. 6, no. 2, pp. 201–206, 2012.

[97] F. Van Dael, J. Van Os, R. De Graaf, M. Ten Have, L. Krabbendam, and I. Myin-Germeys, "Can obsessions drive you mad? Longitudinal evidence that obsessive-compulsive symptoms worsen the outcome of early psychotic experiences," *Acta Psychiatrica Scandinavica*, vol. 123, no. 2, pp. 136–146, 2011.

[98] M. Y. Hwang, S.-W. Kim, S. Y. Yum, and L. A. Opler, "Management of schizophrenia with obsessive-compulsive features," *Psychiatric Clinics of North America*, vol. 32, no. 4, pp. 835–851, 2009.

[99] F. Schirmbeck, F. Rausch, S. Englisch et al., "Differential effects of antipsychotic agents on obsessive-compulsive symptoms in schizophrenia: a longitudinal study," *Journal of Psychopharmacology*, vol. 27, no. 4, pp. 349–357, 2013.

[100] A. Oberbeck, K. Stengler, and H. Steinberg, "Die geschichte der zwangserkrankung: ihre stellung im wandel der psychiatrischen formenlehre bis anfang des 20. jahrhunderts," *Fortschritte der Neurologie-Psychiatrie*, vol. 81, no. 12, pp. 706–714, 2013.

[101] F. G. Dowling, M. T. Pato, and C. N. Pato, "Comorbidity of obsessive-compulsive and psychotic symptoms: a review," *Harvard Review of Psychiatry*, vol. 3, no. 2, pp. 75–83, 1995.

[102] E. Stengel, "A study on some clinical aspects of the relationship between obsessional neurosis and psychotic reaction types," *Journal of Mental Science*, vol. 91, pp. 166–187, 1945.

[103] F. Guillem, J. Satterthwaite, T. Pampoulova, and E. Stip, "Relationship between psychotic and obsessive compulsive symptoms in schizophrenia," *Schizophrenia Research*, vol. 115, no. 2-3, pp. 358–362, 2009.

[104] M. Poyurovsky, S. Faragian, A. Pashinian et al., "Clinical characteristics of schizotypal-related obsessive-compulsive disorder," *Psychiatry Research*, vol. 159, no. 1-2, pp. 254–258, 2008.

[105] M. Poyurovsky and L. M. Koran, "Obsessive-compulsive disorder (OCD) with schizotypy vs. schizophrenia with OCD: diagnostic dilemmas and therapeutic implications," *Journal of Psychiatric Research*, vol. 39, no. 4, pp. 399–408, 2005.

[106] F. Catapano, F. Perris, M. Fabrazzo et al., "Obsessive-compulsive disorder with poor insight: a three-year prospective study," *Progress in Neuro-Psychopharmacology and Biological Psychiatry*, vol. 34, no. 2, pp. 323–330, 2010.

[107] S. Tumkaya, F. Karadag, N. K. Oguzhanoglu et al., "Schizophrenia with obsessive-compulsive disorder and obsessive-compulsive disorder with poor insight: a neuropsychological comparison," *Psychiatry Research*, vol. 165, no. 1-2, pp. 38–46, 2009.

[108] M. Poyurovsky, *Schizo-Obsessive Disorder*, Cambridge University Press, Cambridge, Mass, USA, 2013.

[109] M. Y. Hwang, J. E. Morgan, and M. F. Losconzcy, "Clinical and neuropsychological profiles of obsessive-compulsive schizophrenia: a pilot study," *Journal of Neuropsychiatry and Clinical Neurosciences*, vol. 12, no. 1, pp. 91–94, 2000.

[110] A. Bottas, R. G. Cooke, and M. A. Richter, "Comorbidity and pathophysiology of obsessive-compulsive disorder in schizophrenia: is there evidence for a schizo-obsessive subtype

of schizophrenia?" *Journal of Psychiatry and Neuroscience*, vol. 30, no. 3, pp. 187–193, 2005.

[111] I. Reznik, M. Kotler, A. Weizman, and P. H. Lysaker, "Obsessive and compulsive symptoms in schizophrenia patients—from neuropsychology to clinical typology and classification," *Journal of Neuropsychiatry and Clinical Neurosciences*, vol. 17, no. 2, pp. 254–256, 2005.

[112] I. Reznik, R. Mester, M. Kotler et al., "Obsessive-compulsive schizophrenia: a new diagnostic entity?" *Journal of Neuropsychiatry and Clinical Neurosciences*, vol. 13, no. 1, pp. 115–116, 2001.

[113] M. Poyurovsky, S. Faragiae, A. Pashinian et al., "Neurological soft signs in schizophrenia patients with obsessive-compulsive disorder," *Journal of Neuropsychiatry and Clinical Neurosciences*, vol. 19, no. 2, pp. 145–150, 2007.

[114] L. Sevincok, A. Akoglu, and H. Arslantas, "Schizo-obsessive and obsessive-compulsive disorder: comparison of clinical characteristics and neurological soft signs," *Psychiatry Research*, vol. 145, no. 2-3, pp. 241–248, 2006.

[115] P. H. Lysaker, K. A. Whitney, and L. W. Davis, "Associations of executive function with concurrent and prospective reports of obsessive-compulsive symptoms in schizophrenia," *Journal of Neuropsychiatry and Clinical Neurosciences*, vol. 21, no. 1, pp. 38–42, 2009.

[116] P. H. Lysaker, G. J. Bryson, K. A. Marks, T. C. Greig, and M. D. Bell, "Association of obsessions and compulsions in schizophrenia with neurocognition and negative symptoms," *Journal of Neuropsychiatry and Clinical Neurosciences*, vol. 14, no. 4, pp. 449–453, 2002.

[117] R. Gross-Isseroff, H. Hermesh, J. Zohar, and A. Weizman, "Neuroimaging communality between schizophrenia and obsessive compulsive disorder: a putative basis for schizo-obsessive disorder?" *World Journal of Biological Psychiatry*, vol. 4, no. 3, pp. 129–134, 2003.

[118] H. Ebel, G. Gross, J. Klosterkotter, and G. Huber, "Basic symptoms in schizophrenic and affective psychoses," *Psychopathology*, vol. 22, no. 4, pp. 224–232, 1989.

[119] L. Süllwold and G. Huber, "Basic schizophrenic disorders," *Monographien aus dem Gesamtgebiete der Psychiatrie*, vol. 42, pp. 1–177, 1986.

[120] F. Schirmbeck, D. Mier, C. Esslinger et al., "Increased orbitofrontal cortex activation during treatment with pro-obsessive antipsychotic drugs," submitted to *Neuropsychopharmacology*.

[121] A. K. Kuelz, F. Hohagen, and U. Voderholzer, "Neuropsychological performance in obsessive-compulsive disorder: a critical review," *Biological Psychology*, vol. 65, no. 3, pp. 185–236, 2004.

[122] H. Hermesh, A. Weizman, S. Gur et al., "Alternation learning in OCD/schizophrenia patients," *European Neuropsychopharmacology*, vol. 13, no. 2, pp. 87–91, 2003.

[123] J. H. Meijer, M. Swets, S. Keeman, D. H. Nieman, C. J. Meijer, and L. De Haan, "Is a schizo-obsessive subtype associated with cognitive impairment?: results from a large cross-sectional study in patients with psychosis and their unaffected relatives," *Journal of Nervous and Mental Disease*, vol. 201, no. 1, pp. 30–35, 2013.

[124] P. G. Michalopoulou, G. Konstantakopoulos, M. Typaldou et al., "Can cognitive deficits differentiate between schizophrenia with and without obsessive-compulsive symptoms?" *Comprehensive Psychiatry*, vol. 55, no. 4, pp. 1015–1021, 2014.

[125] A. Tiryaki and E. Özkorumak, "Do the obsessive-compulsive symptoms have an effect in schizophrenia?" *Comprehensive Psychiatry*, vol. 51, no. 4, pp. 357–362, 2010.

[126] K. A. Whitney, P. S. Fastenau, J. D. Evans, and P. H. Lysaker, "Comparative neuropsychological function in obsessive-compulsive disorder and schizophrenia with and without obsessive-compulsive symptoms," *Schizophrenia Research*, vol. 69, no. 1, pp. 75–83, 2004.

[127] A. Borkowska, E. Pilaczyñska, and J. K. Rybakowski, "The frontal lobe neuropsychological tests in patients with schizophrenia and/or obsessive-compulsive disorder," *Journal of Neuropsychiatry and Clinical Neurosciences*, vol. 15, no. 3, pp. 359–362, 2003.

[128] M.-J. Lee, Y.-B. Shin, Y.-K. Sunwoo et al., "Comparative analysis of cognitive function in schizophrenia with and without obsessive compulsive disorder," *Psychiatry Investigation*, vol. 6, no. 4, pp. 286–293, 2009.

[129] R. Cunill, E. Huerta-Ramos, and X. Castells, "The effect of obsessive-compulsive symptomatology on executive functions in schizophrenia: a systematic review and meta-analysis," *Psychiatry Research*, vol. 210, no. 1, pp. 21–28, 2013.

[130] S. R. Kumbhani, R. M. Roth, C. L. Kruck, L. A. Flashman, and T. W. McAllister, "Nonclinical obsessive-compulsive symptoms and executive functions in schizophrenia," *Journal of Neuropsychiatry and Clinical Neurosciences*, vol. 22, no. 3, pp. 304–312, 2010.

[131] D. D. Patel, K. R. Laws, A. Padhi et al., "The neuropsychology of the schizo-obsessive subtype of schizophrenia: a new analysis," *Psychological Medicine*, vol. 40, no. 6, pp. 921–933, 2010.

[132] I. Berman, A. Merson, B. Viegner, M. F. Losonczy, D. Pappas, and A. I. Green, "Obsessions and compulsions as a distinct cluster of symptoms in schizophrenia: a neuropsychological study," *Journal of Nervous and Mental Disease*, vol. 186, no. 3, pp. 150–156, 1998.

[133] F. Schirmbeck, C. Esslinger, F. Rausch, S. Englisch, A. Meyer-Lindenberg, and M. Zink, "Antiserotonergic antipsychotics are associated with obsessive-compulsive symptoms in schizophrenia," *Psychological Medicine*, vol. 41, no. 11, pp. 2361–2373, 2011.

[134] G. Rajender, M. S. Bhatia, K. Kanwal, S. Malhotra, T. B. Singh, and D. Chaudhary, "Study of neurocognitive endophenotypes in drug-naïve obsessive-compulsive disorder patients, their first-degree relatives and healthy controls," *Acta Psychiatrica Scandinavica*, vol. 124, no. 2, pp. 152–161, 2011.

[135] L. Friedlander and M. Desrocher, "Neuroimaging studies of obsessive-compulsive disorder in adults and children," *Clinical Psychology Review*, vol. 26, no. 1, pp. 32–49, 2006.

[136] S. P. Whiteside, J. D. Port, and J. S. Abramowitz, "A meta-analysis of functional neuroimaging in obsessive-compulsive disorder," *Psychiatry Research*, vol. 132, no. 1, pp. 69–79, 2004.

[137] A. Del Casale, G. D. Kotzalidis, C. Rapinesi et al., "Functional neuroimaging in obsessive-compulsive disorder," *Neuropsychobiology*, vol. 64, no. 2, pp. 61–85, 2011.

[138] A. Meyer-Lindenberg, "From maps to mechanisms through neuroimaging of schizophrenia," *Nature*, vol. 468, no. 7321, pp. 194–202, 2010.

[139] F. Aoyama, J. Iida, M. Inoue et al., "Brain imaging in childhood- and adolescence-onset schizophrenia associated with obsessive-compulsive symptoms," *Acta Psychiatrica Scandinavica*, vol. 102, no. 1, pp. 32–37, 2000.

[140] J. B. Levine, S. A. Gruber, A. A. Baird, and D. Yurgelun-Todd, "Obsessive-compulsive disorder among schizophrenic patients: an exploratory study using functional magnetic resonance imaging data," *Comprehensive Psychiatry*, vol. 39, no. 5, pp. 308–311, 1998.

[141] M. Bleich-Cohen, T. Hendler, R. Weizman, S. Faragian, A. Weizman, and M. Poyurovsky, "Working memory dysfunction in schizophrenia patients with obsessive-compulsive symptoms: an fMRI study," *European Psychiatry*, vol. 29, no. 3, pp. 160–166, 2013.

[142] D. M. Coward, "General pharmacology of clozapine," *British Journal of Psychiatry*, vol. 160, no. 17, pp. 5–11, 1992.

[143] H. Y. Meltzer and M. Huang, "In vivo actions of atypical antipsychotic drug on serotonergic and dopaminergic systems," *Progress in Brain Research*, vol. 172, pp. 177–197, 2008.

[144] H. Y. Meltzer, "Clozapine: balancing safety with superior antipsychotic efficacy," *Clinical Schizophrenia and Related Psychoses*, vol. 6, no. 3, pp. 134–144, 2012.

[145] L. Duggan, M. Fenton, R. M. Dardennes, A. El-Dosoky, and S. Indran, "Olanzapine for schizophrenia," *Cochrane Database of Systematic Reviews*, no. 1, 2003.

[146] N. J. Van Der Wee, H. Stevens, J. A. Hardeman et al., "Enhanced dopamine transporter density in psychotropic-naive patients with obsessive-compulsive disorder shown by $[^{123}I]\beta$-CIT SPECT," *American Journal of Psychiatry*, vol. 161, no. 12, pp. 2201–2206, 2004.

[147] A. Meyer-Lindenberg, "Imaging genetics of schizophrenia," *Dialogues in Clinical Neuroscience*, vol. 12, no. 4, pp. 449–456, 2010.

[148] J. Van Os, B. P. F. Rutten, and R. Poulton, "Gene-environment interactions in schizophrenia: review of epidemiological findings and future directions," *Schizophrenia Bulletin*, vol. 34, no. 6, pp. 1066–1082, 2008.

[149] P. D. Arnold, T. Sicard, E. Burroughs, M. A. Richter, and J. L. Kennedy, "Glutamate transporter gene SLC1A1 associated with obsessive-compulsive disorder," *Archives of General Psychiatry*, vol. 63, no. 7, pp. 769–776, 2006.

[150] D. E. Dickel, J. Veenstra-VanderWeele, N. J. Cox et al., "Association testing of the positional and functional candidate gene SLC1A1/EAAC1 in early-onset obsessive-compulsive disorder," *Archives of General Psychiatry*, vol. 63, no. 7, pp. 778–785, 2006.

[151] Y. Y. Shugart, Y. Wang, J. F. Samuels et al., "A family-based association study of the glutamate transporter gene SLC1A1 in obsessive-compulsive disorder in 378 families," *American Journal of Medical Genetics B: Neuropsychiatric Genetics*, vol. 150, no. 6, pp. 886–892, 2009.

[152] S. E. Stewart, J. A. Fagerness, J. Platko et al., "Association of the SLC1A1 glutamate transporter gene and obsessive-compulsive disorder," *American Journal of Medical Genetics B: Neuropsychiatric Genetics*, vol. 144, no. 8, pp. 1027–1033, 2007.

[153] J. R. Wendland, P. R. Moya, K. R. Timpano et al., "A haplotype containing quantitative trait loci for SLC1A1 gene expression and its association with obsessive-compulsive disorder," *Archives of General Psychiatry*, vol. 66, no. 4, pp. 408–416, 2009.

[154] L. Lykouras, B. Alevizos, P. Michalopoulou, and A. Rabavilas, "Obsessive-compulsive symptoms induced by atypical antipsychotics. A review of the reported cases," *Progress in Neuro-Psychopharmacology and Biological Psychiatry*, vol. 27, no. 3, pp. 333–346, 2003.

[155] F. Schirmbeck and M. Zink, "Clozapine-induced obsessive-compulsive symptoms in schizophrenia: a critical review," *Current Neuropharmacology*, vol. 10, no. 1, pp. 88–95, 2012.

[156] H. Y. Meltzer, "Role of serotonin in the action of atypical antipsychotic drugs," *Clinical Neuroscience*, vol. 3, no. 2, pp. 64–75, 1995.

[157] H. Y. Meltzer, Z. Li, Y. Kaneda, and J. Ichikawa, "Serotonin receptors: their key role in drugs to treat schizophrenia," *Progress in Neuro-Psychopharmacology and Biological Psychiatry*, vol. 27, no. 7, pp. 1159–1172, 2003.

[158] X. López-Gil, F. Artigas, and A. Adell, "Unraveling monoamine receptors involved in the action of typical and atypical antipsychotics on glutamatergic and serotonergic transmission in prefrontal cortex," *Current Pharmaceutical Design*, vol. 16, no. 5, pp. 502–515, 2010.

[159] M. Zink, S. Englisch, and A. Schmitt, "Antipsychotic treatment modulates glutamate neurotransmission: From animal models to innovative treatment of schizophrenia," *European Archives of Psychiatry & Clinical Neuroscience*. Submitted.

[160] J. S. Kwon, Y. H. Joo, H. J. Nam et al., "Association of the glutamate transporter gene SLC1A1 with atypical antipsychotics-induced obsessive-compulsive symptoms," *Archives of General Psychiatry*, vol. 66, no. 11, pp. 1233–1241, 2009.

[161] R. W. Baker, K. N. R. Chengappa, J. W. Baird, S. Steingard, M. A. G. Christ, and N. R. Schooler, "Emergence of obsessive compulsive symptoms during treatment with clozapine," *Journal of Clinical Psychiatry*, vol. 53, no. 12, pp. 439–442, 1992.

[162] L. De Haan, D. H. Linszen, and R. Gorsira, "Clozapine and obsessions in patients with recent-onset schizophrenia and other psychotic disorders," *Journal of Clinical Psychiatry*, vol. 60, no. 6, pp. 364–365, 1999.

[163] I. Reznik, I. Yavin, R. Stryjer et al., "Clozapine in the treatment of obsessive-compulsive symptoms in schizophrenia patients: a case series study," *Pharmacopsychiatry*, vol. 37, no. 2, pp. 52–56, 2004.

[164] R. Joober and P. Boksa, "Clozapine: a distinct, poorly understood and under-used molecule," *Journal of Psychiatry and Neuroscience*, vol. 35, no. 3, pp. 147–149, 2010.

[165] J. M. Kane, "A user's guide to clozapine," *Acta Psychiatrica Scandinavica*, vol. 123, no. 6, pp. 407–408, 2011.

[166] X. Kang and G. M. Simpson, "Clozapine: more side effects but still the best antipsychotic," *Journal of Clinical Psychiatry*, vol. 71, no. 8, pp. 982–983, 2010.

[167] J. Kane, G. Honigfeld, J. Singer, and H. Meltzer, "Clozapine for the treatment-resistant schizophrenic. A double-blind comparison with chlorpromazine," *Archives of General Psychiatry*, vol. 45, no. 9, pp. 789–796, 1988.

[168] J. P. McEvoy, J. A. Lieberman, T. S. Stroup et al., "Effectiveness of clozapine versus olanzapine, quetiapine, and risperidone in patients with chronic schizophrenia who did not respond to prior atypical antipsychotic treatment," *American Journal of Psychiatry*, vol. 163, no. 4, pp. 600–610, 2006.

[169] C. A. Lobos, K. Komossa, C. Rummel-Kluge et al., "Clozapine versus other atypical antipsychotics for schizophrenia," *Cochrane Database of Systematic Reviews*, vol. 11, 2010.

[170] S. Gupta and D. G. Daniel, "Cautions in the clozapine-to-risperidone switch," *Annals of Clinical Psychiatry*, vol. 7, no. 3, p. 149, 1995.

[171] R. R. Conley, D. L. Kelly, C. M. Richardson, C. A. Tamminga, and W. T. Carpenter Jr., "The efficacy of high-dose olanzapine versus clozapine in treatment-resistant schizophrenia: a double-blind, crossover study," *Journal of Clinical Psychopharmacology*, vol. 23, no. 6, pp. 668–671, 2003.

[172] D. J. Still, P. G. Dorson, M. L. Crismon, and C. Pousson, "Effects of switching inpatients with treatment-resistant schizophrenia from clozapine to risperidone," *Psychiatric Services*, vol. 47, no. 12, pp. 1382–1384, 1996.

[173] J. Tiihonen, J. Lönnqvist, K. Wahlbeck et al., "11-year follow-up of mortality in patients with schizophrenia: a population-based cohort study (FIN11 study)," *The Lancet*, vol. 374, no. 9690, pp. 620–627, 2009.

[174] A. B. Hill, "The environment and disease: association or causation?" *Bulletin of the World Health Organization*, vol. 58, no. 5, pp. 295–300, 2011.

[175] I. Berman, B. L. Sapers, H. H. J. Chang, M. F. Losonczy, J. Schmildler, and A. I. Green, "Treatment of obsessive-compulsive symptoms in schizophrenic patients with clomipramine," *Journal of Clinical Psychopharmacology*, vol. 15, no. 3, pp. 206–210, 1995.

[176] G. Nolfe, W. Milano, G. Zontini et al., "Obsessive-compulsive symptoms in schizophrenia: their relationship with clinical features and pharmacological treatment," *Journal of Psychiatric Practice*, vol. 16, no. 4, pp. 235–242, 2010.

[177] H. Hippius, "The history of clozapine," *Psychopharmacology*, vol. 99, pp. S3–S5, 1989.

[178] S.-K. Lin, S.-F. Su, and C.-H. Pan, "Higher plasma drug concentration in clozapine-treated schizophrenic patients with side effects of obsessive/compulsive symptoms," *Therapeutic Drug Monitoring*, vol. 28, no. 3, pp. 303–307, 2006.

[179] M. Lim, D. Y. Park, J. S. Kwon, Y. H. Joo, and K. S. Hong, "Prevalence and clinical characteristics of obsessive-compulsive symptoms associated with atypical antipsychotics," *Journal of Clinical Psychopharmacology*, vol. 27, no. 6, pp. 712–713, 2007.

[180] F. Schirmbeck, V. Nieratschker, J. Frank et al., "Polymorphisms in the glutamate transporter gene SLC1A1 and obsessive-compulsive symptoms induced by second-generation antipsychotic agents," *Psychiatric Genetics*, vol. 22, no. 5, pp. 245–252, 2012.

[181] A. Ertugrul, A. E. A. Yagcioglu, N. Eni, and K. M. Yazici, "Obsessive-compulsive symptoms in clozapine-treated schizophrenic patients," *Psychiatry and Clinical Neurosciences*, vol. 59, no. 2, pp. 219–222, 2005.

[182] H. Y. Meltzer and T. Sumiyoshi, "Does stimulation of 5-HT1A receptors improve cognition in schizophrenia?" *Behavioural Brain Research*, vol. 195, no. 1, pp. 98–102, 2008.

[183] G. Remington, "Alterations of dopamine and serotonin transmission in schizophrenia," *Progress in Brain Research*, vol. 172, pp. 117–140, 2008.

[184] D. A. Shapiro, S. Renock, E. Arrington et al., "Aripiprazole, a novel atypical antipsychotic drug with a unique and robust pharmacology," *Neuropsychopharmacology*, vol. 28, no. 8, pp. 1400–1411, 2003.

[185] J. S. Chang, Y. M. Ahn, H. J. Park et al., "Aripiprazole augmentation in clozapine-treated patients with refractory schizophrenia: an 8-week, randomized, double-blind, placebo-controlled trial," *Journal of Clinical Psychiatry*, vol. 69, no. 5, pp. 720–731, 2008.

[186] K. M. Connor, V. M. Payne, K. M. Gadde, W. Zhang, and J. R. T. Davidson, "The use of aripiprazole in obsessive-compulsive disorder: preliminary observations in 8 patients," *The Journal of clinical psychiatry*, vol. 66, no. 1, pp. 49–51, 2005.

[187] S. Englisch, C. Esslinger, D. Inta et al., "Clozapine-induced obsessive-compulsive syndromes improve in combination with aripiprazole," *Clinical Neuropharmacology*, vol. 32, no. 4, pp. 227–229, 2009.

[188] S. Englisch and M. Zink, "Combined antipsychotic treatment involving clozapine and aripiprazole," *Progress in Neuro-Psychopharmacology and Biological Psychiatry*, vol. 32, no. 6, pp. 1386–1392, 2008.

[189] M. Zink, U. Knopf, and A. Kuwilsky, "Management of clozapine-induced obsessive-compulsive symptoms in a man with schizophrenia," *Australian and New Zealand Journal of Psychiatry*, vol. 41, no. 3, pp. 293–294, 2007.

[190] S.-W. Kim, I.-S. Shin, J.-M. Kim, S.-J. Yang, M. Y. Hwang, and J.-S. Yoon, "Amisulpride improves obsessive-compulsive symptoms in schizophrenia patients taking atypical antipsychotics: an open-label switch study," *Journal of Clinical Psychopharmacology*, vol. 28, no. 3, pp. 349–352, 2008.

[191] L. Pani, J. M. Villagrán, V. P. Kontaxakis, and K. Alptekin, "Practical issues with amisulpride in the management of patients with schizophrenia," *Clinical Drug Investigation*, vol. 28, no. 8, pp. 465–477, 2008.

[192] L. De Haan, N. Beuk, B. Hoogenboom, P. Dingemans, and D. Linszen, "Obsessive-compulsive symptoms during treatment with olanzapine and risperidone: a prospective study of 113 patients with recent-onset schizophrenia or related disorders," *Journal of Clinical Psychiatry*, vol. 63, no. 2, pp. 104–107, 2002.

[193] F. L. Rocha and C. Hara, "Benefits of combining aripiprazole to clozapine: three case reports," *Progress in Neuro-Psychopharmacology and Biological Psychiatry*, vol. 30, no. 6, pp. 1167–1169, 2006.

[194] B. Peters and L. de Haan, "Remission of schizophrenia psychosis and strong reduction of obsessive-compulsive disorder after adding clozapine to aripiprazole," *Progress in Neuro-Psychopharmacology and Biological Psychiatry*, vol. 33, no. 8, pp. 1576–1577, 2009.

[195] L. Van Nimwegen, L. De Haan, N. Van Beveren, W. Laan, W. Van Den Brink, and D. Linszen, "Obsessive-compulsive symptoms in a randomized, double-blind study with olanzapine or risperidone in young patients with early psychosis," *Journal of Clinical Psychopharmacology*, vol. 28, no. 2, pp. 214–218, 2008.

[196] M. R. A. Muscatello, A. Bruno, G. Pandolfo et al., "Effect of aripiprazole augmentation of serotonin reuptake inhibitors or clomipramine in treatment-resistant obsessive-compulsive disorder: a double-blind, placebo-controlled study," *Journal of Clinical Psychopharmacology*, vol. 31, no. 2, pp. 174–179, 2011.

[197] S. Steingard, K. N. R. Chengappa, R. W. Baker et al., "Clozapine, obsessive symptoms, and serotonergic mechanisms," *American Journal of Psychiatry*, vol. 150, no. 9, p. 1435, 1993.

[198] H. Y. Meltzer, "An overview of the mechanism of action of clozapine," *Journal of Clinical Psychiatry*, vol. 55, no. 9, pp. 47–52, 1994.

[199] C. U. Correll, "Antipsychotic polypharmacy, Part 2: why use 2 antipsychotics when 1 is not good enough?" *Journal of Clinical Psychiatry*, vol. 69, no. 5, pp. 860–861, 2008.

[200] B. Scatton, Y. Claustre, A. Cudennec et al., "Amisulpride: from animal pharmacology to therapeutic action," *International Clinical Psychopharmacology*, vol. 12, no. 2, pp. S29–S36, 1997.

[201] S. Ryu, S. Oh, E.-Y. Cho et al., "Interaction between genetic variants of DLGAP3 and SLC1A1 affecting the risk of atypical antipsychotics-induced obsessive-compulsive symptoms," *American Journal of Medical Genetics B: Neuropsychiatric Genetics*, vol. 156, no. 8, pp. 949–959, 2011.

[202] J. Cai, W. Zhang, Z. Yi et al., "Influence of polymorphisms in genes SLC1A1, GRIN2B, and GRIK2 on clozapine-induced obsessive-compulsive symptoms," *Psychopharmacology*, vol. 230, no. 1, pp. 49–55, 2013.

[203] H. M. Hashim, N. Fawzy, M. M. Fawzi, and R. A. Karam, "Brain-derived neurotrophic factor Val66Met polymorphism and obsessive-compulsive symptoms in Egyptian schizophrenia

patients," *Journal of Psychiatric Research*, vol. 46, no. 6, pp. 762–766, 2012.

[204] F. Schirmbeck and M. Zink, "Comorbid obsessive-compulsive symptoms in schizophrenia: contributions of pharmacological and genetic factors," *Frontiers in Pharmacology*, vol. 4, Article ID Article 99, 2013.

[205] M. Doyle, A. N. Chorcorain, E. Griffith, T. Trimble, and E. O'Callaghan, "Obsessive compulsive symptoms in patients with Schizophrenia on Clozapine and with Obsessive Compulsive disorder: a comparison study," *Comprehensive Psychiatry*, vol. 55, no. 1, pp. 130–136, 2013.

[206] J. Van Os, G. Kenis, and B. P. F. Rutten, "The environment and schizophrenia," *Nature*, vol. 468, no. 7321, pp. 203–212, 2010.

[207] R. Keers and R. Uher, "Gene-environment interaction in major depression and antidepressant treatment response," *Current Psychiatry Reports*, vol. 14, no. 2, pp. 129–137, 2012.

[208] A. M. Gregory, J. Y. F. Lau, and T. C. Eley, "Finding gene-environment interactions for generalised anxiety disorder," *European Archives of Psychiatry and Clinical Neuroscience*, vol. 258, no. 2, pp. 69–75, 2008.

[209] N. R. Nugent, A. R. Tyrka, L. L. Carpenter, and L. H. Price, "Gene-environment interactions: early life stress and risk for depressive and anxiety disorders," *Psychopharmacology*, vol. 214, no. 1, pp. 175–196, 2011.

[210] G. Eryilmaz, G. H. Sayar, E. Ozten, I. Gögcegöz, and O. Karamustafalioglu, "Aripirazole augmentation in clozapine-associated obsessive-compulsive symptoms in schizophrenia," *Annals of General Psychiatry*, vol. 12, p. 40, 2013.

[211] K.-C. Yang, T.-P. Su, and Y.-H. Chou, "Effectiveness of aripiprazole in treating obsessive compulsive symptoms," *Progress in Neuro-Psychopharmacology and Biological Psychiatry*, vol. 32, no. 2, pp. 585–586, 2008.

[212] M. Poyurovsky, V. Isakov, S. Hromnikov et al., "Fluvoxamine treatment of obsessive-compulsive symptoms in schizophrenic patients: an add-on open study," *International Clinical Psychopharmacology*, vol. 14, no. 2, pp. 95–100, 1999.

[213] I. Reznik and P. Sirota, "Obsessive and compulsive symptoms in schizophrenia: a randomized controlled trial with fluvoxamine and neuroleptics," *Journal of Clinical Psychopharmacology*, vol. 20, no. 4, pp. 410–416, 2000.

[214] F. Canan, U. Aydinoglu, and G. Sinani, "Valproic acid augmentation in clozapine-associated hand-washing compulsion," *Psychiatry and Clinical Neurosciences*, vol. 66, no. 5, pp. 463–464, 2012.

[215] M. Zink, S. Englisch, U. Knopf, A. Kuwilsky, and H. Dressing, "Augmentation of clozapine with valproic acid for clozapine-induced obsessive-compulsive symptoms," *Pharmacopsychiatry*, vol. 40, no. 5, pp. 202–203, 2007.

[216] C. I. Rodriguez, C. Corcoran, and H. B. Simpson, "Diagnosis and treatment of a patient with both psychotic and obsessive-compulsive symptoms," *American Journal of Psychiatry*, vol. 167, no. 7, pp. 754–761, 2010.

[217] A. Tundo, L. Salvati, D. Di Spigno et al., "Cognitive-behavioral therapy for obsessive-compulsive disorder as a comorbidity with schizophrenia or schizoaffective disorder," *Psychotherapy and Psychosomatics*, vol. 81, no. 1, pp. 58–60, 2011.

[218] P. M. G. Emmelkamp and P. van Oppen, *Zwangsstörungen*, Hogrefe, Göttingen, Germany, 2000.

[219] U. Foerstner, A. M. Kuelz, and U. Voderholzer, *Störungsspezifische Behandlung Der Zwangsstörungen: Ein Therapiemanual*, Kohlhammer, Stuttgart, Germany, 2011.

[220] A. Lakatos and H. Reinecker, *Kognitive Verhaltenstherapie Bei Zwangsstörungen: Ein Therapiemanual*, Hogrefe, Göttingen, Germany, 2007.

[221] C. Oelkers, M. Hautzinger, and M. Bleibel, *Zwangsst+Ârungen: Ein Kognitiv-Verhaltenstherapeutisches Behandlungsmanual*, Beltz Psychologie Verlags Union, Weinheim, Germany, 2007.

CYP4F2 (rs2108622) Gene Polymorphism Association with Age-Related Macular Degeneration

Ruta Sakiene,[1] **Alvita Vilkeviciute,**[2] **Loresa Kriauciuniene,**[2,3] **Vilma Jurate Balciuniene,**[3]
Dovile Buteikiene,[3] **Goda Miniauskiene,**[3] **and Rasa Liutkeviciene**[2,3]

[1]*Lithuanian University of Health Sciences, Medical Academy, Eiveniu 2, LT-50009 Kaunas, Lithuania*
[2]*Neuroscience Institute, Lithuanian University of Health Sciences, Medical Academy, Eiveniu 2, LT-50009 Kaunas, Lithuania*
[3]*Department of Ophthalmology, Lithuanian University of Health Sciences, Medical Academy, Eiveniu 2,*
LT-50009 Kaunas, Lithuania

Correspondence should be addressed to Ruta Sakiene; sakiene.ruta@gmail.com

Academic Editor: Xinhua Shu

Background. Age-related macular degeneration is the leading cause of blindness in elderly individuals where aetiology and pathophysiology of age-related macular degeneration are not absolutely clear. *Purpose.* To determine the frequency of the genotype of rs2108622 in patients with early and exudative age-related macular degeneration. *Methods.* The study enrolled 190 patients with early age-related macular degeneration, 181 patients with exudative age-related macular degeneration (eAMD), and a random sample of 210 subjects from the general population (control group). The genotyping of rs2108622 was carried out using the real-time polymerase chain reaction method. *Results.* The analysis of rs2108622 gene polymorphism did not reveal any differences in the distribution of C/C, C/T, and T/T genotypes between the early AMD group, the eAMD group, and the control group. The *CYP4F2* (1347C>T) *T/T* genotype was more frequent in males with eAMD compared to females (10.2% versus 0.8%; $p = 0.0052$); also *T/T* genotype was less frequently present in eAMD females compared to healthy control females (0.8% versus 6.2%; $p = 0.027$). *Conclusion.* Rs2108622 gene polymorphism had no predominant effect on the development of early AMD and eAMD. The *T/T* genotype was more frequent in males with eAMD compared to females and less frequently present in eAMD females compared to healthy females.

1. Introduction

Age-related macular degeneration (AMD) is a progressive neurodegenerative disease and the leading cause of irreversible blindness among individuals aged 65 and older, particularly in western countries [1]. With the ageing population, the number of people with AMD is estimated to increase by approximately 50% by the year 2020 and the burden of this disease is set to grow [2]. Macular degenerative lesions are manifested by drusen formation, retinal pigment epithelium (RPE) changes, retinal pigment epithelium and choroid capillary layer, Bruch's membrane lesion, geographic atrophy of the central fovea, exudative AMD with choroidal neovascularization, retinal pigmentary epithelium detachment, or submacular disciform scarring changes. The pathological hallmark of the disease is amorphous deposits

of protein and lipid, termed drusen [3]. Drusen—colloid material (lipids, phospholipids, and collagen) excrescences, similar to hyaline—accumulate in the retina, in Bruch's membrane underlying the retinal pigment epithelium. This process is associated with retinal pigment epithelium and progressive degeneration of photoreceptors [4]. Drusen disturb oxygenous metabolism and determine the degeneration of photoreceptors, while visual function impairment is associated with the quantity of damaged photoreceptors. In the fovea, where there is the largest quantity of photoreceptors, cones dominate, whereas the parafoveal region, where rods dominate, surrounds the fovea. In the early stages, photoreceptors are mostly damaged in the parafovea.

AMD is a complex disease to which many factors contribute: body ageing together with pathological changes, such as pathogenic oxidative stress, inflammatory processes, changes of the extracellular matrix, biological activity changes in the retinal pigment epithelium, and genetic factors—all of them are important in the pathogenesis of this disease [5]. With advancing age, there is a deposit of lipid particles in a normal Bruch's membrane leading to the creation of a lipid wall, external to the RPE basal lamina, impairing nutrient exchange between the choriocapillaris and the RPE and compromising retinal function [6, 7]. The observation that the location of the lipid wall is the same as and precedes the basal linear deposits and drusen suggests its contribution to drusen formation [8]. Indeed, lipids (both esterified and unesterified cholesterol and phosphatidylcholine) represent at most less than fifty percent of the volume of drusen [9]. Koskela et al. state that the accumulation of oxidized lipids seems to play a pivotal role in the development of AMD [10]. For instance, CYP4F2 is involved in the production of 20-hydroxyeicosatetraenoic acid (20-HETE), a molecule that is proinflammatory and can induce hyperlipidemia [11, 12]. CYP4F2 is also an important endobiotic metabolizing enzyme involved in the metabolism of fatty acids such as arachidonic acid, medium and very long polyunsaturated fatty acids, eicosanoids such as leukotriene B4 (LTB4), prostaglandins, and lipoxins implicating its importance in maintaining liver polyunsaturated fatty acids (PUFA) levels and inflammatory status [13]. The polymorphism (rs2108622, V433M) in the CYP4F2 gene with a valine to methionine substitution at amino acid 433 was found to be associated with changes in all these processes and, for instance, Fava et al. [14] found that CYP4F2 M433 (V433M) carriers had significantly higher levels of waist, triglycerides, blood pressure (BP), and a composite sum of metabolic syndrome (MetS) phenotypes (MetS score) beside lower high density lipoprotein (HDL) cholesterol with respect to V-homozygotes.

Knowing that the main pathological changes of age-related macular degeneration are drusen, which include about 40% lipids, the attempts to find a relation between age-related macular degeneration and the gene rs2108622 controlling lipid metabolism have been made.

2. Materials and Methods

Permission to undertake the study was obtained from the Ethics Committee for Biomedical Research. The study was conducted in the Lithuanian University of Health Sciences (LUHS), Neuroscience Institute, Ophthalmology laboratory (Number BE-2-/13).

The study included patients ($n = 190$) with early age-related macular degeneration and patients ($n = 181$) with exudative age-related macular degeneration and a random sample of the population $n = 210$ (control group).

2.1. Control Group Formation.
The control group consisted of subjects who had no ophthalmologic pathology on examination and who agreed to take part in this study. The control group involved 210 subjects, who matched the early AMD and eAMD group structure according to their age and gender. Thus it comprised 161 women and 49 men with their ages ranging from 50 to 90 years.

TABLE 1: Demographic characteristics of the study population.

| Characteristic | Group | | | p value |
	Early AMD $n = 190$	eAMD $n = 181$	Control $n = 210$	
Men, n (%)	57 (30.0)	59 (32.6)	49 (23.3)	NS
Women, n (%)	133 (70.0)	122 (67.4)	161 (76.7)	NS
Age median (min; max)	66 (50; 93)	76 (50; 90)	52 (20; 90)	NS

NS: nonsignificant.

The control group was created by taking into consideration the distribution of age and gender in the early AMD and eAMD group (Table 1). Therefore, the medians of the patient age of the control group and the early and eAMD group did not differ statistically significantly (NS).

During analysis of data, study subjects were grouped according to their age (younger than 65 years and 65 years and older).

2.2. Ophthalmological Evaluation.
All study subjects were evaluated by slit-lamp biomicroscopy to assess corneal and lenticular transparency. Classification and grading of lens opacities were performed according to the Lens Opacities Classification System III. Best corrected visual acuity (BCVA) was measured using the standard procedure adapted for the Age-Related Eye Disease Study (AREDS) at a 5-meter distance from the chart (letters on the ETDRS logMAR chart), for subjects with sufficiently reduced vision, at 1 meter. At each examination, intraocular pressure was measured. Pupils were dilated with tropicamide 1%, after which fundoscopy, using slit-lamp biomicroscopy with a double aspheric lens of +78 diopters, was performed. For detailed analysis of the macula, colour fundus photographs of the macula, centred at 30° to the fovea, were obtained with a Visucam NM Digital camera (Carl Zeiss Meditec AG, Germany).

The classification system of AMD formulated by the Age-Related Eye Disease Study [15] was used: early AMD consisted of a combination of multiple small drusen and several intermediate drusen (63–124 μm in diameter) or retinal pigment epithelial abnormalities; intermediate AMD was characterized by the presence of extensive intermediate drusen and at least one large drusen (≥125 μm in diameter) or geographic atrophy (GA) not involving the centre of the fovea; and advanced AMD was characterized by GA involving the fovea and/or any of the features of neovascular AMD [16]. Early AMD and eAMD were diagnosed by two ophthalmologists. Simultaneous spectral-domain optical coherence tomography (SD OCT; 870 nm, 40 000 A-scans/sec) and/or fluorescein angiography (FA) were performed for all AMD patients. SD OCT was carried out with Nidek RS 3000 advanced. FA, following fundus photography, patients underwent intravenous retinal fluorescein angiography. According to our standard technique, 5 mL of a 20% solution of sodium fluorescein was rapidly injected into the antecubital vein; then all phases of fluorescein transit in the posterior pole

TABLE 2: Frequency of the CYP4F2 rs2108622 genotypes in the patients with early AMD and in the control group.

Genotype/allele	Frequency (%)				
	Control group n (%) ($n = 210$)	p value HWE	Early AMD group n (%) ($n = 190$)	p value HWE	p value
Genotype		0.854		0.277	
T/T	16 (7.62)		11 (5.8)		
T/C	82 (39.05)		81 (42.6)		
C/C	112 (53.33)		98 (51.6)		$\chi^2 = 0.8676$
Total	210 (100)		190 (100)		$p = 0.6481$
Allele					
T	114 (25.33)		103 (31.21)		
C	336 (74.67)		277 (68.79)		

p value: significance level (alpha = 0.05); p value HWE: significance level (alpha = 0.05) by Hardy-Weinberg equilibrium.

of the study eye were photographically recorded. Some late angiograms of the fellow eye were taken to confirm or exclude exudative AMD.

The following subject exclusion criteria were used: (i) unrelated eye disorders, for example, high refractive error, cloudy cornea, lens opacity (nuclear, cortical, or posterior subcapsular cataract) except minor opacities, keratitis, acute or chronic uveitis, glaucoma, or diseases of the optic nerve; (ii) systemic illnesses, for example, diabetes mellitus, malignant tumours, systemic connective tissue disorders, chronic infectious diseases, or conditions following organ or tissue transplantation; (iii) ungraded colour fundus photographs resulting from obscuration of the ocular optic system or because of fundus photograph quality.

2.3. DNA Extraction and Genotyping. The DNA extraction and analysis of the gene polymorphism of *CYP4F2* (rs2108622) were carried out at the Laboratory of Ophthalmology at the Institute of Neuroscience of LUHS. DNA was extracted from 200 μL venous blood (white blood cells) using a DNA purification kit based on the magnetic beads method (MagJET Genomic DNA Kit, Thermo Scientific) or the silica-based membrane technology utilizing a genomic DNA extraction kit (GeneJET Genomic DNA Purification Kit, Thermo Scientific), according to the manufacturer's recommendations.

The genotyping of *CYP4F2* (rs2108622) was carried out using the real-time polymerase chain reaction (PCR) method. Single-nucleotide polymorphism was determined using TaqMan® Drug Metabolism assay (Thermo Scientific).

The genotyping was performed using a Rotor-Gene Q real-time PCR quantification system (Qiagen, USA). The real-time PCR reagents (2x TaqMan® Universal Master Mix, TaqMan® Drug Metabolism assay, nuclease-free water) were taken out from an environment of −20°C and were thawed at room temperature. The thawed reagents were centrifuged (10 000 rpm) and stored in an ice tub. Appropriate real-time PCR mixtures of *CYP4F2* (rs2108622) were prepared for determining a single-nucleotide polymorphism.

A PCR reaction mixture (9 μL) was poured into the 72 wells of the Rotor-Disc, and then 1 μL of matrix DNA of the samples (~10 ng) and 1 μL of negative control (−K) were added.

The Allelic Discrimination program was used during the real-time PCR. Then, the assay was continued following the manual provided by the manufacturer (http://www.qiagen .com/, Allelic Discrimination). After that, the Allelic Discrimination program was completed, and the genotyping results were received. The program determined the individual genotypes according to the fluorescence intensity rate of different detectors (VIC and FAM).

2.4. Statistical Analysis. Statistical analysis was performed using the SPSS/W 20.0 software (Statistical Package for the Social Sciences for Windows, Inc., Chicago, Illinois, USA). The data are presented as absolute numbers with percentages in brackets, average values, and standard deviations (SD). The frequencies of genotypes (in percentage) are presented in Table 2.

Hardy-Weinberg analysis was performed to compare the observed and expected frequencies of rs2108622 using the χ^2 test in all groups. The distribution of the rs2108622 single-nucleotide polymorphism (SNP) in the AMD and control groups was compared using the χ^2 test or the Fisher exact test. Binomial logistic regression analysis was performed to estimate the impact of genotypes on AMD development. Odds ratios and 95% confidence intervals are presented. The selection of the best genetic model was based on the Akaike Information Criterion (AIC); therefore, the best genetic models were those with the lowest AIC values.

Differences were considered statistically significant when $p < 0.05$.

3. Results

A total of 190 patients with early AMD and 181 patients with eAMD were enrolled into the analysis according to the subject inclusion and exclusion criteria. The control group comprised 210 persons. There were 76.7% ($n = 161$) of women in the control group, 70% ($n = 133$) of women in the early AMD group, and 67.4% ($n = 122$) of women in the eAMD group.

TABLE 3: Frequency of the CYP4F2 rs2108622 genotypes in the patients with eAMD and in the control group.

Genotype/allele	Control group n (%) (n = 210)	p value HWE	eAMD group n (%) (n = 181)	p value HWE	p value
		Frequency (%)			
Genotype		0.854		0.187	
T/T	16 (7.62)		7 (3.87)		
T/C	82 (39.05)		72 (39.78)		
C/C	112 (53.33)		102 (56.35)		$\chi^2 = 2.5012$
Total	210 T (1000)		181 (100)		$p = 0.2863$
Allele					
T	114 (25.33)		86 (23.75)		
C	336 (74.67)		276 (76.25)		

p value: significance level (alpha = 0.05); p value HWE: significance level (alpha = 0.05) by Hardy-Weinberg equilibrium.

TABLE 4: Frequency of CYP4F2 rs2108622 genotype in early AMD patients, in eAMD patients and controls by age.

Genotype	<65 years AMD group n (%)	<65 years Control group n (%)	p value	≥65 years AMD group n (%)	≥65 years Control group n (%)	p value
Frequency of CYP4F2 (1347C>T; V433M) rs2108622 genotype in the patients with early AMD and the control subjects by age						
TT	4 (4.5)	11 (7.1)		7 (6.9)	5 (9.3)	
TC	39 (43.8)	59 (37.8)		42 (41.6)	23 (42.6)	
CC	46 (51.7)	86 (55.1)	0.538	52 (51.5)	26 (48.1)	0.847
Allele						
T	47 (26.4)	81 (25.96)		56 (27.72)	33 (30.55)	
C	131 (73.6)	231 (74.04)		146 (72.28)	75 (69.45)	
Frequency of CYP4F2 (1347C>T; V433M) rs2108622 genotype in the patients with eAMD and the control subjects by age						
TT	1 (3.8)	11 (7.1)		6 (3.9)	5 (9.3)	
TC	9 (34.6)	59 (37.8)		63 (40.6)	23 (42.6)	
CC	16 (61.5)	86 (55.1)	0.751	86 (55.5)	26 (48.1)	0.266
Allele						
T	11 (21.15)	81 (25.96)		75 (24.19)	33 (30.55)	
C	41 (78.85)	231 (74.04)		235 (75.81)	75 (69.45)	

p value: significance level (alpha = 0.05); p value HWE: significance level (alpha = 0.05) by Hardy-Weinberg equilibrium.

The genotyping of rs2108622 was performed in patients with early AMD and eAMD and in the control group subjects (Tables 2 and 3).

The distribution of the analyzed rs2108622 genotype and allele frequencies in early AMD patients, eAMD patients, and controls matched the Hardy-Weinberg equilibrium. rs2108622 gene polymorphism analysis in the overall group did not reveal any differences in the genotypes distribution between patients with AMD and control group subjects.

The comparison of the rs2108622 genotype frequency by age groups did not reveal significant differences as well (Table 4).

The comparison of the rs2108622 genotype in males and females between patients with early AMD and the control group did not show statistically significant differences but revealed statistically significant differences between males and females with eAMD. The CYP4F2 (1347C>T) T/T genotype was more frequent in males with eAMD (10.2% versus 0.8%; $p = 0.0052$). When comparing the CYP4F2 genotype distribution in females with eAMD and healthy females significant differences were also revealed. The CYP4F2 (1347C>T) T/T genotype was less frequently present in eAMD females compared to healthy controls (0.8% versus 6.2%; $p = 0.027$) (Table 5).

Binomial logistic regression analysis in the patients with NeAMD and in the control group was performed (Table 6). Similarly, binomial logistic regression analysis in the patients with eAMD and in the control group was carried out (Table 7). These analyses did not detect any differences in the models between patients with AMD and control group subjects.

Binomial logistic regression analysis in males and females with AMD and in the control group was performed (Table 8). In the female AMD group this analysis revealed that the recessive (p value = 0.049) variables were statistically significant (Table 8).

TABLE 5: Frequency of CYP4F2 rs2108622 genotype in the patients with early AMD and eAMD and the control subjects by gender.

Genotype	Males			Females		
	AMD group n (%)	Control group n (%)	p value	AMD group n (%)	Control group n (%)	p value
Frequency of CYP4F2 (1347C>T; V433M) rs2108622 genotype in the patients with early age-related macular degeneration (AMD) and the control subjects by gender						
TT	6 (10.5)	6 (12.2)	0.149	5 (3.8)	10 (6.2)	0.429
TC	27 (47.4)	23 (46.9)	1	54 (40.6)	59 (36.6)	0.547
CC	24 (42.1)	20 (40.8)	1	74 (55.6)	92 (57.1)	0.814
Allele						
T	39 (34.51)	35 (35.71)		64 (24.06)	79 (24.53)	
C	75 (65.49)	63 (64.29)		202 (75.94)	243 (75.47)	
Frequency of CYP4F2 (1347C>T; V433M) rs2108622 genotype in the patients with exudative age-related macular degeneration (AMD) and the control subjects by gender						
TT	*6 (10.2)**	6 (12.2)	0.767	*1 (0.8)**	*10 (6.2)*	*0.027*
TC	22 (37.7)	23 (46.9)	0.333	50 (41.0)	59 (36.6)	0.462
CC	31 (52.5)	20 (40.8)	0.250	71 (58.2)	92 (57.1)	0.904
Allele						
T	34 (28.81)	35 (35.71)		50 (20.66)	79 (24.53)	
C	84 (71.19)	63 (64.29)		192 (79.34)	243 (75.47)	

*$p = 0.0052$.
p value: significance level (alpha = 0.05); p value HWE: significance level (alpha = 0.05) by Hardy-Weinberg equilibrium.

TABLE 6: Binomial logistic regression analysis of the *CYP4F2 (1347C>T; V433M) rs2108622* in the patients with early AMD and in the control group.

Model	Genotype	OR (95% CI)	p value	AIC
Codominant	T/T	0.786 (0.348; 1.774)	0.562	558.646
	T/C	1.129 (0.750; 1.700)	0.562	
Dominant	T/C + T/T	1.073 (0.724; 1.589)	0.726	557.394
Recessive	T/T	0.745 (0.337; 1.649)	0.468	556.983
Overdominant	T/C	1.160 (0.778; 1.729)	0.466	556.987
Additive	—	1.002 (0.730; 1.376)	0.990	557.517

TABLE 7: Binomial logistic regression analysis of the *CYP4F2 (1347C>T; V433M) rs2108622* in the patients with eAMD and in the control group.

Model	Genotype	OR (95% CI)	p value	AIC
Codominant	T/T	0.480 (0.190; 1.215)	0.121	543.306
	T/C	0.964 (0.637; 1.460)	0.863	
Dominant	T/C + T/T	0.885 (0.593; 1.320)	0.550	543.530
Recessive	T/T	0.488 (0.196; 1.214)	0.123	541.336
Overdominant	T/C	1.031 (0.687; 1.549)	0.883	543.866
Additive	—	1.204 (0.865; 1.675)	0.271	542.671

TABLE 8: Binomial logistic regression analysis of the *CYP4F2 (1347C>T; V433M) rs2108622* in males and females with eAMD and in the control group.

Model	Genotype	OR (95% CI)	p value	AIC
Female				
Codominant	T/T	0.130 (0.016; 1.036)	0.054	386.317
	T/C	1.098 (0.674; 1.788)	0.707	
Dominant	T/C + T/T	0.958 (0.595; 1.542)	0.859	390.898
Recessive	*T/T*	*0.125 (0.016; 0.988)*	*0.049*	*384.458*
Overdominant	T/C	1.201 (0.741; 1.945)	0.458	390.379
Additive	—	1.220 (0.805; 1.850)	0.348	390.041
Male				
Codominant	T/T	0.645 (0.182; 2.282)	0.497	153.306
	T/C	0.617 (0.274; 1.389)	0.243	
Dominant	T/C + T/T	0.623 (0.290; 1.339)	0.225	151.311
Recessive	T/T	0.811 (0.244; 2.696)	0.733	152.676
Overdominant	T/C	0.672 (0.311; 1.452)	0.312	151.767
Additive	—	1.357 (0.770; 2.392)	0.291	151.666

Binomial logistic regression analysis in the males with early AMD and in the control group by age was performed (Table 9). This analysis found that the additive ($p = 0.041$) variables were statistically significant in the group aged over 65 years.

Binomial logistic regression analysis in the males with eAMD and in the control group by age was performed (Table 10). This analysis displayed that the codominant ($p = 0.026$) variables in the group under 65 years old were statistically significant (Table 10). Moreover, the dominant ($p = 0.037$) and additive ($p = 0.015$) variables were statistically significant in the group of over 65 years (Table 10).

4. Discussion

It is known that changes in the metabolism of cholesterol, particularly of HDL, may influence drusen accumulation and

TABLE 9: Binomial logistic regression analysis of the *CYP4F2* *(1347C>T; V433M) rs2108622* in the males with early AMD and in the control group by age.

Model	Genotype	OR (95% CI)	p value	AIC
<65				
Codominant	T/T	1.727 (0.296; 10.082)	0.544	97.984
	T/C	1.524 (0.551; 4.212)	0.417	
Dominant	T/C + T/T	1.555 (0.584; 4.135)	0.377	96.003
Recessive	T/T	1.385 (0.259; 7.414)	0.704	96.648
Overdominant	T/C	1.387 (0.528; 3.639)	0.507	96.350
Additive	—	0.717 (0.335; 1.533)	0.391	96.050
≥65				
Codominant	T/T	0.077 (0.006; 1.023)	0.052	44.437
	T/C	0.154 (0.016; 1.471)	0.104	
Dominant	T/C + T/T	0.128 (0.014; 1.152)	0.067	42.960
Recessive	T/T	0.280 (0.046; 1.705)	0.167	45.938
Overdominant	T/C	0.500 (0.115; 2.175)	0.355	46.931
Additive	—	*3.422 (1.052; 11.130)*	*0.041*	42.961

TABLE 10: Binomial logistic regression analysis of the *CYP4F2* *(1347C>T; V433M) rs2108622* in the males with eAMD and in the control group by age.

Model	Genotype	OR (95% CI)	p value	AIC
<65				
Codominant	T/T	1.583 (0.129; 19.422)	0.719	44.539
	T/C	0.559 (0.091; 3.446)	0.531	
Dominant	T/C + T/T	0.713 (0.141; 3.612)	0.682	43.065
Recessive	T/T	2.00 (0.177; 22.550)	0.575	42.948
Overdominant	T/C	0.518 (0.089; 3.002)	0.463	42.662
Additive	—	1.045 (0.298; 3.667)	0.945	43.230
≥65				
Codominant	T/T	0.062 (0.005; 0.720)	*0.026*	53.304
	T/C	0.123 (0.014; 1.108)	0.062	
Dominant	T/C + T/T	0.103 (0.012; 0.871)	*0.037*	51.927
Recessive	T/T	0.248 (0.048; 1.276)	0.095	56.239
Overdominant	T/C	0.417 (0.105; 1.661)	0.215	57.207
Additive	—	*3.670 (1.282; 10.502)*	*0.015*	52.149

consequently promote AMD development [17]. Cholesterol can be obtained from systemic sources or recycled in the retina, through the circulation of blood lipids. Thus, the retinal rod cells are capable of using both lipids from the liver and those recycled from RPE [18]. With advancing age, there is a deposit of lipid particles in a normal BrM leading to the creation of a lipid wall, external to the RPE basal lamina, impairing nutrient exchange between the choriocapillaris and the RPE which compromises retinal function; thus that accumulation of lipids seems to play a pivotal role in the development of AMD [6, 7, 10]. In addition to genetic predisposition, which accounts for 70% of the risk of the disease development [19], advanced age is also considered a risk factor, which results in the deposition of lipid particles and formation of drusen in the retina, thereby affecting retinal function [18]. The study done by Björkhem et al. states that the most important enzymatic oxidation of

cholesterol takes place with the involvement of the *CYP46A1* and *CYP27A1* loci of cytochrome P450 family which forms 24-hydroxycholesterol (24-Hch) and 27-hydroxycholesterol (27-Hch), respectively [19]. High levels of 27-Kch have been reported in macrophages foam cells and in atherosclerotic plaque but have not been documented in the retina [20, 21]. These population-based genetic studies coupled with animal experiments indicate the prominent role of cholesterol metabolism in the AMD pathology [20, 21]. The rs754203 SNP in the *CYP46A1* gene was evaluated by Fourgeux et al. and no significant difference between the *CYP46A1* genotypes in the AMD and control groups was observed [22]. At the same time, the data from three studies are controversial, due to conflicting results. Therefore, we aimed to determine the frequency of the genotype of 1347C>T (rs2108622) in *CYP4F2* (which is involved in lipid metabolism) in patients with early and exudative AMD. The data of our analysis of rs2108622 polymorphism did not reveal any differences in the distribution of C/C, C/T, and T/T genotypes between the early AMD group, exudative AMD group, and the control group (51.6%, 42.6%, and 5.8% in early AMD group, 56.35%, 39.78%, and 3.87% in the exudative AMD group, and 53.33%, 39.05%, and 7.62%, in the control group, resp.). The *CYP4F2* (1347C>T) *T/T* genotype was more frequent in males with exudative AMD (10.2% versus 0.8%; *p* = 0.0052), and the comparison of the *CYP4F2* genotype distribution in females with exudative AMD and healthy females determined significant differences. The *CYP4F2* (1347C>T) *T/T* genotype was less frequently present in exudative AMD females compared to healthy control females (0.8% versus 6.2%; *p* = 0.027). To interpret our results, the research should be repeated with a larger sample size. However, exposure to environmental hazards has been associated with diseases in humans. The identification of single-nucleotide polymorphism (SNP) in human populations exposed to different environmental hazards is vital for detecting the genetic risks of some important human diseases [23]. Yang et al. study sought to structure a genetic score for smoking behaviour in a Chinese population. They tested GWAS-significant SNPs associated with smoking behaviour in a Chinese population and structured three types of genetic scores. They found that the effects of the three types of genetic score were similar; however, to best extrapolate and understand these types of results, the unweighted genetic score represents the ideal choice. Furthermore, the genetic score was significantly associated with smoking behaviour (smoking status and SI at ≤18 years of age). The results of this study may guide relevant health education for those with a high genetic score and promote smoking control to improve the health of the population [24]. It is possible that the genotype distribution of rs2108622 in the patients with exudative age-related macular degeneration (AMD) and the control subjects by gender can result from gene-environment interactions. One of the environmental risk factors could be smoking.

We found no studies analyzing the *CYP4F2* (1347C>T, rs2108622) gene polymorphism in patients with age-related macular degeneration; thus we can only compare the genotyping results in our control group with results obtained in other studies.

TABLE 11: Frequency of CYP4F2 rs2108622 genotypes in the control groups from other studies.

	Study	Country	VV%	VM%	MM%	Total
1	Our study	Lithuania	53.33	39.05	7.62	
2	Ivashchenko et al. 2013 [41]	Russia	57.1	34.1	7.7	—
3	Cen et al. 2010 [42]	China	52.0	41.0	7.0	—
4	Teichert et al. 2009 [43]	Caucasian	54.4	37.1	8.4	—
5	Zeng et al. 2012 [44]	China	55.1	40.5	4.4	370

Results of the control groups with rs2108622 polymorphism distribution in the other studies are shown in Table 11. It shows quite similar results to our study except for one study in Saudi Arabia [25] but it remains unclear if the reason for this is ethnicity, the size of control group, or something else.

There are many studies analyzing genes that take part in lipid metabolism and about systemic lipoproteins, but results are conflicting. Moreover, conflicting results have been reported with regard to the associations of AMD with serum HDL concentration and the genes involved in lipid metabolism. Some authors agree that increased serum cholesterol levels increase AMD development [16, 26]; however, other authors disagree [27] and some others reported no significant associations [28–31]. Ebrahimi and Handa suggested that before excluding the role of systemic lipids in AMD, the role of plasma lipids in the context of genotype could be examined to identify predisposition in a subset of patients at risk of developing AMD due to genotype and plasma lipid levels [32]. As the major SNPs involved in the HDL pathway, CETP rs3764261, LPL rs12678919, and LIPC rs10468017 have been shown to be associated with AMD in a genome-wide association studies (GWAS) [33]. However, previous studies on the reported HDL cholesterol metabolism genes showed contradictory results, especially in several GWAS; moreover, their genetic susceptibility to AMD varied in diverse populations [34–36]. On the other hand, different studies have found an inverse correlation with HDL and AMD risk. Reynolds et al. [37] recently demonstrated that elevated HDL is associated with a reduced risk of advanced AMD, especially the neovascular (NV) subtype (p value < 0.05, 0.03, resp.), and that higher low density lipoprotein (LDL) is associated with an increased risk of advanced AMD and the NV subtype (p value < 0.03, 0.04, resp.). When looking for an association of serum lipids with advanced AMD in multivariate modeling, Reynolds et al. also found significant trends with a higher quartile of LDL and increasing AMD risk (p for trend <0.03, 0.01). Higher total cholesterol was also associated with AMD risk when controlling for all covariates and genotypes [37].

A Klein et al. study [38] examined 6950 participants from the Beaver Dam Eye Study (BDES), Blue Mountains Eye Study (BMES), and Rotterdam Study (RS). There were few associations among total cholesterol, HDL-C, total cholesterol/HDL-C ratio, and non-HDL-C and the incidence of early AMD, soft indistinct (SI) drusen, large area of drusen, pigmentary abnormalities, late AMD, and exudative AMD. Direct associations of HDL-C with the incidence of pure geographic atrophy (GA) were present in the BDES and RS cohorts but not the BMES cohort. The use of statins was not associated with any incidence of an AMD outcome in any of the cohorts. In the BDES, CETP rs1864163 and LPL rs281 were protective against the development of large drusen area in the macula and CETP rs3764261 was protective against the development of pure GA. In the RS, CETP rs3764261 was linked to an increased risk of late AMD, pure GA, and exudative AMD. CETP rs1864163 was related to a decreased risk of the incidence of early AMD and large drusen area. ABCA1 rs1883025 was associated with a decreased risk of large SI drusen. LPL rs281 was associated with a decreased risk of a large drusen area in the macula. In the BMES, none of these SNPs were found to be significantly associated with any AMD outcomes, although marginally nonsignificant associations were found between ABCA1 rs1883025/T and pure GA and between LIPC rs7163555 and exudative AMD. Mean HDL-C increased in each of the three cohorts with each additional risk allele for CETP rs376426 and decreased with each additional risk allele for CETP rs1864163 and ABCA1 rs1883025 (all $p < 0.05$). There were no consistent statistically significant associations between LIPC or LPL and HDL-C or between any of the lipid genes and total cholesterol [38]. In a meta-analysis, after correction for multiple testing, they did not find an association between serum lipids or lipid pathway genes and the incidence or progression of AMD over a 20-year period using data from three population-based cohort studies, the BDES, BMES, and RS [38].

In addition to being one of the major AMD-susceptibility genes, perhaps accounting for approximately 30%–50% of AMD patients, CFH might interact with lipid metabolism to affect the disease risk [39]. Such interactions among genes in the complement system and HDL metabolism pathway might be proposed as one potential explanation for the lack of heritability [40]. However, whether the interaction is present or not and whether or not these interactions occur with different genes in the HDL metabolism pathway remain unclear [40].

In conclusion, our results suggest that the CYP4F2 (rs2108622) gene polymorphism had no predominant effect on the development of early and eAMD when compared to the control group. But the CYP4F2 (1347C>T) T/T genotype was more frequent in males with eAMD compared to females (10.2% versus 0.8%; $p = 0.0052$), and the comparison of the CYP4F2 genotype distribution in females with eAMD and healthy females did not reveal significant difference. The CYP4F2 (1347C>T) T/T genotype was less frequently present in eAMD females compared to healthy control females (0.8% versus 6.2%; $p = 0.027$), but this must be replicated with a larger sample size to prove these results, as we know that T/T genotype is wild and very rare.

Competing Interests

None of the authors has any proprietary interests or competing interests related to this submission.

References

[1] L. S. Lim, P. Mitchell, J. M. Seddon, F. G. Holz, and T. Y. Wong, "Age-related macular degeneration," *The Lancet*, vol. 379, no. 9827, pp. 1728–1738, 2012.

[2] R. D. Jager, W. F. Mieler, and J. W. Miller, "Age-related macular degeneration," *The New England Journal of Medicine*, vol. 358, no. 24, pp. 2544–2617, 2008.

[3] Y.-F. Wang, Y. Han, R. Zhang, L. Qin, M.-X. Wang, and L. Ma, "CETP/LPL/LIPC gene polymorphisms and susceptibility to age-related macular degeneration," *Scientific Reports*, vol. 5, Article ID 15711, 2015.

[4] R. W. Young, "Pathophysiology of age-related macular degeneration," *Survey of Ophthalmology*, vol. 31, no. 5, pp. 291–306, 1987.

[5] M. A. Zarbin, "Current concepts in the pathogenesis of age-related macular degeneration," *Archives of Ophthalmology*, vol. 122, no. 4, pp. 598–614, 2004.

[6] R. Loebstein, H. Yonath, D. Peleg et al., "Pharmacoepidemiology and drug utilization: interindividual variability in sensitivity to warfarin—nature or nurture?" *Clinical Pharmacology and Therapeutics*, vol. 70, no. 2, pp. 159–164, 2001.

[7] J. Taube, D. Halsall, and T. Baglin, "Influence of cytochrome P-450 CYP2C9 polymorphisms on warfarin sensitivity and risk of over-anticoagulation in patients on long-term treatment," *Blood*, vol. 96, no. 5, pp. 1816–1819, 2000.

[8] G. D'Andrea, R. L. D'Ambrosio, P. Di Perna et al., "A polymorphism in the VKORC1 gene is associated with an interindividual variability in the dose-anticoagulant effect of warfarin," *Blood*, vol. 105, no. 2, pp. 645–649, 2005.

[9] M. D. Caldwell, T. Awad, J. A. Johnson et al., "CYK4F-2 genetic variant alters required warfarin dose," *Blood*, vol. 111, no. 8, pp. 4106–4112, 2008.

[10] A. Koskela, M. Reinisalo, J. M. T. Hyttinen, K. Kaarniranta, and R. O. Karjalainen, "Pinosylvin-mediated protection against oxidative stress in human retinal pigment epithelial cells," *Molecular Vision*, vol. 20, pp. 760–769, 2014.

[11] G. Lai, J. Wu, X. Liu, and Y. Zhao, "20-HETE induces hyperglycemia through the cAMP/ PKA-PhK-GP pathway," *Molecular Endocrinology*, vol. 26, no. 11, pp. 1907–1916, 2012.

[12] K. N. Theken, Y. Deng, M. Alison Kannon, T. M. Miller, S. M. Poloyac, and C. R. Lee, "Activation of the acute inflammatory response alters cytochrome P450 expression and eicosanoid metabolism," *Drug Metabolism and Disposition*, vol. 39, no. 1, pp. 22–29, 2011.

[13] J. P. Hardwick, "Cytochrome P450 omega hydroxylase (CYP4) function in fatty acid metabolism and metabolic diseases," *Biochemical Pharmacology*, vol. 75, no. 12, pp. 2263–2275, 2008.

[14] C. Fava, M. Montagnana, E. Danese et al., "The functional variant V433M of the CYP4F2 and the metabolic syndrome in Swedes," *Prostaglandins and Other Lipid Mediators*, vol. 98, no. 1-2, pp. 31–36, 2012.

[15] Age-Related Eye Disease Study Research Group, "The age-related eye disease study system for classifying age-related macular degeneration from stereoscopic color fundus photographs: the age-related eye disease study report number," *American Journal of Ophthalmology*, vol. 132, no. 5, pp. 668–681, 2001.

[16] K. L. Spencer, L. M. Olson, N. Schnetz-Boutaud et al., "Using genetic variation and environmental risk factor data to identify individuals at high risk for age-related macular degeneration," *PLoS ONE*, vol. 6, no. 3, Article ID e17784, 2011.

[17] S. M. Cezario, M. C. Calastri, C. I. Oliveira et al., "Association of high-density lipoprotein and apolipoprotein E genetic variants with age-related maculardegeneration," *Arquivos Brasileiros de Oftalmologia*, vol. 78, no. 2, pp. 85–88, 2015.

[18] C. A. Curcio, M. Johnson, M. Rudolf, and J.-D. Huang, "The oil spill in ageing Bruch membrane," *British Journal of Ophthalmology*, vol. 95, no. 12, pp. 1638–1645, 2011.

[19] I. Björkhem, A. Cedazo-Minguez, V. Leoni, and S. Meaney, "Oxysterols and neurodegenerative diseases," *Molecular Aspects of Medicine*, vol. 30, no. 3, pp. 171–179, 2009.

[20] I. Björkhem, O. Andersson, U. Diczfalusy et al., "Atherosclerosis and sterol 27-hydroxylase: evidence for a role of this enzyme in elimination of cholesterol from human macrophages," *Proceedings of the National Academy of Sciences of the United States of America*, vol. 91, no. 18, pp. 8592–8596, 1994.

[21] P. V. Luoma, "Cytochrome P450 and gene activation—from pharmacology to cholesterol elimination and regression of atherosclerosis," *European Journal of Clinical Pharmacology*, vol. 64, no. 9, pp. 841–850, 2008.

[22] C. Fourgeux, B. Dugas, F. Richard et al., "Single nucleotide polymorphism in the cholesterol-24SHydroxylase (CYP46A1) hene and Its association with CFH and LOC387715 gene polymorphisms in age-related macular degeneration," *Investigative Ophthalmology and Visual Science*, vol. 53, no. 11, pp. 7026–7033, 2012.

[23] A. L. Hollman, P. B. Tchounwou, and H. C. Huang, "The Association between gene-environment interactions and diseases involving the human GST superfamily with SNP variants," *International Journal of Environmental Research and Public Health*, vol. 13, no. 4, p. 379, 2016.

[24] S. Yang, Y. He, J. Wang et al., "Genetic scores of smoking behaviour in a Chinese population," *Scientific Reports*, vol. 6, Article ID 22799, 2016.

[25] A. Munshi, V. Sharma, S. Kaul et al., "Association of 1347 G/A cytochrome P450 4F2 (CYP4F2) gene variant with hypertension and stroke," *Molecular Biology Reports*, vol. 39, no. 2, pp. 1677–1682, 2012.

[26] A. Cougnard-Grégoire, M.-N. Delyfer, J.-F. Korobelnik et al., "Elevated high-density lipoprotein cholesterol and age-related macular degeneration: the Alienor study," *PLoS ONE*, vol. 9, no. 3, Article ID e90973, 2014.

[27] U. Chakravarthy, T. Y. Wong, A. Fletcher et al., "Clinical risk factors for age-related macular degeneration: a systematic review and meta-analysis," *BMC Ophthalmology*, vol. 10, article 31, 2010.

[28] F. Ulas, M. Balbaba, S. Ozmen, S. Celebi, and U. Dogan, "Association of dehydroepiandrosterone sulfate, serum lipids, C-reactive protein and body mass index with age-related macular degeneration," *International Ophthalmology*, vol. 33, no. 5, pp. 485–491, 2013.

[29] P. Cackett, T. Y. Wong, T. Aung et al., "Smoking, cardiovascular risk factors, and age-related macular degeneration in asians: the singapore malay eye study," *American Journal of Ophthalmology*, vol. 146, no. 6, pp. 960–967.e1, 2008.

[30] W. Smith, P. Mitchell, S. R. Leeder, and J. J. Wang, "Plasma fibrinogen levels, other cardiovascular risk factors, and age-related maculopathy: the Blue Mountains Eye Study," *Archives of Ophthalmology*, vol. 116, no. 5, pp. 583–587, 1998.

[31] S. C. Tomany, J. J. Wang, R. Van Leeuwen et al., "Risk factors for incident age-related macular degeneration: pooled findings from 3 continents," *Ophthalmology*, vol. 111, no. 7, pp. 1280–1287, 2004.

[32] K. B. Ebrahimi and J. T. Handa, "Lipids, lipoproteins, and age-related macular degeneration," *Journal of Lipids*, vol. 2011, Article ID 802059, 14 pages, 2011.

[33] B. M. Neale, J. Fagerness, R. Reynolds et al., "Genome-wide association study of advanced age-related macular degeneration identifies a role of the hepatic lipase gene (LIPC)," *Proceedings of the National Academy of Sciences of the United States of America*, vol. 107, no. 16, pp. 7395–7400, 2010.

[34] V. Cipriani, H.-T. Leung, V. Plagnol et al., "Genome-wide association study of age-related macular degeneration identifies associated variants in the TNXB-FKBPL-NOTCH4 region of chromosome 6p21.3," *Human Molecular Genetics*, vol. 21, no. 18, pp. 4138–4150, 2012.

[35] W. Chen, D. Stambolian, A. O. Edwards et al., "Genetic variants near TIMP3 and high-density lipoprotein-associated loci influence susceptibility to age-related macular degeneration," *Proceedings of the National Academy of Sciences of the United States of America*, vol. 107, no. 16, pp. 7401–7406, 2010.

[36] N. A. Restrepo, K. L. Spencer, R. Goodloe et al., "Genetic determinants of age-related macular degeneration in diverse populations from the PAGE study," *Investigative Ophthalmology & Visual Science*, vol. 55, no. 10, pp. 6839–6850, 2014.

[37] R. Reynolds, B. Rosner, and J. M. Seddon, "Serum lipid biomarkers and hepatic lipase gene associations with age-related macular degeneration," *Ophthalmology*, vol. 117, no. 10, pp. 1989–1995, 2010.

[38] R. Klein, C. E. Myers, G. H. S. Buitendijk et al., "Lipids, lipid genes, and incident age-related macular degeneration: the three continent age-related macular degeneration consortium," *American Journal of Ophthalmology*, vol. 158, no. 3, pp. 513–524.e3, 2014.

[39] J. L. Haines, M. A. Hauser, S. Schmidt et al., "Complement factor H variant increases the risk of age-related macular degeneration," *Science*, vol. 308, no. 5720, pp. 419–421, 2005.

[40] O. Zuk, E. Hechter, S. R. Sunyaev, and E. S. Lander, "The mystery of missing heritability: genetic interactions create phantom heritability," *Proceedings of the National Academy of Sciences of the United States of America*, vol. 109, no. 4, pp. 1193–1198, 2012.

[41] D. Ivashchenko, I. Rusin, D. Sychev, and A. Grachev, "The frequency of CYP2C9, VKORC1, and CYP4F2 polymorphisms in Russian patients with high thrombotic risk," *Medicina*, vol. 49, no. 12, pp. 517–521, 2013.

[42] H.-J. Cen, W.-T. Zeng, X.-Y. Leng et al., "*CYP4F2* rs2108622: a minor significant genetic factor of warfarin dose in Han Chinese patients with mechanical heart valve replacement," *British Journal of Clinical Pharmacology*, vol. 70, no. 2, pp. 234–240, 2010.

[43] M. Teichert, M. Eijgelsheim, F. Rivadeneira et al., "A genome-wide association study of acenocoumarol maintenance dosage," *Human Molecular Genetics*, vol. 18, no. 19, pp. 3758–3768, 2009.

[44] W. T. Zeng, Q. S. Zheng, M. Huang et al., "Genetic polymorphisms of VKORC1, CYP2C9, CYP4F2 in Bai, Tibetan Chinese," *Pharmazie*, vol. 67, no. 1, pp. 69–73, 2012.

3

Chemokines Referee Inflammation within the Central Nervous System during Infection and Disease

Douglas M. Durrant,[1] Jessica L. Williams,[1] Brian P. Daniels,[1] and Robyn S. Klein[1,2,3]

[1] *Department of Internal Medicine, Washington University School of Medicine, Campus Box 8051, 660 S. Euclid Avenue, St. Louis, MO 63110, USA*

[2] *Department of Anatomy and Neurobiology, Washington University School of Medicine, Campus Box 8051, 660 S. Euclid Avenue, St. Louis, MO 63110, USA*

[3] *Department of Pathology and Immunology, Washington University School of Medicine, Campus Box 8051, 660 S. Euclid Avenue, St. Louis, MO 63110, USA*

Correspondence should be addressed to Robyn S. Klein; rklein@dom.wustl.edu

Academic Editor: Cinthia Farina

The discovery that chemokines and their receptors are expressed by a variety of cell types within the normal adult central nervous system (CNS) has led to an expansion of their repertoire as molecular interfaces between the immune and nervous systems. Thus, CNS chemokines are now divided into those molecules that regulate inflammatory cell migration into the CNS and those that initiate CNS repair from inflammation-mediated tissue damage. Work in our laboratory throughout the past decade has sought to elucidate how chemokines coordinate leukocyte entry and interactions at CNS endothelial barriers, under both homeostatic and inflammatory conditions, and how they promote repair within the CNS parenchyma. These studies have identified several chemokines, including CXCL12 and CXCL10, as critical regulators of leukocyte migration from perivascular locations. CXCL12 additionally plays an essential role in promoting remyelination of injured white matter. In both scenarios we have shown that chemokines serve as molecular links between inflammatory mediators and other effector molecules involved in neuroprotective processes.

1. Introduction

Chemokines are small, secreted proteins originally shown to promote the migration of leukocytes both during immune surveillance and in response to inflammation. Chemokine have been classified into CXC, CC, C, or CX_3C subfamilies, according to the positions of conserved cysteine residues at their N-termini, and promiscuously bind receptor members of the G protein-coupled receptor superfamily [1]. Each chemokine or its receptor is named based on their subfamily designation with "L" indicating ligand and "R" indicating receptor plus a number, which corresponds to the same numbers used in the corresponding gene nomenclature. Binding of chemokines to their receptors generally results in calcium mobilization and cytoskeletal rearrangements required for cell motility in response to a signal of increasing chemokine concentration [2, 3]. Their initial discovery by immunologists led to an explosion of studies demonstrating their far-reaching roles in all aspects of immune function from immune surveillance and leukocyte interactions within lymph nodes to orchestration of innate and adaptive immune responses against invading pathogens.

The identification of two chemokine receptors, CCR5 and CXCR4, as critical coreceptors for the entry of HIV-1 into $CD4^+$ T cells [4–6] heralded an intense period of chemokine research leading to the detection of these molecules on multiple cell types within the CNS in both homeostatic and inflammatory conditions. CXCR4, in particular, is expressed by neural progenitors, mature neurons, and endothelial cells in the normal adult CNS [7–10]. CXCR4 is the most highly conserved chemokine receptor throughout evolution [11, 12] with functional origins in the development of multiple organ systems, including the immune and central nervous systems (CNS) [13]. Its primary ligand, CXCL12, is also expressed by neurons and epithelium [14]. CXCL12 is the second most highly conserved chemokine ligand; CXCL14, another CNS chemokine, is the first and a natural inhibitor of CXCL12-CXCR4 interactions [15]. An additional receptor for CXCL12, CXCR7, functions to scavenge the chemokine and heterodimerize with CXCR4 in order to regulate CXCR4 signaling [16–18]. The identification of CXCL12/CXCR4/CXCR7 as primordial is consistent with their critical roles in the development of multiple organ systems and in their physiologic, pleiotropic functions in both immune and nervous systems. CXCL12 was first identified for its role in the homing of hematopoietic progenitor cells to the bone marrow and later as a facilitator of lymphocyte entry into lymph nodes during immune surveillance [19–22], the latter due to it expression along the lumenal surfaces of high endothelial venules. The detection of high levels of CXCL12 expressed by CNS endothelium was curious, as this site is normally regarded for its stringent regulation of lymphocyte entry. However, our laboratory soon discovered that the polarity of CXCL12 expression in the CNS was reversed compared to its expression within lymphoid tissues and ultimately established CXCL12 and its scavenger receptor, CXCR7, as critical molecular components of immune privilege and as orchestrators of efficacious antiviral responses, promoting requisite interactions between leukocytes that localize to perivascular spaces [23–27]. These interactions are critical for limiting the entry of immune cells into the CNS parenchyma to those that may swiftly eliminate pathogen and preserve CNS function.

Studies in chemokine neurobiology also shifted our understanding of the role of proinflammatory chemokine expression during neurologic diseases. Early studies had cast these molecules as immunopathologic targets whose inactivation would ameliorate disease by limiting inflammation. Investigations using both infectious and autoimmune models of neuroinflammation have since demonstrated that chemokine expression within the CNS may be neuroprotective. For example, our laboratory demonstrated that neurons infected with the neurotropic flavivirus West Nile virus (WNV) express T lymphocyte chemoattractants, such as CXCL10, to promote adaptive immune responses within the CNS to clear virus [28, 29]. These studies were also the first to delineate differences in innate immune responses of the hindbrain and forebrain as WNV-infected cerebellar granule cell neurons exhibit brisk upregulation of CXCL10 expression compared with infected cortical neurons, which protects the cerebellum from extensive viral infection. We also demonstrated that while CXCL12 does not mediate leukocyte recruitment into the CNS, increased parenchymal expression of this chemokine during neuroinflammatory states promotes CNS repair, harkening back to its developmental roles in neural progenitor cell proliferation and differentiation [30–32]. In this review, we discuss studies

from our laboratory that have established fundamental and functional roles for chemokines at CNS endothelial barriers and in the protection and repair of the CNS parenchyma.

2. Chemokines Function as Molecular Components of Immune Privilege at the Blood-Brain Barrier

Among the most influential sites of regulation for chemokine signaling in the CNS is the blood-brain barrier (BBB). The BBB is a complex physiological interface between the hematogenous circulation and parenchymal CNS tissues, composed of brain microvascular endothelial cells (BMECs) joined by a network of tight junctions (TJs) and adherens junctions (AJs) [33]. BMECs are ensheathed by pericytes and the endfeet processes of adjacent astrocytes, both of which contribute to TJ and AJ formation and enhance the barrier properties of BMECs [34]. Chemokine signaling at the BBB occurs in all neurovascular cell types, though their actions in endothelial cells and astrocytes are most well understood. Immune cells that infiltrate the CNS via the circulation first enter a space between vascular endothelia and glial endfeet known as the perivascular space, in which they are subject to the regulatory actions of chemokines and other CNS immune factors.

In BMECs, the expression and localized display of CXCL12 is known to be a major regulator of CNS immune privilege. Under homeostatic conditions, CXCL12 is expressed exclusively along basolateral/ablumenal surfaces of BMECs [24, 25]. Upon extravasation into the perivascular space, CXCR4$^+$ leukocytes are captured by endothelial CXCL12, restricting them to the perivascular space and preventing their parenchymal infiltration [24, 25]. This process is responsible for much of the "perivascular cuffing" that occurs during inflammatory episodes of the CNS, as large numbers of infiltrating leukocytes accumulate on the basolateral surfaces of vascular endothelium. This restriction of leukocyte access to the CNS parenchyma is essential to limit immunopathology and bystander injury of neurons, which have limited capacity for repair in comparison to peripheral tissues [35, 36].

Due to this essential function, disease states that alter CXCL12 expression and localization at the BBB can lead to uncontrolled neuroinflammation, resulting in axonal injury, demyelination, and neuronal death. In the CNS autoimmune disease multiple sclerosis (MS) and its mouse model experimental autoimmune encephalomyelitis (EAE), myelin-specific T lymphocytes invade the CNS parenchyma, forming lesions characterized by demyelinated and injured axons. In both MS and EAE, the homeostatic localization of CXCL12 is disturbed, with loss of polarized expression along basolateral surfaces of BMECs. Loss of CXCL12 polarity results in impaired perivascular capture of infiltrating leukocytes, with subsequent accumulations of CXCR4$^+$ cells in parenchymal tissues leading to progressive neuropathology. In mouse studies, blockade of CXCL12-CXCR4 interactions at the BBB via administration of the CXCR4 antagonist AMD3100 resulted in enhanced clinical disease severity during EAE, associated with enhanced parenchymal immune infiltrates, increased microglial activation, and increased CNS expression of Th1 inflammatory mediators [25]. In studies of tissue from MS patients, uninflamed vessels exhibited normal basolateral vascular expression of CXCL12, while inflammatory lesions contained vessels with CXCL12 expression that was redistributed to vessel lumena. Of note, the extent of pathological CXCL12 expression within MS lesions positively correlated with levels of neuroinflammation and demyelination [24]. Together, these studies established a critical role for CXCL12 at the BBB in the orchestration of leukocyte trafficking during CNS autoimmunity.

3. Mediators of CXCL12 Signaling during CNS Autoimmunity

Given the central role of CXCL12 at the BBB during homeostasis and neuroinflammation, understanding the mechanisms by which CXCL12 is regulated at this site is crucial in the development of targeted therapeutics. Endothelial CXCL12 is subject to regulation by a number of factors, including reciprocal regulation by infiltrating immune cells. In particular, mouse studies have established that expression of the inflammatory cytokine IL-1β contributes to loss of CXCL12 polarity in vascular endothelium during the induction of EAE, facilitating later CNS parenchymal invasion by autoreactive leukocytes [37]. During EAE, infiltrating CD4$^+$, CD8$^+$, and $\gamma\delta$ T cells are sources of IL-1β within the CNS. IL1R$^{-/-}$ mice are resistant to EAE, and, in contrast to WT controls, exhibit intact CXCL12 polarity at the BBB following myelin oligodendrocyte glycoprotein- (MOG-) immunization. Administration of recombinant IL-1β also potently induced the relocalization of CXCL12 to vessel lumena in spinal cords of naïve WT mice. Bone marrow chimera experiments revealed that IL1R signaling on both leukocytes and resident CNS cells contributed to changes in CXCL12 polarity at the BBB during EAE, suggesting that IL1R signaling is a key systemic regulator of CXCL12 within the inflamed CNS.

While leukocyte-derived factors play a role in regulating CXCL12 at the BBB, endothelial cells, themselves, express key regulators of CXCL12 expression and polarity that contribute to autoimmune pathogenesis. A key CXCL12 regulatory protein is the atypical chemokine receptor CXCR7/ACKR3 (CXCR7). CXCR7 has key regulatory functions in the CNS during development and homeostasis, regulating the migration of leukocytes, neural precursor cells, and immature neurons via signaling pathways distinct from those of CXCR4 [38, 39]. BMECs are among the primary expressers of CXCR7 within the CNS [23]. Endothelial CXCR7 serves as a scavenging receptor for CXCL12, sequestering the chemokine into lysosomal compartments, thereby negatively regulating CXCL12-CXCR4 signaling. Studies in mice demonstrated that CXCR7 expression was upregulated in vascular endothelium during EAE [23]. This was due, in part, to the actions of the T-cell cytokines IL-1β and IL-17, which enhanced CXCR7 expression and CXCL12 internalization in BMECs *in vitro*. Administration of the CXCR7 antagonist CCX771

diminished the clinical symptoms of EAE by preserving CXCL12 polarity at the BBB, thereby reducing parenchymal infiltration of autoreactive leukocytes. This preservation of CNS immune privilege was further shown via *in vivo* diffusion tensor imaging to prevent axonal injury during EAE [40].

In addition to direct regulation via CXCR7, CXCL12 is also indirectly regulated at the BBB by mediators of endothelial cell biology. In particular, we recently reported that sphingosine-phosphate-1 receptor 2 (S1PR2) signaling in neurovascular cells contributed to BBB dysregulation during CNS autoimmunity [41]. S1PRs at the BBB respond to the bioactive lipid metabolite S1P, which is expressed broadly by endothelial cells, erythrocytes, and neuronal lineage cells. In BMECs, S1PRs regulate a variety of cytoskeletal processes that influence intercellular junctions, paracellular permeability, and apicobasal polarity. In our study, S1PR2 signaling in CNS vascular endothelium was associated with increased BBB permeability and loss of CXCL12 polarity in mice with EAE and in a human *in vitro* BBB model [27, 41]. Pharmacological blockade or genetic deletion of S1PR2 ameliorated clinical symptoms and parenchymal leukocyte infiltrates and was shown to preserve BBB integrity and CXCL12 polarity in CNS microvessels. S1PR2 dysregulation of endothelial barrier integrity was associated with disassembly of endothelial AJs and was dependent on signaling through the cytoskeletal regulatory GTPases RhoA and CDC42, as well as the caveolin-mediated endocytic pathway. Of note, changes to BBB permeability and adherens junction formation were always associated with loss of CXCL12 polarity, indicating that CXCL12 display on basolateral surfaces of BMECs can be controlled both directly via CXCR7-mediated relocation and by general disruption of AJ-mediated apicobasal polarity via cytoskeletal and endocytic regulatory pathways.

S1PR2 signaling at the BBB may prove to be a particularly attractive therapeutic target, due to its recently discovered contribution to sexually dimorphic patterns of CNS autoimmunity. MS exhibits a strong sexual bias in humans; women comprise the majority of patients and are more susceptible to remitting-relapsing forms of the disease. The EAE model in the SJL mouse strain exhibits similar sexual dimorphism, with female mice exhibiting enhanced susceptibility to EAE and experiencing a remitting-relapsing course of clinical disease. In contrast, males do not develop remitting-relapsing disease and instead exhibit variable disease courses, including complete resistance to EAE or standard monophasic disease progression, depending on such factors as method of EAE induction or age of experimental animals [42–44]. Our recent study found sexually dimorphic expression of S1PR2 in the SJL mouse strain, with increased expression in the cerebella of naïve female SJL and in cerebella and spinal cords of female SJL with EAE compared to males. In addition, we reported enhanced expression of S1PR2 in cerebella of female patients with MS compared to males. Remarkably, the enhanced expression of S1PR2 in EAE-susceptible CNS regions of female SJL mice was associated with similarly sexually dimorphic pathological expression of CXCL12. Naïve female SJL mice exhibited dysregulated CXCL12 polarity in lower CNS regions, contributing to their enhanced susceptibility to EAE, and this dysregulation was further exacerbated compared to males during disease. S1PR2 was found to contribute significantly to sexually dimorphic differences in CXCL12 expression and localization, as pharmacological blockade and genetic deletion of S1PR2 signaling preserved CXCL12 polarity during EAE, resulting in ameliorated disease. Together, these findings suggest that targeting S1PR2 signaling may be a powerful tool in addressing sex-specific disease processes in MS, including the dysregulation of chemokine signals that regulate CNS immune privilege.

4. Chemokine-Mediated Repair in the Adult CNS

In MS, myelin destruction and loss of oligodendrocytes lead to motor and sensory disability. A majority of MS patients present with a remitting-relapsing form of the disease, in which periods of inflammation and demyelination are followed by partial recovery [45]. Following neuroinflammation, mechanisms that parallel developmental pathways are activated to facilitate repair. Neural precursors expressing NG2 chondroitin sulfate proteoglycan that give rise to mature oligodendrocytes are found in the ventricular zones of the CNS by embryonic days 12–14. In the final stages of differentiation, oligodendrocyte precursor cells (OPCs) begin to express maturation markers including myelin basic protein (MBP) and myelin oligodendrocyte glycoprotein (MOG) [46]. Similarly, using a model of cuprizone- (CPZ-) mediated demyelination, Patel et al. demonstrated that astrocyte-expressed CXCL12 was necessary for maturation of $NG2^+$ OPCs that express CXCR4 during remyelination in adult mice [30, 31]. Following 6 weeks of CPZ exposure, CXCL12 and CXCR4 mRNA were significantly elevated in the corpus callosum (CC), the primary CNS region affected by CPZ intoxication. Additionally, $CXCL12^+GFAP^+$ astrocytes and $CXCR4^+NG2^+$ OPCs were highest in areas with the most extensive demyelination, the caudal CC [30, 47]. Inhibition of CXCR4 signaling, either via pharmacologic antagonism with AMD3100 or via *in vivo* RNA silencing, prevented OPC maturation and remyelination [30], suggesting that CXCL12-CXCR4 signaling is required for the development of mature oligodendrocytes and repair following CNS injury.

During CNS tissue damage, many inflammatory cytokines are rapidly induced and have diverse roles, with potentially detrimental acute consequences but beneficial effects in CNS recovery [48]. While inflammation and repair are two distinct processes, they are both regulated by inflammatory cytokines, like tumor necrosis factor (TNF-α), which influences tissue-infiltrating leukocytes and development of OPCs. Targeting of TNF-α has been successful in treating peripheral autoimmune diseases like rheumatoid arthritis [49], psoriasis [50], and inflammatory bowel disease [51]; however, administration of a recombinant TNF receptor immunoglobulin fusion protein worsened MS exacerbations [52]. Shortly after this study was completed, it was shown that TNF-α signaling through TNFR2 is essential for proliferation and differentiation of OPCs during remyelination in the CPZ model, perhaps explaining the failure of anti-TNF-α strategies for treating MS [53]. Our follow up study revealed that several CNS cells express both TNFR1 and TNFR2 following CPZ-induced demyelination and that TNFR2 signaling, specifically in astrocytes, was critical for CXCL12 expression. Mice deficient in TNFR2 had reduced CXCL12 expression in astrocytes during demyelination, leading to a reduction in $CXCR4^+$ OPCs due to a lack of CXCL12-mediated proliferation. In rescue experiments, lentiviral delivery of CXCL12 to the demyelinated CC restored OPC proliferation and remyelination in TNFR2-deficient mice. Further, stereotactic injection of postnatal astrocytes infected with a lentivirus expressing CXCL12 restored MBP expression in the CC following chronic demyelination, suggesting astrocyte CXCL12 is sufficient for myelin production [31]. These data indicate that activated astrocytes express TNFR2, which binds TNF-α to increase the levels of CXCL12 and promote OPC proliferation and differentiation.

While CXCL12 is indispensable for the plasticity of the demyelinated adult CNS, there are several factors that regulate CXCL12 expression during neuroinflammation (Figure 1). In addition to soluble factors, CXCR7, an alternative scavenger receptor, works to sequester and degrade CXCL12 [17, 54], regulating activation of CXCR4. CXCR7 is highly expressed during CPZ-mediated demyelination and expression subsides during remyelination, while levels of CXCR4 and CXCL12 remain elevated. This suggests that downregulation of CXCR7 is necessary for CXCL12-CXCR4 binding during repair. To determine if high levels of CXCR7 might regulate CXCL12 expression during demyelination, Williams et al. administered a small molecule inhibitor of CXCR7, CCX771, versus a vehicle control and found that antagonism of CXCR7 during late CPZ-mediated demyelination resulted in increased expression of CXCL12 and an upregulation of activated CXCR4 in OPCs [32]. *In vitro* experiments determined that CCX771-mediated regulation of CXCL12 was due to a decrease in CXCL12 internalization, suggesting that CCX771 works to limit CXCL12 targeting to lysosomal compartments for degradation. *In vivo* CXCR7 antagonism during demyelination led to an increase in OPC proliferation and in mature oligodendrocytes within demyelinated lesions. Further, CCX771 treatment during CPZ-induced demyelination enhanced remyelination, which, through the use of AMD3100, was shown to be CXCR4-dependent suggesting that the CCX771-mediate increase in CXCL12 expression during demyelination has potentially beneficial consequences [32]. These findings are significant as current treatment strategies for MS employ immunosuppressive compounds and do not promote repair. Further, while OPCs are found in MS lesions they are developmentally arrested [55, 56], remyelination gradually fails, and demyelination persists, which leads to progression of clinical disease [57]. Since CXCR7 regulates CXCL12-CXCR4-mediated CNS myelin repair, it may, therefore, serve as a therapeutic target to promote OPC differentiation and remyelination in the adult CNS.

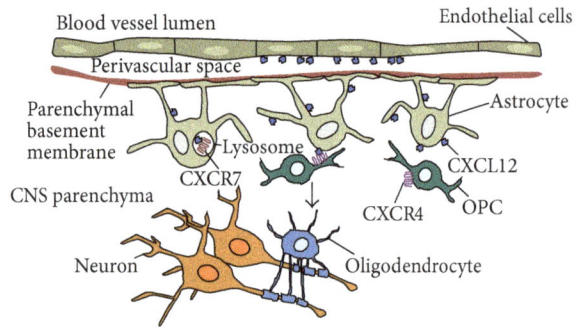

FIGURE 1: Chemokines mediate repair in the adult CNS. Following demyelination, CXCL12 and its receptors, CXCR4 and CXCR7, are upregulated on astrocytes and endothelial cells. CXCL12 binding to CXCR4 on OPCs induces proliferation and maturation into myelin-producing oligodendrocytes. CXCR7 regulates CXCR4 activation by sequestering CXCL12 into lysosomal compartments for degradation.

5. Chemokines Mediate Neuroprotective T-Cell Recruitment and Activation during West Nile Viral Infections of the CNS

Lymphocyte recruitment into the CNS following viral infections is necessary to control viral replication and, in many cases, prevent death. However, viral infections of the CNS pose unique challenges to the immune system with regards to controlling and eliminating the invading pathogen. First, lymphocyte trafficking to the CNS during inflammation is complicated by the BBB, which prevents most lymphocytes from entering the CNS, and second, the CNS contains terminally differentiated cells that are susceptible to injury caused by the infiltration of pathogen-specific as well as bystander T lymphocytes. Thus, regulatory mechanisms are essential to ensure the appropriate CNS entry of virus-specific T cells and that their presence within the CNS does not induce immunopathology. Chemokines have been recognized as key regulators of leukocyte trafficking from the microvasculature into the CNS and are crucial in coordinating protective immune responses during CNS viral infection [58].

WNV, a neurotropic flavivirus, has emerged globally as a significant cause of viral encephalitis [59]. In the CNS, WNV targets neurons, including cortical, midbrain, cerebellar, and spinal cord neurons, leading to their injury or death [60–62]. The clearance of WNV within the CNS relies heavily on cell-mediated immune responses that promote the migration and effector function of T cells in the CNS parenchyma. Shortly after local viral replication begins, virus-specific CD8+ T cells traffic into WNV-infected CNS. Initially, studies suggested that the infiltrating CD8+ T cells may have both a neuroprotective and a neuropathologic role due to injury of WNV-infected neurons [63]; however, studies using targeted deletion of T-cell chemoattractants to inhibit leukocyte trafficking indicate that the CNS entry of virus-specific CD8+ T cells is essential for clearance of WNV within the CNS.

Proinflammatory chemokine expression is strongly induced within the CNS of WNV-infected mice and coincides with the infiltration of mononuclear leukocytes [28, 64]. The chemokines CCL3-5 bind to the chemokine receptor CCR5, which is upregulated within the CNS after WNV infection. The deletion of CCR5, which is expressed on activated T cells and macrophages, decreases efficient leukocyte trafficking and viral clearance within the CNS during WNV infection [64]. CXCL10 expression is also induced following WNV infection by virally infected neurons [28]. Cerebellar neurons express higher levels of CXCL10 compared with cortical neurons, which results in enhanced trafficking of CXCR3-expressing WNV-specific T cells into the hindbrain versus the forebrain [29]. During EAE, neuronal precursor cells also express CXCL10 within the subventricular zone (SvZ) which results in the preferential localization of activated T cells [65] confirming the potent ability of neuronal cells to direct inflammatory cell infiltration. However, this differential pattern in CXCL10 expression during WNV infection may be due to differences in innate neuronal expression of viral sensing proteins [66]. The loss of CXCL10 or CXCR3 via targeted deletion or antibody administration results in decreased recruitment of WNV-specific CD8+ T cells in the CNS, especially within the cerebellum, increased viral loads, and enhanced mortality [28, 29], establishing that WNV-infected neurons directly induce the recruitment of virus-specific T cells in a region-specific manner for the purpose of viral clearance.

CXCL10 is also involved in neuronal apoptosis pathways via activation of CXCR3 by neurons. Previous studies demonstrated that treatment of CXCR3-expressing neurons with CXCL10 results in a caspase-3 dependent apoptotic cell death [67]. Therefore, the chemokine required for the recruitment of effector immune cells by virally infected neurons for their survival might also promote their death. Thus, virally infected neurons, in addition to CXCL10, also express TNF-α, which down-regulates CXCR3 expression in both infected and uninfected neurons [68]. TNF-α-mediated loss of CXCR3 interferes with caspase-3 activation and apoptotic death [68]. Thus, neurons can both facilitate an appropriate antiviral inflammatory response and prevent injury from the proapoptotic effects of the required inflammatory chemokine.

Constitutive chemokines, which are normally expressed by secondary lymphoid tissues as well as the CNS, function in regulating immune surveillance and primary immune responses. As described above, CXCL12, which is expressed by endothelial cells of the CNS microvasculature, regulates the trafficking of leukocytes into the CNS parenchyma during neuroinflammatory diseases [24–26, 37, 40]. Infiltrating lymphocytes cross endothelial barriers within the leptomeninges and enter the CNS via crawling along abluminal surfaces, generating the dense perivascular infiltrates typically observed during neuroinflammatory diseases [69–71]. CXCL12 expression at the microvasculature localizes immune cells, promoting their interaction within perivascular spaces, regulating the entry of fully activated WNV-specific T lymphocytes during WNV encephalitis [25, 26].

Within lymph node tissues, CXCL12 expression mediates the homing and localization of mononuclear cells to lymphoid compartments [72, 73] from which effector lymphocytes are released via changes in CXCR4 expression, the receptor for CXCL12 [74–76]. Similar to its role within the periphery, CXCL12 expression within the CNS functions to retain leukocytes that have migrated into the perivascular spaces of the CNS microvasculature. During WNV encephalitis, levels of abluminal CXCL12 along the microvasculature drop when compared with uninfected counterparts suggesting a mechanism for promoting leukocyte entry for viral clearance [26]. Consistent with this, the blockade of CXCL12 signaling with a CXCR4 antagonist promotes leukocyte entry into the CNS parenchyma and results in improved viral clearance, decreased immunopathology, and enhanced survival during WNV infection [26]. These data provide evidence that the parenchymal location of virus-specific T cells is essential to effectively clear virus and reduce pathology. In addition, they suggest that contrary to the role of CXCL12 within secondary lymphoid tissues, the movement of leukocytes into and out of CNS perivascular spaces relies on regulation of CXCL12 expression rather than CXCR4, which may have an important role in antigen recognition within the CNS.

How CXCL12 expression is regulated is not completely understood. Several studies have demonstrated that members of the TNF superfamily, including TNFα/TNFR and CD40/CD40L, interact and upregulate CXCL12 in various cell types [77, 78]. CD40 is a cell surface receptor that is expressed by numerous immune cells, including dendritic cells, B cells, and macrophages as well as endothelial cells [79]. Ligand binding of CD40 within CNS microvasculature is associated with the retention of myelin-specific T cells in EAE [80, 81]. During WNV infection, the targeted deletion of either CD40 or TNFR-1 decreases CD8$^+$ T-cell trafficking into the CNS parenchyma [82, 83]. These studies suggest that TNF ligand/receptor superfamily interactions facilitate T-cell migration across the BBB to control WNV infection; however, further studies are needed to determine whether these molecules exert their T-cell trafficking effects via regulation of CXL12 expression.

CXCL12-mediated retention of leukocytes within the perivascular compartment promotes leukocyte interactions that ensure the full activation of virus-specific lymphocytes and improves their ability to migrate out of the perivascular space into the CNS parenchyma (Figure 2). CD4$^+$ T cells assist the full activation, migration, and positioning of virus-specific CD8$^+$ T cells within the CNS, which are essential to effectively clear virus [84–86]. In the absence of IL-1 signaling, antigen presenting cells fail to be fully activated, which is required for CD4$^+$ T-cell help to restimulate infiltrating, virus-specific CD8$^+$ T cells [84, 87]. In addition to inefficient viral clearance, the loss of IL-1 signaling results in increased leukocyte entry into the CNS parenchyma, including bystander, nonspecific T cells, increased immunopathology, and enhanced mortality during WNV infection [84, 88]. Proinflammatory chemokines including CCL2, CCL5, and CXCL10 were significantly upregulated following infection yet were ineffective in recruiting leukocytes that mediated viral clearance. Infiltrating macrophages produce IL-1 within the CNS promoting increased expression of CXCL12 along

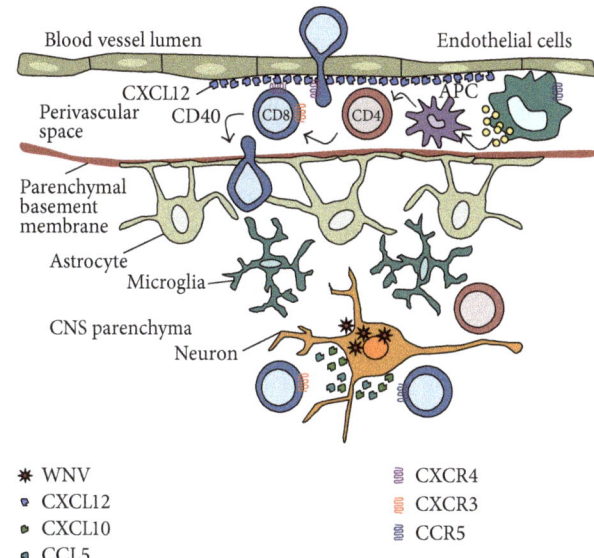

FIGURE 2: Neuroprotective roles of chemokines in response to viral infection of the CNS. Functional roles of chemokines in attracting and activating lymphocytes into the CNS during acute viral infection. Monocytes are attracted into the CNS via the chemokine CCL5 and its receptor CCR5. Macrophages produce IL-1β within the CNS and ensure full activation and CXCL12-mediated interactions of infiltrating leukocytes. CXCR4-expressing lymphocytes are captured by endothelial expression of CXCL12 within the perivascular spaces, which promotes CD4$^+$ T-cell help to infiltrate CD8$^+$ T lymphocytes. In addition to full activation, lymphocyte egress from perivascular spaces requires CD40. During the acute stage of disease, virally infected neurons secrete CXCL10 and CCL5 that attract activated T lymphocytes bearing the receptor CXCR3 and/or CCR5 into the parenchyma. CD8$^+$ and CD4$^+$ T lymphocytes mediate viral control through direct cytolytic activity and/or cytokine secretion.

the microvasculature. This in turn enables leukocyte accumulation to ensure the selective entry of fully activated virus-specific T cells into the parenchyma, which imparts protective CNS inflammation during WNV infection.

Within the CNS there are multiple regulatory mechanisms that govern leukocyte trafficking from the microvasculature into the CNS parenchyma. Chemokines are critical coordinators of these particular immune responses during CNS infection by neurotropic viruses. Taken together, these molecular and cellular events are exceedingly efficient in clearing viral pathogen while limiting CNS immunopathology.

6. Concluding Statements

The hallmark of neuroinflammation is an influx of leukocytes through the BBB. Depending on the disease, the presence of leukocytes can have beneficial or detrimental effects on disease outcome. Chemokines have a protective role within the CNS through their ability to orchestrate leukocyte entry and interactions at the endothelial barriers of the CNS and initiate CNS repair of damaged tissue within the CNS parenchyma. CXCL12 expression along the CNS microvasculature leads to neuroprotection by limiting the parenchymal infiltration of autoreactive leukocytes and ensuring successful interactions for the release of fully activated virus-specific leukocytes necessary for swift viral clearance. Following neuroinflammation, CXCL12 expression, within the white matter of the CNS parenchyma, is critical in promoting OPC maturation and remyelination. The ability of CXCL12, and other proinflammatory chemokines, to mediate leukocyte influx and repair from inflammation mediated tissue damage suggests that chemokines act as an interpreter of an immune reaction and transform the information in neuroprotective mechanisms during infection and disease. However, the protective and immunomodulatory role of chemokines within the CNS during neuroinflammation is still not fully elucidated. For instance, in neurodegenerative diseases such as Alzheimer's disease, recent reports indicate that chemokines accelerate amyloidosis via regulation of resident microglia [89]. Moreover, chemokines may orchestrate intercellular interactions within the CNS, specifically T lymphocyte and APC interactions, which may achieve immune skewing at the microvasculature or other CNS barriers. These chemokine-mediated leukocyte interactions may promote the activation or expansion of functionally precommitted immune cells with the desired phenotype or the suppression of cells with an inappropriate phenotype at the border of the CNS. Additionally, chemokine receptor signaling may modulate the downstream expression of appropriate growth factors necessary for repair within the parenchyma following inflammation. Finally, the protective and immunomodulatory role of chemokines within the CNS may extend beyond this immune-privileged site and be relevant for the immune regulation within other systems such as the eye, intestine, lung, tumor, and chronic infection.

Conflict of Interests

The authors declare that there is no conflict of interests regarding the publication of this paper.

References

[1] A. Zlotnik and O. Yoshie, "The chemokine superfamily revisited," *Immunity*, vol. 36, no. 5, pp. 705–716, 2012.

[2] R. Fredriksson, M. C. Lagerström, L.-G. Lundin, and H. B. Schiöth, "The G-protein-coupled receptors in the human genome form five main families. Phylogenetic analysis, paralogon groups, and fingerprints," *Molecular Pharmacology*, vol. 63, no. 6, pp. 1256–1272, 2003.

[3] A. Rot and U. H. von Andrian, "Chemokines in innate and adaptive host defense: basic chemokinese grammar for immune cells," *Annual Review of Immunology*, vol. 22, pp. 891–928, 2004.

[4] C. C. Bleul, M. Farzan, H. Choe et al., "The lymphocyte chemoattractant SDF-1 is a ligand for LESTR/fusin and blocks HIV-1 entry," *Nature*, vol. 382, no. 6594, pp. 829–833, 1996.

[5] E. Oberlin, A. Amara, F. Bachelerie et al., "The CXC chemokine SDF-1 is the ligand for LESTR/fusin and prevents infection by T-cell-line-adapted HIV-1," *Nature*, vol. 382, no. 6594, pp. 833–835, 1996.

[6] Y. Feng, C. C. Broder, P. E. Kennedy, and E. A. Berger, "HIV-1 entry cofactor: functional cDNA cloning of a seven-transmembrane, G protein-coupled receptor," *Science*, vol. 272, no. 5263, pp. 872–877, 1996.

[7] Y.-R. Zou, A. H. Kottman, M. Kuroda, I. Taniuchi, and D. R. Littman, "Function of the chemokine receptor CXCR4 in heaematopolesis and in cerebellar development," *Nature*, vol. 393, no. 6685, pp. 595–599, 1998.

[8] M. Lu, E. A. Grove, and R. J. Miller, "Abnormal development of the hippocampal dentate gyrus in mice lacking the CXCR4 chemokine receptor," *Proceedings of the National Academy of Sciences of the United States of America*, vol. 99, no. 10, pp. 7090–7095, 2002.

[9] I. Lieberam, D. Agalliu, T. Nagasawa, J. Ericson, and T. M. Jessell, "A Cxcl12-Cxcr4 chemokine signaling pathway defines the initial trajectory of mammalian motor axons," *Neuron*, vol. 47, no. 5, pp. 667–679, 2005.

[10] L. Izikson, R. S. Klein, A. D. Luster, and H. L. Weiner, "Targeting monocyte recruitment in CNS autoimmune disease," *Clinical Immunology*, vol. 103, no. 2, pp. 125–131, 2002.

[11] A. Zlotnik, "Involvement of chemokine receptors in organ-specific metastasis," *Contributions to Microbiology*, vol. 13, pp. 191–199, 2006.

[12] M. E. deVries, A. A. Kelvin, L. Xu, L. Ran, J. Robinson, and D. J. Kelvin, "Defining the origins and evolution of the chemokine/chemokine receptor system," *Journal of Immunology*, vol. 176, no. 1, pp. 401–415, 2006.

[13] R. S. Klein and J. B. Rubin, "Immune and nervous system CXCL12 and CXCR4: parallel roles in patterning and plasticity," *Trends in Immunology*, vol. 25, no. 6, pp. 306–314, 2004.

[14] G. A. Schwarting, T. R. Henion, J. D. Nugent, B. Caplan, and S. Tobet, "Stromal cell-derived factor-1 (chemokine C-X-C motif ligand 12) and chemokine C-X-C motif receptor 4 are required for migration of gonadotropin-releasing hormone neurons to the forebrain," *Journal of Neuroscience*, vol. 26, no. 25, pp. 6834–6840, 2006.

[15] K. Tanegashima, K. Suzuki, Y. Nakayama et al., "CXCL14 is a natural inhibitor of the CXCL12-CXCR4 signaling axis," *FEBS Letters*, vol. 587, no. 12, pp. 1731–1735, 2013.

[16] J. M. Burns, B. C. Summers, Y. Wang et al., "A novel chemokine receptor for SDF-1 and I-TAC involved in cell survival, cell adhesion, and tumor development," *Journal of Experimental Medicine*, vol. 203, no. 9, pp. 2201–2213, 2006.

[17] U. Naumann, E. Cameroni, M. Pruenster et al., "CXCR7 functions as a scavenger for CXCL12 and CXCL11," *PLoS ONE*, vol. 5, no. 2, Article ID e9175, 2010.

[18] A. Levoye, K. Balabanian, F. Baleux, F. Bachelerie, and B. Lagane, "CXCR7 heterodimerizes with CXCR4 and regulates CXCL12-mediated G protein signaling," *Blood*, vol. 113, no. 24, pp. 6085–6093, 2009.

[19] K. Tashiro, H. Tada, R. Heilker, M. Shirozu, T. Nakano, and T. Honjo, "Signal sequence trap: a cloning strategy for secreted proteins and type I membrane proteins," *Science*, vol. 261, no. 5121, pp. 600–603, 1993.

[20] T. Lapidot, A. Dar, and O. Kollet, "How do stem cells find their way home?" *Blood*, vol. 106, no. 6, pp. 1901–1910, 2005.

[21] B. Dubois, C. Massacrier, and C. Caux, "Selective attraction of naive and memory B cells by dendritic cells," *Journal of Leukocyte Biology*, vol. 70, no. 4, pp. 633–641, 2001.

[22] R. Phillips and A. Ager, "Activation of pertussis toxin-sensitive CXCL12 (SDF-1) receptors mediates transendothelial migration

of T lymphocytes across lymph node high endothelial cells," *European Journal of Immunology*, vol. 32, no. 3, pp. 837–847, 2002.

[23] L. Cruz-Orengo, D. W. Holman, D. Dorsey et al., "CXCR7 influences leukocyte entry into the CNS parenchyma by controlling abluminal CXCL12 abundance during autoimmunity," *Journal of Experimental Medicine*, vol. 208, no. 2, pp. 327–339, 2011.

[24] E. E. McCandless, L. Piccio, B. M. Woerner et al., "Pathological expression of CXCL12 at the blood-brain barrier correlates with severity of multiple sclerosis," *The American Journal of Pathology*, vol. 172, no. 3, pp. 799–808, 2008.

[25] E. E. McCandless, Q. Wang, B. M. Woerner, J. M. Harper, and R. S. Klein, "CXCL12 limits inflammation by localizing mononuclear infiltrates to the perivascular space during experimental autoimmune encephalomyelitis," *The Journal of Immunology*, vol. 177, no. 11, pp. 8053–8064, 2006.

[26] E. E. McCandless, B. Zhang, M. S. Diamond, and R. S. Klein, "CXCR4 antagonism increases T cell trafficking in the central nervous system and improves survival from West Nile virus encephalitis," *Proceedings of the National Academy of Sciences of the United States of America*, vol. 105, no. 32, pp. 11270–11275, 2008.

[27] B. P. Daniels, L. Cruz-Orengo, T. J. Pasieka et al., "Immortalized human cerebral microvascular endothelial cells maintain the properties of primary cells in an *in vitro* model of immune migration across the blood brain barrier," *Journal of Neuroscience Methods*, vol. 212, no. 1, pp. 173–179, 2013.

[28] R. S. Klein, E. Lin, B. Zhang et al., "Neuronal CXCL10 directs CD8+ T-cell recruitment and control of West Nile virus encephalitis," *Journal of Virology*, vol. 79, no. 17, pp. 11457–11466, 2005.

[29] B. Zhang, K. C. Ying, B. Lu, M. S. Diamond, and R. S. Klein, "CXCR3 mediates region-specific antiviral T cell trafficking within the central nervous system during west nile virus encephalitis," *Journal of Immunology*, vol. 180, no. 4, pp. 2641–2649, 2008.

[30] J. R. Patel, E. E. McCandless, D. Dorsey, and R. S. Klein, "CXCR4 promotes differentiation of oligodendrocyte progenitors and remyelination," *Proceedings of the National Academy of Sciences of the United States of America*, vol. 107, no. 24, pp. 11062–11067, 2010.

[31] J. R. Patel, J. L. Williams, M. M. Muccigrosso et al., "Astrocyte TNFR2 is required for CXCL12-mediated regulation of oligodendrocyte progenitor proliferation and differentiation within the adult CNS," *Acta Neuropathologica*, vol. 124, no. 6, pp. 847–860, 2012.

[32] J. L. Williams, J. R. Patel, B. P. Daniels, and R. S. Klein, "Targeting CXCR7/ACKR3 as a therapeutic strategy to promote remyelination in the adult central nervous system," *Journal of Experimental Medicine*, vol. 211, no. 5, pp. 791–799, 2014.

[33] P. Ballabh, A. Braun, and M. Nedergaard, "The blood-brain barrier: an overview: structure, regulation, and clinical implications," *Neurobiology of Disease*, vol. 16, no. 1, pp. 1–13, 2004.

[34] N. J. Abbott, L. Rönnbäck, and E. Hansson, "Astrocyte-endothelial interactions at the blood-brain barrier," *Nature Reviews Neuroscience*, vol. 7, no. 1, pp. 41–53, 2006.

[35] G. Yiu and Z. He, "Glial inhibition of CNS axon regeneration," *Nature Reviews Neuroscience*, vol. 7, no. 8, pp. 617–627, 2006.

[36] H. Sabelström, M. Stenudd, P. Réu et al., "Resident neural stem cells restrict tissue damage and neuronal loss after spinal cord injury in mice," *Science*, vol. 342, no. 6158, pp. 637–640, 2013.

[37] E. E. McCandless, M. Budde, J. R. Lees, D. Dorsey, E. Lyng, and R. S. Klein, "IL-1R signaling within the central nervous system regulates CXCL12 expression at the blood-brain barrier and disease severity during experimental autoimmune encephalomyelitis," *The Journal of Immunology*, vol. 183, no. 1, pp. 613–620, 2009.

[38] Y. Wang, G. Li, A. Stanco et al., "CXCR4 and CXCR7 have distinct functions in regulating interneuron migration," *Neuron*, vol. 69, no. 1, pp. 61–76, 2011.

[39] J. L. Williams, D. W. Holman, and R. S. Klein, "Chemokines in the balance: maintenance of homeostasis and protection at CNS barriers," *Frontiers in Cellular Neuroscience*, vol. 8, p. 154, 2014.

[40] L. Cruz-Orengo, Y.-J. Chen, J. H. Kim, D. Dorsey, S.-K. Song, and R. S. Klein, "CXCR7 antagonism prevents axonal injury during experimental autoimmune encephalomyelitis as revealed by *in vivo* axial diffusivity," *Journal of Neuroinflammation*, vol. 8, article 170, 2011.

[41] L. D. Cruz-Orengo, B. P. Dorsey, and D. A. Klein, "Sexually dimorphic S1PR2 expression enhances susceptibility to CNS autoimmunity," *Journal of Clinical Investigation*, 2014.

[42] B. F. Bebo Jr., A. A. Vandenbark, and H. Offner, "Male SJL mice do not relapse after induction of EAE with PLP 139–151," *Journal of Neuroscience Research*, vol. 45, no. 6, pp. 680–689, 1996.

[43] P. D. Fillmore, M. Brace, S. A. Troutman et al., "Genetic analysis of the influence of neuroantigen-complete Freund's adjuvant emulsion structures on the sexual dimorphism and susceptibility to experimental allergic encephalomyelitis," *The American Journal of Pathology*, vol. 163, no. 4, pp. 1623–1632, 2003.

[44] K. M. Spach, M. Blake, J. Y. Bunn et al., "Cutting edge: the Y chromosome controls the age-dependent experimental allergic encephalomyelitis sexual dimorphism in SJL/J mice," *The Journal of Immunology*, vol. 182, no. 4, pp. 1789–1793, 2009.

[45] L. Steinman, "A molecular trio in relapse and remission in multiple sclerosis," *Nature Reviews Immunology*, vol. 9, no. 6, pp. 440–447, 2009.

[46] A. Polito and R. Reynolds, "NG2-expressing cells as oligodendrocyte progenitors in the normal and demyelinated adult central nervous system," *Journal of Anatomy*, vol. 207, no. 6, pp. 707–716, 2005.

[47] Q.-Z. Wu, Q. Yang, H. S. Cate et al., "MRI identification of the rostral-caudal pattern of pathology within the corpus callosum in the cuprizone mouse model," *Journal of Magnetic Resonance Imaging*, vol. 27, no. 3, pp. 446–453, 2008.

[48] S.-M. Lucas, N. J. Rothwell, and R. M. Gibson, "The role of inflammation in CNS injury and disease," *The British Journal of Pharmacology*, vol. 147, supplement 1, pp. S232–S240, 2006.

[49] J. Jin, Y. Chang, and W. Wei, "Clinical application and evaluation of anti-TNF-alpha agents for the treatment of rheumatoid arthritis," *Acta Pharmacologica Sinica*, vol. 31, no. 9, pp. 1133–1140, 2010.

[50] L. H. Kircik and J. Q. Del Rosso, "Anti-TNF agents for the treatment of psoriasis," *Journal of Drugs in Dermatology*, vol. 8, no. 6, pp. 546–559, 2009.

[51] S. Nikolaus and S. Schreiber, "Anti-TNF biologics in the treatment of chronic inflammatory bowel disease," *Der Internist*, vol. 49, no. 8, pp. 947–954, 2008.

[52] "TNF neutralization in MS: results of a randomized, placebo-controlled multicenter study. The Lenercept Multiple Sclerosis Study Group and The University of British Columbia MS/MRI Analysis Group," *Neurology*, vol. 53, no. 3, pp. 457–465, 1999.

[53] H. A. Arnett, J. Mason, M. Marino, K. Suzuki, G. K. Matsushima, and J. P.-Y. Ting, "TNFα promotes proliferation of oligodendrocyte progenitors and remyelination," *Nature Neuroscience*, vol. 4, no. 11, pp. 1116–1122, 2001.

[54] B. Boldajipour, H. Mahabaleshwar, E. Kardash et al., "Control of chemokine-guided cell migration by ligand sequestration," *Cell*, vol. 132, no. 3, pp. 463–473, 2008.

[55] A. Chang, A. Nishiyama, J. Peterson, J. Prineas, and B. D. Trapp, "NG2-positive oligodendrocyte progenitor cells in adult human brain and multiple sclerosis lesions," *Journal of Neuroscience*, vol. 20, no. 17, pp. 6404–6412, 2000.

[56] A. Chang, W. W. Tourtellotte, R. Rudick, and B. D. Trapp, "Premyelinating oligodendrocytes in chronic lesions of multiple sclerosis," *The New England Journal of Medicine*, vol. 346, no. 3, pp. 165–173, 2002.

[57] A. Compston and A. Coles, "Multiple sclerosis," *The Lancet*, vol. 359, no. 9313, pp. 1221–1231, 2002.

[58] S. Man, E. E. Ubogu, and R. M. Ransohoff, "Inflammatory cell migration into the central nervous system: a few new twists on an old tale," *Brain Pathology*, vol. 17, no. 2, pp. 243–250, 2007.

[59] M. A. Samuel and M. S. Diamond, "Pathogenesis of West Nile virus infection: a balance between virulence, innate and adaptive immunity, and viral evasion," *Journal of Virology*, vol. 80, no. 19, pp. 9349–9360, 2006.

[60] B. Shrestha, D. Gottlieb, and M. S. Diamond, "Infection and injury of neurons by West Nile encephalitis virus," *Journal of Virology*, vol. 77, no. 24, pp. 13203–13213, 2003.

[61] J. D. Fratkin, A. A. Leis, D. S. Stokic, S. A. Slavinski, and R. W. Geiss, "Spinal cord neuropathology in human West Nile virus infection," *Archives of Pathology and Laboratory Medicine*, vol. 128, no. 5, pp. 533–537, 2004.

[62] E. A. Hunsperger and J. T. Roehrig, "Temporal analyses of the neuropathogenesis of a West Nile virus infection in mice," *Journal of NeuroVirology*, vol. 12, no. 2, pp. 129–139, 2006.

[63] Y. Wang, M. Lobigs, E. Lee, and A. Müllbacher, "CD8+ T cells mediate recovery and immunopathology in West Nile virus encephalitis," *Journal of Virology*, vol. 77, no. 24, pp. 13323–13334, 2003.

[64] W. G. Glass, J. K. Lim, R. Cholera, A. G. Pletnev, J.-L. Gao, and P. M. Murphy, "Chemokine receptor CCR5 promotes leukocyte trafficking to the brain and survival in West Nile virus infection," *Journal of Experimental Medicine*, vol. 202, no. 8, pp. 1087–1098, 2005.

[65] L. Muzio, F. Cavasinni, C. Marinaro et al., "Cxcl10 enhances blood cells migration in the sub-ventricular zone of mice affected by experimental autoimmune encephalomyelitis," *Molecular and Cellular Neuroscience*, vol. 43, no. 3, pp. 268–280, 2010.

[66] H. Cho, S. C. Proll, K. J. Szretter, M. G. Katze, M. Gale, and M. S. Diamond, "Differential innate immune response programs in neuronal subtypes determine susceptibility to infection in the brain by positive-stranded RNA viruses," *Nature Medicine*, vol. 19, no. 4, pp. 458–464, 2013.

[67] Y. Sui, L. Stehno-Bittel, S. Li et al., "CXCL10-induced cell death in neurons: role of calcium dysregulation," *European Journal of Neuroscience*, vol. 23, no. 4, pp. 957–964, 2006.

[68] B. Zhang, J. Patel, M. Croyle, M. S. Diamond, and R. S. Klein, "TNF-α-dependent regulation of CXCR3 expression modulates neuronal survival during West Nile virus encephalitis," *Journal of Neuroimmunology*, vol. 224, no. 1-2, pp. 28–38, 2010.

[69] J.-P. Bouffard, M. A. Riudavets, R. Holman, and E. J. Rushing, "Neuropathology of the brain and spinal cord in human West Nile virus infection," *Clinical Neuropathology*, vol. 23, no. 2, pp. 59–61, 2004.

[70] I. Bartholomaus, N. Kawakami, F. Odoardi et al., "Effector T cell interactions with meningeal vascular structures in nascent autoimmune CNS lesions," *Nature*, vol. 462, no. 7269, pp. 94–98, 2009.

[71] D. Lodygin, F. Odoardi, C. Schläger et al., "A combination of fluorescent NFAT and H2B sensors uncovers dynamics of T cell activation in real time during CNS autoimmunity," *Nature Medicine*, vol. 19, no. 6, pp. 784–790, 2013.

[72] T. Okada, V. N. Ngo, E. H. Ekland et al., "Chemokine requirements for b cell entry to lymph nodes and Peyer's patches," *The Journal of Experimental Medicine*, vol. 196, no. 1, pp. 65–75, 2002.

[73] M. L. Scimone, T. W. Felbinger, I. B. Mazo, J. V. Stein, U. H. Von Andrian, and W. Weninger, "CXCL12 mediates CCR7-independent homing of central memory cells, but not naive T cells, in peripheral lymph nodes," *Journal of Experimental Medicine*, vol. 199, no. 8, pp. 1113–1120, 2004.

[74] C. Nombela-Arrieta, T. R. Mempel, S. F. Soriano et al., "A central role for DOCK2 during interstitial lymphocyte motility and sphingosine-1-phosphate-mediated egress," *The Journal of Experimental Medicine*, vol. 204, no. 3, pp. 497–510, 2007.

[75] A. C. Yopp, S. Fu, S. M. Honig et al., "FTY720-enhanced T cell homing is dependent on CCR2, CCR5, CCR7, and CXCR4: evidence for distinct chemokine compartments," *The Journal of Immunology*, vol. 173, no. 2, pp. 855–865, 2004.

[76] A. C. Yopp, J. C. Ochando, M. Mao, L. Ledgerwood, Y. Ding, and J. S. Bromberg, "Sphingosine 1-phosphate receptors regulate chemokine-driven transendothelial migration of lymph node but not splenic T cells," *The Journal of Immunology*, vol. 175, no. 5, pp. 2913–2924, 2005.

[77] Y. Jung, J. Wang, A. Schneider et al., "Regulation of SDF-1 (CXCL12) production by osteoblasts; a possible mechanism for stem cell homing," *Bone*, vol. 38, no. 4, pp. 497–508, 2006.

[78] T. Nanki, K. Hayashida, H. S. El-Gabalawy et al., "Stromal cell-derived factor-1-CXC chemokine receptor 4 interactions play a central role in CD4+ T cell accumulation in rheumatoid arthritis synovium," *The Journal of Immunology*, vol. 165, no. 11, pp. 6590–6598, 2000.

[79] K. M. Omari and K. Dorovini-Zis, "CD40 expressed by human brain endothelial cells regulates CD4+ T cell adhesion to endothelium," *Journal of Neuroimmunology*, vol. 134, no. 1-2, pp. 166–178, 2003.

[80] L. M. Howard, A. J. Miga, C. L. Vanderlugt et al., "Mechanisms of immunotherapeutic intervention by anti-CD40L (CD154) antibody in an animal model of multiple sclerosis," *Journal of Clinical Investigation*, vol. 103, no. 2, pp. 281–290, 1999.

[81] L. M. Howard and S. D. Miller, "Autoimmune intervention by CD154 blockade prevents T cell retention and effector function in the target organ," *Journal of Immunology*, vol. 166, no. 3, pp. 1547–1553, 2001.

[82] E. Sitati, E. E. McCandless, R. S. Klein, and M. S. Diamond, "CD40-CD40 ligand interactions promote trafficking of CD8+ T cells into the brain and protection against west Nile virus encephalitis," *Journal of Virology*, vol. 81, no. 18, pp. 9801–9811, 2007.

[83] B. Shrestha, B. Zhang, W. E. Purtha, R. S. Klein, and M. S. Diamond, "Tumor necrosis factor alpha protects against lethal West Nile virus infection by promoting trafficking of mononuclear

leukocytes into the central nervous system," *Journal of Virology*, vol. 82, no. 18, pp. 8956–8964, 2008.

[84] D. M. Durrant, M. L. Robinette, and R. S. Klein, "IL-1R1 is required for dendritic cell-mediated T cell reactivation within the CNS during west nile virus encephalitis," *Journal of Experimental Medicine*, vol. 210, no. 3, pp. 503–516, 2013.

[85] S. A. Stohlman, C. C. Bergmann, M. T. Lin, D. J. Cua, and D. R. Hinton, "CTL effector function within the central nervous system requires CD4$^+$ T cells," *Journal of Immunology*, vol. 160, no. 6, pp. 2896–2904, 1998.

[86] T. W. Phares, S. A. Stohlman, M. Hwang, B. Min, D. R. Hinton, and C. C. Bergmann, "CD4 T cells promote CD8 T cell immunity at the priming and effector site during viral encephalitis," *Journal of Virology*, vol. 86, no. 5, pp. 2416–2427, 2012.

[87] H. J. Ramos, M. C. Lanteri, G. Blahnik et al., "IL-1beta signaling promotes CNS-intrinsic immune control of West Nile viru s infection," *PLoS Pathogens*, vol. 8, no. 11, Article ID e1003039, 2012.

[88] D. M. Durrant, B. P. Daniels, and R. S. Klein, "IL-1R1 signaling regulates CXCL12-mediated T cell localization and fate within the central nervous system during West Nile virus encephalitis," *The Journal of immunology*, Article ID 1401192, 2014.

[89] T. Kiyota, M. Yamamoto, H. Xiong et al., "CCL2 accelerates microglia-mediated Aβ oligomer formation and progression of neurocognitive dysfunction," *PLoS ONE*, vol. 4, no. 7, Article ID e6197, 2009.

4

Targeting BCL2-Proteins for the Treatment of Solid Tumours

Meike Vogler

Department of Biochemistry, University of Leicester, Henry-Wellcome Building, Lancaster Road, Leicester LE19HN, UK

Correspondence should be addressed to Meike Vogler; mv62@leicester.ac.uk

Academic Editor: Teresa Marafioti

Due to their central role in the regulation of apoptosis, the antiapoptotic BCL2-proteins are highly promising targets for the development of novel anticancer treatments. To this end, several strategies have been developed to inhibit BCL2, BCL-X_L, BCL-w, and MCL1. While early clinical trials in haematological malignancies demonstrated exciting single-agent activity of BCL2-inhibitors, the response in solid tumours was limited, indicating that, in solid tumours, different strategies have to be developed in order to successfully treat patients with BCL2-inhibitors. In this review, the function of the different antiapoptotic BCL2-proteins and their role in solid tumours will be discussed. In addition, a comprehensive analysis of current small molecules targeting these antiapoptotic BCL2-proteins (e.g., ABT-737, ABT-263, ABT-199, TW-37, sabutoclax, obatoclax, and MIM1) will be provided including a discussion of the results of any clinical trials. This analysis will summarise the potential of BCL2-inhibitors for the treatment of solid tumours and will unravel novel approaches to utilise these inhibitors in clinical applications.

1. Mechanisms of Apoptosis

Evasion of cell death or apoptosis is a key hallmark of cancer [1]. Generally, cells can die by apoptosis, a form of programmed cell death, or after acute injury by necrosis and cell lysis, which initiates an inflammatory response. Apoptosis was first described as a unique process associated with typical morphological changes by Carl Vogt as early as 1842 and was named apoptosis in 1972 [2]. It is a common property of multicellular organisms and is present in virtually all cell types throughout the body. Apoptosis plays a fundamental role in physiological processes, especially in mammalian development and the immune system [3, 4]. In addition, apoptosis represents a major barrier to cancer cells that must be circumvented. Therefore, many tumours acquire resistance to apoptosis through a variety of strategies. The most commonly occurring loss of a proapoptotic regulator involves the p53 tumour suppressor gene [5]. In addition to the activation of proapoptotic factors, resistance to apoptosis is often due to upregulation of antiapoptotic factors. Thus, a number of genes that encode components of the apoptotic machinery are directly targeted by activating or inactivating genetic lesions in cancer cells.

In many tumours, deregulation of cell death underlies drug resistance and is a major reason for failure of conventional anticancer therapy. Upon activation, apoptosis unfolds in a precisely organised series of steps, resulting in characteristic cellular changes, including chromatin condensation, nuclear fragmentation, breakdown of the cytoskeleton, and cell shrinkage. Most of the morphological changes associated with apoptosis are caused by a set of proteases that are specifically activated in apoptotic cells [6]. These homologous endopeptidases belong to the large family of proteins called caspases (cysteine-dependent aspartate-specific protease). Caspases are among the most specific of proteases, recognizing at least four contiguous amino acids. Although the preferred tetrapeptide motif differs among caspases, the preferred specificity of cleavage for caspases can be described as X-Glu-X-Asp [7]. Besides their function in apoptosis, some members of the caspase family participate in the processing of proinflammatory cytokines [8]. Caspases involved in apoptosis are generally divided into two categories: the initiator caspases, which include caspase-2, caspase-8, caspase-9, and caspase-10, and the effector caspases, consisting of caspase-3, caspase-6, and caspase-7. An initiator caspase is characterized by an extended N-terminal prodomain of >90 amino acids,

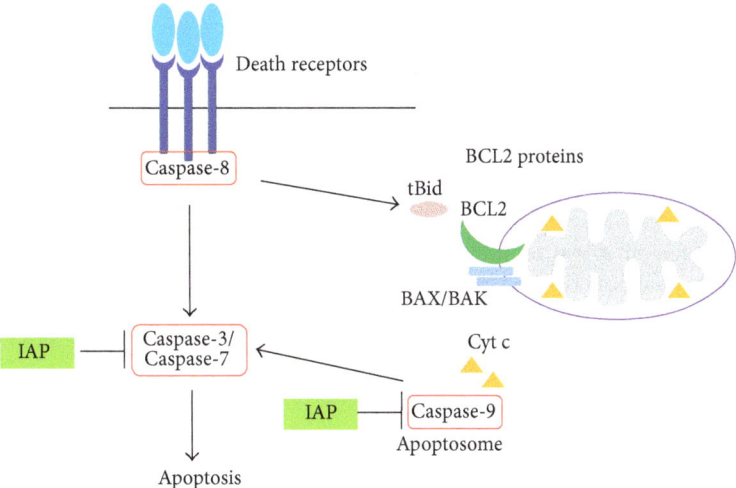

FIGURE 1: Apoptotic signalling pathways. In the extrinsic pathway, apoptosis can be initiated at the cell surface by ligation of death receptors. This results in the activation of caspase-8 at the death inducing signalling complex (DISC) and, in some circumstances, cleavage of the BH3-only protein BID. In the intrinsic pathway, apoptosis is initiated at the mitochondria and is regulated by BCL2-proteins. Activation of the intrinsic pathway, for example, by cellular stress, results in loss of mitochondrial membrane potential, release of cytochrome c, and activation of caspase-9 in the Apaf-1 containing apoptosome. Both pathways converge into the activation of the executioner caspases, for example, caspase-3. Caspases may be inhibited by the Inhibitor of apoptosis proteins (IAPs).

whereas an effector caspase contains only 20–30 residues in its prodomain [9]. In addition, only initiator caspases contain a caspase recruitment domain (CARD) or death effector domain (DED) preceding the catalytic domain. All caspases are synthesized in cells as catalytically inactive zymogens. During apoptosis, they are usually converted to the active form by proteolytic processing. The activation of an effector caspase is performed by an initiator caspase through cleavage at specific internal Asp residues that separate the large and the small subunits of the effector caspase. The initiator caspases, however, are autoactivated. Since the activation of an initiator caspase in cells inevitably triggers a cascade of downstream caspase activation, it has to be tightly regulated and it often requires the assembly of a multicomponent complex under apoptotic conditions. Once activated, effector caspases are responsible for the proteolytic cleavage of a broad spectrum of cellular targets, leading ultimately to cell death. Besides caspases, the cellular substrates include structural components, regulatory proteins, inhibitors of DNAses, and other proapoptotic proteins.

Apoptosis can be triggered either by activating receptors on the cell surface (the extrinsic pathway) or by the perturbation of mitochondria (the intrinsic pathway) (Figure 1).

2. The Extrinsic or Death Receptor Pathway of Apoptosis

In the death receptor pathway, caspase-8 is the key initiator caspase. Death receptors are members of the tumor necrosis factor (TNF) receptor superfamily and comprise a subfamily that is characterized by the intracellular death domain (DD) [10]. The most prominent death ligands are CD95-ligand/Fas-ligand, TNFα, and TNF-related apoptosis inducing ligand (TRAIL). Upon ligand binding, receptors oligomerize and

their death domains attract the intracellular adaptor protein FADD (Fas-associated death domain protein), which, in turn, recruits the inactive proform of caspase-8 or caspase-10 via their DED. The formed multiprotein complex is called DISC (death-inducing signaling complex) [11]. The DISC contains high local concentrations of the zymogene, which leads according to the induced proximity model to autoprocessing of caspase-8. This model posits that, under crowded conditions, the low intrinsic protease activity of caspase-8 is sufficient to allow the various proenzyme molecules to mutually cleave and activate each other. In some cells, known as type I cells, the amount of active caspase-8 formed at the DISC is sufficient to initiate caspase cascade and apoptosis directly, but in type II cells, mitochondria are required to amplify the apoptotic signal [12]. Notably, the activation of caspase-8 is antagonized by FLICE-like inhibitory protein (FLIP), and caspase-9 may be inhibited by the inhibitor of apoptosis proteins (IAPs), thus providing additional levels of regulation. Both pathways result in the activation of effector caspases, proteases that are responsible for most of the morphological and biochemical changes associated with apoptosis.

3. The Intrinsic or Mitochondrial Pathway of Apoptosis

In the intrinsic apoptotic pathway, cytochrome c is released from the mitochondrial intermembrane space into the cytosol, initiating the formation of the apoptosome complex and the activation of caspase-9 as the apical caspase. Therefore, outer mitochondrial membrane (OMM) permeabilisation and release of cytochrome c are considered critical steps in apoptosis induction. OMM permeabilisation is regulated by members of the BCL2-protein family, which act directly, and in concert, on the OMM [13, 14].

4. The BCL2-Family

The BCL2-family is a group of 20 proteins that are characterised by the presence of up to four sequence motifs termed BCL2 homology (BH) domains (Figure 2). The founding member, BCL2, was first identified from the t (14; 18) chromosomal translocation in follicular lymphoma, which brings BCL2 under the control of the immunoglobulin heavy chain promoter [15]. Later on it was identified as a mitochondria-localised protein that functions in apoptosis regulation [16]. BCL2-proteins can be divided into three groups, the antiapoptotic BCL2-proteins, the multidomain proapoptotic proteins (BAX and BAK), and proapoptotic BH3-only proteins [17]. Cells express multiple pro- and antiapoptotic BCL2-proteins, and their interactions regulate cell survival or cell death. Several models explain how the BCL2-proteins interact to regulate apoptosis. In the OMM, BAX and BAK can oligomerise and induce formation of a pore through which cytochrome c can be released into cytosol [18]. The antiapoptotic proteins, comprising BCL2, BCL-X$_L$, MCL1, BCL-B, BCL-w, and BCL2A1, are generally integrated in the OMM. Their main function is to protect the OMM and to prevent cytochrome c release. The different models to explain how the BCL2-proteins interact contain some controversy as to how the antiapoptotic BCL2-proteins prevent the activation of BAX and BAK. The surface structure of the antiapoptotic BCL2-proteins contains a hydrophobic pocket into which BH3-containing proteins bind. In the direct activation model, the main function of the antiapoptotic BCL2-proteins is to sequester BH3-only proteins. Thereby, the sequestration of the BH3-only proteins BIM, BID, and perhaps PUMA is critical for apoptosis inhibition, since if released, these proteins can directly bind to BAX or BAK to initiate their activation [19]. Notably, BID is activated upon the activation of the extrinsic pathway and cleavage by caspase-8 to form tBid. The other BH3-only proteins (NOXA, BIK, BNIP1, HRK, BMF, and BAD) are called sensitizers and can displace the direct activators from the antiapoptotic BCL2-proteins, thus contributing to the initiation of apoptosis. In the indirect activation model, apart from the BH3-only proteins, also BAK and BAX can be directly sequestered and inhibited by the antiapoptotic BCL2-proteins [20–22]. Notably, due to structural differences, certain BH3-only proteins only bind to a subset of antiapoptotic BCL2-proteins, while some BH3-only proteins like BIM, PUMA, and tBid can bind all antiapoptotic BCL2-proteins. Thus, BAD and BMF bind to BCL2, BCL-X$_L$, and BCL-w but not to MCL1 and BCL2A1, whereas NOXA binds to MCL1 and BCL2A1 but not to BCL2, BCL-X$_L$, and BCL-w [22, 23]. This binding pattern has important therapeutic implications, since efficient apoptosis may require the simultaneous neutralisation of all antiapoptotic BCL2-proteins [24].

5. Expression of Antiapoptotic BCL2-Proteins in Solid Tumours

5.1. BCL2. BCL2 was first discovered as an oncogene in B-cell malignancies [15, 25]. However, it is also expressed in

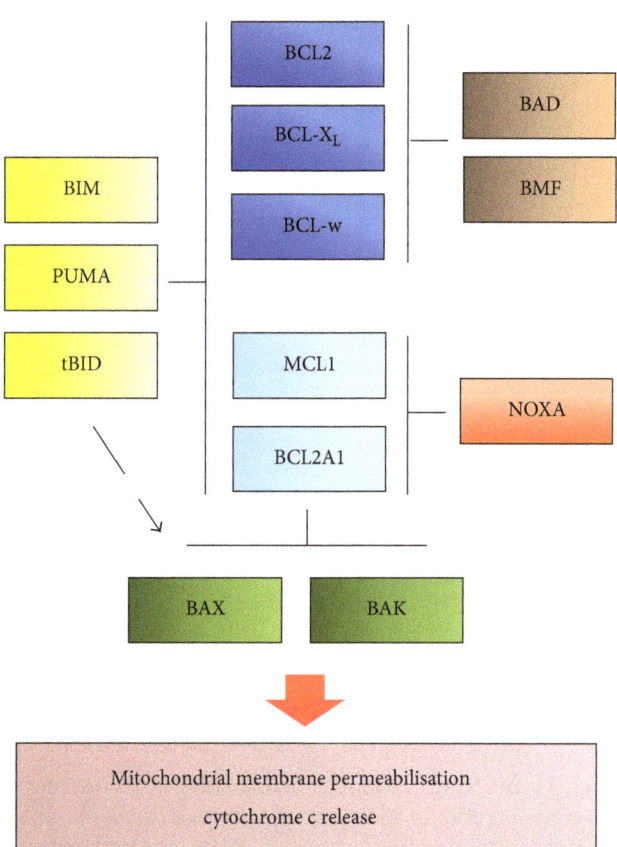

FIGURE 2: The BCL2-family. The multidomain proapoptotic proteins BAX and BAK mediate the release of cytochrome c from mitochondria into cytosol. They are inhibited by the antiapoptotic BCL2-proteins (BCL2, BCL-X$_L$, BCL-w, MCL1, and BCL2A1). BH3-only proteins (e.g., BIM, BID, PUMA, BAD, BMF, and NOXA) can neutralize the function of the antiapoptotic BCL2-proteins and may also directly activate BAX and BAK.

normal lymphoid cells including T-cells [26]. The importance of BCL2 for lymphoid development is highlighted by the phenotype of *Bcl2* knockout mice, which display accelerated lymphocyte apoptosis four weeks after birth [27]. Interestingly, BCL2 is also expressed in nonlymphoid tissues like the nerve system [28, 29] and epithelium [28]. A potential function of BCL2 in neuronal tumours has first been described by Reed et al. [30]. The expression of BCL2 in normal epithelium suggests that BCL2 may also be expressed in carcinoma. Evidence that BCL2 may have oncogenic potential in carcinoma was first provided in prostate cancer, where high expression of BCL2 was found in androgen-independent tumours [31]. Since then, high BCL2 expression has been reported in many different tumour types including lung cancer [32, 33], ovary cancer [34], and breast cancer [35]. The function of BCL2 in inhibiting apoptosis has been proven in many independent studies, for example, by overexpression or knockdown [36]. Paradoxically, several studies have reported that high expression of BCL2 is not associated with the level of malignancies but may even be associated with favourable prognosis, indicating that, in solid tumours, the role of BCL2 as an antiapoptotic gatekeeper is less clear than in haematological malignancies [37, 38].

5.2. MCL1. The second antiapoptotic BCL2-protein discovered was MCL1. It was isolated from the myeloid leukemia cell line ML-1 when undergoing differentiation and was classified as an early response gene [39]. Many reports have demonstrated that MCL1 is a highly regulated protein with a high turn-over linked to rapid proteasomal degradation [40]. Its expression can be induced by different stimuli including cytokines [41] or DNA-damage [42]. Genetic deletion of *Mcl1* results in peri-implantation embryonic lethality, suggesting that MCL1 may have a function beyond the control of apoptosis [43].

MCL1 is an important antiapoptotic oncogene that is overexpressed in the majority of cancers. In particular, multiple myeloma cells display high expression of MCL1 and appear to be dependent on MCL1 for survival [44]. Notably, gene alterations around the locus of MCL1 on 1q21 have been identified as early as 1994, when it was discovered that 1q21 is duplicated or rearranged in many types of cancer [45]. Since then, many studies have identified MCL1 as highly amplified in cancer, emphasizing its importance for carcinogenesis. With the development of next-generation sequencing, gene alterations in cancer are now investigated on a large scale with the aim of identifying driver mutations. Using next-generation sequencing, MCL1 has been identified as the most amplified gene in a screen of 3,000 individual cancers, highlighting its importance for cancer and suggesting a unique function of MCL1 amongst the antiapoptotic BCL2-proteins [46].

5.3. BCL-X$_L$. The antiapoptotic protein BCL-X$_L$ was identified only a few months after MCL1 as a BCL2-related protein isolated from chicken lymphoid cells [47]. Interestingly, the underlying gene *Bcl2l1* can be expressed in two different isoforms, encoding BCL-X$_L$ and BCL-X$_S$. While BCL-X$_L$ has a well-described antiapoptotic function, BCL-X$_S$ may be proapoptotic and its expression may counteract the antiapoptotic function of BCL2. BCL-X$_L$ displays a wider tissue distribution than BCL2, and besides lymphocytes, neuronal cells and epithelium high expression is found in reproductive tissues [48]. Its importance in neuronal tissue is emphasized by the phenotype of *Bcl2l1* deficient mice, which is embryonic lethal due to massive apoptosis in the brain [49]. Elevated expression of BCL-X$_L$ was found in many solid tumours including neuronal tumours [50], adenocarcinoma [51, 52], bladder cancer [53], and gastric cancer [54]. Generally, BCL-X$_L$ appears to be more frequently overexpressed in solid tumours than BCL2. The importance of BCL-X$_L$ in solid tumours was highlighted by a bioinformatics screen to identify markers of chemosensitivity. In this screen, mRNA expression was compared in 60 tumour cell lines and correlated with sensitivity to a panel of 122 standard chemotherapeutic drugs. The most striking relationship observed was a strong negative correlation between basal expression of BCL-X$_L$ and sensitivity to drugs [55]. In addition, BCL-X$_L$ was identified as one of the key genes frequently amplified in cancer [46].

5.4. BCL2A1. In 1993, another antiapoptotic BCL2 protein was discovered and named BCL2A1 or Bfl1 [56]. In contrast to other antiapoptotic BCL2-proteins, BCL2A1 does not display a well-defined C-terminal transmembrane domain [57] and its function in apoptosis inhibition is less well established [58]. The phenotype of *Bcl2a1* knockout mice is less severe than that of other BCL2-proteins with *Bcl2a1* deletion only resulting in hair loss during ageing [59]. However, this may be explained by the existence of multiple gene copies, and loss of BCL2A1 using *in vivo* RNAi has revealed a more severe phenotype in leukocyte development [60].

BCL2A1 is mainly expressed in lymphoid malignancies and appears to play only a minor role in solid tumours [58]. When first identified, human *BCL2A1* mRNA was found overexpressed in stomach cancer compared to normal tissue, indicating a possible function of BCL2A1 also in solid tumours [61]. Amongst a panel of different solid tumour tissues, the highest expression of *BCL2A1* mRNA was detected in breast cancer samples [62]. Interestingly, in advanced breast cancer a higher expression of *BCL2A1* mRNA was found when compared to less advanced tumours [63], suggesting an association of BCL2A1 expression with later and more severe disease stages. Furthermore, *BCL2A1* expression was associated with metastatic disease in melanoma [64] and hepatocellular carcinoma [65]. Interestingly, expression data collected in Oncomine (https://www.oncomine.org) indicate that melanoma may display higher expression of *BCL2A1* than other solid tumours, and its function in inhibiting apoptosis has recently been demonstrated using siRNA mediated knockdown, which was sufficient to induce apoptosis in the melanoma cell line 1205Lu [66]. Transcriptional profiling indicated that *BCL2A1* is highly expressed in squamous cell carcinoma of the skin [67] and that, later on, *BCL2A1* was observed to be overexpressed in oral squamous cell carcinoma [68]. In summary, BCL2A1 has been identified as overexpressed in a variety of haematological malignancies as well as solid tumours and appears to be predominantly associated with advanced or metastatic disease stages.

5.5. BCL-w. BCL-w was identified as an antiapoptotic BCL2 protein in 1996 by Suzanne Cory's laboratory [69]. A study in mice lacking BCL-w indicated that, unlike other BCL2-proteins, BCL-w does not have an important function in lymphoid cells but, instead, appears to be essential for spermatogenesis [70]. However, a function of BCL-w in testicular cancer has not yet been described. Later, studies have found expression of BCL-w in the small intestine as well as epithelial tumours and established a function for BCL-w in protecting epithelial cells from apoptosis induced upon DNA-damage [71].

5.6. BCL-B. The last antiapoptotic BCL2-protein discovered was BCL-B in 2001 [72]. Interestingly, BCL-B binds and inhibits BAX but not BAK. Its mRNA appears to be widely expressed in human tissues. Tumour specific overexpression of BCL-B was observed in breast, gastric, colorectal, and lung adenocarcinoma and correlates with poor prognosis, indicating that BCL-B may play a prominent role in inhibiting apoptosis in solid tumours [73].

6. Targeting of BCL2-Protein as a Novel Anticancer Treatment

Due to their prominent role in inhibiting apoptosis, the BCL2-proteins have been recognised as promising targets for the development of novel anticancer therapeutics. The first approach to target BCL2 itself was based on an antisense RNA [74]. The resulting compound, oblimersen/genasense, was studied in clinical trials for multiple malignancies including solid tumours [75–77]. Genta, the company behind the drug, filed for FDA approval of genasense for the treatment of melanoma and chronic lymphocytic leukemia in 2003 and 2006, respectively, but the drug was rejected in both cases for lack of efficacy. The clinical failure of oblimersen may have been due to the inability of antisense molecules to efficiently inhibit protein synthesis *in vivo*.

Following up on the initial antisense method, the field subsequently advanced to use high-throughput screening of chemical libraries to identify compounds capable of binding to BCL2-proteins. Gossypol, isolated from cotton seeds and used as a male contraceptive, was recognized as binding and interacting with antiapoptotic BCL2 family members as well as inducing apoptosis [78]. The R-state of gossypol (AT-101) was licensed by Ascenta Therapeutics and tested in clinical trials. Initially described as a potent and selective inhibitor of protein kinase C [79], chelerythrine, a naturally occurring benzophenanthridine alkaloid, was subsequently identified by high-throughput screening as an inhibitor of BCL-X_L [80]. EM20-25, which binds to the BH3 domain of BCL2, is a derivative of HA14-1, but it lacks its effects on mitochondrial respiration [81]. However, despite the use of these inhibitors in preclinical mechanistic studies, proof for their specificity for BCL2-proteins has so far been limited [24, 82, 83]. Specific inhibitors of BCL2-proteins should induce apoptosis in a BAX/BAK-dependent manner with subsequent release of cytochrome c and activation of caspase-9. Although it has been shown that several BCL2 inhibitors might activate the intrinsic apoptotic pathway, there is little evidence that activation of this pathway is required for cell death induction.

More recent approaches to target BCL2-protein utilise small molecule inhibitors which mimic BH3-containing proteins and bind specifically into the hydrophobic groove on the antiapoptotic BCL2-proteins (Figure 3). These small molecules are therefore also called BH3-mimetics and will be further described in the following section.

6.1. ABT-737. In 2005 Oltersdorf et al. published the development of ABT-737, a highly potent inhibitor of BCL2, BCL-X_L, and BCL-w [84]. This hallmark paper, which has been cited more than 1,800 times in 2014, described how structure-activity relationship (SAR) by nuclear magnetic resonance (NMR), a technique pioneered by Shuker to identify protein ligands [85], was used to screen a chemical library for fragments that bind into the hydrophobic groove of BCL-X_L. To achieve high-affinity binding, the proximal fragments binding to different sites in the hydrophobic groove of BCL-X_L have subsequently been linked, and lead compounds

were developed. The final compound, ABT-737, binds with very high affinity (Ki < 1 nM) to BCL-X_L, but due to their similar structure also to BCL2 and BCL-w. Notably, MCL1, BCL-B, and BCL2A1 have a less homologous structure and, therefore, are not inhibited by ABT-737. The potential of ABT-737 as an anticancer agent has further been demonstrated in a set of cancer cells including lung cancer cell lines. As a single agent, ABT-737 was mainly active in haematological malignancies but less active in solid tumours. A notable exception was small cell lung cancer (SCLC), where some cell lines were found to be highly sensitive to ABT-737. Additional studies have investigated the effect of ABT-737 in SCLC and identified an essential role of MCL1 in determining resistance to ABT-737 [86–88]. To this end, SCLC cell lines that have low expression of MCL1 were more sensitive to ABT-737 than those with high expression of MCL1. This relationship can be explained by the similar function of MCL1 and BCL2/BCL-X_L/BCL-w. All of these antiapoptotic BCL2-proteins inhibit apoptosis by sequestering proapoptotic BH3-containing BCL2-proteins. In situations where the activity of BCL2/BCL-X_L/BCL-w is inhibited due to the binding of a small molecule inhibitor (ABT-737) into their hydrophobic groove, this binding will displace any bound proapoptotic BH3-containing proteins, for example, BIM or BAX and BAK. These proapoptotic proteins are subsequently free to induce release of cytochrome c, but, in the presence of high levels of MCL1, this may now take over the function of BCL2/BCL-X_L/BCL-w and sequester the proapoptotic BCL2-proteins previously displaced from BCL2/BCL-X_L/BCL-w.

6.2. ABT-263. A major limitation of ABT-737 as an anti-cancer drug is that it is not orally bioavailable, which can limit the dosing regimens particularly in chronic therapy. To this end, Abbott developed a related compound, ABT-263 (Navitoclax), which is orally bioavailable and also binds to BCL2, BCL-X_L, and BCL-w but not to MCL1, BCL2A1, and Bcl-B [89]. The biological activity of ABT-737 and ABT-263 appears to be comparable, although ABT-263 has been shown to be more readily sequestered by human serum albumin than ABT-737 [90]. ABT-263 entered clinical trials for lymphoid malignancies as well as solid tumours. While the results in haematological malignancies were encouraging and single-agent activity was reported [91], the efficacy of ABT-263 as a single agent in solid tumours was a bit disappointing. In the phase I dose-escalation study, 47 patients were enrolled, of whom 27 had SCLC [92]. In line with the preclinical data, SCLC patients appeared to respond better than the other malignancies which were not further described. In the phase II study patients with relapsed SCLC received a lead-in dose of 150 mg daily for one week followed by 325 mg of ABT-263 daily [93]. This lead-in dose was given to circumvent thrombocytopenia caused by a depletion of platelets due to their dependency on BCL-X_L [94]. Partial response to ABT-263 was observed in 1/39 patients (3%) while stable disease was observed in 9/37 patients (23%). Since these were chemotherapy-resistant relapsed tumour patients, the overall survival was very poor (3 months). However, the authors concluded that ABT-263 shows limited single-agent activity

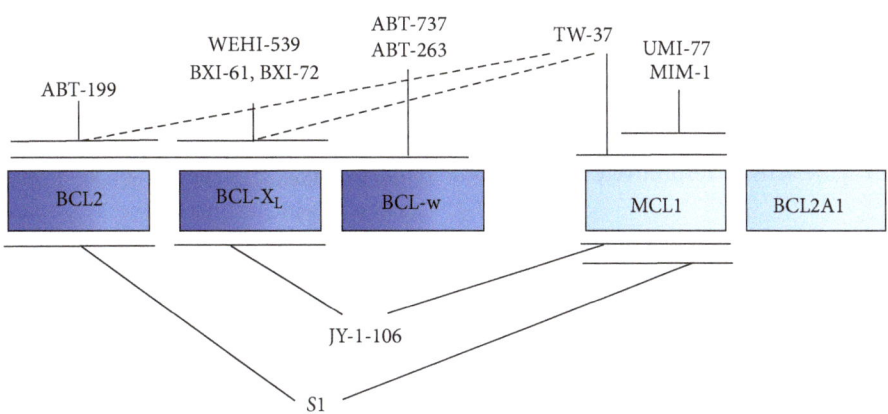

FIGURE 3: Small molecule BCL2-inhibitors. Inhibition of multiple or individual antiapoptotic BCL2-proteins by small molecule antagonists.

against advanced and recurrent SCLC [93]. Interestingly, this study also suggested a potential biomarker of clinical benefit that is based on gene amplification and copy number gain of BCL2 and colocalised genes. This highlights the potential for stratified clinical trials into which only SCLC patients with amplified BCL2 gene could be recruited.

6.3. ABT-199.

The major toxicity of ABT-263 was an on-target effect on BCL-X_L expressed in platelets [94–96]. The discovery that thrombocytopenia was a major mechanism-based effect of ABT-263 led to studies that elegantly demonstrated the importance of BCL-X_L as a molecular clock in platelets [94]. In order to prevent this dose-limiting toxicity, Abbott reengineered ABT-263 and developed ABT-199, a small molecule inhibitor that specifically maintains binding to BCL2 but does not inhibit BCL-X_L or BCL-w [97]. ABT-199 efficiently induces apoptosis in BCL2-dependent tumours without causing thrombocytopenia. Impressively, a single dose of ABT-199 induced tumour lysis syndrome in three patients with leukaemia, indicating potent antitumour activity *in vivo* in humans. Therefore, ABT-199 is currently one of the most exciting agents in the clinical development for haematological malignancies. Due to the prominent role of BCL2 in B-cells, clinical trials with ABT-199 currently concentrate entirely on haematological malignancies. In solid tumours, BCL-X_L appears to be more important for apoptosis inhibition than BCL2, making it unlikely that a selective inhibitor of BCL2 may induce cell death. However, some tumours including SCLC display high expression of BCL2 and may be susceptible to single-agent treatment with ABT-199. Despite high expression of BCL-X_L, ABT-199 displays preclinical activity in breast cancer cells [98]. However, a thorough analysis of the potential of ABT-199, a selective inhibitor of BCL2, or a side-by-side comparison of ABT-199 with ABT-263 or ABT-737 in solid tumours is currently lacking.

6.4. WEHI-539.

To induce apoptosis in solid tumours, a selective inhibitor of BCL-X_L may be advantageous over a selective inhibitor of BCL2. Any true BCL-X_L inhibitor will induce platelet toxicity, but this may be manageable by applying a lead-in dosing schedule and by preselecting patients who display a low risk of developing thrombocytopenia. A specific inhibitor of BCL-X_L, WEHI-539, was developed by experts at the Walter and Eliza Hall Institute of Medical Research (WEHI) in Australia using high-throughput screening [99]. Despite its similar function, WEHI-539 is chemically not closely related to ABT-737 and analogous compounds. It has subnanomolar binding affinity for BCL-X_L and induces cell death in BCL-X_L-dependent tumour cells. To further advance in the clinical development of selective BCL-X_L-inhibitors, Genentech and WEHI are currently collaborating to develop improved analogues of WEHI-539 [100]. These may prove particularly promising for the treatment of solid tumours, but as yet little data has been published. Support for the hypothesis that BCL-X_L is more relevant for solid tumours than BCL2 was provided by a recent study comparing the effect of ABT-737 (the dual BCL2/BCL-X_L-inhibitor), ABT-199 (the selective inhibitor of BCL2), and WEHI-539 (the selective inhibitor of BCL-X_L) in colon cancer stem cells. This study elegantly showed that ABT-737 and WEHI-539 lower the apoptotic threshold of colon cancer cells, while ABT-199 had no effect, indicating that BCL-X_L is the more relevant target [101].

6.5. BXI-61 and BXI-72.

In a similar approach that was used to develop WEHI-539, another set of selective inhibitors of BCL-X_L were developed by screening of the National Cancer Institute (NCI) chemical library, namely, BXI-61 and BXI-72 [102]. These compounds also display subnanomolar binding affinity to BCL-X_L but do not bind any of the other antiapoptotic BCL2-proteins. Their efficiency as anticancer agents was investigated in lung cancer cell lines, and impressive inhibition of tumour cell growth was demonstrated *in vitro* and also *in vivo* in xenograft animal models [102]. Unfortunately, no cellular data on the specificity of the compounds was provided, and experience has shown that a lot of compounds that were originally identified as strong binders of BCL2-proteins have later on been shown to induce cell death independently of BCL2-proteins [82]. With this in mind, it is a bit worrying that, in two completely unrelated high-throughput screens, one of these compounds, BXI-61 or NSC354961, was also identified as a potential binding partner of the enzyme S-adenosylmethionine decarboxylase or an inhibitor of Hdm2 E3 ligase activity, respectively.

6.6. *Obatoclax.* In contrast to the more selective molecules described above, obatoclax or GX15-070 appears to be a pan-BCL2 inhibitor, meaning that it binds to all of the antiapoptotic BCL2-proteins [103]. Preclinical data indicate that obatoclax is not a very specific compound and induces cell death even in the absence of BAX and BAK [82]. Generally, an inhibitor that can neutralise all antiapoptotic BCL2-proteins may have therapeutic advantages, since the function of the antiapoptotic BCL2-proteins is partially redundant and efficient apoptosis may require the neutralisation of all BCL2-proteins [24]. However, such a compound is also bound to have higher toxicities. Early clinical trials with obatoclax have indicated neuronal toxicity which was not observed with more specific compounds [104]. Notably, this toxicity may depend on the dosing schedule. Due to its ability to bind MCL1, obatoclax may be particularly promising for the treatment of solid tumours. To this end, its ability as an anticancer agent was investigated in clinical trials for SCLC [105]. Results were disappointing, and obatoclax mesylate added to topotecan did not exceed the historic response rate seen with topotecan alone in patients with relapsed SCLC following the first-line platinum-based therapy. Currently, there are no open clinical trials with obatoclax in solid tumours.

6.7. *S1.* The small molecule S1 was discovered by screening of organic compound libraries for anticancer agents [106]. By binding to BCL2 and MCL1, it displaces BAK and induces apoptosis. Interestingly, S1 appears to induce cell death dependent on BAX/BAK and knockdown of BAX and BAK prevented apoptosis, indicating that S1 could be a specific inhibitor of BCL2-proteins [107]. Antitumour activity of S1 was shown in a mouse liver carcinoma xenograft model [108]. Resistance to S1 has been reported in SCLC by the activation of the MAPK/ERK pathway and the subsequent phosphorylation of BCL2 [109]. Further investigations into the biological activity of S1 would be highly desirable to determine whether this molecule could be a promising drug candidate.

6.8. *JY-1-106.* Another pan-inhibitor of antiapoptotic BCL2-proteins was published in 2013 and is called JY-1-106 [110]. This inhibitor is based on a trisacrylamide framework and reproduces the chemical nature and relative spatial projections of the key hydrophobic side chains on one face of the BH3 α-helix. Therefore, it can inhibit both BCL-X$_L$ and MCL1. In cells, it induces the displacement of BAK from both BCL-X$_L$ and MCL1 followed by apoptosis. However, data on the specificity of JY-1-106 have not yet been published and its toxicity to cells lacking BAK and BAX has not been investigated. Notably, JY-1-106 was able to suppress tumour growth in a lung cancer xenograft model, indicating that it may be a promising lead compound to treat cancer.

6.9. *Apogossypol, Apogossypolone, and Its Derivatives.* Removal of the toxic aldehyde groups in the naturally occurring polyphenol, gossypol, resulted in the synthesis of apogossypol, which binds to the hydrophobic groove of BCL2 and BCL-X$_L$ [78, 111]. Further substitution of the isopropyl side groups in apogossypol yielded BI97C1 (sabutoclax or ONT-701), which targets multiple antiapoptotic members, including BCL2, BCL-X$_L$, MCL1, and BCL2A1. Apogossypolone is a third-generation gossypol derivative, designed to effectively target MCL1, with reduced toxicity and nonspecific reactivity. Structural derivatives of apogossypolone include BI97C10 and BI112D1 (also called BI97D6), which were designed to display a higher selectivity for MCL1 over BCL2 or BCL-X$_L$ [112–114]. Both BI97C1 and BI112D1 were selective in killing cells in a BAX/BAK- and caspase-9-dependent manner [115]. However, the inhibitors lacked the potency to induce similar extents of death in BCL2-, BCL-X$_L$-, or MCL1-dependent cells, indicating that these are specific but rather weak inhibitors of BCL2-proteins. Further investigations have shown that BI97C1 and BI112D1 induce mitochondrial fragmentation rather than apoptosis [116]. In particular, BI97C1 was proposed as a promising pan-BCL2 inhibitor for further clinical development and licensed by Oncothyreon Inc. This was mainly based on a study indicating that BI97C1 may sensitise leukaemia stem cells to receptor tyrosine kinase inhibition [117]. Its potential in treating solid tumours has been shown in murine models of prostate cancer, where BI97C1 reduced tumourigenesis. Notably, in this study BI97C1 was found to block c-Met activation rather than inducing apoptosis, confirming that its main mode of action may not be via specific inhibition of BCL2-proteins and induction of apoptosis [118].

TW-37 is a second-generation benzenesulphonyl derivative of gossypol developed through computational screening and NMR that binds to MCL1 with higher affinity than to BCL2 and BCL-X$_L$ [119]. Its potential as an anticancer agent has been demonstrated in prostate cancer cells and pancreatic cancer [119, 120]. In murine embryonic fibroblasts lacking BAX and BAK TW-37 did not induce cell death, whereas wild-type fibroblasts underwent apoptosis, indicating that TW-37 induces cell death in a BCL2-protein family specific manner [115]. While cellular experiments have demonstrated that TW-37 is not a very potent inhibitor of BCL2, it may have potential in targeting MCL1 since it induces cell death in MCL1-dependent lung cancer cells [115]. Therefore, TW-37 deserves further exploration to determine its potential as anticancer agent.

6.10. *Selective MCL1-Inhibitors.* Using a library of stabilised alpha-helix of BCL2 domains, the BH3 helix of MCL1 on its own was identified as a potent and exclusive MCL1 inhibitor [121]. Such stapled peptides exhibit selectivity in disrupting specific BH3-mediated interactions *in vitro*, and their sequence-dependent proapoptotic activity has been documented *in vivo* [122, 123]. The interaction of an MCL1 stapled peptide with the BH3-binding groove was employed in a competitive screen to identify MIM-1, a novel molecule that selectively targets the BH3 binding groove of MCL-1 [124]. Whereas MIM-1 exhibits BAK-dependent apoptotic activity, its potency may be limited and cell-type dependent, as it failed to induce apoptosis in two MCL1-dependent cell lines [115]. The molecule ML311 was discovered by ultrahigh-throughput screening coupled with hit optimisation [125]. This screen was designed to identify compounds that can disrupt the interaction of MCL1 with the BH3-domain of BIM. Interestingly, a secondary screen was added to identify compounds that selectively bind to MCL1 as compared to BCL-X_L. To this end, ML311 displays 100-fold higher affinity to MCL1 than to BCL-X_L. Some selectivity of ML311 was also indicated by the reduced activity of ML311 in BAX/BAK-deficient cells. More recently, the selective MCL1-inhibitor UMI-77 was developed by modification of the lead compound UMI-59 [126]. UMI-77 binds to the BH3-binding groove of MCL1 with Ki of 490 nmol/L and inhibits pancreatic cancer cells growth *in vitro* and *in vivo*. Specificity of UMI-77 was further demonstrated by its inability to induce cell death in cells lacking BAX and BAK expression.

Possibly the most promising lead compounds with selective binding of MCL1 have been identified by Stephen Fesik, who was leading in the chemical development of ABT-737. In contrast to other screening approaches, Fesik and colleagues used NMR-based screening of a large fragment library to identify compounds that bind to MCL1 and identified two chemically distinct hit series that bind to different sites on MCL1 [127]. Members of the two fragment classes (benzothiophene and the indole series) were merged together to produce lead compounds that bind to MCL1 with a dissociation constant of <100 nM with selectivity for MCL1 over BCL-X_L and BCL2. X-ray crystallography demonstrated that the hydrophobic unit of the first fragments binds in the lower part of the BH3-binding pocket of MCL1 while the core units derived from the second fragments are positioned in the upper part of the pocket. A similar fragment-based screening approach had previously led to the development of ABT-737 [84], demonstrating the potential of fragment-based drug discovery to target BCL2-proteins.

7. Combination of BCL2-Inhibitors with Chemotherapy

With some notable exceptions, solid tumour cells appear to be resistant to single agent treatment with BCL2-inhibitors. This lack of efficiency may partially be explained by the lack of potent pan-BCL2 inhibitors, which could simultaneously neutralise all antiapoptotic BCL2-proteins. Support for this hypothesis is provided by studies that have identified MCL1 as the major resistance factor for ABT-737 [24, 128]. Only limited data is available on selective inhibitors of MCL1, and instead many approaches have targeted the transcriptional regulation of MCL1. To this end, anthracyclines as well as inhibitors of histone deacetylases or cyclin-dependent

kinases have all been shown to suppress MCL1 expression and thus sensitise ABT-737 induced apoptosis [129, 130]. However, it remains to be seen in which tumour types the simultaneous inhibition of all expressed antiapoptotic BCL2-proteins is sufficient to induce cell death and inhibit tumour growth.

Another approach to utilise BCL2-inhibitors is to combine them either with other targeted agents or with conventional chemotherapy. The rationale for the combination of BCL2-inhibitors with chemotherapy is that the toxic insults induced by chemotherapeutic agents can lead to apoptosis if the threshold to undergo apoptosis is sufficiently low [131]. Since small cell lung cancer appears to be the most susceptible to BCL2-inhibitors and some single-agent activity was observed in cell lines [84], most clinical trials with BCL2-inhibitors have concentrated on small cell lung cancer. To this end, obatoclax has been combined with carboplatin and etoposide in a phase I study in small cell lung cancer [132]. Though patient numbers were small, there was a suggestion of improved efficacy in the obatoclax-treated group. Combination of obatoclax with topotecan in a phase II trial, however, concluded that obatoclax added to topotecan did not exceed the historic response rate seen with topotecan alone in patients with relapsed small cell lung cancer following the first-line platinum-based therapy [133].

Clinical trials investigating gossypol (AT-101) in small cell lung cancer concluded that gossypol alone is not active in patients with recurrent chemosensitive disease, which may be linked to the poor potency of this inhibitor [134]. When combined with topotecan or docetaxel in relapsed or refractory small cell lung cancer, the response was limited and further enrolment of patients was not justified [135, 136]. Besides small cell lung cancer, gossypol was also investigated in prostate cancer where it was combined with docetaxel and prednisone [137]. Gossypol was well tolerated but did not extend survival. However, a potential benefit was observed in high-risk patients, indicating the potential to further explore this compound in clinical trials.

The potential of ABT-263 to sensitise to chemotherapy was demonstrated in many studies in multiple cell lines [138–140]. The combination of ABT-263 with docetaxel and gemcitabine in solid tumours has been investigated in clinical trials, but results have not been disclosed yet. The related compound, ABT-199, is currently only tested in haematological malignancies, with outstanding single-agent activity reported particularly in chronic lymphocytic leukaemia and other non-Hodgkin lymphomas. Due to the high expression of BCL-X_L, it is not clear whether a molecule like ABT-199 that selectively targets BCL2 would be beneficial in solid tumours. The importance of BCL-X_L is highlighted by the observation that colon cancer stem cells can be sensitised by ABT-737 or WEHI-539, but not by ABT-199 [101]. However, overexpression and addiction to BCL2 has been reported in small cell lung cancer [33, 141] and therefore a stratified clinical trial investigating ABT-199 in patients with high BCL2-expression may be justified. Treatment of small cell lung cancer with the potent inhibitor ABT-199 may be particularly promising if combined with chemotherapy.

8. Combination of BCL2-Inhibitors with Other Targeted Agents

A more rational approach to utilise BCL2-inhibitors in clinical applications is the combination with other targeted agents. In contrast to standard chemotherapy which interferes with all dividing cells, these are agents specifically designed to inhibit key survival signalling pathways activated in tumour cells. The most successful targeted therapies include imatinib (a tyrosine kinase inhibitor), gefitinib (an inhibitor of epidermal growth factor receptors), sunitinib (an inhibitor of vascular endothelial growth factor), and bortezomib (a proteasome inhibitor). To this end, ABT-263 has been combined with erlotinib, a tyrosine kinase inhibitor, in a clinical trial for solid tumours. Unfortunately, results of this study have not been published yet.

Apart from the inhibition of survival signalling, BCL2-inhibitors could also be combined with other targeted agents that induce apoptosis in tumour cells. To this end, obatoclax and ABT-737 sensitize hepatoblastoma cells to death-receptor-induced apoptosis [142]. However, the potential of simultaneously targeting different arms of apoptosis signalling and combining a BCL2-inhibitor with other apoptosis-inducing agents needs to be further investigated in order to determine the potential of this approach for solid tumours.

One of the most prominent survival pathways mutated in cancer is regulated by RAF (rapidly accelerated fibrosarcoma) kinases. They participate in the RAS-RAF-MEK (Mitogen-activated protein kinase kinase)-ERK signalling cascade which is frequently hyperactivated in cancer due to mutations in BRAF or RAS. Upon hyperactivation, this pathway induces the expression of proapoptotic BH3-only proteins such as BIM, BMF, and PUMA. While inhibitors of MEK and BRAF typically induce minimal apoptosis, their predominant response is a G1 cell cycle arrest [143]. However, the BH3-only proteins induced by ERK inhibition may prime tumour cells for apoptosis, thus providing a rationale for combining an ERK or MEK inhibitor with BCL2-inhibitors. To this end, addition of ABT-737 converted the predominantly cytostatic effect of MEK inhibition to a cytotoxic effect, causing long-term tumour regression in mice xenografted with human tumour cell lines [144]. Interestingly, a synthetic lethal screen to identify genes that, when inhibited, cooperate with MEK inhibitors to effectively treat KRAS mutant tumours identified BCL-X_L as the most prominent target [145]. In this study, combination of the MEK inhibitor with ABT-263 led to a dramatic reduction of tumour growth in xenograft models of KRAS mutant tumours, supporting combined BCL-X_L/MEK inhibition as a potential therapeutic approach for KRAS mutant cancers and providing a basis for stratified clinical trials. To this end, a clinical trial has recently been initiated to investigate ABT-263 in combination with the MEK-inhibitor Trametinib in KRAS mutant tumours.

Similarly, ABT-737 has been shown to sensitize melanoma cells to BRAF inhibitors only when the V600E activating mutation of BRAF is present [146]. This indicates that combination of selective BRAF inhibitors with ABT-737 or ABT-263 may increase the degree and rate of responses in previously untreated patients with V600E melanoma but not in those with acquired resistance to these agents. To follow up on these preclinical studies, a clinical trial is currently underway to investigate the potential of ABT-263 in combination with Trametinib and the BRAF-inhibitor Dabrafenib as a treatment for BRAF mutant melanoma. Taken together, these studies strongly support the investigation of BCL2-inhibitors in combination with MEK, ERK, or RAF-inhibitors, and the results of the first stratified clinical trials are eagerly awaited.

9. Conclusions

BCL2-proteins are one of the most prominent antiapoptotic proteins deregulated in cancer. They contribute to tumourigenesis and mediate resistance to current anticancer treatments. In recent years, several promising inhibitors of BCL2-proteins have been developed and thus the great challenge now is to explore how to best utilise these compounds in which tumour types. BCL2-inhibitors are unlikely to be as efficient as single agents, but they may be very beneficial when combined with other targeted agents. Therefore, future personalised cancer treatment will include BCL2-inhibitors in those tumours that express addiction to BCL2-proteins.

Conflict of Interests

The author declares that there is no conflict of interests regarding the publication of this paper.

References

[1] D. Hanahan and R. A. Weinberg, "The hallmarks of cancer," *Cell*, vol. 100, no. 1, pp. 57–70, 2000.

[2] J. F. Kerr, A. H. Wyllie, and A. R. Currie, "Apoptosis: a basic biological phenomenon with wide-ranging implications in tissue kinetics," *British Journal of Cancer*, vol. 26, no. 4, pp. 239–257, 1972.

[3] D. L. Vaux, "Caspases and apoptosis—biology and terminology," *Cell Death & Differentiation*, vol. 6, no. 6, pp. 493–494, 1999.

[4] P. H. Krammer, "CD95's deadly mission in the immune system," *Nature*, vol. 407, no. 6805, pp. 789–795, 2000.

[5] P. A. J. Muller and K. H. Vousden, "P53 mutations in cancer," *Nature Cell Biology*, vol. 15, no. 1, pp. 2–8, 2013.

[6] D. R. McIlwain, T. Berger, and T. W. Mak, "Caspase functions in cell death and disease," *Cold Spring Harbor Perspectives in Biology*, vol. 5, no. 4, Article ID a008656, 2013.

[7] G. M. Cohen, "Caspases: the executioners of apoptosis," *Biochemical Journal*, vol. 326, no. 1, pp. 1–16, 1997.

[8] I. G. Rodrigue-Gervais and M. Saleh, "Caspases and immunity in a deadly grip," *Trends in Immunology*, vol. 34, no. 2, pp. 41–49, 2013.

[9] M. Drag and G. S. Salvesen, "Emerging principles in protease-based drug discovery," *Nature Reviews Drug Discovery*, vol. 9, no. 9, pp. 690–701, 2010.

[10] M. E. Peter and P. H. Krammer, "Mechanisms of CD95 (APO-1/Fas)-mediated apoptosis," *Current Opinion in Immunology*, vol. 10, no. 5, pp. 545–551, 1998.

[11] L. S. Dickens, I. R. Powley, M. A. Hughes, and M. MacFarlane, "The 'complexities' of life and death: death receptor signalling

platforms," *Experimental Cell Research*, vol. 318, no. 11, pp. 1269–1277, 2012.

[12] C. Scaffidi, S. Fulda, A. Srinivasan et al., "Two CD95 (APO-1/Fas) signaling pathways," *The EMBO Journal*, vol. 17, no. 6, pp. 1675–1687, 1998.

[13] T. Bender and J. Martinou, "Where killers meet–permeabilization of the outer mitochondrial membrane during apoptosis," *Cold Spring Harbor perspectives in biology*, vol. 5, no. 1, 2013.

[14] A. Shamas-Din, J. Kale, B. Leber, and D. W. Andrews, "Mechanisms of action of Bcl-2 family proteins," *Cold Spring Harbor Perspectives in Biology*, vol. 5, no. 4, Article ID a008714, 2013.

[15] L. Pegoraro, A. Palumbo, J. Erikson et al., "A 14;18 and an 8;14 chromosome translocation in a cell line derived from an acute B-cell leukemia," *Proceedings of the National Academy of Sciences of the United States of America*, vol. 81, no. 22, pp. 7166–7170, 1984.

[16] D. Hockenbery, G. Nunez, C. Milliman, R. D. Schreiber, and S. J. Korsmeyer, "Bcl-2 is an inner mitochondrial membrane protein that blocks programmed cell death," *Nature*, vol. 348, no. 6299, pp. 334–336, 1990.

[17] S. Cory and J. M. Adams, "The BCL2 family: regulators of the cellular life-or-death switch," *Nature Reviews Cancer*, vol. 2, no. 9, pp. 647–656, 2002.

[18] J. E. Chipuk and D. R. Green, "How do BCL-2 proteins induce mitochondrial outer membrane permeabilization?" *Trends in Cell Biology*, vol. 18, no. 4, pp. 157–164, 2008.

[19] A. Letai, M. C. Bassik, L. D. Walensky, M. D. Sorcinelli, S. Weiler, and S. J. Korsmeyer, "Distinct BH3 domains either sensitize or activate mitochondrial apoptosis, serving as prototype cancer therapeutics," *Cancer Cell*, vol. 2, no. 3, pp. 183–192, 2002.

[20] S. N. Willis, J. I. Fletcher, T. Kaufmann et al., "Apoptosis initiated when BH3 ligands engage multiple Bcl-2 homologs, not Bax or Bak," *Science*, vol. 315, no. 5813, pp. 856–859, 2007.

[21] S. N. Willis, L. Chen, G. Dewson et al., "Proapoptotic Bak is sequestered by Mcl-1 and Bcl-xL, but not Bcl-2, until displaced by BH3-only proteins," *Genes & Development*, vol. 19, no. 11, pp. 1294–1305, 2005.

[22] L. Chen, S. N. Willis, A. Wei et al., "Differential targeting of prosurvival Bcl-2 proteins by their BH3-only ligands allows complementary apoptotic function," *Molecular Cell*, vol. 17, no. 3, pp. 393–403, 2005.

[23] J. Deng, N. Carlson, K. Takeyama, P. Dal Cin, M. Shipp, and A. Letai, "BH3 profiling identifies three distinct classes of apoptotic blocks to predict response to ABT-737 and conventional chemotherapeutic agents," *Cancer Cell*, vol. 12, no. 2, pp. 171–185, 2007.

[24] M. F. van Delft, A. H. Wei, K. D. Mason et al., "The BH3 mimetic ABT-737 targets selective Bcl-2 proteins and efficiently induces apoptosis via Bak/Bax if Mcl-1 is neutralized," *Cancer Cell*, vol. 10, no. 5, pp. 389–399, 2006.

[25] Y. Tsujimoto, N. Ikegaki, and C. M. Croce, "Characterization of the protein product of bcl-2, the gene involved in human follicular lymphoma," *Oncogene*, vol. 2, no. 1, pp. 3–7, 1987.

[26] W. B. Graninger, M. Seto, B. Boutain, P. Goldman, and S. J. Korsmeyer, "Expression of Bcl-2 and Bcl-2-Ig fusion transcripts in normal and neoplastic cells," *The Journal of Clinical Investigation*, vol. 80, no. 5, pp. 1512–1515, 1987.

[27] D. J. Veis, C. M. Sorenson, J. R. Shutter, and S. J. Korsmeyer, "Bcl-2-deficient mice demonstrate fulminant lymphoid apoptosis, polycystic kidneys, and hypopigmented hair," *Cell*, vol. 75, no. 2, pp. 229–240, 1993.

[28] D. M. Hockenbery, M. Zutter, W. Hickey, M. Nahm, and S. J. Korsmeyer, "BCL2 protein is topographically restricted in tissues characterized by apoptotic cell death," *Proceedings of the National Academy of Sciences of the United States of America*, vol. 88, no. 16, pp. 6961–6965, 1991.

[29] I. Garcia, I. Martinou, Y. Tsujimoto, and J. Martinou, "Prevention of programmed cell death of sympathetic neurons by the bcl-2 proto-oncogene," *Science*, vol. 258, no. 5080, pp. 302–304, 1992.

[30] J. C. Reed, L. Meister, S. Tanaka et al., "Differential expression of bcl2 protooncogene in neuroblastoma and other human tumor cell lines of neural origin," *Cancer Research*, vol. 51, no. 24, pp. 6529–6538, 1991.

[31] T. J. McDonnell, P. Troncoso, S. M. Brisbay et al., "Expression of the protooncogene bcl-2 in the prostate and its association with emergence of androgen-independent prostate cancer," *Cancer Research*, vol. 52, no. 24, pp. 6940–6944, 1992.

[32] F. Pezzella, H. Turley, I. Kuzu et al., "bcl-2 protein in non-small-cell lung carcinoma," *The New England Journal of Medicine*, vol. 329, no. 10, pp. 690–694, 1993.

[33] N. Ikegaki, M. Katsumata, J. Minna, and Y. Tsujimoto, "Expression of bcl-2 in small cell lung carcinoma cells," *Cancer Research*, vol. 54, no. 1, pp. 6–8, 1994.

[34] Y. Kuwashima, T. Uehara, K. Kishi, K. Shiromizu, M. Matsuzawa, and S. Takayama, "Immunohistochemical characterization of undifferentiated carcinomas of the ovary," *Journal of Cancer Research and Clinical Oncology*, vol. 120, no. 11, pp. 672–677, 1994.

[35] P. Monaghan, D. Robertson, T. A. S. Amos, M. J. S. Dyer, D. Y. Mason, and M. F. Greaves, "Ultrastructural localization of BCL-2 protein," *Journal of Histochemistry and Cytochemistry*, vol. 40, no. 12, pp. 1819–1825, 1992.

[36] R. X.-D. Song, Z. Zhang, G. Mor, and R. J. Santen, "Down-regulation of Bcl-2 enhances estrogen apoptotic action in long-term estradiol-depleted ER^+ breast cancer cells," *Apoptosis*, vol. 10, no. 3, pp. 667–678, 2005.

[37] M. Krishna, T. W. Smith, and L. D. Recht, "Expression of bcl-2 in reactive and neoplastic astrocytes: lack of correlation with presence or degree of malignancy," *Journal of Neurosurgery*, vol. 83, no. 6, pp. 1017–1022, 1995.

[38] H. Joensuu, L. Pylkkänen, and S. Toikkanen, "Bcl-2 protein expression and long-term survival in breast cancer," *The American Journal of Pathology*, vol. 145, no. 5, pp. 1191–1198, 1994.

[39] K. M. Kozopas, T. Yang, H. L. Buchan, P. Zhou, and R. W. Craig, "MCL1, a gene expressed in programmed myeloid cell differentiation, has sequence similarity to BCL2," *Proceedings of the National Academy of Sciences of the United States of America*, vol. 90, no. 8, pp. 3516–3520, 1993.

[40] T. Yang, H. L. Buchan, K. J. Townsend, and R. W. Craig, "MCL-1, a member of the BLC-2 family, is induced rapidly in response to signals for cell differentiation or death, but not to signals for cell proliferation," *Journal of Cellular Physiology*, vol. 166, no. 3, pp. 523–536, 1996.

[41] D. A. Moulding, J. A. Quayle, C. Anthony Hart, and S. W. Edwards, "Mcl-1 expression in human neutrophils: regulation by cytokines and correlation with cell survival," *Blood*, vol. 92, no. 7, pp. 2495–2502, 1998.

[42] Q. Zhan, C. K. Bieszczad, I. Bae, A. J. Fornace Jr., and R. W. Craig, "Induction of BCL2 family member MCL1 as an early response to DNA damage," *Oncogene*, vol. 14, no. 9, pp. 1031–1039, 1997.

[43] J. L. Rinkenberger, S. Horning, B. Klocke, K. Roth, and S. J. Korsmeyer, "Mcl-1 deficiency results in peri-implantation embryonic lethality," *Genes & Development*, vol. 14, no. 1, pp. 23–27, 2000.

[44] B. Zhang, I. Gojo, and R. G. Fenton, "Myeloid cell factor-1 is a critical survival factor for multiple myeloma," *Blood*, vol. 99, no. 6, pp. 1885–1893, 2002.

[45] R. W. Craig, E. W. Jabs, P. Zhou et al., "Human and mouse chromosomal mapping of the myeloid cell leukemia-1 gene: MCL1 maps to human chromosome 1q21, a region that is frequently altered in preneoplastic and neoplastic disease," *Genomics*, vol. 23, no. 2, pp. 457–463, 1994.

[46] R. Beroukhim, C. H. Mermel, D. Porter et al., "The landscape of somatic copy-number alteration across human cancers," *Nature*, vol. 463, no. 7283, pp. 899–905, 2010.

[47] L. H. Boise, M. Gonzalez-Garcia, C. E. Postema et al., "bcl-x, A bcl-2-related gene that functions as a dominant regulator of apoptotic cell death," *Cell*, vol. 74, no. 4, pp. 597–608, 1993.

[48] S. Krajewski, M. Krajewska, A. Shabaik et al., "Immunohistochemical analysis of in vivo patterns of Bcl-X expression," *Cancer Research*, vol. 54, no. 21, pp. 5501–5507, 1994.

[49] N. Motoyama, F. Wang, K. A. Roth et al., "Massive cell death of immature hematopoietic cells and neurons in bcl-x-deficient mice," *Science*, vol. 267, no. 5203, pp. 1506–1510, 1995.

[50] S. Krajewski, M. Krajewska, J. Ehrmann et al., "Immunohistochemical analysis of Bcl-2, Bcl-X, Mcl-1, and Bax in tumors of central and peripheral nervous system origin," *The American Journal of Pathology*, vol. 150, no. 3, pp. 805–814, 1997.

[51] M. Krajewska, C. M. Fenoglio-Preiser, S. Krajewski et al., "Immunohistochemical analysis of Bcl-2 family proteins in adenocarcinomas of the stomach," *The American Journal of Pathology*, vol. 149, no. 5, pp. 1449–1457, 1996.

[52] M. Krajewska, S. F. Moss, S. Krajewski, K. Song, P. R. Holt, and J. C. Reed, "Elevated expression of Bcl-X and reduced Bak in primary colorectal adenocarcinomas," *Cancer Research*, vol. 56, no. 10, pp. 2422–2427, 1996.

[53] E. J. Kirsh, D. A. Baunoch, and W. M. Stadler, "Expression of bcl-2 and bcl-X in bladder cancer," *The Journal of Urology*, vol. 159, no. 4, pp. 1348–1353, 1998.

[54] S. Kondo, Y. Shinomura, S. Kanayama et al., "Over-expression of bcl-xL gene in human gastric adenomas and carcinomas," *International Journal of Cancer*, vol. 68, no. 6, pp. 727–730, 1996.

[55] S. A. Amundson, T. G. Myers, D. Scudiero, S. Kitada, J. C. Reed, and J. Fornace A.J., "An informatics approach identifying markers of chemosensitivity in human cancer cell lines," *Cancer Research*, vol. 60, no. 21, pp. 6101–6110, 2000.

[56] E. Y. Lin, A. Orlofsky, M. S. Berger, and M. B. Prystowsky, "Characterization of A1, a novel hemopoietic-specific early-response gene with sequence similarity to bcl-2," *Journal of Immunology*, vol. 151, no. 4, pp. 1979–1988, 1993.

[57] G. Brien, A. Debaud, X. Robert et al., "C-terminal residues regulate localization and function of the antiapoptotic protein Bfl-1," *The Journal of Biological Chemistry*, vol. 284, no. 44, pp. 30257–30263, 2009.

[58] M. Vogler, "BCL2A1: the underdog in the BCL2 family," *Cell Death & Differentiation*, vol. 19, no. 1, pp. 67–74, 2012.

[59] A. Hamasaki, F. Sendo, K. Nakayama et al., "Accelerated neutrophil apoptosis in mice lacking A1-a, a subtype of the bcl-2-related A1 gene," *Journal of Experimental Medicine*, vol. 188, no. 11, pp. 1985–1992, 1998.

[60] E. Ottina, F. Grespi, D. Tischner et al., "Targeting antiapoptotic A1/Bfl-1 by in vivo RNAi reveals multiple roles in leukocyte development in mice," *Blood*, vol. 119, no. 25, pp. 6032–6042, 2012.

[61] S. S. Choi, I. C. Park, J. W. Yun, Y. C. Sung, S. I. Hong, and H. S. Shin, "A novel Bcl-2 related gene, Bfl-1, is overexpressed in stomach cancer and preferentially expressed in bone marrow," *Oncogene*, vol. 11, no. 9, pp. 1693–1698, 1995.

[62] L. J. Beverly and H. E. Varmus, "MYC-induced myeloid leukemogenesis is accelerated by all six members of the antiapoptotic BCL family," *Oncogene*, vol. 28, no. 9, pp. 1274–1279, 2009.

[63] H. S. Yoon, S. H. Hong, H. J. Kang, B. K. Ko, S. H. Ahn, and J. R. Huh, "Bfl-1 gene expression in breast cancer: its relationship with other prognostic factors," *Journal of Korean Medical Science*, vol. 18, no. 2, pp. 225–230, 2003.

[64] A. I. Riker, S. A. Enkemann, O. Fodstad et al., "The gene expression profiles of primary and metastatic melanoma yields a transition point of tumor progression and metastasis," *BMC Medical Genomics*, vol. 1, article 13, 2008.

[65] C. Lee, Z. Ling, T. Zhao et al., "Genomic-wide analysis of lymphatic metastasis-associated genes in human hepatocellular carcinoma," *World Journal of Gastroenterology*, vol. 15, no. 3, pp. 356–365, 2009.

[66] D. Senft, C. Berking, S. A. Graf, C. Kammerbauer, T. Ruzicka, and R. Besch, "Selective induction of cell death in melanoma cell lines through targeting of Mcl-1 and A1," *PLoS ONE*, vol. 7, no. 1, Article ID e30821, 2012.

[67] V. P. Kathpalia, E. N. Mussak, S. S. Chow et al., "Genome-wide transcriptional profiling in human squamous cell carcinoma of the skin identifies unique tumor-associated signatures," *Journal of Dermatology*, vol. 33, no. 5, pp. 309–318, 2006.

[68] A. Saleh, R. B. Zain, H. Hussaini et al., "Transcriptional profiling of oral squamous cell carcinoma using formalin-fixed paraffin-embedded samples," *Oral Oncology*, vol. 46, no. 5, pp. 379–386, 2010.

[69] L. Gibson, S. P. Holmgreen, D. C. S. Huang et al., "bcl-w, a novel member of the bcl-2 family, promotes cell survival," *Oncogene*, vol. 13, no. 4, pp. 665–675, 1996.

[70] C. G. Print, K. L. Loveland, L. Gibson et al., "Apoptosis regulator Bcl-w is essential for spermatogenesis but appears otherwise redundant," *Proceedings of the National Academy of Sciences of the United States of America*, vol. 95, no. 21, pp. 12424–12431, 1998.

[71] D. M. Pritchard, C. Print, L. O'Reilly, J. M. Adams, C. S. Potten, and J. A. Hickman, "Bcl-w is an important determinant of damage-induced apoptosis in epithelia of small and large intestine," *Oncogene*, vol. 19, no. 34, pp. 3955–3959, 2000.

[72] N. Ke, A. Godzik, and J. C. Reed, "Bcl-B, a novel Bcl-2 family member that differentially binds and regulates Bax and Bak," *The Journal of Biological Chemistry*, vol. 276, no. 16, pp. 12481–12484, 2001.

[73] M. Krajewska, S. Kitada, J. N. Winter et al., "Bcl-B expression in human epithelial and nonepithelial malignancies," *Clinical Cancer Research*, vol. 14, no. 10, pp. 3011–3021, 2008.

[74] J. C. Reed, M. Cuddy, S. Haldar et al., "BCL2-mediated tumorigenicity of a human T-lymphoid cell line: synergy with MYC and inhibiton by BCL2 antisense," *Proceedings of the National Academy of Sciences of the United States of America*, vol. 87, no. 10, pp. 3660–3664, 1990.

[75] R. Raab, J. A. Sparano, A. J. Ocean et al., "A phase I trial of oblimersen sodium in combination with cisplatin and 5-fluorouracil in patients with advanced esophageal, gastroesophageal junction, and gastric carcinoma," *The American Journal of Clinical Oncology: Cancer Clinical Trials*, vol. 33, no. 1, pp. 61–65, 2010.

[76] C. N. Sternberg, H. Dumez, H. van Poppel et al., "Docetaxel plus oblimersen sodium (Bcl-2 antisense oligonucleotide): an EORTC multicenter, randomized phase II study in patients with castration-resistant prostate cancer," *Annals of Oncology*, vol. 20, no. 7, pp. 1264–1269, 2009.

[77] P. A. Ott, J. Chang, K. Madden et al., "Oblimersen in combination with temozolomide and albumin-bound paclitaxel in patients with advanced melanoma: a phase i trial," *Cancer Chemotherapy and Pharmacology*, vol. 71, no. 1, pp. 183–191, 2013.

[78] S. Kitada, M. Leone, S. Sareth, D. Zhai, J. C. Reed, and M. Pellecchia, "Discovery, characterization, and structure-activity relationships studies of proapoptotic polyphenols targeting B-cell lymphocyte/leukemia-2 proteins," *Journal of Medicinal Chemistry*, vol. 46, no. 20, pp. 4259–4264, 2003.

[79] J. M. Herbert, J. M. Augereau, J. Gleye, and J. P. Maffrand, "Chelerythrine is a potent and specific inhibitor of protein kinase C," *Biochemical and Biophysical Research Communications*, vol. 172, no. 3, pp. 993–999, 1990.

[80] S. Chan, M. C. Lee, K. O. Tan et al., "Identification of chelerythrine as an inhibitor of BclXL function," *Journal of Biological Chemistry*, vol. 278, no. 23, pp. 20453–20456, 2003.

[81] E. Milanesi, P. Costantini, A. Gambalunga et al., "The mitochondrial effects of small organic ligands of BCL-2: sensitization of BCL-2-overexpressing cells to apoptosis by a pyrimidine-2,4,6-trione derivative," *The Journal of Biological Chemistry*, vol. 281, no. 15, pp. 10066–10072, 2006.

[82] M. Vogler, K. Weber, D. Dinsdale et al., "Different forms of cell death induced by putative BCL2 inhibitors," *Cell Death and Differentiation*, vol. 16, no. 7, pp. 1030–1039, 2009.

[83] F. W. Kah, S. Chan, S. K. Sukumaran, M. Lee, and V. C. Yu, "Chelerythrine induces apoptosis through a Bax/Bak-independent mitochondrial mechanism," *Journal of Biological Chemistry*, vol. 283, no. 13, pp. 8423–8433, 2008.

[84] T. Oltersdorf, S. W. Elmore, A. R. Shoemaker et al., "An inhibitor of Bcl-2 family proteins induces regression of solid tumours," *Nature*, vol. 435, no. 7042, pp. 677–681, 2005.

[85] S. B. Shuker, P. J. Hajduk, R. P. Meadows, and S. W. Fesik, "Discovering high-affinity ligands for proteins: SAR by NMR," *Science*, vol. 274, no. 5292, pp. 1531–1534, 1996.

[86] S. K. Tahir, X. Yang, M. G. Anderson et al., "Influence of Bcl-2 family members on the cellular response of small-cell lung cancer cell lines to ABT-737," *Cancer Research*, vol. 67, no. 3, pp. 1176–1183, 2007.

[87] X. Lin, S. Morgan-Lappe, X. Huang et al., "'Seed' analysis of off-target siRNAs reveals an essential role of Mcl-1 in resistance to the small-molecule Bcl-2/Bcl-XL inhibitor ABT-737," *Oncogene*, vol. 26, no. 27, pp. 3972–3979, 2007.

[88] C. L. Hann, V. C. Daniel, E. A. Sugar et al., "Therapeutic efficacy of ABT-737, a selective inhibitor of BCL-2, in small cell lung cancer," *Cancer Research*, vol. 68, no. 7, pp. 2321–2328, 2008.

[89] C. Tse, A. R. Shoemaker, J. Adickes et al., "ABT-263: a potent and orally bioavailable Bcl-2 family inhibitor," *Cancer Research*, vol. 68, no. 9, pp. 3421–3428, 2008.

[90] M. Vogler, S. D. Furdas, M. Jung, T. Kuwana, M. J. S. Dyer, and G. M. Cohen, "Diminished sensitivity of chronic lymphocytic leukemia cells to ABT-737 and ABT-263 due to albumin binding in blood," *Clinical Cancer Research*, vol. 16, no. 16, pp. 4217–4225, 2010.

[91] A. W. Roberts, J. F. Seymour, J. R. Brown et al., "Substantial susceptibility of chronic lymphocytic leukemia to BCL2 inhibition: results of a phase I study of navitoclax in patients with relapsed or refractory disease," *Journal of Clinical Oncology*, vol. 30, no. 5, pp. 488–496, 2012.

[92] L. Gandhi, D. R. Camidge, M. R. de Oliveira et al., "Phase I study of navitoclax (ABT-263), a novel bcl-2 family inhibitor, in patients with small-cell lung cancer and other solid tumors," *Journal of Clinical Oncology*, vol. 29, no. 7, pp. 909–916, 2011.

[93] C. M. Rudin, C. L. Hann, E. B. Garon et al., "Phase II study of single-agent navitoclax (ABT-263) and biomarker correlates in patients with relapsed small cell lung cancer," *Clinical Cancer Research*, vol. 18, no. 11, pp. 3163–3169, 2012.

[94] K. D. Mason, M. R. Carpinelli, J. I. Fletcher et al., "Programmed anuclear cell death delimits platelet life span," *Cell*, vol. 128, no. 6, pp. 1173–1186, 2007.

[95] M. Vogler, H. A. Hamali, X. Sun et al., "BCL2/BCL-XL inhibition induces apoptosis, disrupts cellular calcium homeostasis, and prevents platelet activation," *Blood*, vol. 117, no. 26, pp. 7145–7154, 2011.

[96] S. M. Schoenwaelder, Y. Yuan, E. C. Josefsson et al., "Two distinct pathways regulate platelet phosphatidylserine exposure and procoagulant function," *Blood*, vol. 114, no. 3, pp. 663–666, 2009.

[97] A. J. Souers, J. D. Leverson, E. R. Boghaert et al., "ABT-199, a potent and selective BCL-2 inhibitor, achieves antitumor activity while sparing platelets," *Nature Medicine*, vol. 19, no. 2, pp. 202–208, 2013.

[98] F. Vaillant, D. Merino, L. Lee et al., "Targeting BCL-2 with the BH3 mimetic ABT-199 in estrogen receptor-positive breast cancer," *Cancer Cell*, vol. 24, no. 1, pp. 120–129, 2013.

[99] G. Lessene, P. E. Czabotar, B. E. Sleebs et al., "Structure-guided design of a selective BCL-XL inhibitor," *Nature Chemical Biology*, vol. 9, no. 6, pp. 390–397, 2013.

[100] G. Lessene, P. E. Czabotar, B. E. Sleebs et al., "Novel, potent and selective inhibitors of the pro-survival BCL-2 family member BCL-XL," in *Keystone Symposia on The Chemistry and Biology of Cell Death*, p. Q6:2017, 2014.

[101] S. Colak, C. D. Zimberlin, E. Fessler et al., "Decreased mitochondrial priming determines chemoresistance of colon cancer stem cells," *Cell Death and Differentiation*, vol. 21, no. 7, pp. 1170–1177, 2014.

[102] D. Park, A. T. Magis, R. Li et al., "Novel small-molecule inhibitors of Bcl-XL to treat lung cancer," *Cancer Research*, vol. 73, no. 17, pp. 5485–5496, 2013.

[103] M. Nguyen, R. C. Marcellus, A. Roulston et al., "Small molecule obatoclax (GX15-070) antagonizes MCL-1 and overcomes MCL-1-mediated resistance to apoptosis," *Proceedings of the National Academy of Sciences of the United States of America*, vol. 104, no. 49, pp. 19512–19517, 2007.

[104] J. J. Hwang, J. Kuruvilla, D. Mendelson et al., "Phase I dose finding studies of obatoclax (GX15-070), a small molecule Pan-BCL-2 family antagonist, in patients with advanced solid tumors or lymphoma," *Clinical Cancer Research*, vol. 16, no. 15, pp. 4038–4045, 2010.

[105] P. K. Paik, C. M. Rudin, A. Brown et al., "A phase i study of obatoclax mesylate, a Bcl-2 antagonist, plus topotecan in solid tumor malignancies," *Cancer Chemotherapy and Pharmacology*, vol. 66, no. 6, pp. 1079–1085, 2010.

[106] Z. Zhang, L. Jin, X. Qian et al., "Novel Bcl-2 inhibitors: discovery and mechanism study of small organic apoptosis-inducing agents," *ChemBioChem*, vol. 8, no. 1, pp. 113–121, 2007.

[107] Z. Zhang, T. Song, T. Zhang et al., "A novel BH3 mimetic S1 potently induces Bax/Bak-dependent apoptosis by targeting both Bcl-2 and Mcl-1," *International Journal of Cancer*, vol. 128, no. 7, pp. 1724–1735, 2011.

[108] T. Song, X. Chang, Z. Zhang, Y. Liu, and X. Shen, "S1, a novel pan-BH3 mimetic, induces apoptosis in Mcl-1-overexpressing cells through bak," *Journal of Pharmacological Sciences*, vol. 119, no. 4, pp. 330–340, 2012.

[109] Y. Liu, Z. Zhang, T. Song, F. Liang, M. Xie, and H. Sheng, "Resistance to BH3 mimetic S1 in SCLC cells that up-regulate and phosphorylate Bcl-2 through ERK1/2," *British Journal of Pharmacology*, vol. 169, no. 7, pp. 1612–1623, 2013.

[110] X. Cao, J. L. Yap, M. K. Newell-Rogers et al., "The novel BH3 α-helix mimetic JY-1-106 induces apoptosis in a subset of cancer cells (lung cancer, colon cancer and mesothelioma) by disrupting Bcl-xL and Mcl-1 protein–protein interactions with Bak," *Molecular Cancer*, vol. 12, article 42, 2013.

[111] S. Kitada, C. L. Kress, M. Krajewska, L. Jia, M. Pellecchia, and J. C. Reed, "Bcl-2 antagonist apogossypol (NSC736630) displays single-agent activity in Bcl-2 transgenic mice and has superior efficacy with less toxicity compared with gossypol (NSC19048)," *Blood*, vol. 111, no. 6, pp. 3211–3219, 2008.

[112] J. Wei, J. L. Stebbins, S. Kitada et al., "An optically pure apogossypolone derivative as potent pan-active inhibitor of anti-apoptotic bcl-2 family proteins," *Frontiers in Oncology*, vol. 1, article 28, 2011.

[113] J. Wei, J. L. Stebbins, S. Kitada et al., "BI-97C1, an optically pure apogossypol derivative as pan-active inhibitor of antiapoptotic B-cell lymphoma/Leukemia-2 (Bcl-2) family proteins," *Journal of Medicinal Chemistry*, vol. 53, no. 10, pp. 4166–4176, 2010.

[114] J. Wei, S. Kitada, M. F. Rega et al., "Apogossypol derivatives as pan-active inhibitors of antiapoptotic B-cell lymphoma/leukemia-2 (Bcl-2) family proteins," *Journal of Medicinal Chemistry*, vol. 52, no. 14, pp. 4511–4523, 2009.

[115] S. Varadarajan, M. Vogler, M. Butterworth, D. Dinsdale, L. D. Walensky, and G. M. Cohen, "Evaluation and critical assessment of putative MCL-1 inhibitors," *Cell Death & Differentiation*, vol. 20, no. 11, pp. 1475–1484, 2013.

[116] S. Varadarajan, M. Butterworth, J. Wei, M. Pellecchia, D. Dinsdale, and G. M. Cohen, "Sabutoclax (BI97C1) and BI112D1, putative inhibitors of MCL-1, induce mitochondrial fragmentation either upstream of or independent of apoptosis," *Neoplasia*, vol. 15, no. 5, pp. 568–578, 2013.

[117] D. J. Goff, A. C. Recart, A. Sadarangani et al., "A Pan-BCL2 inhibitor renders bone-marrow-resident human leukemia stem cells sensitive to tyrosine kinase inhibition," *Cell Stem Cell*, vol. 12, no. 3, pp. 316–328, 2013.

[118] R. S. Jackson II, W. Placzek, A. Fernandez et al., "Sabutoclax, a Mcl-1 antagonist, inhibits tumorigenesis in transgenic mouse and human xenograft models of prostate cancer," *Neoplasia*, vol. 14, no. 7, pp. 656–665, 2012.

[119] G. Wang, Z. Nikolovska-Coleska, C. Yang et al., "Structure-based design of potent small-molecule inhibitors of antiapoptotic Bcl-2 proteins," *Journal of Medicinal Chemistry*, vol. 49, no. 21, pp. 6139–6142, 2006.

[120] Z. Wang, W. Song, A. Aboukameel et al., "TW-37, a small-molecule inhibitor of Bcl-2, inhibits cell growth and invasion in pancreatic cancer," *International Journal of Cancer*, vol. 123, no. 4, pp. 958–966, 2008.

[121] M. L. Stewart, E. Fire, A. E. Keating, and L. D. Walensky, "The MCL-1 BH3 helix is an exclusive MCL-1 inhibitor and apoptosis sensitizer," *Nature Chemical Biology*, vol. 6, no. 8, pp. 595–601, 2010.

[122] L. D. Walensky, A. L. Kung, I. Escher et al., "Activation of apoptosis in vivo by a hydrocarbon-stapled BH3 helix," *Science*, vol. 305, no. 5689, pp. 1466–1470, 2004.

[123] J. L. LaBelle, S. G. Katz, G. H. Bird et al., "A stapled BIM peptide overcomes apoptotic resistance in hematologic cancers," *Journal of Clinical Investigation*, vol. 122, no. 6, pp. 2018–2031, 2012.

[124] N. A. Cohen, M. L. Stewart, E. Gavathiotis et al., "A competitive stapled peptide screen identifies a selective small molecule that overcomes MCL-1-dependent leukemia cell survival," *Chemistry and Biology*, vol. 19, no. 9, pp. 1175–1186, 2012.

[125] T. Bannister, M. Koenig, Y. He et al., "Small Molecule that Potently and Selectively Disrupts the Protein-Protein Interaction of Mcl-1 and Bim: A Probe for Studying Lymphoid Tumorigenesis," Probe Reports from the NIH Molecular Libraries Program, Bethesda, Md, USA, 2010.

[126] F. Abulwerdi, C. Liao, M. Liu et al., "A novel small-molecule inhibitor of mcl-1 blocks pancreatic cancer growth in vitro and in vivo," *Molecular Cancer Therapeutics*, vol. 13, no. 3, pp. 565–575, 2014.

[127] A. Friberg, D. Vigil, B. Zhao et al., "Discovery of potent myeloid cell leukemia 1 (Mcl-1) inhibitors using fragment-based methods and structure-based design," *Journal of Medicinal Chemistry*, vol. 56, no. 1, pp. 15–30, 2013.

[128] E. Varin, C. Denoyelle, E. Brotin et al., "Downregulation of Bcl-xL and Mcl-1 is sufficient to induce cell death in mesothelioma cells highly refractory to conventional chemotherapy," *Carcinogenesis*, vol. 31, no. 6, pp. 984–993, 2010.

[129] E. Choi, J. Jung, J. Lee, J. Park, N. Cho, and S. Cho, "Myeloid cell leukemia-1 is a key molecular target for mithramycin A-induced apoptosis in androgen-independent prostate cancer cells and a tumor xenograft animal model," *Cancer Letters*, vol. 328, no. 1, pp. 65–72, 2013.

[130] G. Wei, A. A. Margolin, L. Haery et al., "Chemical Genomics Identifies Small-Molecule MCL1 Repressors and BCL-xL as a Predictor of MCL1 Dependency," *Cancer Cell*, vol. 21, no. 4, pp. 547–562, 2012.

[131] T. N. Chonghaile, K. A. Sarosiek, T. Vo et al., "Pretreatment mitochondrial priming correlates with clinical response to cytotoxic chemotherapy," *Science*, vol. 334, no. 6059, pp. 1129–1133, 2011.

[132] A. A. Chiappori, M. T. Schreeder, M. M. Moezi et al., "A phase i trial of pan-Bcl-2 antagonist obatoclax administered as a 3-h or a 24-h infusion in combination with carboplatin and etoposide in patients with extensive-stage small cell lung cancer," *British Journal of Cancer*, vol. 106, no. 5, pp. 839–845, 2012.

[133] P. K. Paik, C. M. Rudin, M. C. Pietanza et al., "A phase II study of obatoclax mesylate, a Bcl-2 antagonist, plus topotecan in relapsed small cell lung cancer," *Lung Cancer*, vol. 74, no. 3, pp. 481–485, 2011.

[134] M. Q. Baggstrom, Y. Qi, M. Koczywas et al., "A phase II study of AT-101 (Gossypol) in chemotherapy-sensitive recurrent extensive-stage small cell lung cancer," *Journal of Thoracic Oncology*, vol. 6, no. 10, pp. 1757–1760, 2011.

[135] N. Ready, N. A. Karaseva, S. V. Orlov et al., "Double-blind, placebo-controlled, randomized phase 2 study of the proapoptotic agent AT-101 plus docetaxel, in second-line non-small cell lung cancer," *Journal of Thoracic Oncology*, vol. 6, no. 4, pp. 781–785, 2011.

[136] R. Suk Heist, J. Fain, B. Chinnasami et al., "Phase I/II study of AT-101 with topotecan in relapsed and refractory small cell lung cancer," *Journal of Thoracic Oncology*, vol. 5, no. 10, pp. 1637–1643, 2010.

[137] G. Sonpavde, V. Matveev, J. M. Burke et al., "Randomized phase II trial of docetaxel plus prednisone in combination with placebo or AT-101, an oral small molecule Bcl-2 family antagonist, as first-line therapy for metastatic castration-resistant prostate cancer," *Annals of Oncology*, vol. 23, no. 7, pp. 1803–1808, 2012.

[138] V. A. Stamelos, E. Robinson, C. W. Redman, and A. Richardson, "Navitoclax augments the activity of carboplatin and paclitaxel combinations in ovarian cancer cells," *Gynecologic Oncology*, vol. 128, no. 2, pp. 377–382, 2013.

[139] K. D. Mason, S. L. Khaw, K. C. Rayeroux et al., "The BH3 mimetic compound, ABT-737, synergizes with a range of cytotoxic chemotherapy agents in chronic lymphocytic leukemia," *Leukemia*, vol. 23, no. 11, pp. 2034–2041, 2009.

[140] J. Chen, S. Jin, V. Abraham et al., "The Bcl-2/Bcl-X L/Bcl-w inhibitor, navitoclax, enhances the activity of chemotherapeutic agents *in vitro* and *in vivo*," *Molecular Cancer Therapeutics*, vol. 10, no. 12, pp. 2340–2349, 2011.

[141] E. T. Olejniczak, C. van Sant, M. G. Anderson et al., "Integrative genomic analysis of small-cell lung carcinoma reveals correlates of sensitivity to Bcl-2 antagonists and uncovers novel chromosomal gains," *Molecular Cancer Research*, vol. 5, no. 4, pp. 331–339, 2007.

[142] F. Vogt, J. Lieber, A. Dewerth, A. Hoh, J. Fuchs, and S. Armeanu-Ebinger, "BH3 mimetics reduce adhesion and migration of hepatoblastoma and hepatocellular carcinoma cells," *Experimental Cell Research*, vol. 319, no. 10, pp. 1443–1450, 2013.

[143] M. J. Sale and S. J. Cook, "That which does not kill me makes me stronger; combining ERK1/2 pathway inhibitors and BH3 mimetics to kill tumour cells and prevent acquired resistance," *British Journal of Pharmacology*, vol. 169, no. 8, pp. 1708–1722, 2013.

[144] M. S. Cragg, E. S. Jansen, M. Cook, C. Harris, A. Strasser, and C. L. Scott, "Treatment of B-RAF mutant human tumor cells with a MEK inhibitor requires Bim and is enhanced by a BH3 mimetic," *Journal of Clinical Investigation*, vol. 118, no. 11, pp. 3651–3659, 2008.

[145] R. B. Corcoran, K. A. Cheng, A. N. Hata et al., "Synthetic lethal interaction of combined BCL-XL and MEK inhibition promotes tumor regressions in KRAS mutant cancer models," *Cancer Cell*, vol. 23, no. 1, pp. 121–128, 2013.

[146] D. Wroblewski, B. Mijatov, N. Mohana-Kumaran et al., "The BH3-mimetic ABT-737 sensitizes human melanoma cells to apoptosis induced by selective BRAF inhibitors but does not reverse acquired resistance," *Carcinogenesis*, vol. 34, no. 2, pp. 237–247, 2013.

5

Efficacy of Synbiotics for Treatment of Bacillary Dysentery in Children: A Double-Blind, Randomized, Placebo-Controlled Study

Manijeh Kahbazi, Marzieh Ebrahimi, Nader Zarinfar, Mohammad Arjomandzadegan, Taha Fereydouni, Fatemeh Karimi, and Amir Reza Najmi

Infectious Diseases Research Centre (IDRC), Arak University of Medical Sciences, Arak, Iran

Correspondence should be addressed to Mohammad Arjomandzadegan; arjomandzadegan@arakmu.ac.ir

Academic Editor: Aliya Naheed

Bacillary dysentery is a major cause of children's admission to hospitals. To assess the probiotic and prebiotic (synbiotics) effects in children with dysentery in a randomized clinical trial, 200 children with dysentery were studied in 2 groups: the synbiotic group received 1 tablet/day of synbiotic for 3–5 days and the placebo group received placebo tablets (identical tablet form like probiotics). The standard treatment was administered for all patients. Duration of hospitalization, dysentery, fever, and the weight loss were assessed in each group. It was concluded that there was no significant difference in both groups in the baseline characteristics. The mean duration of dysentery reduced ($P < 0.05$). The mean duration of fever has been significantly reduced in the synbiotic group (1.64 ± 0.87 days) in comparison to the placebo group (2.13 ± 0.94 days) ($P < 0.001$). Average amount of weight loss was significantly lower in the synbiotic group in comparison to that in the placebo group (129.5 ± 23.388 grams and 278 ± 28.385 grams, resp.; $P < 0.001$). There was no significant difference in the mean duration of hospitalization in both groups ($P > 0.05$). The use of synbiotics as an adjuvant therapy to the standard treatment of dysentery significantly reduces the duration of dysentery, fever, and rate of weight losses. The trial is registered with IRCT201109267647N1.

1. Introduction

Bacillary dysentery is a disease in the category of acute infectious diarrhea. This is mostly spread by the following Gram-negative bacteria: *Shigella flexneri*, *S. dysenteriae*, *S. boydii*, and *S. sonnei* [1]. Shigella is a pathogen transmitted through the fecal-oral route, primarily via person-to-person contact. Shigellosis in children has variable symptoms ranging from a mild, self-limited diarrhea without inflammation to a severe, inflammatory, bloody diarrhea with high fever, abdominal cramps, vomiting, lack of appetite, toxic appearance, painful defecation, and other extraintestinal complications [2]. Shigellosis is estimated to be responsible for about 170 million cases and 14,000 deaths worldwide annually and such a burden is a major health problem with socioeconomic consequences [3]. Estimation of the disease inflictions remains largely speculative because only a small percentage of patients

seek medical treatments and are diagnosed through stool cultures [4]. The most common microorganisms diagnosed in developing countries are *S. flexneri* and *S. dysenteriae*, but *S. sonnei* frequently causes community-wide outbreaks in industrialized countries [5]. The widely accepted definition of probiotics is as follows: "the live microorganisms which when administered in adequate amounts confer a health benefit on the host" [6]. Probiotics are mostly species of the *Lactobacillus*, *Bifidobacterium*, and *Streptococcus* genera. Also, in some studies, yeasts, such as *Saccharomyces boulardii*, have also been suggested and are used as probiotics [7–9]. In some in vitro studies, *Lactobacillus acidophilus* has been effective against some intestinal pathogen elements such as *Shigella*, *Salmonella*, *Staphylococcus*, *Proteus*, *Klebsiella*, *Pseudomonas*, *E. coli*, *Clostridium perfringens*, and *Vibrio*. The positive effects of *Lactobacillus acidophilus* on the gastrointestinal system are due to adhesion and colonization to the intestinal mucosa, competition for adhesion sites on gut, or other tissue surfaces to prevent pathogens colonization, stimulation of mucosal and systemic immunities, production of antibacterial factors, and special bacteriocin, including acidophilin, lactocidin, acidolin, lactolin, organic acids (lactic acid), and the reduction of PH [10–15]. Probiotics have been used for many purposes, but they are most extensively studied in connection with acute infectious diarrhea, but further research in different age groups and various doses of different probiotics is required to evaluate the impact of probiotics on management of infectious dysentery [9, 16, 17]. Prebiotics are dietary fiber which trigger the growth and activate the activity of a limited number of bacteria in the intestinal flora. In addition, prebiotics can increase the effects of probiotics because of their synbiotic relationships. Synbiotics are combinations of probiotics and prebiotics which can synergistically promote the growth of beneficial bacteria or newly added species in the colon [18]. In this study, we investigated the effects of *Lactobacillus* GG (probiotic) plus prebiotic fructooligosaccharides on dysentery in 1-month–5-year-old children.

2. Materials and Methods

The study was conducted between October 2011 and October 2012 at Amirkabir Hospital, Arak, Iran, with a catchment area of 1500000 people.

2.1. Description of Participants. The inclusion criteria were male and female patients between the ages of 1 and 60 months who presented with acute dysentery to the PICU or Pediatric Emergency of the Amirkabir Hospital. Participants were patients at the same level of economic conditions who had experienced loose stools with mucus or blood and frequency of more than three times a day for less than two weeks, white blood cell (WBC) count ≥ 5/high-power-field (HPF) in the stool exam (SE), positive stool culture of *Shigella* spp. with or without the presence of fever, abdominal pain, dehydration, anorexia, and vomiting. The criteria for exclusion from the study were refusal of consent by parents, malnutrition status, chronic or concurrent diseases (sepsis, meningitis, pneumonia, and toxic colitis), previous diagnosed acute dysentery, acute abdomen condition, usage of other probiotics, usage of antibiotics or antidiarrheal agents within last 3 days, immune deficiency or treatment with immunosuppressive drugs during the last 60 days, failure to isolate *Shigella* spp. or presence of erythrophagocytic trophozoite of *Entameba histolytica* or cyst/trophozoites of *Giardia lamblia* in the microbial analysis of the stool, and usage of drugs that may have effects on gastrointestinal motility and/or digestion and absorption. The patients who required intravenous fluids, after receiving the treatment in the emergency rooms or PICU, were included in the study as patients with severe or medium dehydration status.

2.2. Clinical Management. All patients were examined by a pediatrician. The degree of dehydration, stool appearance, stool consistency, stool frequency, weight loss, duration of dysentery, and fever were recorded. All patients in both groups received the same standard routine treatment such as oral and/or intravenous fluid therapy, antibiotic treatment (Ciprofloxacin, 15 mg/kg, twice a day and for 3 days, orally) and nutritional support. And breastfeeding was promoted.

2.3. Randomization, Masking Procedure, and Study Design. In a double-blind manner, the patients were randomized and divided into the placebo and synbiotic groups. Randomization sequence was generated by a computer-generated randomization table in blocks of 4. Except for the study coordinator, all investigators and patients remained blinded to the randomization process until the study was completed. Each patient was given a different code. Parents and the patients were not informed about their allocation status (the synbiotic or placebo group). Placebos and synbiotics were provided by a pharmacist in packages with the same form and were labeled with the code letter A or B. In the production of placebo tablets, the preservative substances and artificial colors had not been used. Also, there was no fermented substance in the tablet. The same as the synbiotic tablets, the placebo tablets did not have any taste. In the PICU or hospital emergency room, the researcher, in a direct and double-blinded manner, supervised the patients to take the tablets properly. The patients in the synbiotic group were given 1 tablet/day of synbiotic tablets (Lactol®), containing probiotic material (bacillus coagulant, 150 million spores per serving) and prebiotic material (fructooligosaccharides, 100 mg per serving) for a period of 3–5 days.

2.4. Ethical Approval. The protocol has been written based on guidelines for good clinical practice (GCP) for trials on pharmaceutical products. The protocol approval was obtained from the clinical human research and ethical review committee at the Arak University of Medical Sciences, Iran. The purpose of the study, its objectives, potential benefits, risks, and inconveniences, alternative treatment that may be available, and the subject's rights and responsibilities were explained to the parents. After reading the consent form to the parents in presence of a third party, written informed consent (in accordance with the current revision of the Declaration of Helsinki) was obtained from every parent who wanted their children to participate in the study [19].

2.5. Data Analysis. At the end of the study, the study coordinator informed the researcher about the content, synbiotics or placebo, of the packages. Statistical analyses were performed using SPSS (version 12.0., Chicago, USA). An independent sample of *t*-test was administered. Mean ± standard deviation, standard error, Chi squared test, and its non-parametric equivalent (Mann-Whitney) were used to analyze the difference between two groups and find the drug efficacy. $P < 0.05$ was considered statistically significant.

3. Results

Out of the patients admitted to the pediatric emergency, 200 patients (out of 961 screened patients) were included in the study. The age of participants was between 1 month and 5 years. The patients were divided into two groups in a double-blind manner; 100 patients were assigned to the synbiotic group and 100 to the placebo group. Before the treatment, there was no difference between the groups in terms of age, gender, degree of dehydration, frequency of stools, or initial period of dysentery. The mean and SD of participants ages were 37.267 ± 22.2 months and 36.933 ± 18.467 in the synbiotic and placebo groups, respectively ($P >$ 0.05). In the synbiotic group, there were 54 females (54%) and 46 males (46%). In the placebo group, there were 62 females and 38 males (62% and 38%, resp.; $P =$ 0.25). Table 1 shows the baseline characteristic information related to both synbiotic and placebo groups. Based on these results, age and sex distributions in both synbiotic and placebo groups were similar and no difference was observed among them. Therefore, it can be said that general characteristics of participants do not have any negative influence on the obtained results of the study.

In this study, a comparison between various levels of dehydration shows that, in both synbiotic and placebo groups, a small portion of patients were affected by acute dehydration. In synbiotic group, 84 participants (84%) were affected by minor dehydration, 15 participants (15%) were affected by medium dehydration, and 1 participant (1%) was affected by severe dehydration. In placebo group, 71 participants (71%) were affected by minor dehydration, 25 participants (25%) were affected by medium dehydration, and 4 participants (4%) were affected by severe dehydration (Table 1). The results show that there is no significant relationship between dehydration mean in synbiotic and placebo groups at the beginning of the study ($P >$ 0.05). The results obtained by Kolmogorov-Smirnov test show that data distribution is normal. So, the use of independent sample t-test is permissible. The demographic findings, mean and standard deviation of duration of dysentery, duration of fever, duration of hospitalization, and the amount of weight loss following the intervention are summarized in Table 2. The mean duration of dysentery was significantly reduced in the synbiotic group when compared to the placebo group (2.5 ± 0.98 days versus 2.9 ± 1.09 days, resp.). Duration of fever after starting treatment was reduced significantly ($P <$ 0.001) in children receiving synbiotics (1.64 ± 0.87 days) compared with those in the placebo group (2.13 ± 0.94 days). There was no statistical difference between groups in the mean of hospitalization (3.6 ± 1.04 in synbiotic group versus 3.7 ± 1.08 in placebo group; $P >$ 0.05). At the end of the study, Patients taking synbiotics were less likely to have weight loss (129.5 ± 23.3 grams in the synbiotic group versus 278 ± 28.3 grams in the placebo group). There was no death or severe clinical complications during the course of the trial and no adverse effects related to synbiotics were observed.

4. Discussion

The present study confirmed the positive effects of probiotics and prebiotics on the treatment of children affected by dysentery. The results of this study showed that routine treatment of dysentery in combination with three to five days of synbiotics reduced the duration of dysentery, duration of fever, and weight changes in children aged between 1 and 60

TABLE 1: General characteristics of patients in both synbiotic and placebo groups.

Characteristic	Synbiotic	Placebo	P value
Age, mean ± SD, months	37.267 ± 22.2	36.933 ± 18.467	0.9
Sex (male/female)	46%/54%	38%/62%	0.25
Dehydration			
Minor	84%	71%	
Medium	15%	25%	0.067
Severe	1%	4%	

TABLE 2: Mean and standard deviation of patient characteristics during the study.

Characteristics	Synbiotic	Placebo	P value
Duration of dysentery (day)	2.5 ± 0.98	2.9 ± 1.09	0.01
Duration of fever (day)	1.64 ± 0.87	2.13 ± 0.94	<0.001
Duration of hospitalization (day)	3.6 ± 1.04	3.7 ± 1.08	0.691
Weight loss (gram)	129.5 ± 23.3	278 ± 28.3	<0.001

months. Treatment of acute infectious dysentery is mainly designed to compensate for the dehydration and the loss of electrolytes [20] and to protect the normal gastrointestinal microenvironment [21, 22].

Probiotics are used for this purpose to retrieve the deteriorated normal intestinal microflora. The most investigated probiotics in this field are *Lactobacilli* and *Saccharomyces boulardii* [9]. In spite of the fact that there are numerous studies about probiotics as a treatment for infectious diarrhea, there are some unsolved problems related to the dysentery description, remission criteria, probiotic type, probiotic potent dose, study quality, and probiotic effectiveness evaluation [23]. Recent studies using different probiotics have shown variable effects and meta-analyses show uncertain results due to inequality of studies [24–26]. This suggests that each probiotic has its unique efficacy, so each probiotic needs to be tested to assess its efficacy in specific conditions [27].

Recent systematic reviews recommend further studies of probiotics in an outpatient setting [24, 28]. There are some meta-analyses which have assessed the results of probiotics in the treatment of AGE. In a recent meta-analysis, in order to evaluate the efficacy of probiotics in the treatment of AGE, data was collected from 63 randomized controlled trials [RCTs] and 8014 subjects. 56 out of all those RCTs were carried out in infants and young children. Forty-six RCTs assessed a single probiotic, and 17 RCTs tested a combination of different probiotics. *Lactobacillus* GG, *S. boulardii*, and *Enterococcus* lactic acid bacteria strain SF68 were the most common probiotics used in studies. The Cochrane Review suggested that *Lactobacillus* GG can reduce the duration of diarrhea about 27 hours, stool frequency on the second day, and the probability of diarrhea lasting 4 days. The authors have suggested that more assessments are needed to help clinicians in the use of particular probiotic regimens in specific patient groups [29].

According to a research on the impact of *Lactobacillus reuteri* DSM 17938 on acute infectious diarrhea in a pediatric outpatient setting, it was shown that probiotics had a positive impact on the length of hospitalization and diarrhea. The positive impact on the length of diarrhea was consistent with the findings of the present study [30]. In another study, Golam H. Rabbani et al. studied the impact of green banana on clinical severity of childhood shigellosis. They found that cooked green banana had a positive impact on the length of hospitalization among all age groups. The impact on diarrhea reduction in treatment group was consistent with the findings of the present study [31]. There was no data of weight changes of participants and the impact on the duration of fever was not consistent with the results obtained in the present study.

Ashraf et al. conducted a clinical trial in 2001. In that study, children with confirmed shigellosis were given hyperimmune bovine colostrums in addition to receiving routine treatment. The impact of hyperimmune bovine colostrum on the duration of fever, duration of anorexia, duration of abdominal pain, duration of tenesmus, duration of diarrhea after inclusion, duration of blood in stool, stool frequency on day 3, stool frequency on day 5, cumulative stool frequency in 5-day therapy, number of positive stool cultures on day 3, and number of positive stool cultures on day 5 was investigated in that study. Values were not significantly different between groups. They concluded that HBC as an adjuvant is unable to show any beneficial effect in reducing the severity of childhood shigellosis [32].

In another recent study conducted by Işlek et al. (2014) in Turkey, the role of *Bifidobacterium lactis* B94 plus Inulin in the treatment of acute infectious diarrhea in children was investigated. Compared to the control group, the duration of diarrhea was significantly reduced in the synbiotic group in comparison to the placebo group (3.9 ± 1.2 days versus 5.2 ± 1.3 days, resp.; $P < 0.001$). These results are consistent with the findings of this study in which the positive impact of probiotics/prebiotics on the shortening of duration of diarrhea was observed (2.5 ± 0.98 in synbiotic group and 2.9±1.09 in placebo group). In Işlek et al.'s study, the durations of fever were similar in interference and control groups which were not consistent with the findings of the present study [23].

Vinh et al. conducted a study in 2009. In that study, the impact of Gatifloxacin on the children affected by shigellosis was compared to that of Ciprofloxacin. The results of the study showed that the duration of symptoms in the group receiving Ciprofloxacin was almost the same as that in the group receiving Ciprofloxacin ($P > 0.05$) [33]. They concluded that Ciprofloxacin and Gatifloxacin are similarly effective for the treatment of acute shigellosis. This was not consistent with the findings of the present study.

There is a randomized double-blinded, placebo-controlled clinical trial study performed by Chen et al. (2010) on 304 children aged 3 months to 6 years with acute infectious diarrhea. The patients received Bio-Three (a mixture of *Bacillus mesentericus*, *Enterococcus faecalis*, and *Clostridium butyricum*) or placebo for one week in Chang Gung Children's Hospital in Northern Taiwan. In comparison to the placebo group, the Bio-Three group presented a significant reduction in the severity and duration of diarrhea and the duration of hospital stay, although no reduction of the duration of fever was observed [34]. The Working Group on Probiotics of the European Society for Pediatric Gastroenterology, Hepatology and Nutrition (ESPGHAN) described that the use of probiotics should be considered as an adjuvant therapy to ORS in the management of acute gastroenteritis [9, 24].

In the literature, the properties of probiotics have been recognized as a safe and beneficial adjunct to many treatments for infections [35–38]. In our study, no adverse effect toward synbiotics has been reported as well; but recently it has been a matter of intense debate so that in a review article it has been concluded that since there may be different strains of different probiotics with different properties it is possible to have different results of efficacy or adverse effects [39].

5. Conclusion

Dysentery is one of the most common diseases among children. This disease has harmful impacts on children, family, and society. Due to harmful consequences in terms of economy, human loss, and also the lack of definite treatment which leads to the resistant form of the disease, using probiotics can be beneficial. The findings of this study indicate the beneficial effects of *Lactobacillus* as an adjunct to standard treatment on the children affected by dysentery, shortening duration of fever and duration of dysentery. Besides, many studies have confirmed the lack of side effects of probiotics. Therefore, it seems that using probiotics/prebiotics as a tool of side treatment in areas affected by dysentery can be beneficial to improve children's health.

Competing Interests

The authors declare that they have no competing interests.

References

[1] S. K. Niyogi, "Shigellosis," *Journal of Microbiology*, vol. 43, no. 2, pp. 133–143, 2005.

[2] A. V. Sangeetha, S. C. Parija, J. Mandal, and S. Krishnamurthy, "Clinical and microbiological profiles of Shigellosis in children," *Journal of Health, Population and Nutrition*, vol. 32, no. 4, pp. 580–586, 2014.

[3] P. Bardhan, A. S. G. Faruque, A. Naheed, and D. A. Sack, "Decrease in shigellosis-related deaths without shigella spp.-specific interventions, Asia," *Emerging Infectious Diseases*, vol. 16, no. 11, pp. 1718–1723, 2010.

[4] E. Scallan, T. F. Jones, A. Cronquist et al., "Factors associated with seeking medical care and submitting a stool sample in estimating the burden of foodborne illness," *Foodborne Pathogens and Disease*, vol. 3, no. 4, pp. 432–438, 2006.

[5] A. L. Shane, N. A. Tucker, J. A. Crump, E. D. Mintz, and J. A. Painter, "Sharing Shigella: risk factors for a multicommunity outbreak of shigellosis," *Archives of Pediatrics & Adolescent Medicine*, vol. 157, no. 6, pp. 601–603, 2003.

[6] A. S. Neish, "Microbes in Gastrointestinal Health and Disease," *Gastroenterology*, vol. 136, no. 1, pp. 65–80, 2009.

[7] M. J. Kullen and J. Bettler, "The delivery of probiotics and prebiotics to infants," *Current Pharmaceutical Design*, vol. 11, no. 1, pp. 55–74, 2005.

[8] S. Michail, F. Sylvester, G. Fuchs, and R. Issenman, "Clinical efficacy of probiotics: review of the evidence with focus on children," *Journal of Pediatric Gastroenterology and Nutrition*, vol. 43, no. 4, pp. 550–557, 2006.

[9] H. Szajewska, A. Guarino, I. Hojsak et al., "Use of probiotics for management of acute gastroenteritis: a position paper by the ESPGHAN working group for probiotics and prebiotics," *Journal of Pediatric Gastroenterology and Nutrition*, vol. 58, no. 4, pp. 531–539, 2014.

[10] K. Arunachalam, H. S. Gill, and R. K. Chandra, "Enhancement of natural immune function by dietary consumption of Bifidobacterium lactis (HN019)," *European Journal of Clinical Nutrition*, vol. 54, no. 3, pp. 263–267, 2000.

[11] M. D. Cabana, A. L. Shane, C. Chao, and M. Oliva-Hemker, "Probiotics in primary care pediatrics," *Clinical Pediatrics*, vol. 45, no. 5, pp. 405–410, 2006.

[12] V. De Preter, T. Vanhoutte, G. Huys, J. Swings, P. Rutgeerts, and K. Verbeke, "Effect of lactulose and Saccharomyces boulardii administration on the colonic urea-nitrogen metabolism and the bifidobacteria concentration in healthy human subjects," *Alimentary Pharmacology and Therapeutics*, vol. 23, no. 7, pp. 963–974, 2006.

[13] R. N. Fedorak and K. L. Madsen, "Probiotics and prebiotics in gastrointestinal disorders," *Current Opinion in Gastroenterology*, vol. 20, no. 2, pp. 146–155, 2004.

[14] H. Link-Amster, F. Rochat, K. Y. Saudan, O. Mignot, and J. M. Aeschlimann, "Modulation of a specific humoral immune response and changes in intestinal flora mediated through fermented milk intake," *FEMS Immunology and Medical Microbiology*, vol. 10, no. 1, pp. 55–63, 1994.

[15] S. Michail and F. Abernathy, "Lactobacillus plantarum reduces the in vitro secretory response of intestinal epithelial cells to enteropathogenic Escherichia coli infection," *Journal of Pediatric Gastroenterology and Nutrition*, vol. 35, no. 3, pp. 350–355, 2002.

[16] S. J. Allen, B. Okoko, E. Martinez, G. Gregorio, and L. F. Dans, "Probiotics for treating infectious diarrhoea," *Cochrane Database of Systematic Reviews*, no. 2, Article ID CD003048, 2004.

[17] H. Szajewska and J. Z. Mrukowicz, "Probiotics in the treatment and prevention of acute infectious diarrhea in infants and children: a systematic review of published randomized, double-blind, placebo-controlled trials," *Journal of Pediatric Gastroenterology and Nutrition*, vol. 33, supplement 2, pp. S17–S25, 2001.

[18] G. T. Macfarlane, H. Steed, and S. Macfarlane, "Bacterial metabolism and health-related effects of galacto-oligosaccharides and other prebiotics," *Journal of Applied Microbiology*, vol. 104, no. 2, pp. 305–344, 2008.

[19] J. E. Idanpaan-Heikkila, "WHO guidelines for good clinical practice (GCP) for trials on pharmaceutical products: responsibilities of the investigator," *Annals of Medicine*, vol. 26, no. 2, pp. 89–94, 1994.

[20] S. Koletzko and S. Osterrieder, "Acute infectious diarrhea in children," *Deutsches Ärzteblatt International*, vol. 106, no. 33, pp. 539–548, 2009.

[21] A. C. Senok, A. Y. Ismaeel, and G. A. Botta, "Probiotics: facts and myths," *Clinical Microbiology and Infection*, vol. 11, no. 12, pp. 958–966, 2005.

[22] B. Wallace, "Clinical use of probiotics in the pediatric population," *Nutrition in Clinical Practice*, vol. 24, no. 1, pp. 50–59, 2009.

[23] A. Işlek, E. Sayar, A. Yilmaz, B. O. Baysan, D. Mutlu, and R. Artan, "The role of Bifidobacterium lactis B94 plus inulin in the treatment of acute infectious diarrhea in children," *The Turkish Journal of Gastroenterology*, vol. 25, no. 6, pp. 628–633, 2014.

[24] S. B. Freedman, D. Pasichnyk, K. J. L. Black et al., "Gastroenteritis therapies in developed countries: systematic review and meta-analysis," *PLoS ONE*, vol. 10, no. 6, article e0128754, 2015.

[25] J. A. Hawrelak, D. L. Whitten, and S. P. Myers, "Is *Lactobacillus rhamnosus* GG effective in preventing the onset of antibiotic-associated diarrhoea: a systematic review," *Digestion*, vol. 72, no. 1, pp. 51–56, 2005.

[26] B. C. Johnston, J. Z. Goldenberg, P. O. Vandvik, X. Sun, and G. H. Guyatt, "Probiotics for the prevention of pediatric antibiotic-associated diarrhea," *The Cochrane Database of Systematic Reviews*, no. 11, Article ID CD004827, 2011.

[27] M. Pham, D. A. Lemberg, and A. S. Day, "Probiotics: sorting the evidence from the myths," *The Medical Journal of Australia*, vol. 188, no. 5, pp. 304–308, 2008.

[28] C. C. Butler, D. Duncan, and K. Hood, "Does taking probiotics routinely with antibiotics prevent antibiotic associated diarrhoea?" *BMJ (Online)*, vol. 344, article e682, 2012.

[29] S. J. Allen, E. G. Martinez, G. V. Gregorio, and L. F. Dans, "Probiotics for treating acute infectious diarrhoea," *The Cochrane Database of Systematic Reviews*, no. 11, Article ID CD003048, 2010.

[30] E. C. Dinleyici, N. Dalgic, S. Guven et al., "*Lactobacillus reuteri* DSM 17938 shortens acute infectious diarrhea in a pediatric outpatient setting," *Jornal de Pediatria*, vol. 91, no. 4, pp. 392–396, 2015.

[31] J.-F. Rossignol, N. Lopez-Chegne, L. M. Julcamoro, M. E. Carrion, and M. C. Bardin, "Nitazoxanide for the empiric treatment of pediatric infectious diarrhea," *Transactions of the Royal Society of Tropical Medicine and Hygiene*, vol. 106, no. 3, pp. 167–173, 2012.

[32] H. Ashraf, D. Mahalanabis, A. K. Mitra, S. Tzipori, and G. J. Fuchs, "Hyperimmune bovine colostrum in the treatment of shigellosis in children: a double-blind, randomized, controlled trial," *Acta Paediatrica*, vol. 90, no. 12, pp. 1373–1378, 2001.

[33] H. Vinh, V. T. C. Anh, N. D. Anh et al., "A multi-center randomized trial to assess the efficacy of gatifloxacin versus ciprofloxacin for the treatment of shigellosis in Vietnamese children," *PLoS Neglected Tropical Diseases*, vol. 5, no. 8, Article ID e1264, 2011.

[34] C.-C. Chen, M.-S. Kong, M.-W. Lai et al., "Probiotics have clinical, microbiologic, and immunologic efficacy in acute infectious diarrhea," *The Pediatric Infectious Disease Journal*, vol. 29, no. 2, pp. 135–138, 2010.

[35] E. C. A. Dinleyici and Y. Vandenplas, "Lactobacillus reuteri DSM 17938 effectively reduces the duration of acute diarrhoea in hospitalised children," *Acta Paediatrica*, vol. 103, no. 7, pp. e300–e305, 2014.

[36] R. Francavilla, L. Polimeno, A. Demichina et al., "*Lactobacillus reuteri* strain combination in *Helicobacter pylori* infection: a randomized, double-blind, placebo-controlled study," *Journal of Clinical Gastroenterology*, vol. 48, no. 5, pp. 407–413, 2014.

[37] S. Guandalini, L. Pensabene, M. A. Zikri et al., "Lactobacillus GG administered in oral rehydration solution to children with acute diarrhea: a multicenter European trial," *Journal of*

Pediatric Gastroenterology and Nutrition, vol. 30, no. 1, pp. 54–60, 2000.

[38] Z. Weizman, G. Asli, and A. Alsheikh, "Effect of a probiotic infant formula on infections in child care centers: comparison of two probiotic agents," *Pediatrics*, vol. 115, no. 1, pp. 5–9, 2005.

[39] G. J. Oudhuis, D. C. J. J. Bergmans, and A. Verbon, "Probiotics for prevention of nosocomial infections: efficacy and adverse effects," *Current Opinion in Critical Care*, vol. 17, no. 5, pp. 487–492, 2011.

6

Mesenchymal Conversion of Mesothelial Cells Is a Key Event in the Pathophysiology of the Peritoneum during Peritoneal Dialysis

Manuel López-Cabrera

Centro de Biología Molecular-Severo Ochoa, CSIC, UAM, Cantoblanco, C/Nicolás Cabrera 1, 28049 Madrid, Spain

Correspondence should be addressed to Manuel López-Cabrera; mlcabrera@cbm.uam.es

Academic Editor: Anjali Satoskar

Peritoneal dialysis (PD) is a therapeutic option for the treatment of end-stage renal disease and is based on the use of the peritoneum as a semipermeable membrane for the exchange of toxic solutes and water. Long-term exposure of the peritoneal membrane to hyperosmotic PD fluids causes inflammation, loss of the mesothelial cells monolayer, fibrosis, vasculopathy, and angiogenesis, which may lead to peritoneal functional decline. Peritonitis may further exacerbate the injury of the peritoneal membrane. In parallel with these peritoneal alterations, mesothelial cells undergo an epithelial to mesenchymal transition (EMT), which has been associated with peritoneal deterioration. Factors contributing to the bioincompatibility of classical PD fluids include the high content of glucose/glucose degradation products (GDPs) and their acidic pH. New generation low-GDPs-neutral pH fluids have improved biocompatibility resulting in better preservation of the peritoneum. However, standard glucose-based fluids are still needed, as biocompatible solutions are expensive for many potential users. An alternative approach to preserve the peritoneal membrane, complementary to the efforts to improve fluid biocompatibility, is the use of pharmacological agents protecting the mesothelium. This paper provides a comprehensive review of recent advances that point to the EMT of mesothelial cells as a potential therapeutic target to preserve membrane function.

1. Introduction

Peritoneal dialysis (PD) is a form of renal replacement therapy that has become an established alternative to hemodialysis [1–3]. During the last years, great effort was made to improve the biocompatibility of the dialysis solutions with the expectancy of diminishing their adverse effects on peritoneal morphology and function [4–12]. The number of patients included in PD programs has increased progressively worldwide and is presently used by approximately 10 to 15% of the total global dialysis population [2, 13]. PD offers major advantages in terms of quality of life, costs, and home-based treatment opportunities. The increase of PD programs could also be attributed to the undoubted improvement of the PD technique, especially in terms of peritonitis prevention and of biocompatibility of the dialysis solutions. At present, PD is a successful treatment for end-stage renal disease, and several studies have confirmed equivalent adequacy, mortality, and fluid balance status when compared with hemodialysis, at least for the first 4-5 years [14–17]. However, the growth of PD continues being limited by the membrane incapacity to perform adequate diffusive and/or convective transports at long term [2, 18]. Peritonitis and ultrafiltration failure, with a clinical result of extracellular volume overload and an increased cardiovascular risk, are still the major factors contributing to technique dropouts [2, 18, 19].

PD technique requires the instillation and periodical renovation, through a permanently installed catheter, of a hyperosmotic PD fluid into the peritoneal cavity. The peritoneum acts as a semipermeable membrane across which ultrafiltration and diffusion take place [1–3]. In consequence, one of the most important goals in PD is the long-term preservation of the peritoneal membrane integrity [2, 18, 19]. The use of solutions with neutral pH and with low content of glucose degradation products (GDPs) may represent a potential strategy to attenuate some of the PD-related adverse effects [20]. The impact of these novel, more biocompatible, solutions on the clinical outcomes is currently being recognized [21, 22]. However, classical glucose-based PD fluids are still needed, because the new-generation biocompatible solutions are expensive and many potential users cannot afford them. One possibility to reduce the adverse effects of classical PD fluids on the peritoneum is by decreasing the dwell time of the dialysate [23, 24]. Another alternative approach to preserve the peritoneal membrane could be the use of pharmacological agents protecting the mesothelium or targeting inflammation and fibrosis [25, 26]. In this review, we discuss two putative long-term pharmacological intervention strategies that have been tested in experimental animal models of PD. One strategy is the addition of pharmacological agents into the PD fluids and the other strategy is the use of drugs that are administrated by oral route. We summarize the current knowledge regarding the therapeutic approaches in experimental PD models directed against the epithelial to mesenchymal transition (EMT) of mesothelial cells (MCs) or against the EMT-promoting stimuli operating *in vivo*.

2. Pathogenesis of Peritoneal Membrane Dysfunction

The structure of the peritoneum is simple and is composed of a single layer of MCs that lines a compact zone of connective tissue that contains few fibroblasts, mast cells, macrophages, and vessels [27, 28]. It was generally believed that the uremic status might affect the architecture of the peritoneal membrane and its transport characteristics. In this context, the peritoneum of partially nephrectomized rats showed altered permeability [29]. Despite these findings in animal models, the effect of uremia itself on the peritoneum in humans is controversial. Two human peritoneal biopsy studies have shown a modest compact zone thickening and vasculopathy in predialysis renal patients [30, 31]. In contrast, in other studies no significant fibrosis or vasculopathy was observed in uremic non-PD patients [32].

The bioincompatible nature of some PD fluids and episodes of bacterial and fungal infection are considered the main etiologic factors of peritoneal deterioration [2, 12, 19, 25, 33]. They induce acute and chronic inflammatory and reparative responses that initiate the structural alterations of the peritoneal membrane including loss of MCs monolayer, fibrosis, angiogenesis, and hyalinizing vasculopathy [30, 31, 34–36] (Figure 1). Such alterations are considered the major cause of ultrafiltration failure and loss of the dialytic capacity of the peritoneum [2, 19, 37, 38]. There is emerging evidence suggesting that the local injury induced by classical glucose-based PD fluids is mediated, at least in part, by the presence of GDPs and by the acidic pH. GDPs through the formation advanced glycation-end products (AGEs) may stimulate the production of extracellular matrix components (ECM) as well as the synthesis of profibrotic and angiogenic factors [2, 19]. Several studies have demonstrated the appearance of AGEs in the peritoneal effluents of PD patients, which

correlated with the time on PD treatment. Biopsy studies have confirmed the accumulation of AGEs in the peritoneal tissues of PD patients. The intensity of AGEs accumulation is associated with fibrosis and ultrafiltration dysfunction [2, 19].

The peritoneal immune response to injury or infection involves, among other cells, MCs and resident macrophages that work in a coordinated manner to recruit other inflammatory cells, including mononuclear phagocytes, lymphocytes, and neutrophils. MCs and infiltrating immune cells can produce a wide number of cytokines, growth factors, and chemokines to establish a complex network that feedbacks resulting in acute or chronic inflammation [2, 25, 39–41]. Sustained inflammation might trigger the fibrogenic and angiogenic processes associated with the ultrafiltration failure that causes PD technique dropout (Figure 1).

There are two different pathologic forms of PD-related fibrosis [42–44]. The most common is simple peritoneal sclerosis (SPS), which occurs in almost all patients. The degree of fibrosis is mild and shows a relation with the time on dialysis. In general terms, SPS ceases when the patient is transplanted or shifted to hemodialysis [28, 31, 38, 42–44]. On the other end of the spectrum is encapsulating peritoneal sclerosis (EPS), which is a rare form of sclerosis that evolves rapidly with intense fibrosis, inflammation, and fibrin deposits [43–46]. It is a life threatening condition that in many cases evolves to visceral encapsulation with a fibrous cocoon and progresses even if the patient is removed from PD. In this context, EPS often becomes apparent after renal transplantation or switching patients to hemodialysis [47–49]. The etiopathogenesis of EPS is still debated, with some sustaining that it is a rare form of progression of SPS and others that it is a primitive form of sclerosis [50–52]. Thus, the main reasons that have led to PD-induced sclerosis to become a subject of active research are the high frequency of mild degree peritoneal fibrosis (SPS) and the severity and poor prognosis of EPS.

However, fibrosis does not appear to be the unique structural alteration of the peritoneal membrane induced by PD. Besides this alteration the peritoneum may also show an increase of capillary number (angiogenesis) and hyalinizing vasculopathy [2, 25] (Figure 1). Vascular endothelial growth factor (VEGF) is a strong angiogenic factor involved, among other molecules, in endothelial cell proliferation and vascular permeability [53]. It has been suggested that local production of VEGF during PD plays a central role in the processes leading to peritoneal angiogenesis and functional decline [54–58]. It has been demonstrated that MCs can produce high amounts of VEGF *in vitro* in response to various stimuli [59–62]. In addition, it has been suggested that MCs, via a mesenchymal conversion, may convert into the major local producer of VEGF during PD, which in turn appears to be associated with peritoneal transport alteration [57, 62, 63]. Some studies of peritoneal biopsies have suggested that angiogenesis and vasculopathy are the most characteristic structural alteration in PD-related peritoneal pathology, at least in patients with severe membrane failure [30, 34]. In contrast, other studies have shown that in stable uncomplicated PD patients vascular density does not increase, while intact vessels decrease with time of treatment and severe

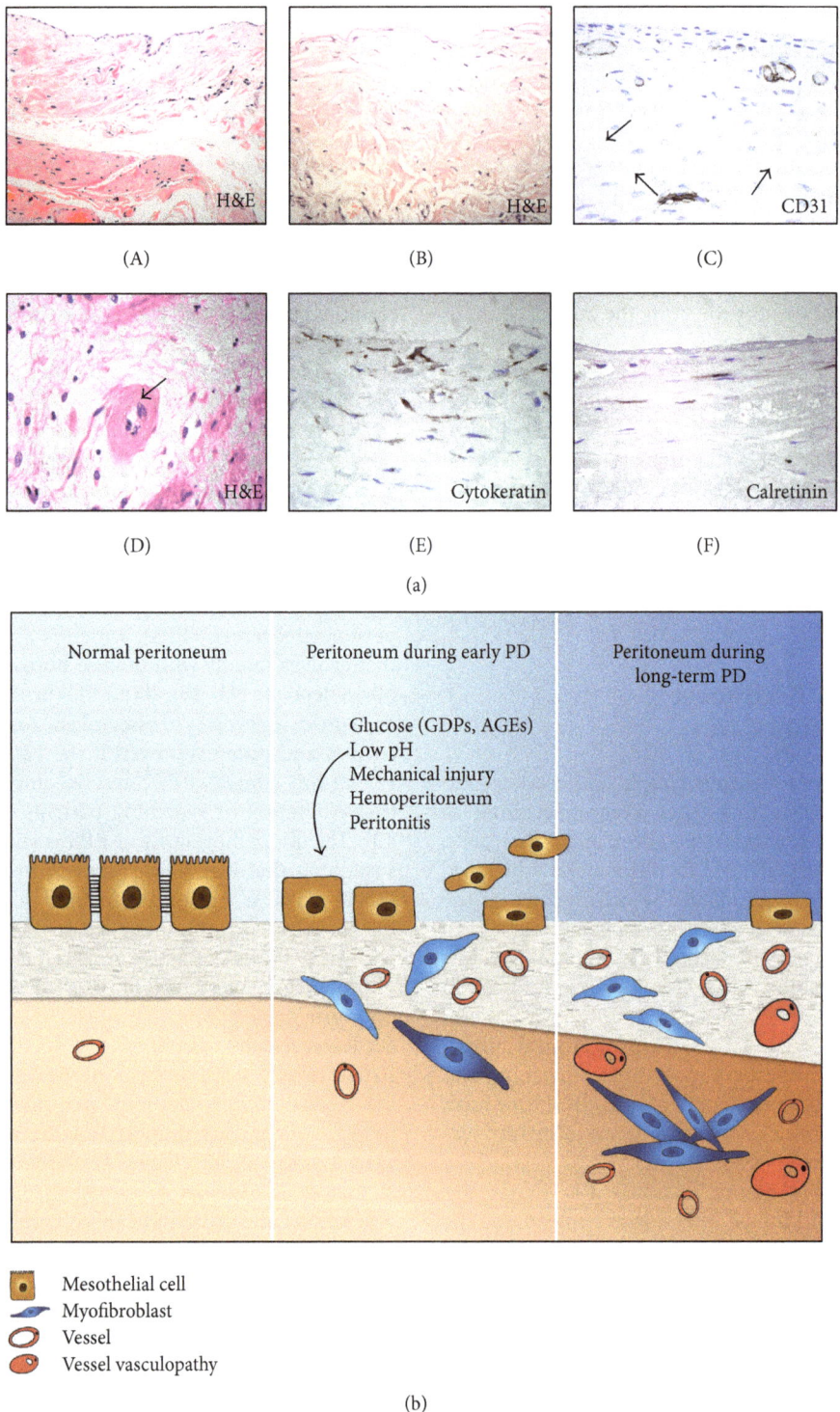

FIGURE 1: Structural alteration of the peritoneal membrane during PD. (a) Normal peritoneal tissue from a healthy donor stained with Haematoxylin-eosin (H&E) shows a preserved MCs monolayer that lines a compact zone of connective tissue (A). Peritoneal membrane from a PD patient stained with H&E shows the loss of the MCs monolayer and increased thickness of the compact zone (B). Magnification ×200. Staining of the peritoneal vessels with anti-CD31 antibody demonstrates an intense angiogenesis in peritoneal membrane from PD patient (C). Hyalinizing vasculopathy can be observed in the peritoneal tissue from PD patient (D). Immunohistochemical analysis of the peritoneal membrane from PD patient reveals the presence of fibroblast-like cells embedded in the fibrotic stroma expressing the mesothelial markers cytokeratins and calretinin (E) and (F). Magnification ×150. (b) Schematic representation of the progressive alterations of the peritoneal membrane in the time course of PD.

vasculopathy predominate mostly in long-term PD [36, 64, 65]. The only change that is constantly found in peritoneal biopsies after a time on PD is submesothelial fibrosis [2, 19, 30–32, 34]. Nevertheless, there is increasing evidence that fibrosis in conjunction with angiogenesis and most probably with augmented vessel permeability are key determinants of ultrafiltration dysfunction [25, 30]. In animal models of PD it has been shown that fibrosis and angiogenesis may be two separate responses to peritoneal injury [66–69]. However, in PD patients, it is possible that fibrosis and angiogenesis are intimately and closely related in the response of the peritoneum to prolonged injury [25].

3. Peritoneal Dialysis Induces the Accumulation of Myofibroblasts

Another characteristic structural alteration of the peritoneum during PD is the loss of the MC monolayer and the progressive accumulation of a particular type of activated fibroblast termed myofibroblast (Figure 1), which, as will be discussed below, derive partially from the local conversion of MCs. The term myofibroblast defines a cell with intermediate features between a fibroblast and a smooth muscle cell. From an immunophenotypic perspective, they are defined by the expression of α-smooth muscle actin (α-SMA). Myofibroblasts were initially described by Gabbiani et al. in the granulation tissue of a cutaneous model of wound repair [70, 71]. Since then, they have been reported as important protagonists of almost all situations of repair and fibrosis that take place in human pathology [72]. Their capacity to synthesize extracellular matrix elements, growth factors, cytokines, and participation in the inflammatory response, as well as their contractile properties, converts them to the most important fibroblastic phenotype. As stated by Phan they must be considered the "reference" fibroblast phenotype to which all others must be related or compared [73]. Myofibroblasts are neither present in the normal peritoneum nor in the peritoneum obtained from uremic non-PD patients [32, 74]. In contrast, they can be easily observed in many patients undergoing PD treatment [32, 34, 75].

The origin of myofibroblasts is still an open question and a matter of intense debate [76–81], but it is generally accepted that these fibroblasts constitute a heterogeneous population that may derive from multiple sources (Figure 2). There is emerging evidence that the origin of myofibroblasts may vary between different organs and within different areas of individual organs. These observations may suggest that tissue- and organ-specific microenvironments dictate the different proportions of myofibroblasts subpopulations [76, 77, 82–87]. The activation of resident fibroblasts has classically been considered the main origin of myofibroblasts in most fibrotic pathologies [70–73, 83, 86]. Other studies have pointed to cells recruited from the bone marrow (fibrocytes) as an important source of myofibroblasts in several fibrotic disorders [76, 87–90]. In addition, it has been shown that the local conversion of epithelial cells and endothelial cells may also contribute to the accumulation of myofibroblasts in some reparative and fibrotic diseases. The conversion

into myofibroblasts by these cells is achieved through two closely related processes termed epithelial to mesenchymal transition (EMT) and endothelial to mesenchymal transition (EndMT), respectively [86, 90–95]. More recently it has been suggested that vessel-associated pericytes may also transdifferentiate into myofibroblasts [77, 96] (Figure 2).

In the peritoneal membrane, the myofibroblasts may have at least a dual origin: (1) from resident fibroblasts through an activation process and (2) from the mesothelium via EMT [25, 32, 97] (Figure 1). The presence of other myofibroblasts subpopulations in the damaged peritoneum during PD has not been described so far in PD patients [25]. However, in a mouse model of PD fluid exposure, it has been shown that myofibroblasts may have different origins including resident fibroblasts, MCs, endothelial cells, and bone marrow-derived cells [82]. As we will discuss below, the identification of the EMT of MCs as a key process in the onset and progression of peritoneal fibrosis and angiogenesis opens new insights for therapeutic intervention.

4. Mesothelial Cells Undergo a Mesenchymal Transition in Response to PD-Induced Damage

The mesothelium is a continuous surface layer formed by flattened, polygonal, and mononuclear MCs [28]. This monolayer shows remarkable fibrinolytic properties and is thought to be involved in the prevention of fibrous adhesion formation in the peritoneum. MCs cells have vast biosynthetic capacity and secrete phospholipids and phosphatidylcholine in the form of lamellar bodies that provide a lubricating surface for the movement of abdominal viscera [98–100]. The presence of MCs that have undergone a mesenchymal conversion *in vivo* in the effluent and in the peritoneal tissue of PD patients was first demonstrated in a landmark paper published in 2003 [97]. The authors described that soon after PD is initiated, peritoneal MCs showed a progressive loss of epithelial phenotype and acquired myofibroblast characteristics [97]. About the same time it was demonstrated that the treatment *in vitro* of omentum-derived MCs with TGF-β1 induced a myofibroblast conversion of these cells that were reminiscent of an EMT-like process [101].

Effluent-derived MCs can be easily isolated from PD patients using standard methods [97, 102]. It was described that *ex vivo* cultures of effluent-derived MCs showed two main morphologies: epithelioid and nonepithelioid (fibroblast-like). After analyzing several hundred MC cultures with growth capacity, it could be determined that the frequencies of the different effluent-derived MC cultures were approximately 53 percent for epithelioid phenotype and 44 percent for nonepithelioid MCs. The prevalence of nonepithelioid MC cultures appeared to be associated with the time the patients have been subjected to PD and with the episodes of acute or recurrent peritonitis or hemoperitoneum [97, 102]. A less frequent cell culture type (less than 6 percent) with mixed morphologies has also been described [97, 102]. In the course of practicing *ex vivo* cultures of effluent-derived cells, it can be observed occasionally hypertrophic MCs,

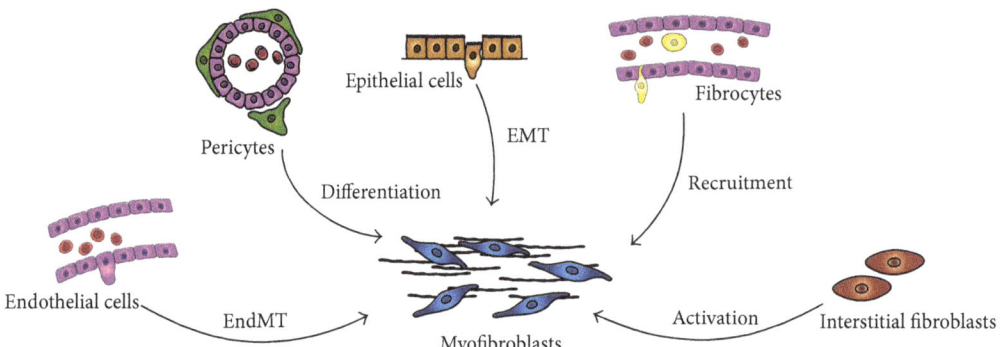

FIGURE 2: Multiple origins of myofibroblasts have been proposed in tissue fibrosis. Myofibroblasts may derive from at least five different sources through various mechanisms: phenotypic activation from interstitial fibroblasts; differentiation from vascular pericytes; recruitment from circulating fibrocytes; capillary endothelial-mesenchymal transition (EndMT); and epithelial-mesenchymal transition (EMT). The relative contribution of each source to the myofibroblast pool in peritoneal fibrosis still requires further studies.

which might appear alone or accompanied by MCs with a normal size [102, 103]. Hypertrophic MCs could be the consequence of an arrest of the cell cycle, since these cells are unable to proliferate [104].

Proliferating MCs from effluents showed high expression of ICAM-1 independently of their morphology, and even mixed cultures were homogeneous in the expression of this marker. On the contrary, ICAM-1 was negligible on fibroblasts from omentum, supporting that effluent non-epitheliod cells have a mesothelial origin [97]. In addition, effluent-derived cells also showed high expression of CA-125, a known mesothelial marker, independently of their shape, whereas fibroblasts were negative for this molecule, reinforcing the concept of a mesothelial origin of these cells and rule out possible fibroblast contaminations [102]. The analysis of the expression of the epithelial markers cytokeratins and E-cadherin was important to determine more precisely the nature of effluent-derived cells. High expression of cytokeratins and E-cadherin was only observed in naïve omentum-derived MC, whereas effluent-derived cells showed a progressive reduction in the expression of these molecules, although even nonepithelioid MCs might maintain a small population of positive cells. Fibroblasts were completely negative for these two markers [97, 102]. The morphological changes and downregulation of cytokeratin and E-cadherin in effluent-derived MCs were indicative of an EMT-like process. However, the definitive prove to demonstrate that the PD-induced phenotype changes of the MCs were related with an EMT process came from the analysis of the expression of several mesenchymal markers including snail, N-cadherin, fibronectin, collagen I, α-smooth-muscle actin (α-SMA), and fibroblast specific protein-1 (FSP-1) that were gradually upregulated in effluent MCs with epithelioid and nonepithelioid phenotypes [19, 25, 97, 102].

MCs that have undergone a mesenchymal phenotype acquire higher migratory and invasive capacities, which allow these cells to invade the submesothelial stroma [25, 58, 97, 105]. Thus, the mesenchymal conversion of MCs may also be observed *in vivo* in the peritoneum as a response to PD. Immunohistochemical analysis of peritoneal biopsies

from PD patients has shown the presence of fibroblast-like cells embedded in the compact zone expressing mesothelial markers such as cytokeratins, E-cadherin, ICAM-1, and calretinin [25, 32, 57, 65, 97] (Figure 1(a)). In addition, these peritoneal biopsies showed expression of α-SMA in the fibrotic stroma, especially in the upper submesothelial level, and in many cases these myofibroblasts showed coexpression of cytokeratins [32, 74]. These results indicated that new myofibroblastic cells could arise from local conversion of MCs by EMT during the repair responses that take place in PD. The myofibroblastic conversion of MC has been confirmed in an *in vivo* animal model based on the injection of an adenovirus vector that transferred active transforming growth factor (TGF)-β1 in rodent peritoneum [106, 107].

MCs have a mesodermal origin and share characteristics with both epithelial cells and endothelial cells, which may undergo EMT and endothelial to mesenchymal transition (EndMT), respectively. Thus, recently several authors have proposed renaming the mesenchymal conversion of MCs, that takes place in different organs such as lung, liver, or peritoneum, with a more appropriate term: mesothelial to mesenchymal transition (MMT) [62, 82, 108–111]. MMT is a complex and step-wise process that requires alterations in cellular architecture and a deep molecular reprogramming with new biochemical instruction [19, 25, 58]. MMT starts with the dissociation of intercellular junctions, due to downregulation of intercellular adhesion molecules, and with the loss of microvilli and apical-basal polarity. Then, the cells adopt a front to back polarity and acquire α-SMA expression and increased migratory capacity. In the latest stages of MMT, the cells increase their capacity to degrade the basement membrane and to invade the fibrotic compact zone (Figure 3). During the end-stages of the myofibroblast conversion, the MCs are able to produce large amount of extracellular matrix components and to synthesize a wide range of inflammatory, profibrotic, and angiogenic factors that may contribute to the structural and functional deterioration of the peritoneal membrane [2, 19, 25, 58]. Other commonly used molecular markers for MMT include the downregulation of cytokeratins, Wilm's tumor protein-1

(WT1), and calretinin and up-regulation of N-cadherin, FSP-1, and transcription factor snail (Figure 3).

MMT process *in vivo* results from an integration of diverse signals triggered by multiple factors, being difficult to assign priorities or hierarchy [25, 58, 63]. Receptors-mediated signaling in response to these factors trigger the activation of a complex network of intracellular effectors such as Smad 2 and 3, integrin-linked kinase (ILK), Notch1, nuclear factor-κB (NF-κB), extracellular-signal regulated kinases 1/2 (ERKs1/2), phosphatidylinositol 3-kinase (PI3-K)/Akt pathway, c-jun-N terminal kinase (JNK), and TGF-β-activated kinase-1 (TAK-1) (Figure 3). These effectors orchestrate the dissociation of intercellular adhesion complexes, the changes in cytoskeletal organization, and the acquisition of migratory and invasive capacities that take place during MMT [25, 63, 105, 106, 112, 113].

It is noteworthy that MMT is a reversible process, at least during the early stages. Therefore, molecules that negatively regulate MMT and promote mesenchymal to mesothelial transition (rMMT) must exist. Two endogenous factors, namely, hepatocyte growth factor (HGF) and bone morphogenetic protein-7 (BMP-7), have been demonstrated to block and reverse MMT [114–116]. Smad7 is another molecule that negatively regulates MMT [117–119]. On the other hand, the MMT process may be modulated by mitogen-activated protein (MAP) kinase p38 to prevent an exacerbated response to MMT-promoting stimuli [120]. Recently, it has been shown that caveolin-1 (CAV-1) impedes the exacerbation of the mesenchymal conversion of endothelial cells [121] and MCs (unpublished data) by promoting the internalization of TGF-β receptor and modulating TGF-β signaling (Figure 3).

5. TGF-β1 Is a Master Molecule in the Pathogenesis of Peritoneal Damage and in the Regulation of MMT

In the complex microenvironment that occurs during PD fluid-induced tissue injury a wide range of cytokines and factors are upregulated making it difficult to assign priorities or hierarchy for their effects on MMT and on the onset and progression of peritoneal damage [25]. Nonetheless, TGF-β1 is considered a master molecule in the development of peritoneal dysfunction, because its overexpression has been correlated with worse PD outcomes [122–124]. The relevance of TGF-β1 in peritoneal damage is further suggested in experimental animal models, in which TGF-β1 gene is overexpressed into the peritoneal cavity with adenovirus vectors, recapitulating the structural and functional alterations observed in PD patients [106, 107, 125]. Overexpression of molecules counteracting TGF-β1-triggered Smad signaling, including Smad7 and BMP-7, prevents and reverses PD fluid induced peritoneal damage in animal PD models [115, 116, 118, 119]. Recently, it has been demonstrated that direct targeting of TGF-β1, by using specific TGF-β1-blocking peptides, preserves the peritoneal membrane from dialysis fluid-induced damage in a mouse PD model [82]. TGF-β1 is a prototypical inducer of EMT in several tissues and organs [126–128]. TGF-β1 is also a key factor for the myofibroblastic conversion of MCs through MMT [58, 82, 97, 101].

5.1. Smad-Dependent Signaling Pathways in TGF-β1-Induced MMT. TGF-β1 belongs to a family of growth factors that includes TGF-βs, activins, and bone morphogenic proteins (BMPs) [126–130]. We will focus on the members TGF-β1 and BMP-7 because the balance between these two factors is a key determinant in the maintaining of the epithelial-like phenotype of MCs, and conversely, in the acquisition of mesenchymal-like characteristics [114, 116]. In fact, BMP-7 is a natural antagonist of TGF-β1 during organ fibrosis [130]. These factors signal via heterodimeric serine/threonine kinase transmembrane receptor complexes [129–131]. The binding of the ligand to its primary receptor (receptor type II) allows the recruitment, transphosphorylation, and activation of the signaling receptor (receptor type I) (Figure 4). The receptor type I of TGF-β1, also known as activin receptor-like kinase 5 (ALK5), is then able to exert its serine-threonine kinase activity to phosphorylate Smad2 and Smad3. The receptor type I of BMP-7 (ALK3) phosphorylate Smad1, Smad5, and Smad8 (Figure 4). These receptor-activated Smads (R-Smads) interact directly with and are phosphorylated by activated TGF-β or BMP receptor type I, respectively. Upon phosphorylation, they form heterodimers with Smad4, a common mediator of all Smad pathways [126, 129–131]. The resulting Smad heterocomplexes are then translocated into the nucleus where they bind directly to DNA and activate target genes involved either in the mesenchymal conversion of MCs (MMT) in the case of Smads2/3 or in the blocking/reversion of the mesenchymal transition (rMMT) in the case of Smads1/5/8 (Figure 4). Members of the third group of Smads, known as inhibitory Smads (Smad6 and Smad7), control BMP-7- and TGF-β1-triggered Smad signaling by preventing the phosphorylation and/or nuclear translocation of R-Smads and by inducing receptor complex degradation through the recruitment of ubiquitin ligases [126, 127, 129, 130].

The necessity of Smad2/3 signaling in TGF-β1-induced MMT is clearly illustrated *in vivo* in Smad3 knockout mice, which are protected from peritoneal fibrosis, show reduced collagen accumulation, and display attenuated MMT [106]. Targeting Smad signaling by inhibitory Smad7 also blocks MMT and reduces peritoneal fibrotic lesions [129–131]. Blockade of Smad2/3 signaling is also linked to the inhibition of MMT by hepatocyte growth factor (HGF) and BMP-7 [115, 116]. Mechanistically, HGF interferes with TGF-β1-mediated MMT by inducing the expression of the transcriptional corepressors such as SnoN and TGIF that interact with activated Smad2/4 complex and block the expression of Smad-dependent genes [132–134]. The mechanism underlying BMP-7 blockade of MMT is by activation of Smad1/5/8 protein that counteracts with TGF-β-activated Smad2/3 [116, 130].

It has been shown that MCs constitutively express BMP-7 and display basal activation of Smad1/5/8, which probably contribute to the maintaining of the epithelial-like phenotype. Induction of MMT with TGF-β1 results in

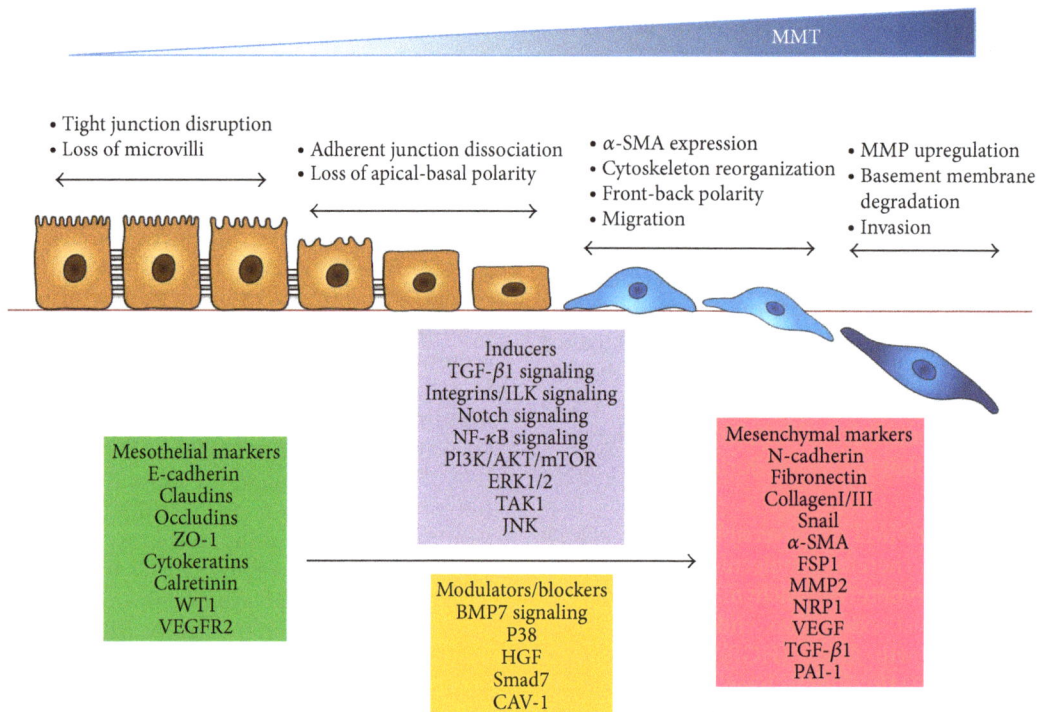

FIGURE 3: Schematic illustration of the key events during MMT. Mesothelial to mesenchymal transition (MMT) occurs when mesothelial cells lose their epithelial-like characteristics, including dissolution of cell-cell junctions, that is, tight junctions, adherens junctions and desmosomes, and loss of apical-basolateral polarity, and acquire a mesenchymal phenotype, characterized by actin reorganization and stress fiber formation, migration, and invasion. The diagram shows four key steps essential for the completion of entire MMT, the most commonly used mesothelial and mesenchymal markers, and the molecules and signal transduction pathways that act either as inducer or modulator of the MMT process. See text for details.

downregulation of BMP-7 and inactivation of BMP-7-specific Smad proteins [116]. Mechanistically, the TGF-β1-mediated inhibition of BMP-7 signaling might be explained by BMP-7 downregulation itself, or alternatively, by the upregulation of modulators of BMP-7 and TGF-β1 pathways. In this context, it has been shown that connective tissue growth factor (CTGF), a cytokine that is induced in MCs upon TGF-β1 treatment [135–138], inhibits BMP-7 and activates TGF-β1 signals by direct binding in the extracellular space [139, 140]. In addition, mesothelial BMP-7 signaling might also be influenced by other BMP-7 modulators such as gremlin-1, kielin/chordin-like protein (KCP), or uterine sensitization-associated gene 1 (USAG-1) [130, 141] (Figure 4). Thus, the relative contribution of these different factors in the inhibition of BMP-7 pathway by TGF-β1 remains to be established and deserves further studies.

5.2. Non-Smad Signaling Pathways in TGF-β1-Induced MMT. The Smad-dependent pathways are not the only ways by which TGF-β1 regulate cellular functions in MCs including the MMT process. Smad-independent pathways including the mitogen-activated protein kinases (MAPKs) ERKs 1/2, JNK, and p38, as well as NF-κB, TAK-1, and PI3-K/Akt pathways, also participate in TGF-β1-induced MMT (Figure 5). These pathways can either potentiate or modulate the outcome of TGF-β1-induced Smad signaling. Emerging evidences suggest that Smad signaling is tightly integrated

within a complex network of signaling pathways with cross-talks that modify the initial Smad signals and allow the pleiotropic activities of TGF-β1 [142, 143]. In this context, it has been shown that the signaling pathways of ERKs 1/2, JNK, NF-κB, and TAK-1 potentiate the TGF-β1-induced MMT [105, 112]. On the contrary, the p38-mediated pathway modulates the mesenchymal conversion of MCs by a feedback mechanism based on the downregulation of ERKs 1/2, NF-κB, and TAK-1 activities [120] (Figure 5).

There are instances in which Smad signaling is not required for TGF-β1 responses, as exemplified by the activation of the PI3-K/Akt pathway in Smad3 deficient mice leading to the stabilization of β-catenin, which in turn promote MMT [106]. A central role in this Smad3-independent signaling pathway is achieved by glycogen-synthase kinase (GSK)-3β, which has been shown to phosphorylate β-catenin and the transcriptional repressor Snail, leading to their ubiquitinization and degradation via the proteasome. The phosphorylation of GSK-3β by PI3-K/Akt leads to its functional inhibition. As a result, β-catenin is stabilized and localizes to the nucleus, where it feeds into the Wnt signaling pathway by interacting with lymphoid enhancer factor-1/T-cell factor (LEF1/TCF) and contributes to the transcription of mesenchymal-related genes. In addition, the inhibition of GSK-3β also drives the stabilization and nuclear translocation of Snail, a potent transcriptional repressor of E-cadherin and other intercellular adhesion molecules

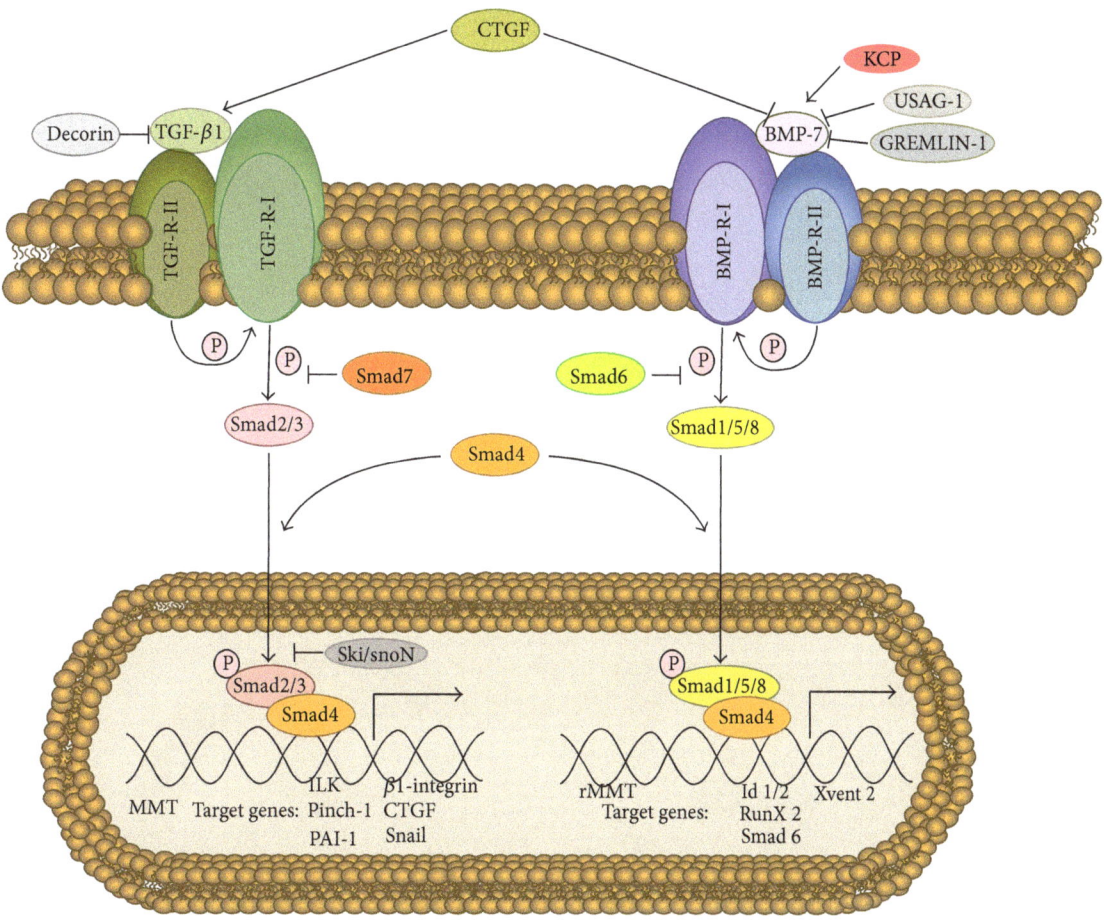

FIGURE 4: Smad-dependent signaling pathways of TGF-β1 and BMP-7. The binding of TGF-β1 and BMP-7 to their primary receptors (receptors type II) allows the recruitment, transphosphorylation, and activation of the signaling receptors (receptors type I). The receptor type I of TGF-β1 phosphorylate Smad2 and Smad3. The receptor type I of BMP-7 phosphorylate Smad1, Smad5, and Smad8. These receptor-activated Smads form heterodimers with Smad4. The resulting Smad complexes are then translocated into the nucleus where they activate target genes involved either in the mesenchymal conversion of MCs (MMT) in the case of Smads2/3 or in the blocking/reversion of the mesenchymal transition (rMMT) in the case of Smads1/5/8. Smad6 and Smad7 control BMP-7- and TGF-β1-triggered Smad signaling by preventing the phosphorylation and/or nuclear translocation and by inducing receptor complex degradation through the recruitment of ubiquitin ligases. Extracellular regulation of TGF-β1 and BMP-7 is achieved by various molecules. CTGF inhibits BMP-7 and activates TGF-β1 signals by direct binding in the extracellular space. BMP-7 signaling might also be influenced by other BMP-7 modulators such as gremlin-1, kielin/chordin-like protein (KCP), or uterine sensitization-associated gene 1 (USAG-1).

[144–147] (Figure 5). Interestingly, *in vivo* inhibition of the mammalian target of rapamycin (mTOR) by rapamycin completely abrogates the MMT response in Smad3-deficient mice [106]. Thus, TGF-β1 causes peritoneal injury through Smad-dependent and Smad-independent pathways suggesting that suppression of both pathways may be necessary to abrogate MMT.

6. Pathologic Significance of MMT in Peritoneal Dysfunction

It has been shown that during the progression of MMT, MCs acquire the ability to synthesize large amounts of components of the matrix such as fibronectin and collagen I [25, 57, 58]. In addition, MCs that undergo a MMT express high levels of cyclooxygenase (COX)-2 [148, 149],

CTGF [135, 136, 138], and VEGF [54, 56, 57], which have been implicated in inflammatory responses as well as in the fibrotic and angiogenic processes [2, 19, 25, 58]. In this context, it has been described that MCs from effluents with non-epitheliod (fibroblast-like) phenotype produced higher levels of COX-2 and VEGF *ex vivo* than MCs with epithelial-like phenotype. Interestingly, the levels of expression of these molecules by cultured effluent MCs correlated with the rate of peritoneal transport in PD patients [57, 148]. In addition, it was observed that patients draining non-epitheliod cells had higher blood VEGF levels than patients with MCs with epithelial-like phenotype in their effluents. Again, a correlation between *in vivo* VEGF levels and the rate of peritoneal transport in PD patients could be demonstrated [57]. A clinical study using peritoneal biopsies from 35 stable patients being on PD for up to 2 years demonstrated that patients in the highest quartile of mass transfer area coefficient of creatinine

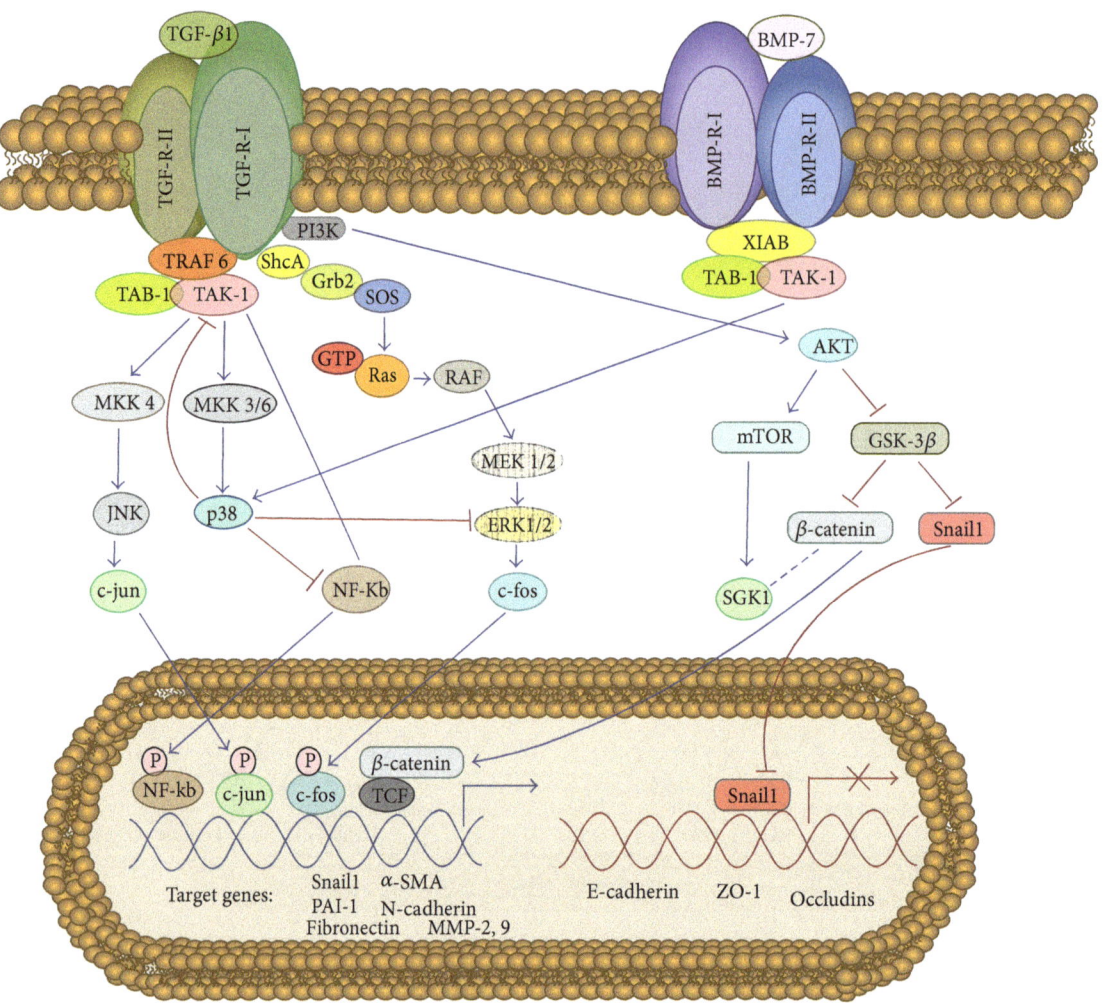

FIGURE 5: Non-Smad signaling in response to TGF-β1 and BMP-7. TGF-β1 activates MAP kinases JNK and p38 signaling and NF-κB through the activation of TAK1 by receptor-associated TRAF6. TGF-β1 also activates MAP kinase ERK 1/2 signaling through recruitment and phosphorylation of Shc by the TGF-β1 type I receptor. In MCs the p38-mediated pathway acts as modulator of the mesenchymal conversion by a feedback mechanism based on the downregulation of ERKs 1/2, NF-κB, and TAK-1 activities. Interestingly, BMP-7 activates p38 signaling by receptor-associated XIAB, which may contribute to the maintaining epithelial-like phenotype. TGF-β1 also induces PI3-K/Akt pathway leading to the activation of mTOR and the stabilization of β-catenin and snail through the inactivation of GSK-3β. As a result, β-catenin localizes to the nucleus, where it feeds into the Wnt signaling pathway by interacting with lymphoid enhancer factor-1/T-cell factor (LEF1/TCF) and contributes to the transcription of mesenchymal-related genes. In addition, the nuclear translocation of snail promotes the transcriptional repression of E-cadherin and other intercellular adhesion molecules.

(Cr-MTAC) showed significantly higher MMT prevalence in the peritoneal compact zone. In the multivariate analysis, the highest quartile of Cr-MTAC remained as an independent factor predicting the presence of MMT after adjusting for fibrosis [65]. These findings indicate that MMT is a frequent morphological change in the peritoneal membrane.

Another study showed that the dialysate-to-plasma ratio for creatinine (D/P Cr) was positively correlated to dialysate CTGF concentration. Furthermore, CTGF mRNA expression was higher in peritoneal tissues with ultrafiltration failure and was correlated with thickness of the peritoneum. Interestingly, the study demonstrated that high peritoneal transport state was associated with increased CTGF production by effluent MCs stimulated with TGF-β1 [138]. Thus, these results suggest that functional alteration of MCs, namely,

acquisition of mesenchymal properties, may be involved in the progression of peritoneal structural alteration and in high transport state.

7. MMT as a Potential Therapeutic Target

Having accepted that MMT is a key event in peritoneal damage induced by PD, during the last years it has been suggested that MMT might be a potential target for therapeutic intervention [25, 58]. The therapeutic strategies may be designed to block or revert the MMT itself because this process can be manipulated with a wide range of agents and pharmaceutical products. Conversely, the therapeutic approaches may be directed to interfere or modify

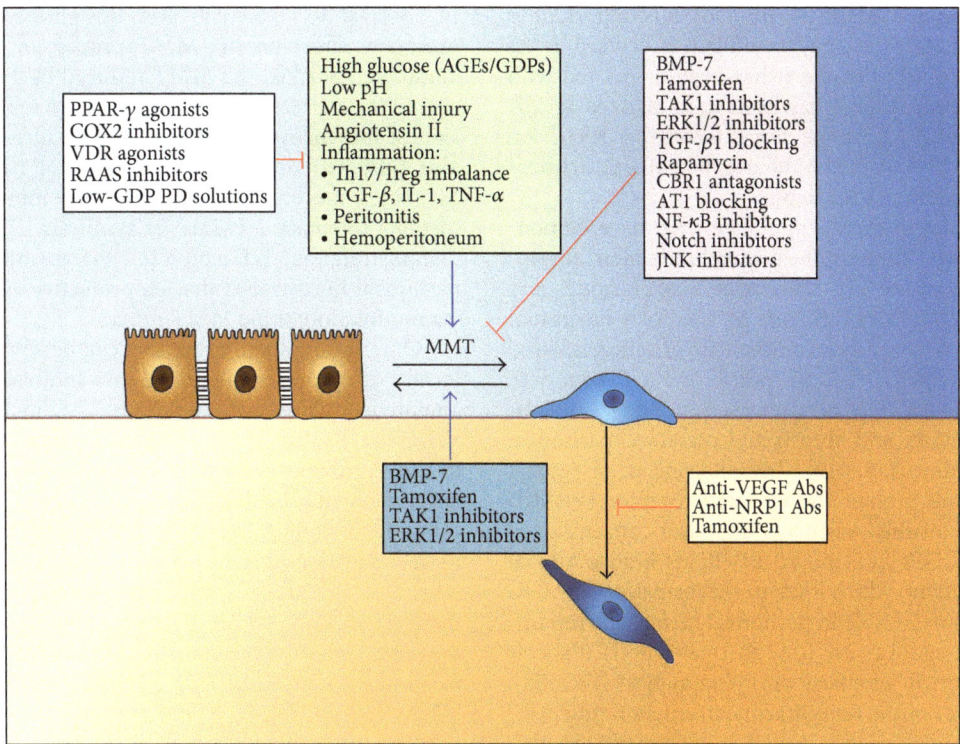

FIGURE 6: Therapeutic strategies for peritoneal membrane failure based on MMT. MMT *in vivo* results from integrated signals induced by multiple stimuli. These include high concentration of glucose and glucose degradation products (GDPs) in the PD fluids, which contribute to the formation of advanced glycation-end products (AGEs) and stimulate the mesenchymal conversion of MCs. The low pH of the dialysates and the mechanical injury during PD fluid exchanges may cause tissue irritation and contribute to chronic inflammation of the peritoneum, which promote MMT. Episodes of bacterial or fungal infections or hemoperitoneum cause acute inflammation and upregulation of cytokines and growth factors such as TGF-β, IL-1, TNF-α, and Angiotensin II, among others, which are strong inducers of MMT. The therapeutic strategies may be designed either to prevent or reverse the MMT itself, to decrease the MMT-promoting stimuli, or to treat MMT-associated effects such as the invasion capacity to avoid their accumulation in the compact zone. The diagram illustrates aspects related with the MMT process that can be clinically managed, alone or in combination, in order to prevent peritoneal membrane failure. See text for details.

the upstream MMT-promoting stimuli operating *in vivo* (e.g., inflammation, low pH, mechanical injury, GDPs content of PD fluids, and accumulation of AGEs) (Figure 6). For the design of the different therapeutic approaches, *in vitro* and *ex vivo* cultures of MCs as well as experimental animal models of PD have been very useful for testing pharmacological agents with potential effects on MMT.

The use of solutions with neutral pH and low GDPs content may represent the first and most obvious approach to attenuate some of the PD-related adverse effects including the mesenchymal conversion of MCs [20–22]. It has been shown that these new-generation low-GDPs fluids have less impact on MMT *in vivo* in PD patients and *in vitro* in cultured MCs [150, 151]. In agreement with these results, it has been demonstrated that low-GDPs fluids induce less inflammatory response and less fibrosis in a mouse PD model [148]. However, completely biocompatible PD fluids will be difficult to develop, at least under cost-effective perspectives. In addition, classical glucose-based PD fluids are still needed, because the new-generation biocompatible solutions are expensive and many potential users cannot afford them. An alternative approach to preserve the peritoneal membrane could be the use of pharmacological agents targeting

inflammation and injury or preserving the mesothelium (Figure 6). Two long-term pharmacological intervention strategies have been tested in experimental animal models of PD. One strategy is the addition of pharmacological agents into the PD fluids and the other strategy is the use of drugs that are administrated by oral route.

As discussed above, TGF-β1 is a master molecule in the pathogenesis of peritoneal damage and in the regulation of MMT. In fact it has been demonstrated that addition to the PD fluid of two specific TGF-β1-blocking peptides preserved the peritoneal membrane from damage in a mouse PD model [82]. However, it should be considered that agents directly blocking TGF-β1 cannot be easily employed in the clinical practice of PD, at least for long-term treatments, because TGF-β1 has important modulating functions of the immune and inflammatory responses [152, 153]. The molecular studies of the TGF-β1 Smad-dependent and Smad-independent signaling pathways involved in MMT provide more specific strategies for the preservation of peritoneal membrane with less side effects (Figure 6). In this context, the endogenous factors HGF and BMP-7 have been demonstrated to block MMT *in vitro*. In addition, intraperitoneal administration of these proteins prevented and reverted peritoneal damage in experimental animal models [115, 116, 154]. It is important to note that the use of BMP-7 may be difficult to be used in the clinical practice of PD because it has been associated with ossification; indeed, BMP-7 has been administered locally into bone lesions to promote bone formation [155]. An alternative to BMP-7 would be the use of synthetic agonists of the BMP-7 receptor ALK3 [156].

Three examples of therapeutic drugs that have demonstrated to preserve the peritoneal membrane after administration by oral route are Celecoxib, Rosiglitazone, and Tamoxifen [108, 111, 148, 149] (Figure 6). Celecoxib is a potent anti-inflammatory drug whose mechanism of action is based on the inhibition of COX-2. In mouse or rat PD models, orally administered Celecoxib decreased peritoneal inflammation, angiogenesis, and fibrosis and preserved peritoneal membrane function [148, 149]. Rosiglitazone is an agonist of the peroxisome proliferator-activated receptor (PPAR)-γ that improves insulin sensitivity. The high concentration of glucose and GDPs in standard PD fluids induce a local diabetic environment, which leads to the formation of AGEs that have an important role in peritoneal membrane inflammation. PPAR-γ agonists are used to treat type II diabetes and they have beneficial effects on inflammation [157, 158]. Hence, the efficacy of the Rosiglitazone in ameliorating peritoneal membrane damage was tested in a mouse PD model. Rosiglitazone reduced peritoneal AGEs accumulation, preserved the mesothelial cell monolayer, reduced fibrosis and angiogenesis, and improved peritoneal ultrafiltration. This was associated with increased peritoneal concentration of the anti-inflammatory cytokine interleukin-10 (IL-10) and with a higher percentage of CD4/CD25/FoxP3 regulatory T cells (Tregs) [108]. These animal experiments provide proof-of-concept evidence for the feasibility and potential efficacy of targeting the inflammation in order to preserve the peritoneal membrane. The clinical use of some of the specific compounds tested so far in animals may encounter several hurdles. Thus, side effects associated with thiazolidinediones including edema, weight gain, bone fracture risk, heart failure, and an adverse lipid profile, have led to the withdrawal from the European market of Rosiglitazone [26, 108]. Prolonged use of COX-2 inhibitors may exert vasoconstrictor and thrombogenic effects, especially worrisome in renal patients, who have a high cardiovascular risk [26]. Immunomodulatory drugs may have an impact on the risk or severity of peritonitis. Further studies are needed in this regard since none of the *in vivo* PD studies addressed infectious complications. Still, independently of any specific drug considerations, preclinical studies support the feasibility of modulating inflammation pharmacologically to improve the response to bioincompatible PD fluids [26, 108, 148].

Tamoxifen is a synthetic modulator of the estrogen receptor that has been used successfully to treat retroperitoneal fibrosis and EPS associated with PD [52, 111]. Thus, the efficacy of Tamoxifen to preserve the peritoneal structure and function was tested in the mouse PD model. Oral administration of Tamoxifen significantly reduced peritoneal thickness, angiogenesis, invasion of the compact zone by mesenchymal MCs, and improved peritoneal function. Tamoxifen also reduced the effluent levels of VEGF and leptin [111].

In contrast to Celecoxib and Rosiglitazone that did not exert any effect on the MMT process *in vitro* [108, 148], Tamoxifen blocked the MMT induced by TGF-β1, as it preserved the expression of E-cadherin and reduced the expression of mesenchymal-associated molecules [111]. Tamoxifen also inhibited the invasion capacity of mesenchymal-like MCs by a mechanism implicating the inhibition of matrix metalloproteinase-2 (MMP-2) synthesis [111]. These results demonstrate that Tamoxifen is a therapeutic option to treat peritoneal fibrosis and that its protective effect is mediated via modulation of the MMT process.

Other examples of drugs that can be administered either locally or by oral route are certain inhibitors of the renin-angiotensin-aldosterone system (RAAS) including Aliskiren, Valsartan, Enalapril, and Lisinopril (Figure 6). Components of the RAAS are constitutively expressed within peritoneal MCs and are upregulated in the presence of acute inflammation and chronic exposure to peritoneal dialysate. Furthermore, activation of the RAAS contributes to MMT, resulting in progressive fibrosis and angiogenesis of the peritoneal membrane [159]. Administration of the RAAS inhibitors by different routes reduced peritoneal thickening and improved peritoneal function in PDF exposure models in rats [159–162].

Activators of vitamin D receptor (VDR) are used to treat secondary hyperparathyroidism in PD patients. VDR activation modulates inflammation, fibrosis, and immune responses, modifying the Th1/Th2 pattern, inducing Tregs, and decreasing NF-κB [163]. It also exerts antiproliferative actions, increases antifibrotic factors such as BMP-7, and decreases renal fibrosis [163]. However, the potential benefit of VDR activators for the peritoneum has not been studied so far.

The molecular characterization of the TGF-β1-mediated signaling and other pathways involved in the regulation of MMT provide a wide range of possible molecular targets such as ERKs-1/2, JNK, TAK 1, NF-κB, and Notch 1, many of which still require to be tested in animal PD models [105, 112, 120] (Figure 6). In this regard, it has been shown that TGF-β1 induced Notch signaling in rat peritoneal MCs. The gamma-secretase inhibitor "DAPT" significantly inhibited *in vitro* the TGF-β1-induced expression of the mesenchymal markers α-SMA, collagen I, and VEGF. Furthermore, it has been demonstrated that intraperitoneal injection of DAPT significantly attenuated peritoneal fibrosis, decreased mass transfer of glucose, and increased ultrafiltration rate in a rat PD model. Thus, the gamma-secretase inhibitor that interferes with Notch signaling prevents biochemical, histological, and functional consequences of peritoneal fibrosis through inhibiting MMT [113].

Finally, an alternative therapeutic approach that still needs to be tested *in vivo* consists of the blocking of the invasive capacity of mesenchymal MCs to avoid their accumulation in the submesothelial compact zone (Figure 6). MMT is accompanied by upregulated expression of matrix metalloproteinases such as MMP-2 and MMP-9, which would degrade the basal membrane and the connective tissue allowing the submesothelial invasion by the mesenchymal-like MCs. It could be expected that MMPs inhibitors, or drugs that inhibit the synthesis of MMPs (e.g., Tamoxifen), may prevent the accumulation MCs-derived myofibroblasts in the submesothelial compartment. Recently, it has been demonstrated that invasion capacity of MCs that have undergone a MMT is governed, at least partially, by the VEGF/VEGF receptors/coreceptors axis [62]. It was shown that blocking antibodies directed against VEGF or the coreceptor neuropilin-1 efficiently interfered the invasion of MCs *in vitro* [62]. It would be interesting to test *in vivo* whether the prevention of the accumulation of MCs-derived myofibroblasts would, in turn, diminish the structural alteration of the peritoneal membrane.

8. Conclusions

During the last years several studies using *ex vivo* cultures of effluent-derived MCs, in conjunction with immunohistochemical analysis of peritoneal biopsies, have allowed the identification of the MMT as a key process in peritoneal membrane failure. In fact, it could be demonstrated that effluent-derived MCs reflect the functional status of the peritoneal tissue of PD patients. It can be expected that different omics approaches applied to the MMT process will provide new biomarkers, with diagnostic and/or prognostic value, for the progressive peritoneal deterioration, and for the identification of master molecules governing the mesenchymal conversion of MCs.

Pharmacological interventions targeting MMT or MMT-promoting stimuli operating *in vivo* (e.g., inflammation) represent interesting approaches to limit peritoneal damage during PD. The feasibility of two pharmacological intervention approaches has been tested in experimental animal models of PD. One was the addition of pharmacological agents to the PD fluids. This approach has been useful for proof-of-concept studies. However, incorporation of new components to the PD solutions requires major changes from a regulatory point of view and will increase the cost of PD. Self-administration of a therapeutic agent into the solution by the patient will also increase the cost of PD and has a potential risk of contamination. The other approach, the use of oral agents, is technically easier. The general response to tissue injury involves inflammation to eliminate the insult as well as damaged tissue in order to restore its architecture and functionality. Sustained inflammation promotes fibrosis and angiogenesis, processes associated with the ultrafiltration failure that causes PD technique dropout. PD patients present a chronic inflammatory state and may suffer acute inflammatory processes induced by infection or "haemoperitoneum." A better understanding of the role and regulation of inflammation in PD-related peritoneal damage is essential to design novel therapeutic strategies to protect the peritoneal membrane.

Careful benefit/risk studies are required. Ideally, we should better understand the potential benefits for the peritoneum of drugs that may serve multiple purposes for PD patients. Since a key market for these approaches is the low-income countries that cannot afford the newer, more biocompatible PD fluids, cost will be an issue and generic drugs are preferable over new compounds. In one scenario, patients may use the drug for as long as they are on PD. In other scenarios, the drugs would be required during especially vulnerable periods, as the peritonitis episodes or when hyperosmotic fluids are needed.

Conflict of Interests

The author declares that there is no conflict of interests regarding the publication of this paper.

Acknowledgments

This work was supported by Grant SAF2010-21249 from the "Ministerio de Economia y Competitividad" and by Grant S2010/BMD-2321 from "Comunidad Autónoma de Madrid" to Manuel López-Cabrera. Manuel López-Cabrera is a member of the Consortium "European Training & Research in Peritoneal Dialysis (EuTRiPD)."

References

[1] C. Chaimovitz, "Peritoneal dialysis," *Kidney International*, vol. 45, no. 4, pp. 1226–1240, 1994.

[2] O. Devuyst, P. J. Margetts, and N. Topley, "The pathophysiology of the peritoneal membrane," *Journal of the American Society of Nephrology*, vol. 21, no. 7, pp. 1077–1085, 2010.

[3] R. T. Krediet, "The peritoneal membrane in chronic peritoneal dialysis," *Kidney International*, vol. 55, no. 1, pp. 341–356, 1999.

[4] A. Breborowicz and D. G. Oreopoulos, "Biocompatibility of peritoneal dialysis solutions," *American Journal of Kidney Diseases*, vol. 27, no. 5, pp. 738–743, 1996.

[5] K. Wieczorowska-Tobis, A. Polubinska, J. Wisniewska et al., "Multidirectional approach to study peritoneal dialysis fluid biocompatibility in a chronic peritoneal dialysis model in the rat," *Nephrology Dialysis Transplantation*, vol. 16, no. 3, pp. 655–656, 2001.

[6] K. Wieczorowska-Tobis, A. Styszynski, A. Breborowicz, and D. G. Oreopoulos, "Comparison of the biocompatibility of phosphate-buffered saline alone, phosphate-buffered saline supplemented with glucose, and dianeal 3.86%," *Peritoneal Dialysis International*, vol. 21, supplement 3, pp. S362–S364, 2001.

[7] M. Krishnan, P. Tam, G. Wu, A. Breborowicz, and D. G. Oreopoulos, "Glucose degradation products (GDP's) and peritoneal changes in patients on chronic peritoneal dialysis: will new dialysis solutions prevent these changes?" *International Urology and Nephrology*, vol. 37, no. 2, pp. 409–418, 2005.

[8] C. J. Holmes, "Biocompatibility of peritoneal dialysis solutions," *Peritoneal Dialysis International*, vol. 13, no. 2, pp. 88–94, 1993.

[9] C. J. Holmes and D. Faict, "Peritoneal dialysis solution biocompatibility: definitions and evaluation strategies," *Kidney International*, vol. 64, no. 88, pp. S50–S56, 2003.

[10] L. A. Cooker, P. Luneburg, C. J. Holmes et al., "Interleukin-6 levels decrease in effluent from patients dialyzed with bicarbonate/lactate-based peritoneal dialysis solutions," *Peritoneal Dialysis International*, vol. 21, supplement 3, pp. S102–S107, 2001.

[11] R. Mackenzie, C. J. Holmes, S. Jones, J. D. Williams, and N. Topley, "Clinical indices of in vivo biocompatibility: the role of

ex vivo cell function studies and effluent markers in peritoneal dialysis patients," *Kidney International*, vol. 64, no. 88, pp. S84–S93, 2003.

[12] E. García-López, B. Lindholm, and S. Davies, "An update on peritoneal dialysis solutions," *Nature Reviews Nephrology*, vol. 8, no. 4, pp. 224–233, 2012.

[13] A. Grassmann, S. Gioberge, S. Moeller, and G. Brown, "ESRD patients in 2004: global overview of patient numbers, treatment modalities and associated trends," *Nephrology Dialysis Transplantation*, vol. 20, no. 12, pp. 2587–2593, 2005.

[14] S. S. A. Fenton, D. E. Schaubel, M. Desmeules et al., "Hemodialysis versus peritoneal dialysis: a comparison of adjusted mortality rates," *American Journal of Kidney Diseases*, vol. 30, no. 3, pp. 334–342, 1997.

[15] A. J. Collins, W. Hao, H. Xia et al., "Mortality risks of peritoneal dialysis and hemodialysis," *American Journal of Kidney Diseases*, vol. 34, no. 6, pp. 1065–1074, 1999.

[16] D. E. Schaubel, H. I. Morrison, and S. S. A. Fenton, "Comparing mortality rates on CAPD/CCPD and hemodialysis. The Canadian experience: fact or fiction?" *Peritoneal Dialysis International*, vol. 18, no. 5, pp. 478–484, 1998.

[17] E. F. Vonesh, J. J. Snyder, R. N. Foley, and A. J. Collins, "Mortality studies comparing peritoneal dialysis and hemodialysis: what do they tell us?" *Kidney International*, vol. 70, no. 103, pp. S3–S7, 2006.

[18] R. Selgas, M.-J. Fernandez-Reyes, E. Bosque et al., "Functional longevity of the human peritoneum: how long is continuous peritoneal dialysis possible? Results of a prospective medium long-term study," *American Journal of Kidney Diseases*, vol. 23, no. 1, pp. 64–73, 1994.

[19] P. J. Margetts and P. Bonniaud, "Basic mechanisms and clinical implications of peritoneal fibrosis," *Peritoneal Dialysis International*, vol. 23, no. 6, pp. 530–541, 2003.

[20] J. Perl, S. J. Nessim, and J. M. Bargman, "The biocompatibility of neutral pH, low-GDP peritoneal dialysis solutions: benefit at bench, bedside, or both," *Kidney International*, vol. 79, no. 8, pp. 814–824, 2011.

[21] J. D. Williams, K. J. Craig, N. Topley, and G. T. Williams, "Peritoneal dialysis: changes to the structure of the peritoneal membrane and potential for biocompatible solutions," *Kidney International*, vol. 63, no. 84, pp. S158–S161, 2003.

[22] J. D. Williams, N. Topley, K. J. Craig et al., "The euro-balance trial: the effect of a new biocompatible peritoneal dialysis fluid (balance) on the peritoneal membrane," *Kidney International*, vol. 66, no. 1, pp. 408–418, 2004.

[23] M. Fischbach, A. Zaloszyc, B. Schaefer, and C. P. Schmitt, "Optimizing peritoneal dialysis prescription for volume control: the importance of varying dwell time and dwell volume," *Pediatric Nephrology*, 2013.

[24] C. P. Schmitt, A. Zaloszyc, B. Schaefer, and M. Fischbach, "Peritoneal dialysis tailored to pediatric needs," *International Journal of Nephrology*, vol. 2011, Article ID 940267, 9 pages, 2011.

[25] L. S. Aroeira, A. Aguilera, J. A. Sánchez-Tomero et al., "Epithelial to mesenchymal transition and peritoneal membrane failure in peritoneal dialysis patients: pathologic significance and potential therapeutic interventions," *Journal of the American Society of Nephrology*, vol. 18, no. 7, pp. 2004–2013, 2007.

[26] G. T. González-Mateo, L. S. Aroeira, M. López-Cabrera, M. Ruiz-Ortega, A. Ortiz, and R. Selgas, "Pharmacological modulation of peritoneal injury induced by dialysis fluids: is it an option?" *Nephrology Dialysis Transplantation*, vol. 27, no. 2, pp. 478–481, 2012.

[27] H. F. H. Brulez and H. A. Verbrugh, "First-line defense mechanisms in the peritoneal cavity during peritoneal dialysis," *Peritoneal Dialysis International*, vol. 15, no. 7, pp. S24–S34, 1995.

[28] N. Di Paolo and G. Sacchi, "Atlas of peritoneal histology," *Peritoneal Dialysis International*, vol. 20, supplement 3, pp. S5–S96, 2000.

[29] S. Combet, M.-L. Ferrier, M. Van Landschoot et al., "Chronic uremia induces permeability changes, increased nitric oxide synthase expression, and structural modifications in the peritoneum," *Journal of the American Society of Nephrology*, vol. 12, no. 10, pp. 2146–2157, 2001.

[30] J. D. Williams, K. J. Craig, N. Topley et al., "Morphologic changes in the peritoneal membrane of patients with renal disease," *Journal of the American Society of Nephrology*, vol. 13, no. 2, pp. 470–479, 2002.

[31] J. Plum, S. Hermann, A. Fusshöller et al., "Peritoneal sclerosis in peritoneal dialysis patients related to dialysis settings and peritoneal transport properties," *Kidney International*, vol. 59, no. 78, pp. S42–S47, 2001.

[32] J. A. Jiménez-Heffernan, A. Aguilera, L. S. Aroeira et al., "Immunohistochemical characterization of fibroblast subpopulations in normal peritoneal tissue and in peritoneal dialysis-induced fibrosis," *Virchows Archiv*, vol. 444, no. 3, pp. 247–256, 2004.

[33] L. W. Morgan, A. Wieslander, M. Davies et al., "Glucose degradation products (GDP) retard remesothelialization independently of D-glucose concentration," *Kidney International*, vol. 64, no. 5, pp. 1854–1866, 2003.

[34] M. A. M. Mateijsen, A. C. Van Der Wal, P. M. E. M. Hendriks et al., "Vascular and interstitial changes in the peritoneum of CAPD patients with peritoneal sclerosis," *Peritoneal Dialysis International*, vol. 19, no. 6, pp. 517–525, 1999.

[35] R. T. Krediet, M. M. Zweers, A. C. van der Wal, and D. G. Struijk, "Neoangiogenesis in the peritoneal membrane," *Peritoneal Dialysis International*, vol. 20, supplement 2, pp. S19–S25, 2000.

[36] A. M. Sherif, M. Nakayama, Y. Maruyama et al., "Quantitative assessment of the peritoneal vessel density and vasculopathy in CAPD patients," *Nephrology Dialysis Transplantation*, vol. 21, no. 6, pp. 1675–1681, 2006.

[37] P. J. Margetts and D. N. Churchill, "Acquired ultrafiltration dysfunction in peritoneal dialysis patients," *Journal of the American Society of Nephrology*, vol. 13, no. 11, pp. 2787–2794, 2002.

[38] R. T. Krediet, B. Lindholm, and B. Rippe, "Pathophysiology of peritoneal membrane failure," *Peritoneal Dialysis International*, vol. 20, supplement 4, pp. S22–S42, 2000.

[39] N. Topley, T. Liberek, A. Davenport, F.-K. Li, H. Fear, and J. D. Williams, "Activation of inflammation and leukocyte recruitment into the peritoneal cavity," *Kidney International*, vol. 50, no. 56, pp. S17–S21, 1996.

[40] K. N. Lai, S. C. Tang, and J. C. Leung, "Mediators of inflammation and fibrosis," *Peritoneal Dialysis International*, vol. 27, supplement 2, pp. S65–S71, 2007.

[41] G. Baroni, A. Schuinski, T. P. de Moraes et al., "Inflammation and the peritoneal membrane: causes and impact on structure and function during peritoneal dialysis," *Mediators of Inflammation*, vol. 2012, Article ID 912595, 4 pages, 2012.

[42] N. Di Paolo and G. Garosi, "Peritoneal sclerosis," *Journal of Nephrology*, vol. 12, no. 6, pp. 347–361, 1999.

[43] G. Garosi, "Different aspects of peritoneal damage: fibrosis and sclerosis," *Contributions to Nephrology*, vol. 163, pp. 45–53, 2009.

[44] A. M. Sherif, H. Yoshida, Y. Maruyama et al., "Comparison between the pathology of encapsulating sclerosis and simple sclerosis of the peritoneal membrane in chronic peritoneal dialysis," *Therapeutic Apheresis and Dialysis*, vol. 12, no. 1, pp. 33–41, 2008.

[45] Y. Kawaguchi, H. Kawanishi, S. Mujais, N. Topley, and D. G. Oreopoulos, "Encapsulating peritoneal sclerosis: definition, etiology, diagnosis, and treatment," *Peritoneal Dialysis International*, vol. 20, no. 4, pp. S43–S55, 2000.

[46] T. Augustine, P. W. Brown, S. D. Davies, A. M. Summers, and M. E. Wilkie, "Encapsulating peritoneal sclerosis: clinical significance and implications," *Nephron Clinical Practice*, vol. 111, no. 2, pp. c149–c154, 2009.

[47] H. Kawanishi, Y. Kawaguchi, H. Fukui et al., "Encapsulating peritoneal sclerosis in Japan: a prospective, controlled, multicenter study," *American Journal of Kidney Diseases*, vol. 44, no. 4, pp. 729–737, 2004.

[48] A. M. Summers, M. J. Clancy, F. Syed et al., "Single-center experience of encapsulating peritoneal sclerosis in patients on peritoneal dialysis for end-stage renal failure," *Kidney International*, vol. 68, no. 5, pp. 2381–2388, 2005.

[49] M. W. J. A. Fieren, M. G. H. Betjes, M. R. Korte, and W. H. Boer, "Posttransplant encapsulating peritoneal sclerosis: a worrying new trend?" *Peritoneal Dialysis International*, vol. 27, no. 6, pp. 619–624, 2007.

[50] N. Di Paolo, G. Sacchi, G. Garosi, P. Taganelli, and E. Gaggiotti, "Simple peritoneal sclerosis and sclerosing peritonitis: related or distinct entities?" *International Journal of Artificial Organs*, vol. 28, no. 2, pp. 117–128, 2005.

[51] C. Goodlad and E. A. Brown, "Encapsulating peritoneal sclerosis: what have we learned?" *Seminars in Nephrology*, vol. 31, no. 2, pp. 183–198, 2011.

[52] J. Loureiro, G. Gonzalez-Mateo, J. Jimenez-Heffernan et al., "Are the mesothelial-to-mesenchymal transition, sclerotic peritonitis syndromes, and encapsulating peritoneal sclerosis part of the same process?" *International Journal of Nephrology*, vol. 2013, Article ID 263285, 7 pages, 2013.

[53] N. Ferrara, H.-P. Gerber, and J. LeCouter, "The biology of VEGF and its receptors," *Nature Medicine*, vol. 9, no. 6, pp. 669–676, 2003.

[54] R. Pecoits-Filho, M. R. T. Araújo, B. Lindholm et al., "Plasma and dialysate IL-6 and VEGF concentrations are associated with high peritoneal solute transport rate," *Nephrology Dialysis Transplantation*, vol. 17, no. 8, pp. 1480–1486, 2002.

[55] M. M. Zweers, D. R. De Waart, W. Smit, D. G. Struijk, and R. T. Krediet, "Growth factors VEGF and TGF-β1 in peritoneal dialysis," *Journal of Laboratory and Clinical Medicine*, vol. 134, no. 2, pp. 124–132, 1999.

[56] M. M. Zweers, D. G. Struijk, W. Smit, and R. T. Krediet, "Vascular endothelial growth factor in peritoneal dialysis: a longitudinal follow-up," *Journal of Laboratory and Clinical Medicine*, vol. 137, no. 2, pp. 125–132, 2001.

[57] L. S. Aroeira, A. Aguilera, R. Selgas et al., "Mesenchymal conversion of mesothelial cells as a mechanism responsible for high solute transport rate in peritoneal dialysis: role of vascular endothelial growth factor," *American Journal of Kidney Diseases*, vol. 46, no. 5, pp. 938–948, 2005.

[58] A. Aguilera, M. Yáñez-Mo, R. Selgas, F. Sánchez-Madrid, and M. López-Cabrera, "Epithelial to mesenchymal transition as a triggering factor of peritoneal membrane fibrosis and angiogenesis in peritoneal dialysis patients," *Current Opinion in Investigational Drugs*, vol. 6, no. 3, pp. 262–268, 2005.

[59] S. Mandl-Weber, C. D. Cohen, B. Haslinger, M. Kretzler, and T. Sitter, "Vascular endothelial growth factor production and regulation in human peritoneal mesothelial cells," *Kidney International*, vol. 61, no. 2, pp. 570–578, 2002.

[60] H. Ha, M. K. Cha, H. N. Choi, and H. B. Lee, "Effects of peritoneal dialysis solutions on the secretion of growth factors and extracellular matrix proteins by human peritoneal mesothelial cells," *Peritoneal Dialysis International*, vol. 22, no. 2, pp. 171–177, 2002.

[61] R. Catar, J. Witowski, P. Wagner et al., "The proto-oncogene c-Fos transcriptionally regulates VEGF production during peritoneal inflammation," *Kidney International*, vol. 84, pp. 1119–1128, 2013.

[62] M. L. Perez-Lozano, P. Sandoval, A. Rynne-Vidal et al., "Functional relevance of the switch of VEGF receptors/co-receptors during peritoneal dialysis-induced mesothelial to mesenchymal transition," *PLoS ONE*, vol. 8, no. 4, Article ID e60776, 2013.

[63] R. Selgas, A. Bajo, J. A. Jiménez-Heffernan et al., "Epithelial-to-mesenchymal transition of the mesothelial cell: its role in the response of the peritoneum to dialysis," *Nephrology Dialysis Transplantation*, vol. 21, supplement 2, pp. ii2–ii7, 2006.

[64] J. A. Jiménez-Heffernan, C. Perna, M. A. Bajo et al., "Tissue distribution of hyalinazing vasculopathy lesions in peritoneal dialysis patients. An autopsy study," *Pathology Research and Practice*, vol. 204, no. 8, pp. 563–567, 2008.

[65] G. Del Peso, J. A. Jiménez-Heffernan, M. A. Bajo et al., "Epithelial-to-mesenchymal transition of mesothelial cells is an early event during peritoneal dialysis and is associated with high peritoneal transport," *Kidney International*, vol. 73, no. 108, pp. S26–S33, 2008.

[66] P. J. Margetts, S. Gyorffy, M. Kolb et al., "Antiangiogenic and antifibrotic gene therapy in a chronic infusion model of peritoneal dialysis in rats," *Journal of the American Society of Nephrology*, vol. 13, no. 3, pp. 721–728, 2002.

[67] P. J. Margetts, M. Kolb, L. Yu et al., "Inflammatory cytokines, angiogenesis, and fibrosis in the rat peritoneum," *The American Journal of Pathology*, vol. 160, no. 6, pp. 2285–2294, 2002.

[68] D. Cina, P. Patel, J. C. Bethune et al., "Peritoneal morphological and functional changes associated with platelet-derived growth factor B," *Nephrology Dialysis Transplantation*, vol. 24, no. 2, pp. 448–457, 2009.

[69] Y. Sekiguchi, J. Zhang, S. Patterson et al., "Rapamycin inhibits transforming growth factor beta-induced peritoneal angiogenesis by blocking the secondary hypoxic response," *Journal of Cellular and Molecular Medicine*, vol. 16, no. 8, pp. 1934–1945, 2012.

[70] G. Gabbiani, B. J. Hirschel, G. B. Ryan, P. R. Statkov, and G. Majno, "Granulation tissue as a contractile organ. A study of structure and function," *Journal of Experimental Medicine*, vol. 135, no. 4, pp. 719–734, 1972.

[71] W. Schürch, T. A. Seemayer, and G. Gabbiani, "The myofibroblast: a quarter century after its discovery," *The American Journal of Surgical Pathology*, vol. 22, no. 2, pp. 141–147, 1998.

[72] D. W. Powell, R. C. Mifflin, J. D. Valentich, S. E. Crowe, J. I. Saada, and A. B. West, "Myofibroblasts. I. Paracrine cells important in health and disease," *The American Journal of Physiology: Cell Physiology*, vol. 277, no. 1, part 1, pp. C1–C19, 1999.

[73] S. H. Phan, "Fibroblast phenotypes in pulmonary fibrosis," *American Journal of Respiratory Cell and Molecular Biology*, vol. 29, no. 3, pp. S87–S92, 2003.

[74] G. Del Peso, J. A. Jiménez-Heffernan, M. A. Bajo et al., "Myofibroblastic differentiation in simple peritoneal sclerosis," *International Journal of Artificial Organs*, vol. 28, no. 2, pp. 135–140, 2005.

[75] S. V. Bertoli, L. Buzzi, D. Ciurlino, M. Maccario, and S. Martino, "Morpho-functional study of peritoneum in peritoneal dialysis patients," *Journal of Nephrology*, vol. 16, no. 3, pp. 373–378, 2003.

[76] V. S. LeBleu, G. Taduri, J. O'Connell et al., "Origin and function of myofibroblasts in kidney fibrosis," *Nature Medicine*, vol. 19, no. 8, pp. 1047–1053, 2013.

[77] B. D. Humphreys, S.-L. Lin, A. Kobayashi et al., "Fate tracing reveals the pericyte and not epithelial origin of myofibroblasts in kidney fibrosis," *The American Journal of Pathology*, vol. 176, no. 1, pp. 85–97, 2010.

[78] M. Zeisberg and J. S. Duffield, "Resolved: EMT produces fibroblasts in the kidney," *Journal of the American Society of Nephrology*, vol. 21, no. 8, pp. 1247–1253, 2010.

[79] S. E. Quaggin and A. Kapus, "Scar wars: mapping the fate of epithelial-mesenchymal-myofibroblast transition," *Kidney International*, vol. 80, no. 1, pp. 41–50, 2011.

[80] M. Fragiadaki and R. M. Mason, "Epithelial-mesenchymal transition in renal fibrosis—evidence for and against," *International Journal of Experimental Pathology*, vol. 92, no. 3, pp. 143–150, 2011.

[81] W. Kriz, B. Kaissling, and M. Le Hir, "Epithelial-mesenchymal transition (EMT) in kidney fibrosis: fact or fantasy?" *Journal of Clinical Investigation*, vol. 121, no. 2, pp. 468–474, 2011.

[82] J. Loureiro, A. Aguilera, R. Selgas et al., "Blocking TGF-β1 protects the peritoneal membrane from dialysate-induced damage," *Journal of the American Society of Nephrology*, vol. 22, no. 9, pp. 1682–1695, 2011.

[83] K. Iwaisako, D. A. Brenner, and T. Kisseleva, "What's new in liver fibrosis? The origin of myofibroblasts in liver fibrosis," *Journal of Gastroenterology and Hepatology*, vol. 27, supplement s2, pp. 65–68, 2012.

[84] A. J. Gilbane, C. P. Denton, and A. M. Holmes, "Scleroderma pathogenesis: a pivotal role for fibroblasts as effector cells," *Arthritis Research & Therapy*, vol. 15, no. 3, article 215, 2013.

[85] K. T. Weber, Y. Sun, S. K. Bhattacharya et al., "Myofibroblast-mediated mechanisms of pathological remodelling of the heart," *Nature Reviews Cardiology*, vol. 10, no. 1, pp. 15–26, 2013.

[86] M. T. Grande and J. M. López-Novoa, "Fibroblast activation and myofibroblast generation in obstructive nephropathy," *Nature Reviews Nephrology*, vol. 5, no. 6, pp. 319–328, 2009.

[87] R. Bucala, L. A. Spiegel, J. Chesney, M. Hogan, and A. Cerami, "Circulating fibrocytes define a new leukocyte subpopulation that mediates tissue repair," *Molecular Medicine*, vol. 1, no. 1, pp. 71–81, 1994.

[88] N. Sakai, T. Wada, H. Yokoyama et al., "Secondary lymphoid tissue chemokine (SLC/CCL21)/CCR7 signaling regulates fibrocytes in renal fibrosis," *Proceedings of the National Academy of Sciences of the USA*, vol. 103, no. 38, pp. 14098–14103, 2006.

[89] A. Bellini and S. Mattoli, "The role of the fibrocyte, a bone marrow-derived mesenchymal progenitor, in reactive and reparative fibroses," *Laboratory Investigation*, vol. 87, no. 9, pp. 858–870, 2007.

[90] M. Iwano, D. Plieth, T. M. Danoff, C. Xue, H. Okada, and E. G. Neilson, "Evidence that fibroblasts derive from epithelium during tissue fibrosis," *Journal of Clinical Investigation*, vol. 110, no. 3, pp. 341–350, 2002.

[91] J. S. Zolak, R. Jagirdar, R. Surolia et al., "Pleural mesothelial cell differentiation and invasion in fibrogenic lung injury," *The American Journal of Pathology*, vol. 182, no. 4, pp. 1239–1247, 2013.

[92] M. Guarino, A. Tosoni, and M. Nebuloni, "Direct contribution of epithelium to organ fibrosis: epithelial-mesenchymal transition," *Human Pathology*, vol. 40, no. 10, pp. 1365–1376, 2009.

[93] E. M. Zeisberg, S. E. Potenta, H. Sugimoto, M. Zeisberg, and R. Kalluri, "Fibroblasts in kidney fibrosis emerge via endothelial-to-mesenchymal transition," *Journal of the American Society of Nephrology*, vol. 19, no. 12, pp. 2282–2287, 2008.

[94] J. Li, X. Qu, and J. F. Bertram, "Endothelial-myofibroblast transition contributes to the early development of diabetic renal interstitial fibrosis in streptozotocin-induced diabetic mice," *The American Journal of Pathology*, vol. 175, no. 4, pp. 1380–1388, 2009.

[95] E. M. Zeisberg, O. Tarnavski, M. Zeisberg et al., "Endothelial-to-mesenchymal transition contributes to cardiac fibrosis," *Nature Medicine*, vol. 13, no. 8, pp. 952–961, 2007.

[96] S.-L. Lin, T. Kisseleva, D. A. Brenner, and J. S. Duffield, "Pericytes and perivascular fibroblasts are the primary source of collagen-producing cells in obstructive fibrosis of the kidney," *The American Journal of Pathology*, vol. 173, no. 6, pp. 1617–1627, 2008.

[97] M. Yáñez-Mó, E. Lara-Pezzi, R. Selgas et al., "Peritoneal dialysis and epithelial-to-mesenchymal transition of mesothelial cells," *The New England Journal of Medicine*, vol. 348, no. 5, pp. 403–413, 2003.

[98] S. E. Mutsaers, "Mesothelial cells: their structure, function and role in serosal repair," *Respirology*, vol. 7, no. 3, pp. 171–191, 2002.

[99] S. E. Mutsaers, "The mesothelial cell," *International Journal of Biochemistry and Cell Biology*, vol. 36, no. 1, pp. 9–16, 2004.

[100] S. Yung and T. M. Chan, "Glycosaminoglycans and proteoglycans: overlooked entities?" *Peritoneal Dialysis International*, vol. 27, supplement 2, pp. S104–S109, 2007.

[101] A. H. Yang, J. Y. Chen, and J. K. Lin, "Myofibroblastic conversion of mesothelial cells," *Kidney International*, vol. 63, no. 4, pp. 1530–1539, 2003.

[102] M. López-Cabrera, A. Aguilera, L. S. Aroeira et al., "Ex vivo analysis of dialysis effluent-derived mesothelial cells as an approach to unveiling the mechanism of peritoneal membrane failure," *Peritoneal Dialysis International*, vol. 26, no. 1, pp. 26–34, 2006.

[103] M. A. Bajo, G. del Peso, M. A. Castro et al., "Pathogenic significance of hypertrophic mesothelial cells in peritoneal effluent and ex vivo culture," *Advances in Peritoneal Dialysis*, vol. 20, pp. 43–46, 2004.

[104] K. Ksiazek, K. Korybalska, A. Jörres, and J. Witowski, "Accelerated senescence of human peritoneal mesothelial cells exposed to high glucose: the role of TGF-β1," *Laboratory Investigation*, vol. 87, no. 4, pp. 345–356, 2007.

[105] R. Strippoli, I. Benedicto, M. L. Perez Lozano et al., "Inhibition of transforming growth factor-activated kinase 1 (TAK1) blocks and reverses epithelial to mesenchymal transition of mesothelial cells," *PLoS ONE*, vol. 7, no. 2, Article ID e31492, 2012.

[106] P. Patel, Y. Sekiguchi, K.-H. Oh, S. E. Patterson, M. R. J. Kolb, and P. J. Margetts, "Smad3-dependent and -independent pathways are involved in peritoneal membrane injury," *Kidney International*, vol. 77, no. 4, pp. 319–328, 2010.

[107] P. J. Margetts, P. Bonniaud, L. Liu et al., "Transient overexpression of TGF-β1 induces epithelial mesenchymal transition

in the rodent peritoneum," *Journal of the American Society of Nephrology*, vol. 16, no. 2, pp. 425–436, 2005.

[108] P. Sandoval, J. Loureiro, G. González-Mateo et al., "PPAR-γ agonist rosiglitazone protects peritoneal membrane from dialysis fluid-induced damage," *Laboratory Investigation*, vol. 90, no. 10, pp. 1517–1532, 2010.

[109] K. K. Mubarak, A. Montes-Worboys, D. Regev et al., "Parenchymal trafficking of pleural mesothelial cells in idiopathic pulmonary fibrosis," *European Respiratory Journal*, vol. 39, no. 1, pp. 133–140, 2012.

[110] Y. Li, J. Wang, and K. Asahina, "Mesothelial cells give rise to hepatic stellate cells and myofibroblasts via mesothelial-mesenchymal transition in liver injury," *Proceedings of the National Academy of Sciences of the USA*, vol. 110, no. 6, pp. 2324–2329, 2013.

[111] J. Loureiro, P. Sandoval, G. del Peso et al., "Tamoxifen ameliorates peritoneal membrane damage by blocking mesothelial to mesenchymal transition in peritoneal dialysis," *PLoS ONE*, vol. 8, no. 4, Article ID e61165, 2013.

[112] R. Strippoli, I. Benedicto, M. L. P. Lozano, A. Cerezo, M. López-Cabrera, and M. A. del Pozo, "Epithelial-to-mesenchymal transition of peritoneal mesothelial cells is regulated by an ERK/NF-κB/Snail1 pathway," *Disease Models and Mechanisms*, vol. 1, no. 4-5, pp. 264–274, 2008.

[113] F. Zhu, T. Li, F. Qiu et al., "Preventive effect of Notch signaling inhibition by a γ-secretase inhibitor on peritoneal dialysis fluid-induced peritoneal fibrosis in rats," *The American Journal of Pathology*, vol. 176, no. 2, pp. 650–659, 2010.

[114] R. Vargha, M. Endemann, K. Kratochwill et al., "Ex vivo reversal of in vivo transdifferentiation in mesothelial cells grown from peritoneal dialysate effluents," *Nephrology Dialysis Transplantation*, vol. 21, no. 10, pp. 2943–2947, 2006.

[115] M.-A. Yu, K.-S. Shin, J. H. Kim et al., "HGF and BMP-7 ameliorate high glucose-induced epithelial-to-mesenchymal transition of peritoneal mesothelium," *Journal of the American Society of Nephrology*, vol. 20, no. 3, pp. 567–581, 2009.

[116] J. Loureiro, M. Schilte, A. Aguilera et al., "BMP-7 blocks mesenchymal conversion of mesothelial cells and prevents peritoneal damage induced by dialysis fluid exposure," *Nephrology Dialysis Transplantation*, vol. 25, no. 4, pp. 1098–1108, 2010.

[117] X. Wang, X. Li, L. Ye et al., "Smad7 inhibits TGF-beta1-induced MCP-1 upregulation through a MAPK/p38 pathway in rat peritoneal mesothelial cells," *International Urology and Nephrology*, vol. 45, no. 3, pp. 899–907, 2013.

[118] H. Guo, J. C. K. Leung, F. L. Man et al., "Smad7 transgene attenuates peritoneal fibrosis in uremic rats treated with peritoneal dialysis," *Journal of the American Society of Nephrology*, vol. 18, no. 10, pp. 2689–2703, 2007.

[119] J. Nie, X. Dou, W. Hao et al., "Smad7 gene transfer inhibits peritoneal fibrosis," *Kidney International*, vol. 72, no. 11, pp. 1336–1344, 2007.

[120] R. Strippoli, I. Benedicto, M. Foronda et al., "p38 maintains E-cadherin expression by modulating TAK1-NF-κB during epithelial-to-mesenchymal transition," *Journal of Cell Science*, vol. 123, no. 24, pp. 4321–4331, 2010.

[121] Z. Li, P. J. Wermuth, B. S. Benn et al., "Caveolin-1 deficiency induces spontaneous endothelial-to-mesenchymal transition in murine pulmonary endothelial cells in vitro," *The American Journal of Pathology*, vol. 182, no. 2, pp. 325–331, 2013.

[122] K. N. Lai, K. B. Lai, C. W. K. Lam, T. M. Chan, F. K. Li, and J. C. K. Leung, "Changes of cytokine profiles during peritonitis in patients on continuous ambulatory peritoneal dialysis," *American Journal of Kidney Diseases*, vol. 35, no. 4, pp. 644–652, 2000.

[123] A. S. Gangji, K. S. Brimble, and P. J. Margetts, "Association between markers of inflammation, fibrosis and hypervolemia in peritoneal dialysis patients," *Blood Purification*, vol. 28, no. 4, pp. 354–358, 2009.

[124] Q. Yao, K. Pawlaczyk, E. R. Ayala et al., "The role of the TGF/Smad signaling pathway in peritoneal fibrosis induced by peritoneal dialysis solutions," *Nephron Experimental Nephrology*, vol. 109, no. 2, pp. e71–e78, 2008.

[125] P. J. Margetts, M. Kolb, T. Galt, C. M. Hoff, T. R. Shockley, and J. Gauldie, "Gene transfer of transforming growth factor-β1 to the rat peritoneum: effects on membrane function," *Journal of the American Society of Nephrology*, vol. 12, no. 10, pp. 2029–2039, 2001.

[126] J. Xu, S. Lamouille, and R. Derynck, "TGF-B-induced epithelial to mesenchymal transition," *Cell Research*, vol. 19, no. 2, pp. 156–172, 2009.

[127] T. Gui, Y. Sun, A. Shimokado, and Y. Muragaki, "The roles of mitogen-activated protein kinase pathways in TGF-β-induced epithelial-mesenchymal transition," *Journal of Signal Transduction*, vol. 2012, Article ID 289243, 10 pages, 2012.

[128] Y. Liu, "New insights into epithelial-mesenchymal transition in kidney fibrosis," *Journal of the American Society of Nephrology*, vol. 21, no. 2, pp. 212–222, 2010.

[129] Y. Shi and J. Massagué, "Mechanisms of TGF-β signaling from cell membrane to the nucleus," *Cell*, vol. 113, no. 6, pp. 685–700, 2003.

[130] R. Weiskirchen and S. K. Meurer, "BMP-7 counteracting TGF-betal activities in organ fibrosis," *Frontiers in Bioscience*, vol. 18, pp. 1407–1434, 2013.

[131] P. Boor, T. Ostendorf, and J. Floege, "Renal fibrosis: novel insights into mechanisms and therapeutic targets," *Nature Reviews Nephrology*, vol. 6, no. 11, pp. 643–656, 2010.

[132] C. Dai and Y. Liu, "Hepatocyte growth factor antagonizes the profibrotic action of TGF-β1 in mesangial cells by stabilizing Smad transcriptional corepressor TGIF," *Journal of the American Society of Nephrology*, vol. 15, no. 6, pp. 1402–1412, 2004.

[133] J. Yang, C. Dai, and Y. Liu, "A novel mechanism by which hepatocyte growth factor blocks tubular epithelial to mesenchymal transition," *Journal of the American Society of Nephrology*, vol. 16, no. 1, pp. 68–78, 2005.

[134] R. Tan, X. Zhang, J. Yang, Y. Li, and Y. Liu, "Molecular basis for the cell type-specific induction of SnoN expression by hepatocyte growth factor," *Journal of the American Society of Nephrology*, vol. 18, no. 8, pp. 2340–2349, 2007.

[135] J. C. K. Leung, L. Y. Y. Chan, K. Y. Tam et al., "Regulation of CCN2/CTGF and related cytokines in cultured peritoneal cells under conditions simulating peritoneal dialysis," *Nephrology Dialysis Transplantation*, vol. 24, no. 2, pp. 458–469, 2009.

[136] K. H. Zarrinkalam, J. M. Stanley, J. Gray, N. Oliver, and R. J. Faull, "Connective tissue growth factor and its regulation in the peritoneal cavity of peritoneal dialysis patients," *Kidney International*, vol. 64, no. 1, pp. 331–338, 2003.

[137] C.-C. Szeto, K.-B. Lai, K.-M. Chow, C. Y.-K. Szeto, T. Y.-H. Wong, and P. K.-T. Li, "Differential effects of transforming growth factor-beta on the synthesis of connective tissue growth factor and vascular endothelial growth factor by peritoneal mesothelial cell," *Nephron Experimental Nephrology*, vol. 99, no. 4, pp. e95–e104, 2005.

[138] M. Mizutani, Y. Ito, M. Mizuno et al., "Connective tissue growth factor (CTGF/CCN2) is increased in peritoneal dialysis patients with high peritoneal solute transport rate," *The American Journal of Physiology: Renal Physiology*, vol. 298, no. 3, pp. F721–F733, 2010.

[139] J. G. Abreu, N. I. Ketpura, B. Reversade, and E. M. De Robertis, "Connective-tissue growth factor (CTGF) modulates cell signalling by BMP and TGF-β," *Nature Cell Biology*, vol. 4, no. 8, pp. 599–604, 2002.

[140] T. Q. Nguyen, P. Roestenberg, F. A. Van Nieuwenhoven et al., "CTGF inhibits BMP-7 signaling in diabetic nephropathy," *Journal of the American Society of Nephrology*, vol. 19, no. 11, pp. 2098–2107, 2008.

[141] M. Zeisberg, "Bone morphogenic protein-7 and the kidney: current concepts and open questions," *Nephrology Dialysis Transplantation*, vol. 21, no. 3, pp. 568–573, 2006.

[142] J. Massague, "How cells read TGF-beta signals," *Nature Reviews Molecular Cell Biology*, vol. 1, no. 3, pp. 169–178, 2000.

[143] R. Derynck and Y. E. Zhang, "Smad-dependent and Smad-independent pathways in TGF-β family signalling," *Nature*, vol. 425, no. 6958, pp. 577–584, 2003.

[144] B. W. Doble and J. R. Woodgett, "Role of glycogen synthase kinase-3 in cell fate and epithelial-mesenchymal transitions," *Cells Tissues Organs*, vol. 185, no. 1–3, pp. 73–84, 2007.

[145] J. P. Thiery and J. P. Sleeman, "Complex networks orchestrate epithelial-mesenchymal transitions," *Nature Reviews Molecular Cell Biology*, vol. 7, no. 2, pp. 131–142, 2006.

[146] R. E. Bachelder, S.-O. Yoon, C. Franci, A. García De Herreros, and A. M. Mercurio, "Glycogen synthase kinase-3 is an endogenous inhibitor of Snail transcription: Implications for the epithelial—mesenchymal transition," *Journal of Cell Biology*, vol. 168, no. 1, pp. 29–33, 2005.

[147] B. P. Zhou, J. Deng, W. Xia et al., "Dual regulation of Snail by GSK-3β-mediated phosphorylation in control of epithelial-mesenchymal transition," *Nature Cell Biology*, vol. 6, no. 10, pp. 931–940, 2004.

[148] L. S. Aroeira, E. Lara-Pezzi, J. Loureiro et al., "Cyclooxygenase-2 mediates dialysate-Lnduced alterations of the peritoneal membrane," *Journal of the American Society of Nephrology*, vol. 20, no. 3, pp. 582–592, 2009.

[149] P. Fabbrini, M. N. Schilte, M. Zareie et al., "Celecoxib treatment reduces peritoneal fibrosis and angiogenesis and prevents ultrafiltration failure in experimental peritoneal dialysis," *Nephrology Dialysis Transplantation*, vol. 24, no. 12, pp. 3669–3676, 2009.

[150] M. A. Bajo, M. L. Príez-Lozano, P. Albar-Vizcaino et al., "Low-GDP peritoneal dialysis fluid ("balance") has less impact in vitro and ex vivo on epithelial-to-mesenchymal transition (EMT) of mesothelial cells than a standard fluid," *Nephrology Dialysis Transplantation*, vol. 26, no. 1, pp. 282–291, 2011.

[151] A. Fernandez-Perpen, M. L. Perez-Lozano, M. A. Bajo et al., "Influence of bicarbonate/low-GDP peritoneal dialysis fluid (BicaVera) on in vitro and ex vivo epithelial-to-mesenchymal transition of mesothelial cells," *Peritoneal Dialysis International*, vol. 32, no. 3, pp. 292–304, 2012.

[152] A. Yoshimura, Y. Wakabayashi, and T. Mori, "Cellular and molecular basis for the regulation of inflammation by TGF-β," *Journal of Biochemistry*, vol. 147, no. 6, pp. 781–792, 2010.

[153] X. Wang, J. Nie, Z. Jia et al., "Impaired TGF-β signalling enhances peritoneal inflammation induced by *E. Coli* in rats," *Nephrology Dialysis Transplantation*, vol. 25, no. 2, pp. 399–412, 2010.

[154] T. Matsuoka, Y. Maeda, K. Matsuo et al., "Hepatocyte growth factor prevents peritoneal fibrosis in an animal model of encapsulating peritoneal sclerosis," *Journal of Nephrology*, vol. 21, no. 1, pp. 64–73, 2008.

[155] G. E. Friedlaender, C. R. Perry, J. D. Cole et al., "Osteogenic protein-1 (bone morphogenetic protein-7) in the treatment of tibial nonunions," *The Journal of Bone and Joint Surgery A*, vol. 83, supplement 1, part 2, pp. S151–S158, 2001.

[156] H. Sugimoto, V. S. LeBleu, D. Bosukonda et al., "Activin-like kinase 3 is important for kidney regeneration and reversal of fibrosis," *Nature Medicine*, vol. 18, no. 3, pp. 396–404, 2012.

[157] R. B. Clark, D. Bishop-Bailey, T. Estrada-Hernandez, T. Hla, L. Puddington, and S. J. Padula, "The nuclear receptor PPARγ and immunoregulation: PPARγ mediates inhibition of helper T cell responses," *Journal of Immunology*, vol. 164, no. 3, pp. 1364–1371, 2000.

[158] M. Ricote, A. C. Li, T. M. Willson, C. J. Kelly, and C. K. Glass, "The peroxisome proliferator-activated receptor-γ is a negative regulator of macrophage activation," *Nature*, vol. 391, no. 6662, pp. 79–82, 1998.

[159] S. J. Nessim, J. Perl, and J. M. Bargman, "The renin-angiotensin-aldosterone system in peritoneal dialysis: is what is good for the kidney also good for the peritoneum," *Kidney International*, vol. 78, no. 1, pp. 23–28, 2010.

[160] J. Perez-Martinez, F. C. Perez-Martinez, B. Carrion et al., "Aliskiren prevents the toxic effects of peritoneal dialysis fluids during chronic dialysis in rats," *PLoS ONE*, vol. 7, no. 4, Article ID e36268, 2012.

[161] G. Koçak, A. Azak, H. M. Astarci et al., "Effects of renin-angiotensin-aldosterone system blockade on chlorhexidine gluconate-induced sclerosing encapsulated peritonitis in rats," *Therapeutic Apheresis and Dialysis*, vol. 16, no. 1, pp. 75–80, 2012.

[162] S. Duman, K. Wieczorowska-Tobis, A. Styszynski, B. Kwiatkowska, A. Breborowicz, and D. G. Oreopoulos, "Intraperitoneal enalapril ameliorates morphologic changes induced by hypertonic peritoneal dialysis solutions in rat peritoneum," *Advances in Peritoneal Dialysis*, vol. 20, pp. 31–36, 2004.

[163] J. Rojas-Rivera, C. de la Piedra, A. Ramos, A. Ortiz, and J. Egido, "The expanding spectrum of biological actions of vitamin D," *Nephrology Dialysis Transplantation*, vol. 25, no. 9, pp. 2850–2865, 2010.

7

Burden and Depression among Caregivers of Visually Impaired Patients in a Canadian Population

Zainab Khan,[1] Puneet S. Braich,[2] Karim Rahim,[1] Jaspreet S. Rayat,[1] Lin Xing,[1] Munir Iqbal,[1] Karim Mohamed,[1] Sanjay Sharma,[1] and David Almeida[3]

[1]*Department of Ophthalmology, Hotel Dieu Hospital, Queen's University, 166 Brock Street, Kingston, ON, Canada K7L 5G2*
[2]*Department of Ophthalmology, Virginia Commonwealth University School of Medicine,*
 401 N. 11th Street, Suite 439, Richmond, VA 23219, USA
[3]*VitreoRetinal Surgery, PA, 7760 France Avenue S., Minneapolis, MN 55435, USA*

Correspondence should be addressed to David Almeida; drpa27@yahoo.com

Academic Editor: Gianfranco Spalletta

Purpose/Background. This study reports the degree of burden and the proportion at risk for depression among individuals who provide care to visually impaired patients. *Study Design*. This is clinic-based, cross-sectional survey in a tertiary care hospital. *Methods*. Caregivers were considered unpaid family members for patients whose sole impairment was visual. Patients were stratified by vision in their better seeing eye into two groups: Group 1 had visual acuity between 6/18 and 6/60 and Group 2 were those who had 6/60 or worse. Burden was evaluated by the Burden Index of Caregivers and the prevalence of being at risk for depression was determined by the Center for Epidemiologic Studies Depression scale. *Results*. 236 caregivers of 236 patients were included. Total mean BIC scores were higher in Group 2. Female caregivers, caregivers providing greater hours of care, and caregivers of patients who have not completed vision rehabilitation programs are at higher risk for depression.

1. Introduction

Burden of care has been defined as the financial physical, psychological, and social discomfort experienced by the principal caregiver of a disabled family member [1]. Care burden has been reported to significantly increase the risk for mortality among caregivers of elderly spouses with at least moderate disability irrespective of etiology [2]. Moreover, depression among caregivers is higher during the period at which they provide care, and burden is positively correlated with depression within this time frame [3].

The majority of the literature on this topic comes from the evaluation of caregivers of patients with intractable neurological diseases (e.g., Alzheimer's and Parkinson disease) [4]. However, recent studies have examined the role of burden in the caregivers of patients with cancer [5], eating disorders [6], and lung transplants [7]. In the ophthalmic literature, prior studies have examined the prevalence of depression and diminished quality of life reported by blind patients themselves [8, 9]. Recently, however, there have been investigations [10] on the quantitative evaluation of burden and depression faced by caregivers of individuals with visual impairment in India and the USA. This study examines this relationship in a Canadian population.

In North America, unipolar depressive disorders are the 2nd leading cause of disability-adjusted life years (DALY) and the 4th cause of DALY worldwide [11]. In Canada alone, it is estimated that 8% of the general adult population will experience a major depressive episode at some point in their lives [12]. Mood disorders such as depression have major economic impact through associated health care costs as well as lost work productivity. According to the Public Health Agency of Canada [13], this impact is dual in nature. Firstly, it comes with the associated loss of productivity in the workplace due to absenteeism and diminished effectiveness. Secondly, it comes with the high health care costs attributable to primary care visits, hospitalizations, and medication. Another aspect of mental health is the burden experienced by individual caregivers which may not directly affect health care costs but is still compelling. A recently published study examining the psychological distress of caregiving and non-caregiving twins found that caregiving was associated with distress as measured by mental health functioning, anxiety, perceived stress, and depression [14]. Bernbaum et al. [15] found that diabetes-related visual impairment was a major stressor in marital relationships. In their sample of either legally blind or no light perception (NLP) patients, 50% were separated or divorced within a mean of 1.6 years of the onset of visual impairment regardless of the length of the relationship prior to vision loss. The risk of separation or divorce was comparatively higher in couples where one partner had no light perception (NLP) vision. A longitudinal study done by Strawbridge et al. [16] found that spouses of patients with vision loss had an increased risk of poorer physical and emotion well-being over 5 years. Researchers postulate that visual impairment results in the loss of unseen gestures and body language thus having an effect on communication between partners [17].

Severe visual impairment is known to impact the social and economic prosperity of the patient, the family, and community in which they reside [18–20]. As the proportion of older adults in Canada rises, the number of Canadians with age related ocular disease and vision impairment is predicted to increase substantially within the next few decades [21, 22]. In light of these facts and the growing attention of public health issues surrounding the burden of disease, we conducted a cross-sectional study to measure the care burden and the proportion of those at risk for depression among caregivers of legally blind and low vision patients in a population receiving care in Kingston, Ontario, Canada. Undoubtedly, caregivers of all patients, regardless of age, with severe visual impairments can presumably experience substantial care burden. Nonetheless, the scope of this study was to assess adult patients from a clinic that is predominantly comprised of patients with advanced macular degeneration and diabetic retinopathy. Furthermore, while there is overlap between depressive symptomatology and depressive disorders, the aim of this study in assessing patients at risk of depression is basing this risk upon the depressive symptomatology. Making a formal diagnosis of depression is beyond the scope of what could be accomplished through questionnaires and would require the aid of psychiatrists. The aims of this study were to (1) report and contrast the burden faced by caregivers of patients who either are legally blind or have low vision, (2) explore factors related to burden faced by caregivers, (3) elucidate the proportion of those at risk for depression among caregivers of these patients, and (4) explore factors related to being at risk for depression in these caregivers.

2. Methods

2.1. Study Design.
This study is clinic-based, cross-sectional survey of caregivers of patients with visual impairment.

2.2. Participants and Procedures.
This study was conducted in accordance with the tenets of the Declaration of Helsinki and all provincial and federal laws. It received approval from the Queen's University (Kingston, Ontario, Canada) research ethics board committee. All participants provided informed consent; this included caregivers as well as patients. When possible, consent forms were signed in person. However, many participants served by the eye clinic travelled from large distances and required phone consent if they were unable to appear in person to sign the appropriate paperwork.

Patients were divided into 2 groups based on their severity of visual impairment: Group 1 had visual acuity better than 6/60 yet still worse than 6/18 (low vision) and Group 2 were those with 6/60 or worse (legally blind). Participants were recruited from the medical retina clinics at one institution (Hotel Dieu Hospital) in Kingston, Ontario, in Canada. While no specific disease related exclusion criteria were outlined, all patients in our clinic had either a diagnosis of diabetic retinopathy secondary to Type 2 diabetes or age related macular degeneration. We included caregivers of all patients with visual impairment requiring aide from a caregiver with either their activities of daily living (ADL) or instrumental activities of daily living (IADL). Caregivers were eligible if they were a family member or a friend that the blind patient identified as the "person they usually turn to for help regarding their care." Caregivers had to be adults who were unpaid for their support, able to converse in English, and provided care at the patients' homes (nursing home and assisted living center patients were excluded). Adults were defined as being over the age of 18 years. All patients or caregivers who were unable to give informed consent were excluded from this study. Caregivers were interviewed by telephone or in person using validated multidimensional instruments. The study period was from September 2011 to April 2012. The formal exclusion criteria consisted of the patient having intractable neurological disease, physical handicap, mental handicap, prior stroke, renal dialysis, cancer, dementia, severe motor deficits, or any condition which rendered the patient unable to ambulate. Examples of patient comorbidities that were not excluded were hypertension, diabetes mellitus, hyperlipidemia, mild inflammatory arthritis, mild degenerative joint disease, osteoporosis, mild to moderate chronic obstructive pulmonary disease (COPD), hearing impairment, obesity (excluding morbid obesity), and congestive heart failure New York Heart Association (NYHA) class I or II (excluding classes III and IV). This criterion was directed to isolate those caregivers that needed to provide care predominantly due to a patient's visual impairment. The same exclusion criteria applied to caregivers.

2.3. Measurements

2.3.1. Burden Index of Caregivers (BIC).
This is a multidimensional scale that measures care burden and has been previously validated [23]. It is composed of five burden domains: (1) time-dependent, (2) emotional, (3) existential, (4) physical, and (5) service-related burden. Each domain consists of 2 questions with each question assessed using a 5-point Likert scale (0 = never, 1 = almost never, 2 = sometimes, 3 = often, and 4 = always). There is one additional item that assesses overall burden, that is, "How burdensome do you

TABLE 1: Caregiver and patient characteristics, $N = 236$.

Mean patient age in years ± SD	76.4 ± 12.1
Patient gender, N (%):	
Male	109 (46)
Female	127 (54)
Group by visual acuity, N (%):	
Group 2 (legally blind)	76 (32)
Group 1 (low vision, but not legally blind)	160 (68)
Completed vision rehabilitation in past, N (%):	
Yes	169 (72)
No	67 (28)
Etiologies of diminished vision, N (%)	
Age related macular degeneration	170 (72)
Secondary to diabetic disease	38 (16)
Prior vascular occlusion	28 (7)
Caregiver gender, N (%):	
Male	97 (41)
Female	139 (59)
Mean caregiver age, years ± SD	64.8 ± 10.2
Relationship with patient, N (%):	
Child	70 (30)
Spouse	122 (52)
Sibling	31 (13)
Other (friend/grandchild)	13 (6)
Caregivers with chronic illness, N (%):	
None	175 (74)
One or more chronic illnesses	61 (26)
Patients with chronic illness, N (%):	
None	126 (52)
One or more chronic illnesses	110 (48)
Duration of caregiving, years, mean ± SD	6.1 ± 5.6
Hours required for close supervision of the patient per day, mean ± SD	2.2 ± 0.7
Number of supplemental caregivers, mean ± SD	0.37 ± 0.68

BCVA: best corrected visual acuity. Group 1: best corrected visual acuity in the better eye > 6/60 yet worse than 6/18. Group 2: best corrected visual acuity in the better eye ≤6/60 (legally blind).

think providing care is to you?" In total, there are 11 questions (Appendix A).

2.3.2. Center for Epidemiologic Studies Depression (CES-D) Scale.

The CES-D scale was developed by the United States' National Institute of Mental Health. This is a scale of 20 questions used to identify individuals at risk for depression [20]. Responses indicate the number of days per week the subject was affected by depressive symptoms (0 days with a score of 0; 1-2 days with a score of 1; 3-4 days with a score of 2; and >5 days with a score of 3). Scores can range from 0 to 60, with a higher score representing a stronger tendency toward depression. As done in multiple prior studies [11, 24–26], a score ≥16 was used to indicate those at risk for major depression (Appendix B).

2.4. Statistical Analysis.

Mean scores of total BIC and personal estimates of overall burden were calculated for the two groups. Independent two-sided t-tests were used with $\alpha = 0.05$ to compare the mean BIC scores between the two groups. The mean scores for the total BIC measure and the personal estimate of overall burden were the dependent variables for the linear regressions models used to determine which factors significantly contributed to caregiver burden. Independent variables were the numerous participant characteristics (see Table 1). With these parameters defined, a backwards selection technique was used.

A Z-test was used to compare the two groups regarding the proportion of patients at risk for depression. To determine the covariates associated with the risk of depression, we used the demographic data (Table 1) as the independent variables for our logistic regression model. The binary dependent variable was risk of depression (yes or no, based on a CES-D score of ≥16). Backwards selection was used to exclude any variables that did not contribute significantly to the fit of the model. All statistical analysis was done with SAS 9.3 (2011 SAS Institute Inc., Cary, NC, USA).

TABLE 2: The modified Burden Index of Caregivers scores among caregivers of patients with varying degrees of visual impairment.

	Group 1	Group 2	P value
Time-dependent burden	0.58 ± 0.37	2.12 ± 0.89	<0.01
Emotional burden	0.37 ± 0.24	1.54 ± 0.63	<0.01
Existential burden	0.20 ± 0.17	1.15 ± 0.52	<0.01
Physical burden	0.21 ± 0.13	1.22 ± 0.58	<0.01
Service-related burden	0.17 ± 0.27	0.95 ± 0.43	<0.01
Personal estimate of overall burden	0.20 ± 0.12	1.32 ± 0.71	<0.01
Total mean BIC	2.03 ± 0.63	8.01 ± 2.25	<0.01

P value calculated using independent two-tailed t-tests showed that values for Group 2 were significantly higher for each domain. Group 1: best corrected visual acuity in the better eye > 6/60 yet worse than 6/18. Group 2: best corrected visual acuity in the better eye ≤6/60 (legally blind).

TABLE 3: Covariates impacting caregiver burden (2 linear regression models).

	Regression coefficient	Standard error	P value
Personal estimate of overall burden ($R^2 = 0.38$)			
Hours of close supervision	0.67	0.34	<0.01
Completion of vision rehabilitation			
Yes (reference)	—	—	—
No	0.59	0.34	0.04
Modified BIC total ($R^2 = 0.33$)			
Hours of close supervision	0.94	0.31	<0.01
Completion of vision rehabilitation			
Yes (reference)	—	—	—
No	0.64	0.36	0.04

BIC: Burden Index of Caregivers.

3. Results

3.1. Participant Characteristics. A total of 236 caregivers completed the survey, all of which were viable for the final analysis. Of the 236 participating caregivers, 160 were from Group 1 (low vision without being legally blind) and 76 were from Group 2 (legally blind). Table 1 shows demographic and other information collected from participants. The mean age of patients and caregivers was 76.4 and 64.8, respectively. The majority of patients and caregivers were female, 54% and 59%, respectively. The majority of the caregivers were either adult children (30%) or spouses (52%). The proportion of patients and caregivers with at least one chronic illness was 48% and 26%, respectively. Nearly three-quarters of the patients were visually impaired due to age related macular degeneration (ARMD) or its sequelae. Moreover, roughly three-quarters of the patients also completed vision rehabilitation at least once in their lifetime.

3.2. Care Burden: Low Vision versus Legally Blind Patients. Mean scores for each of the BIC measures were stratified by group (Table 2). The BIC scores were significantly higher for Group 2 compared to Group 1 for all of the domains as well as the personal estimate of overall burden and the total BIC ($P < 0.01$). Amongst the individual domains, the greatest difference between the groups was seen in time-dependent burden followed by the emotional burden. The smallest difference was noted for service-related burden.

3.3. Covariates Impacting the Fit of the 2 Linear Regression Models. Covariates significantly impacting the fit of the 2 models are shown in Table 3. Daily hours of close supervision were significant for both measures. Examples of close supervision consisted of bathing the patient, grooming the patient, acting as a walking guide, transferring and transporting patient, and so forth. Patients who had not completed a vision rehabilitation program at least once during their lifetime were shown to have caregivers with higher burden scores. The participant characteristics that were not significant in either of these measures were visual acuity, age, relationship to the patient, duration of caregiving years, etiology of vision loss, presence of chronic illness, and the number of supplemental caregivers.

3.4. Prevalence of Caregivers at Risk for Depression. Figure 1 illustrates the prevalence of those at risk for depression, reflected by a CES-D score ≥16. The proportion of caregivers at risk of depression increased from Group 1 to Group 2, although this difference was not statistically significant ($P = 0.11$). Group 2 had 7 caregivers at risk for depression (9.2%) and Group 1 had 6 at risk caregivers (3.8%).

3.5. Factors Related to the Risk of Depression among Caregivers. The covariates significantly correlated to depression risk are shown in Table 4. Caregivers providing close supervision for ≥2.5 hours per day were at 7.45 increased odds of depression compared to those who provided <2.5 hours.

TABLE 4: Covariates impacting the risk of depression among caregivers in the logistic regression model.

	Odds ratio (95% confidence intervals)	P value
Caregiver gender		
Male (reference)	—	
Female	5.39 (2.92–9.14)	<0.01
Completed vision rehabilitation		
Yes (reference)	—	
No	4.23 (1.32–7.32)	<0.01
Hours required for close supervision		
<2.5 hours (reference)	—	
≥2.5 hours	7.45 (3.45–10.34)	<0.01

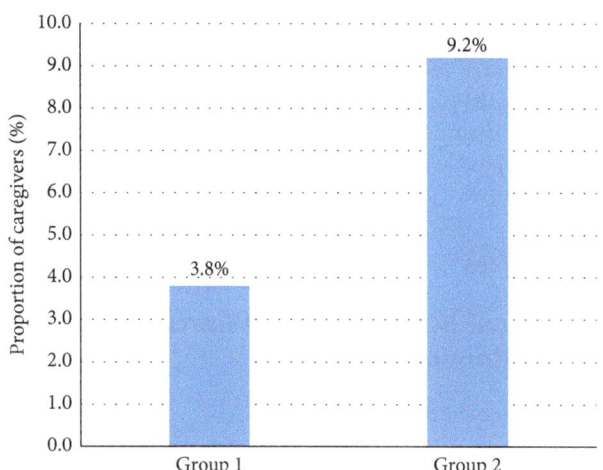

FIGURE 1: Proportion of caregivers at risk for depression (by Center for Epidemiologic Studies Depression [CES-D] scale). Group 1: best corrected visual acuity in the better eye >6/60 yet worse than 6/18. Group 2: best corrected visual acuity in the better eye ≤6/60 (legally blind).

Female caregivers compared to male caregivers had roughly fivefold higher odds of being at risk for depression. Caregivers of patients who did not complete at least one vision rehabilitation program in their lifetime were at 4.23 increased odds of being at risk for depression compared to caregivers of patients who completed at least one vision rehabilitation program.

Caregivers identified as being at risk for depression were contacted by the principal investigator and questioned about suicidal ideation or thoughts of harming oneself. Fortunately, none of the caregivers in this study endorsed such thoughts. However, they were all encouraged to seek an evaluation with a mental health provider or their primary care physician. An appointment was offered at the local university hospitals where the study was conducted.

4. Discussion

The investigation of burden and depression among caregivers has been a popular area of study for patients with disabilities secondary to neurological diseases. The study of this relationship among caregivers of visually impaired patients is an emerging field in public health and an important one since caregivers play a vital role in the well-being of patients. Instrumental assistance (e.g., providing transportation, managing finances) from family members is associated with better adaption to vision loss, fewer depressive symptoms, and greater life satisfaction [27–30].

Previous studies reported the burden and depression risk amongst caregivers in India and the USA. However, a Canadian population has not been evaluated to the same degree. The differences between health care structures, cultures, and patient demographics between these populations have generated an interest in undertaking this study in Canada.

The mean burden scores for each of the 5 domains revealed that individuals providing care to patients who are legally blind experience higher burden than those providing care to patients who are not legally blind but meet the threshold for low vision. We speculate that caregivers of patients with low vision do not experience as much burden because these patients still retain enough vision which can be improved by low vision aids (e.g., magnifying glasses and closed circuit television systems). Perhaps this results in greater independent functioning and a decreased reliance on caregivers. Furthermore, the burden scores for caregivers of the patients with low vision were considerably lower than the caregivers of legally blind patients from studies performed in India and the USA. It appears that being legally blind imparts considerable limitations on an individual compared to having low vision. For example, in the province of Ontario, certain kinds of low vision patients may still be allowed to operate noncommercial motor vehicles, albeit with restrictions, whereas a legally blind patient is not permitted to operate motor vehicles at all. Instances like these are just one example of how a legally blind patient has greater limitations compared to someone with low vision. It is plausible to see how legally blind patients would have some degree of reduction in their personal freedom and capabilities thus increasing their reliance on family members for simple needs. The greatest disparity among the various domain scores was for the time domain burden, revealing that the perceived burden related by the caregivers was due to limitations on their personal time. Given that the maximum score for each domain could be 4, the low scores for the remaining domains imply that caregivers of patients with visual impairment perceive relatively small amounts of burden. Another contributor to the low burden scores could be the widespread use of vision rehabilitation amongst our sample of patients. Vision rehabilitation and low vision programs were completed by 72% of our sample at least once in their lifetime. It is conceivable that skills learned during these programs enable patients with low vision to be more independent and rely less on supplementary support by family members.

The linear regression models revealed that the largest impact on burden scores was the hours of close supervision and the lack of completion of vision rehabilitation services. However, the relatively low R^2 values reveal that there are other potential covariates affecting their burden scores that our models did not account for. How caregivers could endorse greater sentiments of burden with increasing time spent providing close personal care is readily understandable.

Caregivers of patients who are legally blind do not seem to be more at risk for depression than caregivers of low vision patients. Although a larger number of participants may have revealed a statistically significant difference between the two groups, both values are fairly low. Again, we believe the widespread utilization of vision rehabilitation services among patients resulted in the acquisition of greater skills, tools, and coping mechanisms, which in turn translated to less reliance on caregivers. Our data reveals that caregivers of blind patients experience significantly more burden than caregivers of low vision patients. Yet this difference is not seen when it comes to being at risk for depression. It can be speculated that although burden and depression tend to correlate, there exists a spectrum of severity, whereby only high levels of burden may translate to concomitant depression. Since the overall burden in our sample was lower in severity, there was no meaningful difference regarding the proportion of caregivers at risk for depression.

Similar to the regression model for burden, the factors having the greatest impact on the risk of depression were hours of close supervision and the lack of completing vision rehabilitation services. An additional risk factor identified here was female gender among caregivers. Depression has been cited to be more common in females in many landmark studies [31, 32] and perhaps may not reveal anything new about the dynamic of providing care to visually impaired patients. Moreover, this may just be a reflection of our sample of caregivers being predominantly female (59%).

There are some noteworthy limitations in this study. First, we relied on convenience sampling among caregivers who agreed to be interviewed. The caregivers and patients refusing to do the survey may be systematically different from those who completed the study. Second, this cross-sectional design prevents any causal relationship to be implicated between blindness or low vision and caregiver burden or depression. Longitudinal investigations will help elucidate this relationship. Third, psychiatric histories for the caregivers were not obtained and may have been relevant predictors of depression. Caregivers with concurrent psychiatric comorbidities were not formally excluded and this may have also confounded our results. Fourth, we did not look at social problem-solving abilities which have been shown to be correlated with caregiver burden and depression [28], namely, a negative orientation to problem-solving (believing one cannot solve a problem no matter how hard they try), impulsive/careless outlook (proceeding with the first idea that comes to mind when trying to solve a difficult problem), and an avoidant outlook (procrastinating to solve problems that occur in one's life). Fifth, we did not have a comparison group in this study to assess if there were differences specific in this sample regarding burden and depression among caregivers of legally blind or low vision patients and similar caregivers of patients who were not legally blind or did not have low vision. However, it was unrealistic to obtain several hundred controls, given our stringent exclusion criteria for comorbidities.

The major implications of this study for visual health specialists in Canada are threefold: first, to be cognizant that caregivers of legally blind or low vision patients may be at risk for depression as well as burden and these disorders should be considered when assessing the low vision patients; second, to recognize the various risk factors mentioned in this study associated with either higher burden or risk of depression: greater daily hours of close supervision provided, patients not completing a vision rehabilitation program, and female gender among caregivers; third, the use of vision rehabilitation services not only provides skills to patients with low vision but will also mitigate sentiments of burden and depression amongst caregivers. Future directions of this study include introduction of additional surveys that provide insight into the overall quality of life of caregivers despite overall increases in care burden. One such survey is the Quality of Life questionnaire. Furthermore, the addition of questionnaires and scales such as the Cornell Depression Scale, the Hamilton Scale for Depression, or the Beck Depression Inventory could provide valuable clinical information that may assist physicians in the formulation of diagnoses of depressive disorders. They may also be valuable life-saving tools that enable the investigation of suicide ideation that would otherwise go unnoticed.

Appendices

A. Original Burden Index of Caregivers (BIC) Questionnaire

Time-Dependent Burden

(1) I cannot freely leave the house because of care-giving

(2) I do not have enough time for myself because of care-giving

Emotional Burden

(3) I want to delegate the care to someone else

(4) I am completely distressed by care-giving

Existential Burden

(5) I am experiencing hardship because care-giving does not give me a sense of satisfaction

(6) Care-giving is hard because I cannot find the meaning of providing care

Physical Burden

(7) My body aches when providing care to my family member

(8) I have ruined my health in the course of providing care

TABLE 5: Which best describes how often you felt or behaved during the last week?

	Rarely or none of the time (less than 1 day)	Some or a little of the time (1-2 days)	Occasionally or a moderate amount of the time (3-4 days)	Most or all of the time (5–7 days)
During the past week:	0	1	2	3
(1) I was bothered by things that usually don't bother me	0	1	2	3
(2) I did not feel like eating; my appetite was poor	0	1	2	3
(3) I felt that I could not shake off the blues even with help from my family and friends	0	1	2	3
(4) I felt that I was just as good as other people	0	1	2	3
(5) I had trouble keeping my mind on what I was doing	0	1	2	3
(6) I felt depressed	0	1	2	3
(7) I felt that everything I did was an effort	0	1	2	3
(8) I felt hopeful about the future	0	1	2	3
(9) I thought my life had been a failure	0	1	2	3
(10) I felt fearful	0	1	2	3
(11) My sleep was restless	0	1	2	3
(12) I was happy	0	1	2	3
(13) I talked less than usual	0	1	2	3
(14) I felt lonely	0	1	2	3
(15) People were unfriendly	0	1	2	3
(16) I enjoyed life	0	1	2	3
(17) I had crying spells	0	1	2	3
(18) I felt sad	0	1	2	3
(19) I felt that people disliked me	0	1	2	3
(20) I could not get "going"	0	1	2	3

Service-Related Burden

(9) It is a burden that public aid service personnel enter our house

(10) I have a hard time because patients resent receiving public aid care services

Personal Estimate of Overall Burden

(11) How burdensome do you think providing care is to you?

Legend. Each question was rated on a Likert scale: 0, never; 1, almost never; 2, sometimes; 3, often; 4, always.
Adapted from [4].

B. Center for Epidemiologic Studies Depression (CES-D) Scale

See Table 5.

Disclosure

This research received no specific grant from any funding agency in the public, commercial, or not-for-profit sectors. All listed authors have met the criteria for authorship.

Competing Interests

The authors of this study have no personal or financial conflicting interests that bias the work of this study.

References

[1] S. H. Zarit, K. E. Reever, and J. Bach-Peterson, "Relatives of the impaired elderly: correlates of feelings of burden," *Gerontologist*, vol. 20, no. 6, pp. 649–655, 1980.

[2] R. Schulz and S. R. Beach, "Caregiving as a risk factor for mortality: the caregiver health effects study," *The Journal of the American Medical Association*, vol. 282, no. 23, pp. 2215–2219, 1999.

[3] R. Schulz, A. B. Mendelsohn, W. E. Haley et al., "End-of-life care and the effects of bereavement on family caregivers of persons with dementia," *The New England Journal of Medicine*, vol. 349, no. 20, pp. 1936–1942, 2003.

[4] M. Miyashita, Y. Narita, A. Sakamoto et al., "Care burden and depression in caregivers caring for patients with intractable neurological diseases at home in Japan," *Journal of the Neurological Sciences*, vol. 276, no. 1-2, pp. 148–152, 2009.

[5] C. H. van Houtven, S. D. Ramsey, M. C. Hornbrook, A. A. Atienza, and M. van Ryn, "Economic burden for informal caregivers of lung and colorectal cancer patients," *Oncologist*, vol. 15, no. 8, pp. 883–893, 2010.

[6] A. Padierna, J. Martín, U. Aguirre, N. González, P. Muñoz, and J. M. Quintana, "Burden of caregiving amongst family caregivers of patients with eating disorders," *Social Psychiatry and Psychiatric Epidemiology*, vol. 48, no. 1, pp. 151–161, 2013.

[7] J. Xu, O. Adeboyejo, E. Wagley et al., "Daily burdens of recipients and family caregivers after lung transplant," *Progress in Transplantation*, vol. 22, no. 1, pp. 41–47, 2012.

[8] A. Cruess, G. Zlateva, X. Xu, and S. Rochon, "Burden of illness of neovascular age-related macular degeneration in Canada," *Canadian Journal of Ophthalmology*, vol. 42, no. 6, pp. 836–843, 2007.

[9] J. R. Evans, A. E. Fletcher, and R. P. L. Wormald, "Depression and anxiety in visually impaired older people," *Ophthalmology*, vol. 114, no. 2, pp. 283–288, 2007.

[10] P. S. Braich, V. Lal, S. Hollands, and D. R. Almeida, "Burden and depression in the caregivers of blind patients in India," *Ophthalmology*, vol. 119, no. 2, pp. 221–226, 2012.

[11] World Health Organization, "Global Burden of Disease," http://www.who.int/healthinfo/global_burden_disease/gbd/en/.

[12] Canadian Mental Health Association, "Fast Facts About Mental Illness," http://www.cmha.ca/media/fast-facts-about-mental-illness/#.VedIEs4n-jw.

[13] Public Health Agency of Canada, "A Report on Mental Illnesses in Canada," http://www.phac-aspc.gc.ca/publicat/miic-mmac/chap_2-eng.php.

[14] P. P. Vitaliano, E. Strachan, E. Dansie, J. Goldberg, and D. Buchwald, "Does caregiving cause psychological distress? The case for familial and genetic vulnerabilities in female twins," *Annals of Behavioral Medicine*, vol. 47, no. 2, pp. 198–207, 2014.

[15] M. Bernbaum, S. G. Albert, P. N. Duckro, and W. Merkel, "Personal and family stress in individuals with diabetes and vision loss," *Journal of Clinical Psychology*, vol. 49, no. 5, pp. 670–677, 1993.

[16] W. J. Strawbridge, M. I. Wallhagen, and S. J. Shema, "Impact of spouse vision impairment on partner health and well-being: a longitudinal analysis of couples," *Journals of Gerontology B Psychological Sciences and Social Sciences*, vol. 62, no. 5, pp. S315–S322, 2007.

[17] L. Westaway, W. Wittich, and O. Overbury, "Depression and burden in spouses of individuals with sensory impairment," *Insight: Research and Practice in Visual Impairment and Blindness*, vol. 4, no. 1, pp. 29–36, 2011.

[18] M. M. Brown, G. C. Brown, S. Sharma, B. Busbee, and H. Brown, "Quality of life associated with unilateral and bilateral good vision," *Ophthalmology*, vol. 108, no. 4, pp. 643–647, 2001.

[19] G. P. Pokharel, S. Selvaraj, and L. B. Ellwein, "Visual functioning and quality of life outcomes among cataract operated and unoperated blind populations in Nepal," *British Journal of Ophthalmology*, vol. 82, no. 6, pp. 606–610, 1998.

[20] P. S. Braich, D. R. Almeida, S. Hollands, and M. T. Coleman, "Effects of pictograms in educating 3 distinct low-literacy populations on the use of postoperative cataract medication," *Canadian Journal of Ophthalmology*, vol. 46, no. 3, pp. 276–281, 2011.

[21] A. L. Silva-Smith, T. W. Theune, and P. E. Spaid, "Primary support persons for individuals who are visually impaired: who they are and the support they provide," *Journal of Visual Impairment and Blindness*, vol. 101, no. 2, pp. 113–118, 2007.

[22] D. S. Friedman, N. Congdon, J. Kempen, and J. M. Tielsch, *Vision Problems in the U.S. Chicago*, Prevent Blindness America, 2002.

[23] M. Miyashita, A. Yamaguchi, M. Kayama et al., "Validation of the Burden Index of Caregivers (BIC), a multidimensional short care burden scale from Japan," *Health and Quality of Life Outcomes*, vol. 4, article 52, 2006.

[24] S. S. Kazarian, "Validation of the armenian center for epidemiological studies depression scale (Ces-D) among ethnic Armenians in Lebanon," *International Journal of Social Psychiatry*, vol. 55, no. 5, pp. 442–448, 2009.

[25] P. A. Camacho, G. E. Rueda-Jaimes, J. F. Latorre, A. A. Navarro-Mancilla, M. Escobar, and J. A. Franco, "Validity and reliability of the Center for Epidemiologic Studies-Depression scale in Colombian adolescent students," *Biomedica*, vol. 29, no. 2, pp. 260–269, 2009.

[26] D. Stahl, C. F. Sum, S. S. Lum et al., "Screening for depressive symptoms: validation of the center for epidemiologic studies depression scale (CES-D) in a multiethnic group of patients with diabetes in Singapore," *Diabetes Care*, vol. 31, no. 6, pp. 1118–1119, 2008.

[27] J. P. Reinhardt, "Effects of positive and negative support received and provided on adaptation to chronic visual impairment," *Applied Developmental Science*, vol. 5, no. 2, pp. 76–85, 2001.

[28] J. K. Bambara, V. Wadley, C. Owsley, R. C. Martin, C. Porter, and L. E. Dreer, "Family functioning and low vision: a systematic review," *Journal of Visual Impairment and Blindness*, vol. 103, no. 3, pp. 137–149, 2009.

[29] G. Watson, W. De l'Aune, J. Stelmack, J. Maino, and S. Long, "A national survey of veterans' use of low vision devices," *Optometry Vision Science*, vol. 74, no. 5, pp. 249–259, 1997.

[30] W. C. Mann, D. Hurren, and M. Tomita, "Comparison of assistive device use and needs of home-based older persons with different impairments," *The American Journal of Occupational Therapy*, vol. 47, no. 11, pp. 980–987, 1993.

[31] C. M. Mazure, A. H. Weinberger, B. Pittman, I. Sibon, and J. Swendsen, "Gender and stress in predicting depressive symptoms following stroke," *Cerebrovascular Diseases*, vol. 38, no. 4, pp. 240–246, 2014.

[32] I. Rouch, E. Achour-Crawford, F. Roche et al., "Seven-year predictors of self-rated health and life satisfaction in the elderly: the proof study," *Journal of Nutrition, Health and Aging*, vol. 18, no. 9, pp. 840–847, 2014.

8

Osteogenic Potential of Multipotent Adult Progenitor Cells for Calvaria Bone Regeneration

Dong Joon Lee,[1] Yonsil Park,[2] Wei-Shou Hu,[2] and Ching-Chang Ko[1,3]

[1]*Oral and Craniofacial Health Sciences Research, School of Dentistry, University of North Carolina, Chapel Hill, NC 27599-7455, USA*
[2]*Department of Chemical Engineering and Materials Science, University of Minnesota, Minneapolis, MN 55455-0132, USA*
[3]*Department of Orthodontics, School of Dentistry, University of North Carolina, Chapel Hill, NC 27599-7454, USA*

Correspondence should be addressed to Ching-Chang Ko; ching-chang_ko@unc.edu

Academic Editor: Patrizia D'Amelio

Osteogenic cells derived from rat multipotent adult progenitor cells (rMAPCs) were investigated for their potential use in bone regeneration. rMAPCs are adult stem cells derived from bone marrow that have a high proliferation capacity and the differentiation potential to multiple lineages. They may also offer immunomodulatory properties favorable for applications for regenerative medicine. rMAPCs were cultivated as single cells or as 3D aggregates in osteogenic media for up to 38 days, and their differentiation to bone lineage was then assessed by immunostaining of osteocalcin and collagen type I and by mineralization assays. The capability of rMAPCs in facilitating bone regeneration was evaluated *in vivo* by the direct implantation of multipotent adult progenitor cell (MAPC) aggregates in rat calvarial defects. Bone regeneration was examined radiographically, histologically, and histomorphometrically. Results showed that rMAPCs successfully differentiated into osteogenic lineage by demonstrating mineralized extracellular matrix formation *in vitro* and induced new bone formation by the effect of rMAPC aggregates *in vivo*. These outcomes confirm that rMAPCs have a good osteogenic potential and provide insights into rMAPCs as a novel adult stem cell source for bone regeneration.

1. Introduction

For the repair of large bone defects, a bone tissue engineering strategy has to employ osteogenic cells, osteoinductive growth factors, and osteoconductive scaffolds. The key to the success of this strategy is the effectiveness of the cell source. An ideal cell source for bone tissue engineering should have readily available cells, high proliferative potential *in vitro*, and a high osteogenic differentiation potential under *in vitro* culture condition. Various stem cells have been explored as the cell source for tissue engineering applications as they can be expanded and differentiated in culture to meet the demand [1–3]. In particular, adult stem cells are attractive because they can be isolated from patients, and autologous applications are possible. Their differentiation potential in bone lineage makes them promising cell sources in repairing skeletal defects caused by trauma, tumor removal, and congenital malformations [4, 5]. Currently, bone marrow derived mesenchymal stem cells (BMSCs), adipose tissue stem cells (ASCs), amniotic stem cells (ASCs), and multipotent adult stem cells (MAPCs) have been shown to possess osteogenic potential, and their potential use in bone regeneration has been explored [6–9].

Among those adult stem cells, BMSCs have been the most commonly used in bone tissue engineering. In the studies of other types of adult stem cells for bone regeneration, BMSCs have often been used as the control for comparison [10]. However, MSCs usually have less proliferative potential compared to pluripotent stem cells such as embryonic stem cells and induced pluripotent stem cells. Their expansion and differentiation potential may vary depending on the age of donor or patient. Many have reported the aging effects of donor source for MSC, and this effect may have implications in the potential use of autologous MSCs for bone regeneration [11, 12].

MAPC was first isolated from adult bone marrow during the subculturing of mesenchymal cells by Jiang et al. [13, 14].

Within the BMSC population, there was a group of cells that were identified to have an extensive expansion capability with high expression of Oct4, a pluripotent marker. MAPCs do not form teratoma when transplanted into mice and require no feeder layers. They can differentiate into various specialized cell types including mesodermal cells, muscle cells, endothelial cells, liver cells, and neuroectodermal cells under defined experimental conditions. Their wide range of differentiation potentials makes them attractive as a possible cell source for the regeneration of bone tissue. Recently, it was discovered that rMAPCs are similar to rat blastocyst-derived extraembryonic endoderm precursor (rXENP) cells, which showed extensive extraembryonic endodermal differentiation [15]. Under rMAPC culture conditions, rat hypoblast stem cells (rHypoSCs) are similar to rMAPCs and MAPC medium-shifted rXENP cells in their gene expression profiles and developmental potentials. rHypoSCs were derived from rat blastocysts in a more direct and rapid way assigning the lineage identity to rMAPCs, indicating that rMAPCs are originated by environmental reprogramming [16, 17].

Only a few studies have explored the osteogenic differentiation potential of rMAPCs; Ferreira et al. reported that titanium enriched hydroxyapatite scaffold could enhance bone regeneration in calvarial defect sites, and three-dimensional cell seeding method could also help rMAPCs to regenerate bone defects in vivo [18]. Inspired by the study of Ferreira et al. on three-dimensional (3D) culture method of rMAPCs, rMAPCs were also examined for their osteogenic differentiation potential as 3D aggregates [19]. In a recent publication, higher bone regeneration was induced by using a novel biomaterial, hydroxyapatite-gelatin calcium silicate (HGCS), with rMAPCs in a rat model. In the study, HGCS had an osteogenic effect on rMAPCs and stimulated calvarial bone regeneration [20].

Recent studies on immunological characteristics of human multipotent adult stem cells (hMAPCs) revealed that they have comparable immunomodulatory effects to human mesenchymal stem cells (hMSCs) [21]. MHC class I was expressed highly in MSCs but only at a low level in MAPCs. Both hMSCs and hMAPCs do not express MHC class II on the surface. hMAPCs showed strong immunosuppressive effects on T-cell proliferation and were not influenced by MHC compatibility [22]. These findings have clinical relevance of MAPCs for the potential use in bone regeneration. In humans, while hMAPCs can expand over 70 population doublings, hMSCs can only have 20 to 25 population doublings [23]. This extensive growth capability of hMAPCs allows cell banking for better cell supply and quality control. The immunomodulatory property of hMAPCs may allow them to be a universal donor.

In this study, we hypothesized that both rMAPCs in the form of 3D aggregates and single rMAPCs can have osteogenic differentiation potential after osteogenic differentiation, and the rMAPCs can stimulate in vivo bone formation. To test the hypothesis, we examined the osteogenic potential of rMAPCs in monolayer and 3D aggregate culture to determine whether the rMAPCs have in vitro osteogenic differentiation potential or not. The 3D aggregates were further assessed for their in vivo osteogenic potential in bone regeneration.

2. Materials and Methods

2.1. Preparation of HG Scaffolds. The preparation of hydroxyapatite and gelatin (HG) scaffolds and HG coated dishes was described in a previous study [20]. Briefly, HAP-Gel slurry was biomimetically synthesized by the coprecipitation method using in situ hybridization of calcium silicates or titanium oxide with HG powders. The powders of calcium hydroxide and HG were mixed and cross-linked with enT-MOS (bis[3-(trimethoxysilyl)-propyl]ethylenediamine) for 30 seconds before adding a calcium chloride solution to the mixture. As the mixture thickened, the material was quickly transferred into 1 cc syringes with 1 mm inner diameter needles, and the material was extruded to make intertwined structures with macropores. The structures were then dried for 7 days and sterilized with cold ethylene oxide (EO) gas before use.

2.2. MAPCs and Differentiation in 2D and 3D Aggregates. The isolation and culture of rMAPCs from rat have been described in previous studies [13, 14, 18]. For the 2D monolayer cultures, rMAPCs (8×10^4 cells) were seeded with growth media (GM) in 24-well plates (Costar, Corning Inc. Life Sciences, Lowell, MA, USA). Cells were allowed to grow for 5 days until they reach 80 to 90% of confluency. Subsequently, growth media were replaced by osteogenic media (OM, Dulbecco's Modified Eagle's Media, 10% Fetal Bovine serum, 0.2 mM β-glycerophosphate, 0.2 μM ascorbic acid, and 10 nM Dexamethasone). The media were changed every 3 days for up to 42 days.

To prepare the 3D aggregates, rMAPCs (2×10^3 cells) were seeded in suspension with rMAPC growth media in 96-well rounded bottom ultralow attachment plates (Costar, Corning Inc. Life Sciences, Lowell, MA, USA), using a modification of a forced aggregation method reported previously [24–26]. Briefly, rMAPC suspension was centrifuged at 1400 rpm for 4 min to allow cells to form aggregates over time. Aggregates were grown for 5 days. Then, ten aggregates were distributed to each well of 24-well ultralow attachment plates (Costar, Corning Inc. Life Sciences, Lowell, MA, USA) and switched to osteogenic media. Fresh osteogenic media were supplied every 3 days up to 38 days to stop the differentiation.

2.3. Characterization for rMAPCs. A characterization study of rMAPCs was described in previous studies [13, 14, 18]. rMAPCs were provided by Dr. Hu from the University of Minnesota. Briefly, a monolayer culture of rMAPCs was harvested by trypsinization and suspended in phosphate-buffered saline (PBS) with 3% serum at 100,000 cells per Eppendorf tube (1.5 mL). All immunostaining (both osteocalcin and collagen type I) was performed for the rMAPCs on the HG coated dish or the frozen section of rMAPC aggregates except for Oct4 and CD31. Both rMAPCs and 3D aggregates were fixed with 4% paraformaldehyde (PFA), rinsed, treated with 0.3% H_2O_2 for 30 minutes, dehydrated in 100% methanol, rehydrated with water, and transferred to Triton X-100 in PBS solution. Then, avidin/biotin activity was blocked with Avidin-Biotin kit (Dako, CA, USA) and the sample was rinsed three times with PBST (Triton X-100 in PBS) and specific antibody binding sites were blocked for 30 min with 0.4% fish skin gelatin in PBS. Cell/matrix layers were incubated overnight at 4°C with rabbit primary antibody against rat collagen type I (NB600-408, Novus Biologicals, CO), rinsed three times, and incubated with secondary biotinylated goat anti-rabbit IgG antibody (NB730-B, Novus Biologicals, CO) for 30 min at room temperature (RT). The cell/matrix layer was incubated in ABC complex (Vector Laboratories, CA) according to the manufacturer's protocol and rinsed three times, and DAB Chromogen solution (Liquid DAB+Substrate Chromogen System, Dako, CA) was added to the matrix layer for 5 to 20 minutes until a brown color developed. MC3T3-E1 cells were used as positive control and negative controls were without primary antibody.

rMAPCs morphology on the HG coated dish was examined using a scanning electron microscope (SEM) (Hitachi TM3000). rMAPC cultures were fixed in 4% PFA at room temperature (RT) and then analyzed at 15 kV in low vacuum state for nonconductive materials. The HG coated dishes with rMAPCs were cut, embedded in resin blocks, sliced into ultrathin sections with a diamond knife, and stained with a saturated solution of uranyl acetate in methanol, followed by Reynold's lead citrate, and the image was acquired with a Hitachi H-7000 TEM at 120 kV.

2.4. Proliferation of rMAPCs.
rMAPCs (P18) were plated in 96-well plates at a density of 2×10^3 cells per each well using basal osteogenic media. The proliferation of the rMAPCs in growth and osteogenic media was conducted by MTS assay following the company's instruction. Composition and method to prepare growth and osteogenic media for rMAPCs were outlined in the previous publications [18]. The MTS (3-(4,5-dimethylthiazol-2-yl)-5-(3-carboxymethoxyphenyl)-2-(4-sulfophenyl)-2H-tetrazolium (Promega Co., Madison, WI, USA)) reacted with cells at 37°C for 1 hour. After transferring the solution into a 96-well plate, absorbance of growth and osteogenic media group was measured on days 1 and 7, at 490 nm using a plate reader (Bio-Rad, Hercules, CA, USA). The proliferation of 3D aggregates was described in a previous study [19].

2.5. Osteogenic Differentiation of Single rMAPCs and 3D Aggregates.
For the 2D monolayer cultures, rMAPCs (8×10^4 cells) were seeded with growth media in 24-well plates (Costar, Corning Inc. Life Sciences, Lowell, MA, USA). Cells were allowed to grow for 5 days until they reached 80 to 90% of confluency for mesodermal differentiation. Then, growth media were replaced by osteogenic media. Media were changed every 3 days. rMAPCs were differentiated in osteogenic media for 3, 7, 14, 21, and 42 days.

To prepare the 3D aggregates, rMAPCs (2×10^3 cells) were seeded in suspension with rMAPC growth media in 96-well rounded bottom ultralow attachment plates (Costar, Corning Inc. Life Sciences, Lowell, MA, USA), using a modification of the forced aggregation method reported previously [24–26].

Briefly, MAPC suspension was centrifuged at 1400 rpm for 4 min to allow cells to form aggregates over time. Aggregates were grown for 5 days. Then, ten aggregates were distributed to each well of 24-well ultralow attachment plates (Costar, Corning Inc. Life Sciences, Lowell, MA, USA) and switched to osteogenic media. Fresh osteogenic media were supplied every 3 days up to 38 days for osteogenic differentiation.

2.6. Analysis of Single rMAPCs and 3D Aggregates for OCN and Col-1 and Mineralization.
For immunostaining of Col-I and OCN, single rMAPCs and cryosectioned 3D aggregates were fixed with 4% PFA, rinsed, incubated for 30 min with 0.3% H_2O_2 in 100% methanol, rehydrated, and transferred to PBS-Triton solution. After blocking for 30 min with 0.4% fish skin gelatin in PBS, both cells and aggregates were incubated overnight at 4°C with rabbit primary antibody against rat collagen type I (NB600-408, Novus Biologicals, CO), rinsed thrice, and incubated with secondary biotinylated goat anti-rabbit IgG antibody (NB730-B, Novus Biologicals) for 30 min at RT. After incubation in ABC complex (Vector Laboratories, CA) following the manufacturer's instruction, DAB Chromogen solution (Dako, CA) was added for 5–20 minutes until a brown color developed. For the OCN, primary OCN antibody (Santa Cruz) and FITC conjugated secondary antibody (Abcam) were used instead. Images were acquired with a Nikon fluorescence imaging system and a DP70 color digital camera equipped with color image software (DP11, Olympus USA, Center Valley, PA, USA).

Both single rMAPCs on HG coated dish and 3D aggregates were fixed in neutral buffered 10% formalin, and then the aggregates were embedded in optimal cutting temperature (OCT) solution. Five-micrometer sections were cut and stained with Alizarin Red S (ARS) solution (pH 4.2) to observe mineralized extracellular matrices. Mineralization on HG coated dishes by rMAPCs was also stained with ARS on days 3, 7, 14, and 21. After drying, stained dishes were scanned for the images acquisition.

2.7. In Vivo Implantation of MAPC Aggregate and HG Scaffolds.
Differentiated rMAPC aggregates in osteogenic media were seeded onto the HGCS scaffolds ($n = 3$). Two test groups (HG only and HG+MAPCs) were used with three rats in each group for a total of six male Sprague-Dawley rats (Charles River, Wilmington, MA; about 250 to 300 g, 7 weeks). An 8 mm, critical-sized defect (CSD) was created after anesthetization by Ketamine-HCl injection (10 mg/kg: Putney Inc., Portland, ME, USA). Three rats were implanted with HG scaffold only and the other three rats were implanted with HG scaffold and MAPC aggregates. For the mineral apposition rate (MAR) measurement, fluorochrome labels, Alizarin Red S (30 mg/kg, Sigma-Aldrich, St. Louis, MO, USA), and Calcein (20 mg/kg, Sigma-Aldrich, St. Louis, MO, USA) were injected perivascularly into each animal twice during the study. Alizarin Red S was administered 10 days after the surgery and Calcein was given 15 days before sacrifice. The interlabeling periods were 10 and 70 days.

2.8. Micro-CT Analysis.
After 12 weeks, the calvariae were removed and trimmed by preserving the implanted sites

before fixing in 10% formalin for 7 days at 4°C. Then, the specimens were preserved in 70% isopropyl alcohol at 4°C. The calvaria explants were scanned by using a micro-CT system (mCT 40; Scanco Medical, Brüttisellen, Switzerland) at 70 kV and 114 mA with a 200 ms integration time. Detailed setting parameters for acquisition and analysis of the acquired images were described in a previous study [20].

2.9. Fluorescence Microscopy for Mineral Deposition.

The detailed method for the slide preparation was described previously [22]. The fluorescent images of completed sections were acquired by using a fluorescence microscope (Eclipse Ti-U, Nikon Instruments Inc., Melville, NY, USA) with bright field, TRITC and FITC filters, and a digital camera. After fluorescent image acquisition, calvaria specimen slides were further stained with Steven Blue by counterstaining with Van Gieson to visualize the formation of newly formed bone (NFB) tissue for the quantitation as previously described [19]. Briefly, entire images of the medial (central) sagittal histologic section were acquired with a DP70 color digital camera equipped with color image software (DP11, Olympus USA, Center Valley, PA, USA) under 20x magnification and then merged using Adobe Photoshop CS6 (Adobe Systems Inc., San Jose, CA, USA) to recreate as one figure. The new bone surface area (B.Ar.) and the total area of each defect (T.Ar.) were measured in pixels by using an automated image analysis system (ImageJ software version 1.46R, NIH, Bethesda, MD, USA) to calculate the NFB (in %: B.Ar./T.Ar./0.01) based on the standardized protocols of the American Society for Bone and Mineral Research [27]. A one-tailed Student t-test was used to compare the means between the groups.

2.10. Statistical Analysis.

All results were quantified as mean ± standard deviation. ANOVA was used to define whether differences between each group were significant or not. When the p value was less than 0.05, the differences were considered significant.

3. Results and Discussion

For effective bone regeneration using a tissue engineering and regenerative medicine strategy, the stem cells and the scaffold material are the two major components. Because the osteogenic inducing capability of the scaffold materials was already examined in previous studies [18–20], our study was mainly focused on the rMAPCs for their *in vitro* osteogenic differentiation and *in vivo* bone forming potential. The detailed mechanisms by which a component (either stem cell or material) contributes to bone regeneration are not known. Besides, the fate of implanted stem cells and the extent of their direct contribution to bone regeneration remain controversial [28].

rMAPCs are small, elongated, or oval shape cells when grown on the fibronectin coated culture dishes (Figure 1(a)). rMAPCs express a high level of the transcription factors Rex1 [29] and Oct4 [30], which are pluripotency markers for stem cells. In this study, undifferentiated rMAPCs were confirmed by showing the expression of Oct4 and CD31 by immunostaining (Figures 1(b) and 1(c)).

rMAPCs can be differentiated into endothelial, adipogenic, chondrogenic, and osteogenic linage cells, cardiomyocytes, and hepatocytes [13, 31]. In 2D tissue culture plates, rMAPCs do not attach strongly like other mesenchyme origin cells (Figures 1(a) and 1(b)). The morphology of undifferentiated rMAPCs in HG was examined by SEM (Figures 1(d) and 1(e)) and TEM (Figure 1(f)). After 2 days, rMAPCs were weakly attached to the surface of HG compared to the cells on fibronectin coated plates. Most attached cells exhibited round or oval shapes rather than flat ones.

To observe *in vitro* proliferative potential, rMAPCs were tested in either growth or osteogenic medium for MTS assay. In general, when higher numbers of rMAPCs react with MTS, higher formazan activity will be yielded. Using the biochemical reaction, we measured MTS activity of the rMAPCs on days 1 and 7. At day 1, rMAPCs cultured in growth medium had an OD value of 0.06 ± 0.07 and 0.07 ± 0.08 in osteogenic media. The low value of OD is due to the nature of the rMAPC culture, maintaining low cell density to keep the cells undifferentiated. On day 7, rMAPCs in growth and osteogenic media had ODs of 0.35 ± 0.44 and 0.39 ± 0.6, respectively (Figure 1(g)). Both growth and osteogenic media stimulated rMAPC proliferation. In many previous studies, MSCs were used as control to compare the growth potential with new adult stem cell source. However, the differentiation potential of MSCs is largely dependent on the age of the donor so it is recommended to maintain MSCs at low passage number (passage 6 or less for human cells) for their stemness and high proliferative potential [21]. While rMAPCs share characteristics of pluripotent stem cells with high expression of Oct4, rMAPCs can be expanded to more than 70 doublings.

Differentiated cells were immunostained for osteocalcin (OCN) and collagen type I (Col-I) after 21 and 38 days of osteogenic differentiation in 2D and 3D culture, respectively. Osteocalcin, generated by mature osteoblasts, is known to deposit onto the extracellular matrix as an indicator of bone repair [32]. Osteocalcin was detected around and between each differentiated cell (Figure 2(a), white arrows). It appears to show expression of OCN when rMAPCs were differentiated alone (Figure 2(a), top) and also when rMAPCs were differentiated on the HG coated dish (Figure 2(a), bottom). Although OCN expression was not quantified, rMAPCs in osteogenic media could express higher level than that in growth media. rMAPCs under growth media did not express OCN in both control and coated dish (data not shown). The expression of Col-I on differentiated rMAPCs showed a similar trend to OCN expression on the differentiated rMAPCs. HG coating increased the expression level of Col-I in osteogenic differentiation of rMAPCs (Figure 2(b)).

Although we did not quantify the expression level of osteogenic protein and mineralization to compare between 2D and 3D differentiation, we did observe that both single rMAPC culture and 3D aggregate showed clear expression of OCN and Col-I protein as well as mineral formation (Figures 2 and 3). Another advantage for using rMAPC aggregate is to increase the cellular viability during the seeding process by

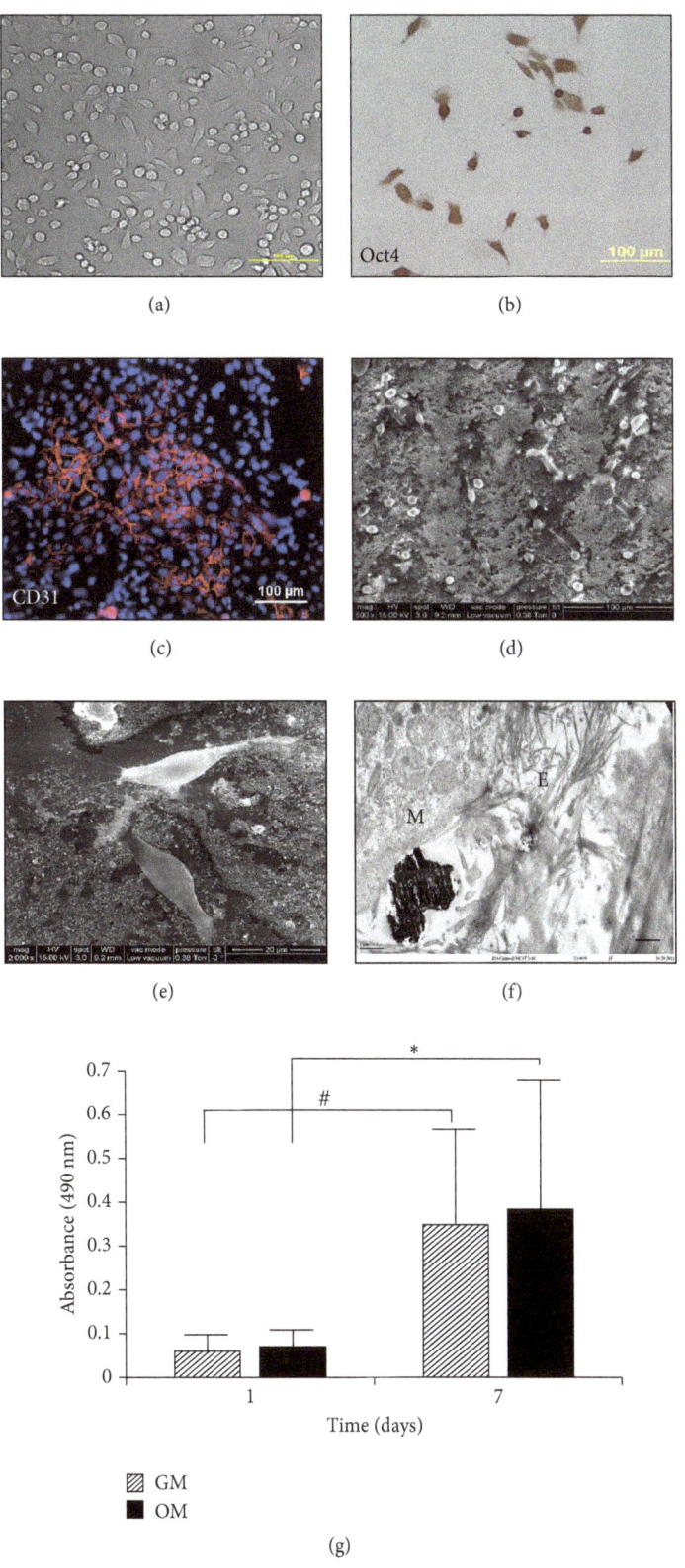

FIGURE 1: Characterization of rat MAPCs. DIC microscopic picture of MAPCs culture on the fibronectin coated dish (a). MAPCs were stained with Oct4 antibody conjugated with chemiluminescent dye (b) and CD31 antibody conjugated with TRITC (c). SEM analysis visualized MAPCs on the HG materials in low power (d) and high power (e). TEM image of MAPCs that interacted with ECM and HG materials (f): hydroxyapatite (HG), MAPCs (M), and extracellular matrix (E). Scale: 5 μm. MAPCs proliferation was assessed at baseline (within 24 h after seeding) and after 7 days in osteogenic media; [*,#]$p < 0.05$.

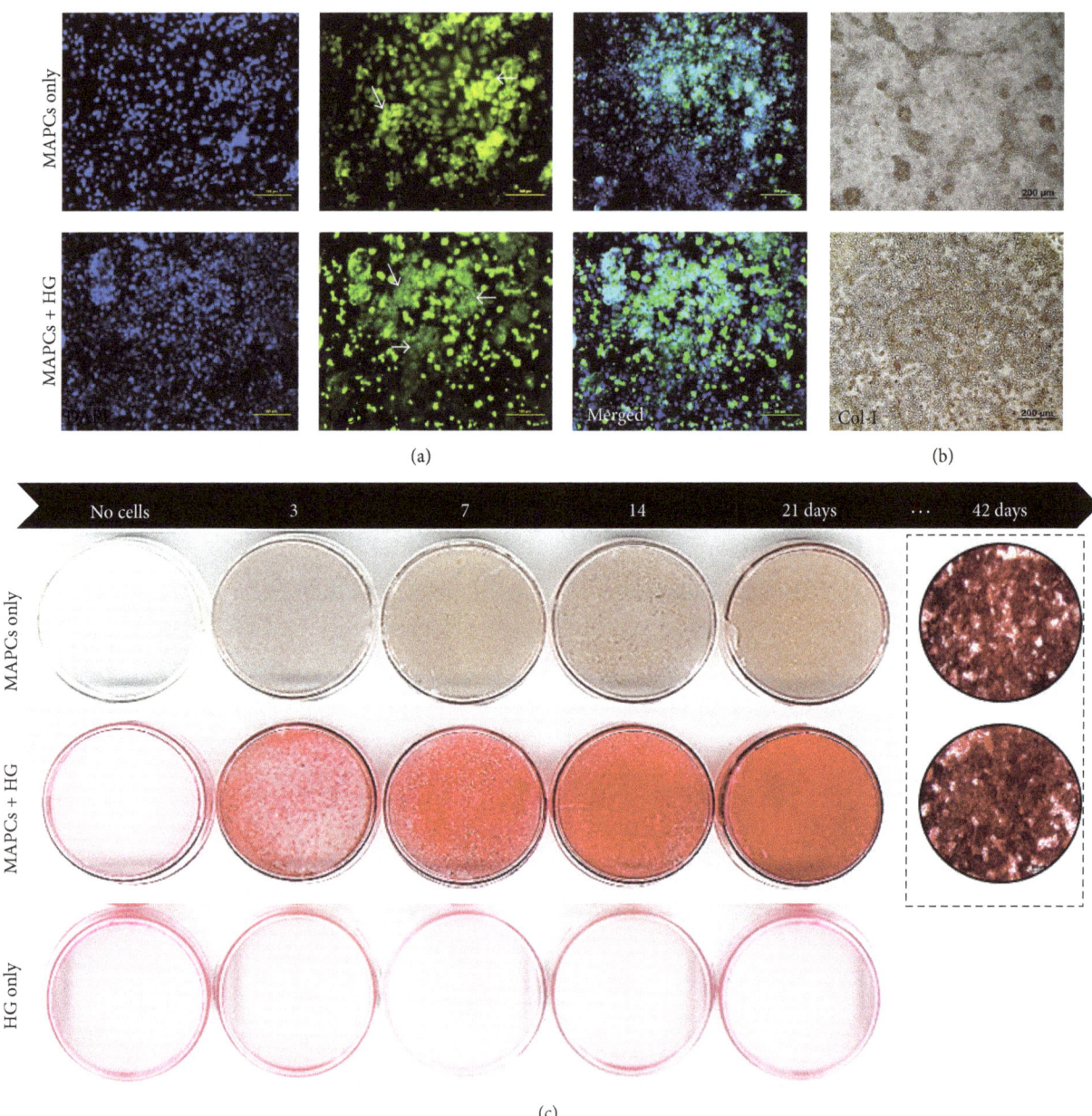

FIGURE 2: *In vitro* assessment of osteogenic differentiation of MAPCs on the HG material-coated dishes. Immunohistochemical staining with osteocalcin (a) and collagen type I (b) antibodies against MAPCs cultured on the HG coated culture plate (bottom) and without a coating as control (top). Mineral formation was detected by Alizarin Red S staining (c) after culturing MAPCs with osteogenic media on the coated dish (middle), no coating as control (top), and coated dish without MAPCs (bottom). Microscopic images further confirmed the ability of mineralization by MAPCs after 42 days of osteogenic differentiation.

sustaining the aggregates in the defect site without absorption (Figure 3(i)). While seeding single cells on the scaffold or defect site, cells can be easily lost by their absorption into the surrounding tissues. Generally, a scaffold plays a role as a carrier to prevent the loss of cells during the seeding process. Still, the poor attachment characteristic makes single rMAPCs even difficult to be successfully retained in the scaffold.

The mineralization of rMAPCs differentiated in a monolayer was tested by staining the calcium deposition after 7, 14, and 21 days of osteogenic differentiation. Mineral deposition in the control plate without HG coating increased over time up to 21 days (Figure 2(c), top) and was visible 7 days after differentiation. Differentiation in the control plate (rMAPC only) showed more intense mineralization by ARS staining than the HG coated dish without rMAPCs (Figure 2(c), bottom). Differentiated aggregates were also tested for the same markers and mineralization as the cells in 2D culture. The *in vitro* osteogenic differentiation study indicated that rMAPCs in both 2D and 3D culture system could differentiate

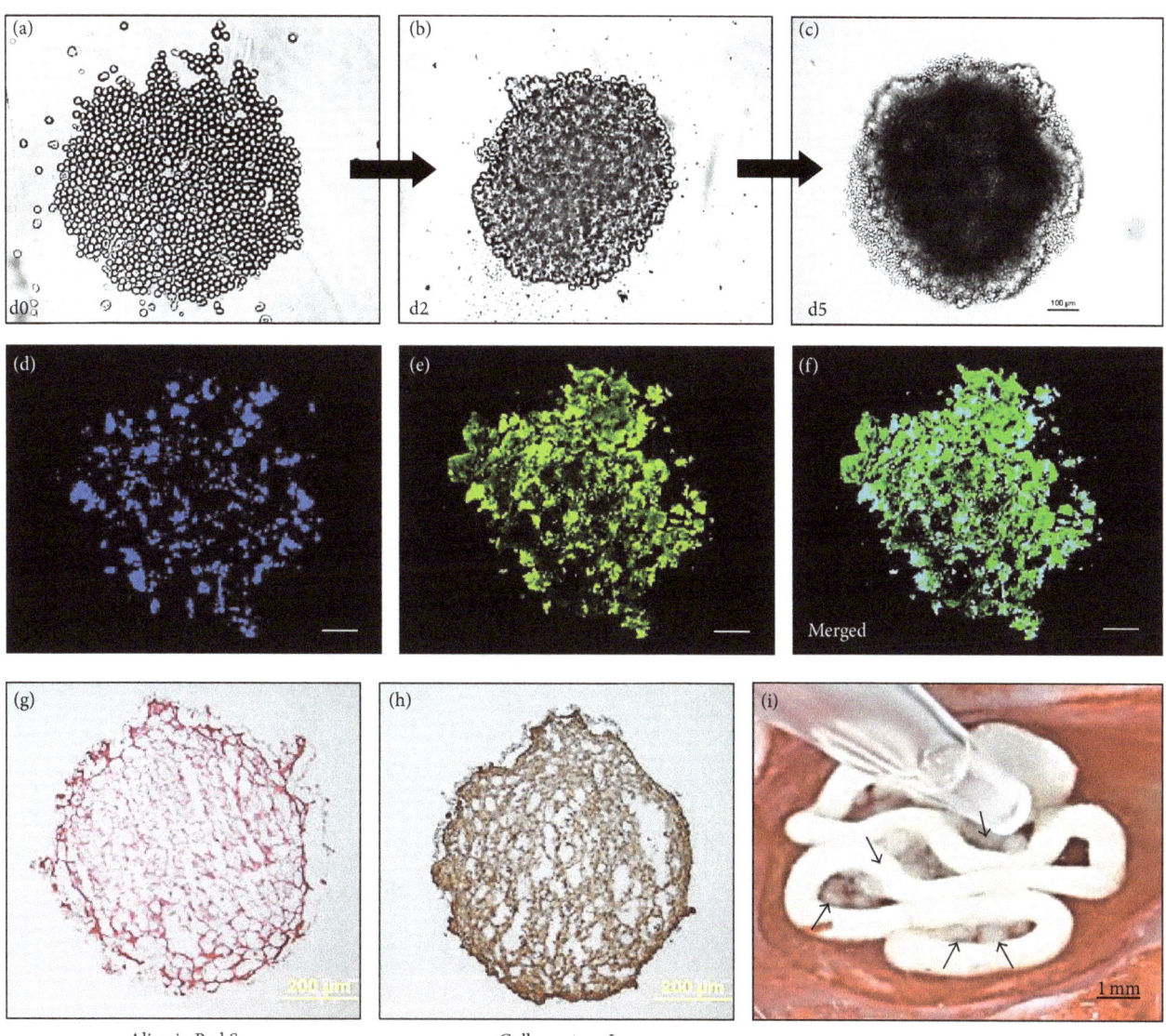

FIGURE 3: Characterization of osteogenic differentiation of MAPCs in 3D aggregate culture. The generation of MAPC aggregates was observed on 0, 2, and 5 days after suspension culture ((a) to (c)). Cell aggregation formed a compact spheroid at day 5 (c). After 28 days, osteogenic potential of 3D aggregates was analyzed by immunostaining with osteocalcin ((d), (e), and (f)) and collagen type I (h) antibodies. Mineralization was also observed by Alizarin Red S staining (g). (i) showed direct aggregates seeding on the scaffold during surgery on rat calvarial defect (arrows indicate 3D aggregates). Scale bars: 100 μm ((a) to (f)), 200 μm ((g) and (h)), and 1 mm (i).

into osteogenic cells. Although the osteogenic effect by HG materials on rMAPCs was not prominent in the 2D culture system, still they may have a critical influence on bone regeneration. Further studies will be needed to provide clarification.

To evaluate whether the bone regeneration potential rMAPC aggregates can stimulate bone formation, the rMAPC aggregates were tested by depositing on HG scaffolds in calvarial critical-sized defects in a rat model. After 12 weeks of implantation, calvariae were resected and evaluated by μCT (Figure 4). The resection procedure must be carried out with great caution because any small errors in the defect site can cause significant misinterpretation of the result. In Figure 4, the HG scaffold with MAPC aggregates regenerated

bone in the defect site better than HG scaffold only. Many times, the micro-CT image from the dorsal and ventral sides showed different degrees of bone formation. Zooming on the ventral side of the calvaria clearly showed that higher bone regeneration was induced by rMAPC aggregates. One possible prediction is that many rMAPC aggregates seeded on the defect site flowed through the HG scaffold to the bottom of the defect site. Without absorption, the 3D aggregates could stimulate the bone regeneration mostly on the dorsal site. Most of all, the regenerated site with rMAPC aggregates with HG had a continuous bridge through the center of the defect. This demonstrated a high degree of bone regeneration in the calvarial defect site and is used as a scoring system by many researchers [33]. On the other hand, bone regeneration

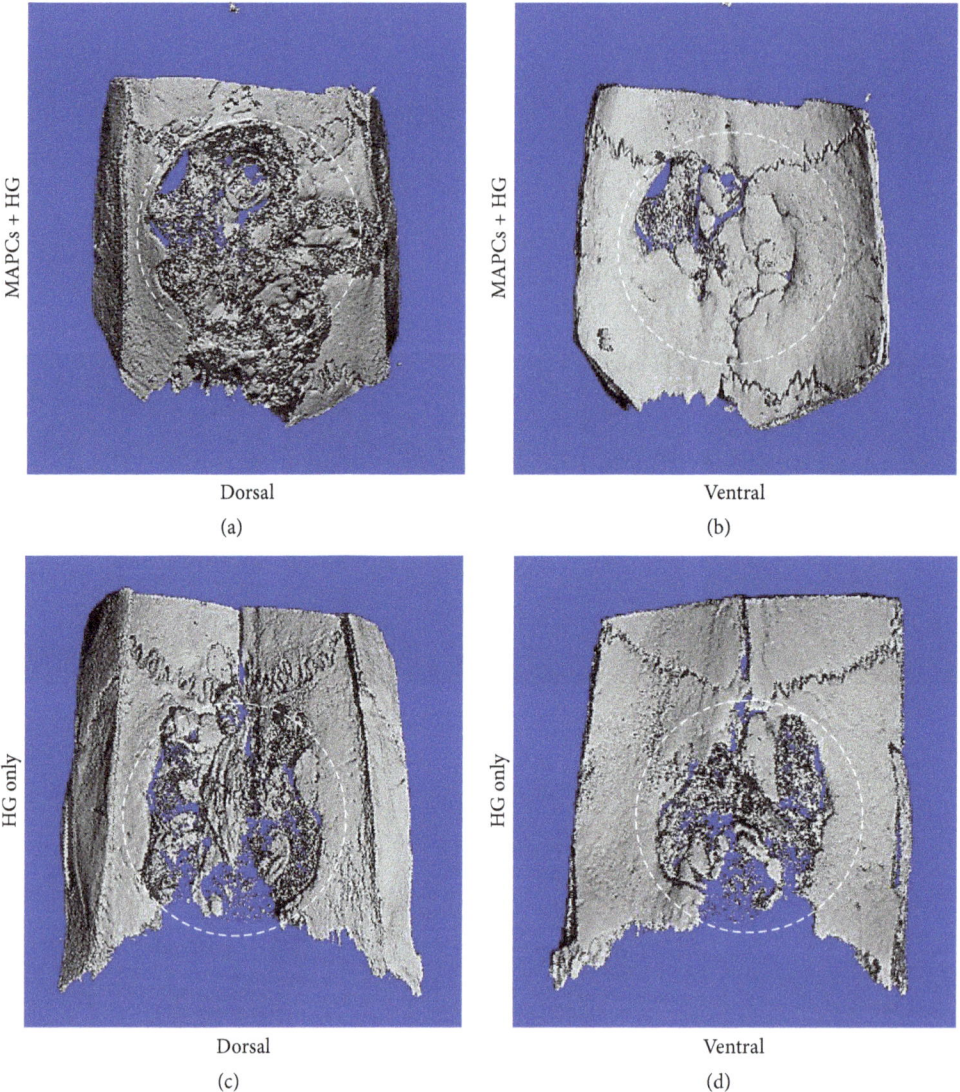

FIGURE 4: Micro-CT images of critical-sized calvarial defects after 12 weeks of implantation. White dotted circle represents defect site (8 mm in diameter). MAPCs with HG group ((a) and (b)) and HG-only group ((c) and (d)).

on the defect site with HG showed less bone formation and a more disintegrated appearance than HG with rMAPC aggregates.

For the analysis of new bone formation, micro-CT image alone is inadequate to distinguish new bones from the surrounding host bone or the radiopaque HG materials. Histological and fluorescent image can provide further information on new bone formation. Undecalcified calvaria sections were stained with Steven Blue and Van Gieson to identify new bone formation (brighter red) in the defect site (Figures 5(a) and 5(b)). New bone formation was calculated to be 66.99 ± 26.44% for rMAPCs with HG group and 34.44 ± 19.62% for the HG-only group (Figure 5(c)). As the higher percentage indicated, more new bones were observed in the center of defect apart from host tissue in rMAPCs with HG group (Figure 5(b)). Unlike the rMAPCs with HG group, HG-only groups relied on the cell source from the host

bone. Most of the new bone was observed near each end (near host bone) without much new bone formation in the center of the defect area (Figure 5(a)). However, whether implanted rMAPCs did differentiate into osteoblasts *in vivo* to create new bone is not clear. There is also a possibility that rMAPCs could induce more repairing capability of host cells by extending its coverage to the center of the defect although rMAPCs themselves did not generate bones. Further studies using a cell tracking method will be necessary to find whether rMAPCs can directly participate in bone regeneration.

Taken together, rMAPC aggregates can be differentiated into osteogenic linage *in vitro* both in 2D monolayer and in 3D aggregate culture systems. *In vivo* bone regeneration using rMAPC aggregates with HG scaffold resulted in higher bone regeneration than using HG scaffold only. This supports our hypothesis that MAPCs can differentiate into osteogenic cells and also promotes bone regeneration.

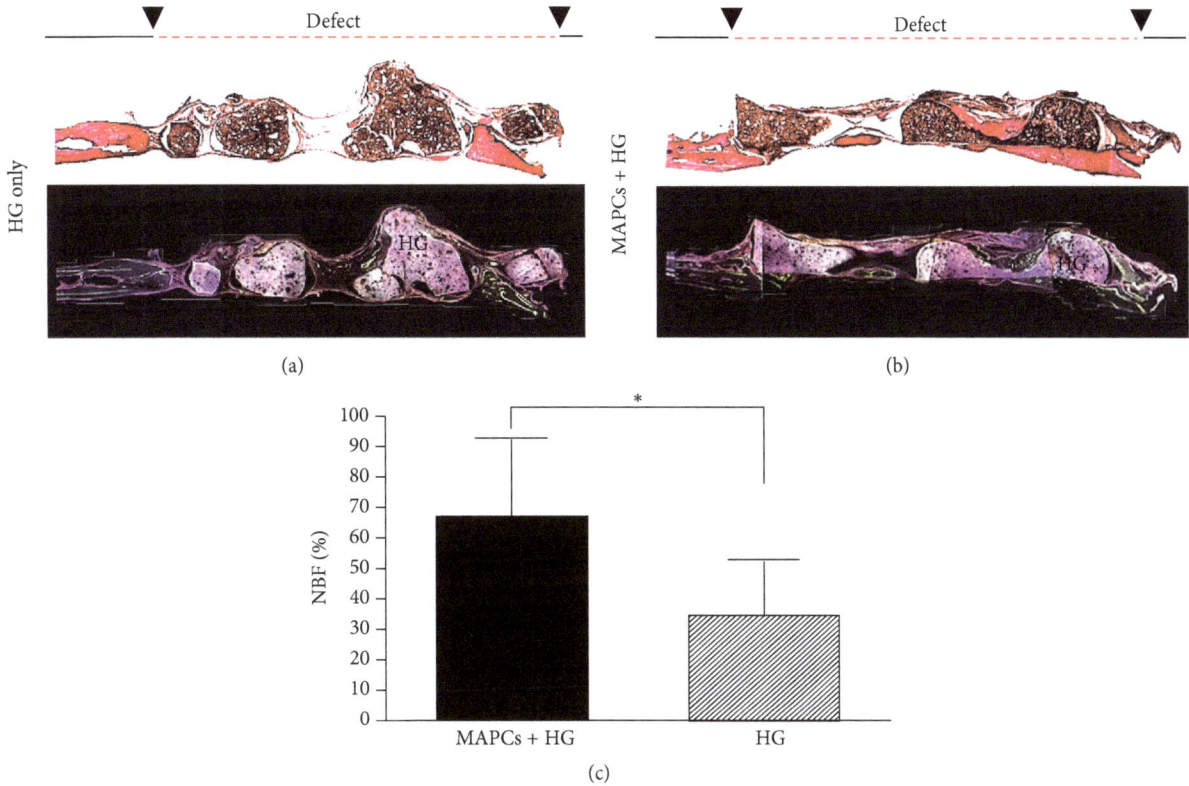

FIGURE 5: Sagittal section of the defect area after 12 weeks of implantation. Sections were stained with Steven Blue and Van Gieson ((a) and (b), top) and fluorescence image was labeled with Calcein and Alizarin Red S dye ((a) and (b), bottom). The area of new bone formation (NFB) was quantified in % using ImageJ software; $^*p < 0.05$ (c).

For possible improvement in bone regeneration using rMAPCs in the future, a study on the mechanism of rMAPC aggregated in terms of osteogenic signal pathways such as Wnt and TGF beta signal transduction may provide crucial factors to modulate the osteogenic differentiation of rMAPCs. Although rMAPCs in this study showed an osteogenic potential both *in vitro* and *in vivo*, whether their bone regenerative capability is superior to other types of adult stem cells is still uncertain. Therefore, a comparative study of rMAPCs with other types of stem cells will also give a better insight into choosing the right cell source for future bone tissue engineering applications.

4. Conclusion

The findings in this study support the osteogenic potential of rMAPCs and the direct effect on bone regeneration both *in vitro* and *in vivo*. rMAPCs showed a good cell proliferation ability in both growth and osteogenic media. Also, *in vitro* osteogenic differentiation was able to be induced in osteogenic media for 28 days and confirmed by expression of osteogenic markers, osteocalcin, and collage type I. rMAPCs formed the moderate mineralization up to 21 days and further differentiation up to 42 days clearly showed the deposition of highly mineralized extracellular matrix by differentiated cells. After examining rMAPCs in 3D aggregate culture in osteogenic media for 39 days, high level of osteocalcin,

collagen type I, and mineralization was observed. The 3D aggregates of rMAPCs showed a significantly higher level of osteogenic differentiation outcome than rMAPCs in 2D monolayer culture *in vitro*. Thus, aggregates were carried by HG scaffold in a construct and implanted into the rat calvarial defect. The *in vivo* osteogenic effect of rMAPCs with HG scaffolds was revealed by the superior bone formation on the defect site. Micro-CT, histology, and histomorphometric analysis also showed much higher bone formation for the group implanted with rMAPC aggregates than HG scaffold only.

In summary, the outcomes confirmed that rMAPCs have superior osteogenic potential in the application of 3D aggregates for both *in vitro* mineralization and *in vivo* bone formation. These results may regard the rMAPCs as a novel adult stem cell source for the future clinical applications in bone regeneration.

Competing Interests

The authors declare that they have no competing interests.

Acknowledgments

The authors would like to thank John Whitley for editorial support and Joao Ferreira and Li Zhang for their technical assistance. The research reported in this paper was supported, in part, by NIH/NIDCR K08DE018695 and R01DE022816.

References

[1] Y. H. T. Liao, C. B. Verchere, and G. L. Warnock, "Adult stem or progenitor cells in treatment for type 1 diabetes: current progress," *Canadian Journal of Surgery*, vol. 50, no. 2, pp. 137–142, 2007.

[2] M. Mimeault, R. Hauke, and S. K. Batra, "Stem cells: a revolution in therapeutics—recent advances in stem cell biology and their therapeutic applications in regenerative medicine and cancer therapies," *Clinical Pharmacology & Therapeutics*, vol. 82, no. 3, pp. 252–264, 2007.

[3] N. Christoforou and J. D. Gearhart, "Stem cells and their potential in cell-based cardiac therapies," *Progress in Cardiovascular Diseases*, vol. 49, no. 6, pp. 396–413, 2007.

[4] J. R. Mauney, V. Volloch, and D. L. Kaplan, "Role of adult mesenchymal stem cells in bone tissue-engineering applications: current status and future prospects," *Tissue Engineering*, vol. 11, no. 5-6, pp. 787–802, 2005.

[5] J. T. Triffitt, "Stem cells and the philosopher's stone," *Journal of Cellular Biochemistry*, vol. 38, pp. 13–19, 2002.

[6] X. Wang, Y. Wang, W. Gou, Q. Lu, J. Peng, and S. Lu, "Role of mesenchymal stem cells in bone regeneration and fracture repair: a review," *International Orthopaedics*, vol. 37, no. 12, pp. 2491–2498, 2013.

[7] C. Pipino and A. Pandolfi, "Osteogenic differentiation of amniotic fluid mesenchymal stromal cells and their bone regeneration potential," *World Journal of Stem Cells*, vol. 7, no. 4, pp. 681–690, 2015.

[8] W. Tsuji, J. P. Rubin, and K. G. Marra, "Adipose-derived stem cells: implications in tissue regeneration," *World Journal of Stem Cells*, vol. 6, no. 3, pp. 312–321, 2014.

[9] S. La Francesca, A. E. Ting, J. Sakamoto et al., "Multipotent adult progenitor cells decrease cold ischemic injury in *ex vivo* perfused human lungs: an initial pilot and feasibility study," *Transplantation Research*, vol. 3, no. 1, article 19, 2014.

[10] A. Peister, M. A. Woodruff, J. J. Prince, D. P. Gray, D. W. Hutmacher, and R. E. Guldberg, "Cell sourcing for bone tissue engineering: amniotic fluid stem cells have a delayed, robust differentiation compared to mesenchymal stem cells," *Stem Cell Research*, vol. 7, no. 1, pp. 17–27, 2011.

[11] C. Raggi and A. C. Berardi, "Mesenchymal stem cells, aging and regenerative medicine," *Muscles, Ligaments and Tendons Journal*, vol. 2, no. 3, pp. 239–242, 2012.

[12] D. L. Jones and T. A. Rando, "Emerging models and paradigms for stem cell ageing," *Nature Cell Biology*, vol. 13, no. 5, pp. 506–512, 2011.

[13] Y. Jiang, B. N. Jahagirdar, R. L. Reinhardt et al., "Pluripotency of mesenchymal stem cells derived from adult marrow," *Nature*, vol. 418, no. 6893, pp. 41–49, 2002.

[14] Y. Jiang, B. N. Jahagirdar, R. L. Reinhardt et al., "Pluripotency of mesenchymal stem cells derived from adult marrow," *Nature*, vol. 447, pp. 880–881, 2007.

[15] B. G. Debeb, V. Galat, J. Epple-Farmer et al., "Isolation of Oct4-expressing extraembryonic endoderm precursor cell lines," *PLoS ONE*, vol. 4, no. 9, Article ID e7216, 2009.

[16] A. Lo Nigro, M. Geraerts, T. Notelaers et al., "MAPC culture conditions support the derivation of cells with nascent hypoblast features from bone marrow and blastocysts," *Journal of Molecular Cell Biology*, vol. 4, no. 6, pp. 423–426, 2012.

[17] B. Binas and C. M. Verfaillie, "Concise review: bone marrow meets blastocyst: Lessons from an unlikely encounter," *Stem Cells*, vol. 31, no. 4, pp. 620–626, 2013.

[18] J. R. Ferreira, R. Padilla, G. Urkasemsin et al., "Titanium-enriched hydroxyapatite-gelatin scaffolds with osteogenically differentiated progenitor cell aggregates for calvaria bone regeneration," *Tissue Engineering Part A*, vol. 19, no. 15-16, pp. 1803–1816, 2013.

[19] J. R. Ferreira, M. L. Hirsch, L. Zhang et al., "Three-dimensional multipotent progenitor cell aggregates for expansion, osteogenic differentiation and 'in vivo' tracing with AAV vector serotype 6," *Gene Therapy*, vol. 20, no. 2, pp. 158–168, 2013.

[20] D. J. Lee, R. Padilla, H. Zhang, W.-S. Hu, and C.-C. Ko, "Biological assessment of a calcium silicate incorporated hydroxyapatite-gelatin nanocomposite: a comparison to decellularized bone matrix," *BioMed Research International*, vol. 2014, Article ID 837524, 12 pages, 2014.

[21] S. A. Jacobs, V. D. Roobrouck, C. M. Verfaillie, and S. W. Van Gool, "Immunological characteristics of human mesenchymal stem cells and multipotent adult progenitor cells," *Immunology and Cell Biology*, vol. 91, no. 1, pp. 32–39, 2013.

[22] S. A. Jacobs, J. Pinxteren, V. D. Roobrouck et al., "Human multipotent adult progenitor cells are nonimmunogenic and exert potent immunomodulatory effects on alloreactive T-cell responses," *Cell Transplantation*, vol. 22, no. 10, pp. 1915–1928, 2013.

[23] V. Roobrouck, C. Clavel, S. A. Jacobs et al., "Differentiation potential of human postnatal mesenchymal stem cells, mesoangioblasts, and multipotent adult progenitor cells reflected in their transcriptome and partially influenced by the culture conditions," *Stem Cells*, vol. 29, no. 5, pp. 871–882, 2011.

[24] K. Subramanian, Y. Park, C. M. Verfaillie, and W. S. Hu, "Scalable expansion of multipotent adult progenitor cells as three-dimensional cell aggregates," *Biotechnology and Bioengineering*, vol. 108, no. 2, pp. 364–375, 2011.

[25] E. S. Ng, R. P. Davis, L. Azzola, E. G. Stanley, and A. G. Elefanty, "Forced aggregation of defined numbers of human embryonic stem cells into embryoid bodies fosters robust, reproducible hematopoietic differentiation," *Blood*, vol. 106, no. 5, pp. 1601–1603, 2005.

[26] K. Subramanian, M. Geraerts, K. A. Pauwelyn et al., "Isolation procedure and characterization of multipotent adult progenitor cells from rat bone marrow," *Methods in Molecular Biology*, vol. 636, pp. 55–78, 2010.

[27] A. M. Parfitt, M. K. Drezner, F. H. Glorieux et al., "Bone histomorphometry: standardization of nomenclature, symbols, and units. Report of the ASBMR Histomorphometry Nomenclature Committee," *Journal of Bone and Mineral Research*, vol. 2, no. 6, pp. 595–610, 1987.

[28] A. J. Salgado, O. P. Coutinho, and R. L. Reis, "Bone tissue engineering: state of the art and future trends," *Macromolecular Bioscience*, vol. 4, no. 8, pp. 743–765, 2004.

[29] E. Ben-Shushan, J. R. Thompson, L. J. Gudas, and Y. Bergman, "Rex-1, a gene encoding a transcription factor expressed in the early embryo, is regulated via Oct-3/4 and Oct-6 binding to an octamer site and a novel protein, Rox-1, binding to an adjacent site," *Molecular and Cellular Biology*, vol. 18, no. 4, pp. 1866–1878, 1998.

[30] H. R. Scholer, A. K. Hatzopoulos, R. Balling, N. Suzuki, and P. Gruss, "A family of octamer-specific proteins present

during mouse embryogenesis: evidence for germline-specific expression of an Oct factor," *The EMBO Journal*, vol. 8, no. 9, pp. 2543–2550, 1989.

[31] Y. Park, K. Subramanian, C. M. Verfaillie, and W. S. Hu, "Expansion and hepatic differentiation of rat multipotent adult progenitor cells in microcarrier suspension culture," *Journal of Biotechnology*, vol. 150, no. 1, pp. 131–139, 2010.

[32] C. Chenu, S. Colucci, M. Grano et al., "Osteocalcin induces chemotaxis, secretion of matrix proteins, and calcium-mediated intracellular signaling in human osteoclast-like cells," *The Journal of Cell Biology*, vol. 127, no. 4, pp. 1149–1158, 1994.

[33] P. P. Spicer, J. D. Kretlow, S. Young, J. A. Jansen, F. K. Kasper, and A. G. Mikos, "Evaluation of bone regeneration using the rat critical size calvarial defect," *Nature Protocols*, vol. 7, no. 10, pp. 1918–1929, 2012.

9

Impact of a Core Ferrule Design on Fracture Resistance of Teeth Restored with Cast Post and Core

Loubna Shamseddine[1] and Farid Chaaban[2]

[1]Department of Prosthodontics, Lebanese University, School of Dentistry, P.O. Box 6573/14, Beirut, Lebanon
[2]Faculty of Engineering and Architecture, American University of Beirut, Mazraa-Daybess Street, Ferdawss Building, First Floor, P.O. Box 11-0236, Beirut 1107 2020, Lebanon

Correspondence should be addressed to Loubna Shamseddine; drloubna1@hotmail.com

Academic Editor: James K. Hartsfield

Objectives. To investigate the influence of a contra bevel on the fracture resistance of teeth restored with cast post and core. *Materials and Methods*. Sixty plastic analogues of an upper incisor were endodontically treated and prepared with 6° internal taper and 2 mm of ferrule in order to receive a cast post and core. The prepared samples were divided into two groups ($n = 30$); the first group serves as control while the second group was prepared with an external 30° bevel on the buccal and lingual walls. All samples crowned were exposed to a compressive load at 130° to their long axis until fractures occurred. Fracture resistance loads were recorded and failure modes were also observed. Mann-Whitney test was carried out to compare the two groups. *Results*. Mean failure loads for the groups were, respectively, 1038.69 N (SD ±243.52 N) and 1078.89 N (SD ±352.21 N). Statistically, there was no significant difference between the two groups ($P = 0.7675 > 0.05$). *Conclusion*. In the presence of a ferrule and a crown in the anterior teeth, adding a secondary ferrule to the cast post and core will not increase the resistance to fracture.

1. Introduction

The prognosis of endodontically treated teeth (ETT) is proven to be affected by the type of the restoration [1, 2], and in this aspect numerous methods of restoring ETT have been advocated. The traditional approach for restoration of ETT with moderate-to-severe tooth loss is to make a post and core and, subsequently, place a crown [3, 4]. Present options include cast metal posts and cores and prefabricated metal or fiber-reinforced composite posts [5]. The purpose of the post is to retain coronal structure restoration with the ability to save severely damaged teeth. Cast posts and cores are considered as the restorative method of choice for anterior teeth with moderate and severe destruction [4, 6]. Custom cast post and core allow for a close adaptation of the post-to-post space preparation and should fit optimally [4].

Common failure types of ETT restored with cast posts vary from post dislodgment to root fracture. The latter is the primary reason for the extraction of such teeth [7]. In fact, ETT often have little coronal tissue remaining due to caries, trauma, cavity preparation, and/or root canal treatment, making them even more susceptible to fracture [8, 9].

Several factors affecting fracture strength of ETTs are found in the literature; some are related to the tooth restored and others to the type of post used. Tooth location is also one of these factors. In fact, the magnitude and direction of functional loads play a major role in stress concentration within the dowel-restored teeth [10]. Anterior teeth undergo nonaxial forces more than posterior teeth that are primarily axially loaded [11]. Nonaxial forces are more detrimental to the tooth restoration interface [8, 12] and increase the frequency of fracture [13]. The preparation of the tooth is another parameter directly related to the fracture resistance. An adequate resistance to displacement of every cast restoration depends largely on the retention and resistance form in the preparation [14]. The ideal taper recommended varies from 2° to 7° per axial wall. This taper is suggested to avoid forming undercuts to the withdrawal axis of a cast post [15, 16]. Clinically, the reported ideal axial wall convergence values for full coverage restorations are ranging from 4° to 20° [17, 18].

Different means as ferrule effect, interlocking devices, grooves, and contra bevel have been suggested to improve retention and enhance the resistance of ETT. Most recent studies agree that the most important factor of success when restoring ETTs with post and core is the ferrule. This encompassing band of cast metal around the coronal surface of the tooth may resist stresses such as functional lever forces, wedging effect of posts, and the lateral forces exerted during the post insertion [19]. To ensure durability, ETTs must have a ferrule height of at least 1.5 to 2 mm [20, 21]. It operates as an anti-rotary device and improves the biomechanical stability of the tooth [9, 22–25]. Ferrule design has been studied and found to produce greater strength when it is circumferential and uniform [26–28]. Various ferrule designs have been suggested but currently there is little research supporting one design over the others [29, 30].

The post type and its adaptation are the major factors affecting the strength of ETTs. Relevant reports and studies have indicated that cast posts are proven to have higher fracture resistance compared to fiber posts [31–33]. Similarly, fracture strength in the anterior teeth has been reported to be higher with cast posts than with fiber posts [34–36] and higher than that of prefabricated titanium post and composite core [37]. Although cast post and cores restored teeth showed higher prevalence of irreparable failures [38], they exhibit a high survival rate up to 19.5 years [39].

The main advantage of using a cast post and core technique is the ability to conform to any canal space and to provide a good fit that would lead to uniform distribution of forces within the root [37, 40]. Moreover, in cast post and core restorations, a balance exists between maximizing retention and maintaining resistance to root fracture [41]. Cast posts would fit passively into the canal and would resist rotation and rocking [41]. Grooves have been advocated as additional retention through the preparation as a means for improving the crown retention [42] with an antirotational mean for the post [14]. However, the incorporation of the antirotational device in cast post and core on the buccal and lingual faces concomitantly was found to increase the stress-strain values [43] but was judged to be insignificant in terms of fracture resistance of the teeth [43–45].

The contra bevel has also been suggested as a secondary ferrule and as an antirotational mechanism incorporated to the cast post and core [14, 28, 44, 46, 47]. It is an external bevel arising from the occlusal surface or edge of a tooth preparation and placed at an angle that opposes or contrasts the angle of the surface it arises from [48]. This contra bevel used as a core ferrule has been found to enhance fracture resistance in several studies [47, 49, 50], while in other studies no significant effects were observed [46, 51]. It should be noted that the fracture resistance studies did not take the full coverage crowns into consideration. An external 30 degrees bevel may be of interest for strengthening ETT because it acts as a positioning guide and as an antirotational device for the post and core.

Based on the positive correlation between the retention of the cast post and core and the resistance to fracture of the

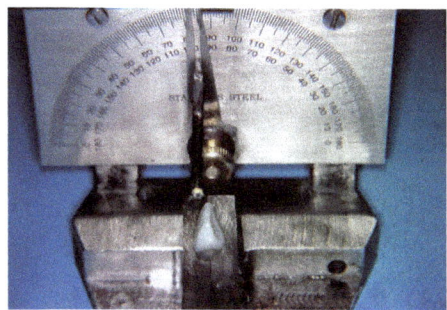

FIGURE 1: Metallic block with protractor used for the experiment.

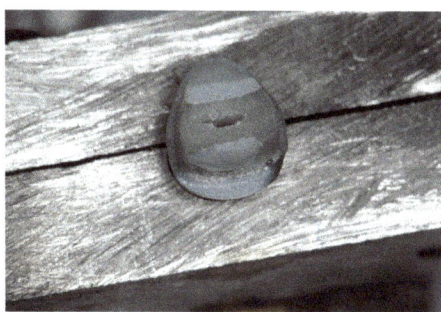

FIGURE 2: Coronal preparation for full coverage crown in both groups.

teeth, the antirotary resistance form, realized by the contra bevel, could modify the load direction and stress distribution within the post/dentin system.

The purpose of this study is to assess the effect of a contra bevel on the fracture resistance of crowned anterior teeth restored with cast posts and core. The null hypothesis being tested was that there is no difference between the two types of teeth prepared with or without a contra bevel.

2. Materials and Methods

Sixty clear acrylic standardized analogues B22X-500 (Kilgore International, Inc., USA) simulating ETT maxillary central incisors and a special metallic device were fabricated to subsequently mount the analogues for this experiment. This device was made of a base and a mounting block with a hinge access having the ability to move in mesiodistal direction thus allowing the axis of analogues to be fixed with different rotational angles. In addition, a protractor instrument related to the base was used for the inclination of the block (Figure 1).

2.1. Preparation of the Crown. Into the block, all specimens were prepared using an electronic surveyor. The crowns were prepared perpendicular to the root axis with an abrasive disc (X928-7 TP, Abrasive Technology, Inc., USA), leaving 5 mm above the cervical area. The axial surfaces of the tooth were prepared with specific burs (facial: 1.5 mm ISO number 806, 104 173 544 031, palatal and proximal: 0.8 mm ISO number 806, 104 173 544 016) following the cement enamel junction to receive a full coverage metal crown (Figure 2). The specimens were divided into two groups of 30 analogues each. A 2 mm

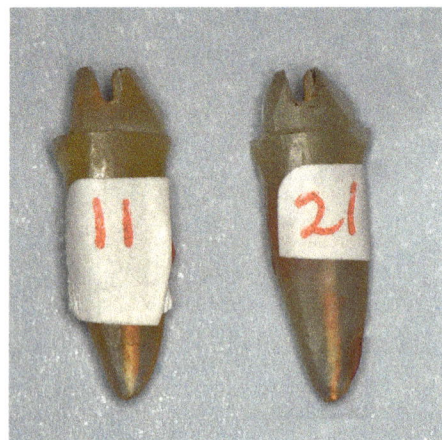

FIGURE 3: Specimen of each group showing the prepared contra bevel in group 2.

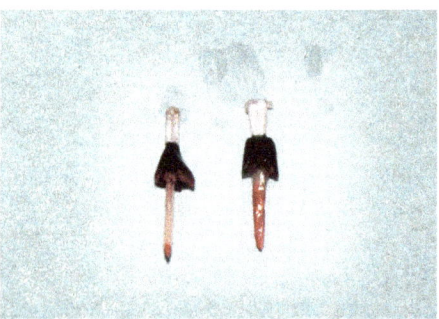

FIGURE 4: Specimens of post and core fabricated with wax patterns.

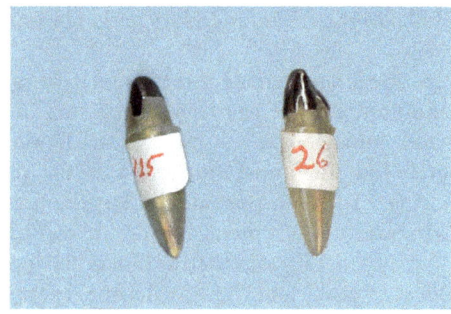

FIGURE 5: Specimen of cemented cast post in each group.

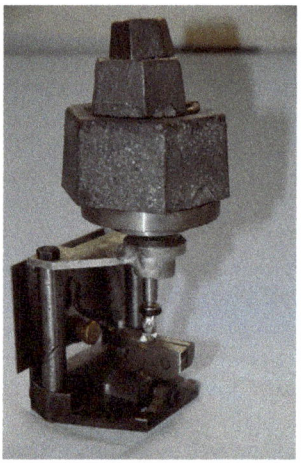

FIGURE 6: Cementation of a crown under static load.

ferrule was left at the proximal sides. Group 1 was considered as control group without modifications, while group 2 was obtained by changing the axis of the analogues to 24° and the facial and palatal walls were prepared to create an external bevel 30° to the long axis of the tooth (Figure 3).

2.2. Endodontic Preparation. Analogues were prepared with an access cavity of 6° taper using the protractor at 0° and burs with 6° taper. Root canal preparation was then executed with the protaper system according to the manufacturer's instructions to a working length of 18 mm. Gutta-percha was then laterally condensed with a manual spreader (Kerr, W 0697840 and W 0693510).

2.3. Post and Cores Fabrication. Gates Glidden drill number 3 (Dentsply Maillefer A0008 240 00500) and 1.1 mm Largo (Dentsply Maillefer A0008 230 002 00 to A0008 230 003 00) were used to prepare the post spaces, leaving 7 mm of apical seal. Post and cores were constructed using 1.25 mm burn-out plastic posts coated in increments with wax patterns to fit the root canal. For the coronal fabrication, a silicone index of the intact tooth and wax were used to standardize the coronal dimension for all specimens. The bevel at the coronal part in group 2 was filled by wax patterns thus becoming a part of the post and core (Figure 4). The post and cores

were cast in a Ni-Cr alloy and cemented using spiral paste filler (Dentsply Maillefer Instrument) under a static load 1.5 Kg for a duration of 15 min with zinc phosphate cement (spofaDental Adhesor®) (Figure 5).

2.4. Cast Crowns Fabrication. After removing cement excess, a crown was waxed and adapted directly to the analogue using the previously prepared silicon index. After investing the wax pattern and casting it with Ni-Cr, the crown was cemented with zinc phosphate under a static load of 1.5 kg, also for 15 min (Figure 6).

2.5. Fracture Testing. Fracture strength testing was then performed on the two groups, in the laboratories of the Mechanical Engineering Department at the American University of Beirut, Lebanon. The testing device is a tension and compression system (YLUTM) and is fully computerized. This testing machine has an error margin of 0.04% for maximal load of 10 000 kg, a margin of 0.01% for repetitive maximal load of 10 000 kg with a resolution of displacement of 0.01 mm (10 μm) and accurate speed of 0.01% of full scale. The crowned analogues were subjected to an inclined compressive load (with a 1-kN cell at a crosshead speed of 0.05 mm/min at 130° to the long axis) divided into a compressive and bending components until fracture occurred (Figure 7).

TABLE 1: Summary of statistical results.

Group	Load means (SD)	Displacement means (SD)	Test of normality (Lilliefors)			Mann-Whitney strength test		Kruskal-Wallis test for displacement	
			Fracture load	Displacement	Load and displacement Judgment 5%	P value Judgment 5%		P value Judgment 5%	
			P values Judgment 5%						
1	1038.69 (243.52)	1.36 (0.31)	0.028	0.053	Absence of normal distribution	0.7675	No significant difference	0.7470	No significant difference
2	1078.89 (335.21)	1.44 (0.58)	0.008	0.003					

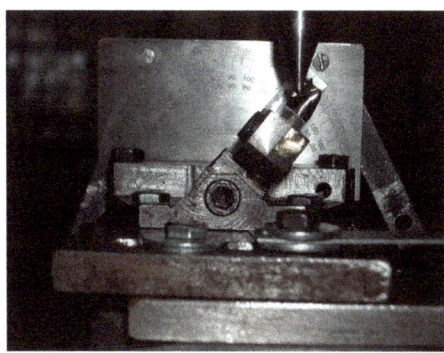

FIGURE 7: Simulating clinical direction in class I occlusion for testing.

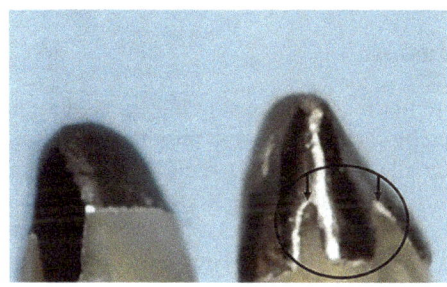

FIGURE 8: Illustration of the incomplete seating of post and cores in group 2.

3. Statistical Analysis

Data from the test results were analyzed using statistical software (SPSS 17; SPSS Inc., USA) and, for each group, load to fracture mean values and standard deviations (SD) were calculated.

Lilliefors test was used to check for normality and subsequently the Mann-Whitney test was used to compare fracture resistance between the groups. For the displacement values, the Kruskal-Wallis test was used to compare the groups. The level of significance (P) was set at 0.05.

4. Results

Incomplete seating of posts for all specimens of group 2 was the first result noticed before fracture testing (Figure 8). Another finding is that all analogues failed with the same

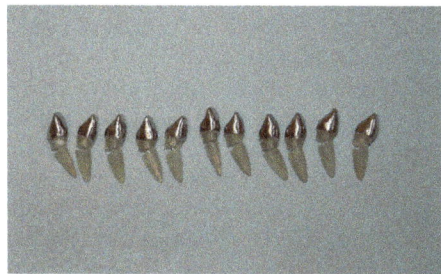

FIGURE 9: Fracture line visualized after testing in all specimens.

line direction and level after fracture testing (Figure 9). Considering the values obtained, the same displacement was observed for both groups. Statistical results are summarized in Table 1. There was no significant difference between the two groups for fracture load ($P = 0.7675$) as well as for the displacement ($P = 0.7470$). Means and standard deviations for the two parameters are also given in Table 1.

5. Discussion

Since fracture load depends on the geometry of teeth [52], this study used acrylic analogue to compare between the tested specimens as human incisors would have had a larger variability in size and morphology. This variability would have been otherwise required to observe significant differences between the two groups.

The localization of fracture lines for all specimens obtained in this study is attributed to the metallic device that holds the specimens during the testing process. The level and direction in the mouth could be different since bone and periodontal ligaments affect the strength of the roots [53, 54]. This metallic device explains the result of almost no difference found in the displacement between the two groups. The major objective of this study was to find which preparation design had a better resistance force to fracture, despite the load values or the failure localization.

The hypothesis that the mechanical behavior of anterior endodontically treated teeth would be affected by the ferrule added to the cast post and core was rejected. A slight increase in the fracture load has been found in group 2 without a significant difference in group 1 (P value = 0.7675).

The results of the present study indicate that a contra bevel incorporated to the custom cast post core did not improve the fracture resistance of ETT. The results of the study are in agreement with previous studies conducted by Sorensen and Engelman in 1990, Kutesa-Mutebi and Osman in 2004, and by Goyal et al. in 2007 [29, 46, 51].

It was stated that as the volume of posts decreases, the absorption of forces by the post system also decreases to a considerable degree [55]. In the study, group 2 with a larger volume of cast post and core demonstrated an equivalent fracture strength compared to the smaller volume of group 1. This could be attributed to the inconvenience of extra coronal additional part and its casting simultaneously to the intracoronal part. In fact, casting an extracoronal restoration differs from that of the post and core. It is necessary to fabricate a slightly undersized cast post to allow for passive fit and cement placement [56, 57], while oversized castings could give a better adapted crown margin upon cementation than an undersized one [58]. The study was carried out to develop undersized cast post and cores to fit passively the shape of the post space, in order to lead to a better transmission of the stresses. The two groups should exhibit the same adaptation of the post into the canal since they have the same root preparation, same post and core fabrication, and same cementation protocols. The similar fracture strength found in both groups could be explained by the cementation technique used in both groups (static load of 1.5 kg for a duration of 15 min) and especially to the equivalent taper of the canal and cavity walls. However, the undersized contra bevel makes it more difficult for air and excess cement to escape from the canal thus increasing the occurring of the filtration phenomenon. This phenomenon could prevent the post from being well placed and could affect the physicochemical properties of the cements and biomechanical behavior of the fixed restauration [37] with a higher film thickness than the ADA spec number 8 Zinc phosphate cement [59]. A similar pattern in the group 2 is possible as extracoronal casted parts can lead to the incomplete seating of posts for all specimens. This finding is supported by Dreyer and Jørgensen 1955 and Dimashkieh et al. 1974 who found that a filtration phenomenon can occur in the cementation onto well-fitted teeth preparations using zinc phosphate cement. When the passage of cement is reduced and large grains of cement powder begin to jam together, cement liquid filtration occurs and this resulted in an uneven distribution of cement powder portion in the phosphate matrix. The solid particles would form a mass that allows passage of the thinner liquid only causing further separation and filtration of the cement [60, 61].

The absence of adequate relief spaces impedes the flow of cement, leading to incomplete seating because of hydraulic pressure [62]. Dreyer and Jørgensen suggested that when the crown carrying the cement is placed on the prepared tooth, cement accumulates on the occlusal surface [60] and when pressure is applied to complete the seating of the crown, the excess cement can escape only through the space at the cervical margin. The flow of noncompressible liquid is inhibited and seating of restoration is resisted [60]. The same phenomenon would have occurred in undersized post and core cementation in group 2. As the post and core approaches its final position, this space becomes smaller. Consequently,

the casting of the external part complicates the proper seating of the post and core as shown in the cementation step. To alleviate this phenomenon, several methods were attempted to reduce the marginal discrepancy of the crown. Internal carving of wax patterns before casting [63], internal grinding of castings [64] venting, vibration during cementation [65], limiting the amount and site of cement placement [66], and adding a layer of die-spacer at the axioocclusal line angle [62] facilitate the drainage of excess cement and reduce the hydrostatic pressure. Additional studies to investigate the fracture resistance in presence of a core ferrule having means of cement escape are needed.

The final analysis in this study verified that fracture resistance is not associated with the cast metal post/core designed with a ferrule. The main limitation of the study is evaluating ferrule design on acrylic analogues. As a consequence, the load fracture found could not reflect the same values as for the mouth since their fracture strengths are different than teeth [67]. Thus, dynamic or fatigue behavior cannot be inferred in clinical situations until proven. However, in the literature, the use of analogues to compare the fracture resistance is valid [68–71].

Another limitation is the usage of a metallic device to hold specimens during fracture test. The fracture line and direction could have been different in the oral environment in the presence of bone and ligaments. Simulated clinical conditions might have affected the results. Further studies that simulate the oral environment are recommended.

6. Conclusion

Given these findings and considering the limitations of this study, it can be concluded that in presence of circumferential 2 mm of ferrule a secondary ferrule added to the cast post and core will not enhance the strength of crowned anterior teeth. A ferrule added to the cast post and core complicates the escape of the zinc phosphate during the cementation procedure.

Competing Interests

The authors declare that there is no conflict of interests regarding the publication of this paper.

Acknowledgments

The contribution of Mr. Helmi El Khatib in providing the labs facilities at the American University of Beirut (AUB) for conducting the fracturing tests is deeply acknowledged.

References

[1] K. H. Alsamadani, E.-S. M. Abdaziz, and E.-S. Gad, "Influence of different restorative techniques on the strength of endodontically treated weakened roots," *International Journal of Dentistry*, vol. 2012, Article ID 343712, 10 pages, 2012.

[2] R. D. Trushkowsky, "Restoration of endodontically treated teeth: criteria and technique considerations," *Quintessence International*, vol. 45, no. 7, pp. 557–567, 2014.

[3] A. Tikku, A. Chandra, and R. Bharti, "Are full cast crowns mandatory after endodontic treatment in posterior teeth?" *Journal of Conservative Dentistry*, vol. 13, no. 4, pp. 246–248, 2010.

[4] P. Ratnakar, R. Bhosgi, K. K. Metta, K. Aggarwal, S. Vinuta, and N. Singh, "Survey on restoration of endodontically treated anterior teeth: a questionnaire based study," *Journal of International Oral Health*, vol. 6, no. 6, pp. 41–45, 2014.

[5] A. Al-Ansari, "Which type of post and core system should you use?" *Evidence-Based Dentistry*, vol. 8, no. 2, p. 42, 2007.

[6] S. Sreedevi, R. Sanjeev, R. Raghavan, A. Abraham, T. Rajamani, and G. K. Govind, "An in vitro study on the effects of post-core design and ferrule on the fracture resistance of endodontically treated maxillary central incisors," *Journal of International Oral Health*, vol. 7, no. 8, pp. 37–41, 2015.

[7] D. Landys Borén, P. Jonasson, and T. Kvist, "Long-term survival of endodontically treated teeth at a public dental specialist clinic," *Journal of Endodontics*, vol. 41, no. 2, pp. 176–181, 2015.

[8] I. Peroz, F. Blankenstein, K.-P. Lange, and M. Naumann, "Restoring endodontically treated teeth with posts and cores- a review," *Quintessence International*, vol. 36, no. 9, pp. 737–746, 2005.

[9] F. Zicari, B. Van Meerbeek, R. Scotti, and I. Naert, "Effect of ferrule and post placement on fracture resistance of endodontically treated teeth after fatigue loading," *Journal of Dentistry*, vol. 41, no. 3, pp. 207–215, 2013.

[10] R. McAndrew and P. H. Jacobsen, "The relationship between crown and post design on root stress—a finite element study," *The European Journal of Prosthodontics and Restorative Dentistry*, vol. 10, no. 1, pp. 9–13, 2002.

[11] J. P. Okeson, "Criteria for optimum functional occlusion," in *Management of Temporomandibular Disorders and Occlusion*, J. P. Okeson, Ed., pp. 97–110, Elsevier, St. Louis, Mo, USA, 6th edition, 2008.

[12] S. Arunpraditkul, S. Saengsanon, and W. Pakviwat, "Fracture fesistance of endodontically treated teeth: three walls versus four walls of remaining coronal tooth structure," *Journal of Prosthodontics*, vol. 18, no. 1, pp. 49–53, 2009.

[13] C. G. Castro, F. R. Santana, M. G. Roscoe, P. C. Simamoto, P. C. F. Santos-Filho, and C. J. Soares, "Fracture resistance and mode of failure of various types of root filled teeth," *International Endodontic Journal*, vol. 45, no. 9, pp. 840–847, 2012.

[14] S. F. Rosenstiel, M. F. Land, and J. Fujimoto, *Contemporary Fixed Prosthodontics*, Elsevier/Mosby, St. Louis, Mo, USA, 5th edition, 2016.

[15] J. E. Noonan Jr. and M. H. Goldfogel, "Convergence of the axial walls of full veneer crown preparations in a dental school environment," *The Journal of Prosthetic Dentistry*, vol. 66, no. 5, pp. 706–708, 1991.

[16] P. B. Robinson and J. W. Lee, "The use of real time video magnification for the pre-clinical teaching of crown preparations," *British Dental Journal*, vol. 190, no. 9, pp. 506–510, 2001.

[17] R. N. Rafeek, W. A. J. Smith, K. G. Seymour, L. F. Zou, and D. Y. D. Samarawickrama, "Taper of full-veneer crown preparations by dental students at the university of the West Indies," *Journal of Prosthodontics*, vol. 19, no. 7, pp. 580–585, 2010.

[18] M. F. Ayad, A. A. Maghrabi, and S. F. Rosenstiel, "Assessment of convergence angles of tooth preparations for complete crowns among dental students," *Journal of Dentistry*, vol. 33, no. 8, pp. 633–638, 2005.

[19] J. A. Sorensen and M. J. Engelman, "Effect of post adaptation on fracture resistance of endodontically treated teeth," *The Journal of Prosthetic Dentistry*, vol. 64, no. 4, pp. 419–424, 1990.

[20] L. Zhi-Yue and Z. Yu-Xing, "Effects of post-core design and ferrule on fracture resistance of endodontically treated maxillary central incisors," *Journal of Prosthetic Dentistry*, vol. 89, no. 4, pp. 368–373, 2003.

[21] B. Carlini-Júnior, D. Cecchin, A. P. Farina, G. D. S. Pereira, L. T. Prieto, and L. A. M. S. Paulillo, "Influence of remaining coronal structure and of the marginal design on the fracture strength of roots restored with cast post and core," *Acta Odontologica Scandinavica*, vol. 71, no. 1, pp. 278–282, 2013.

[22] J. S. Mamoun, "On the ferrule effect and the biomechanical stability of teeth restored with cores, posts, and crowns," *European Journal of Dentistry*, vol. 8, no. 2, pp. 281–286, 2014.

[23] S. Singh and P. Thareja, "Fracture resistance of endodontically treated maxillary central incisors with varying ferrule heights and configurations: in vitro study," *Journal of Conservative Dentistry*, vol. 17, no. 2, pp. 115–118, 2014.

[24] V. Aggarwal, M. Singla, S. Yadav, H. Yadav, V. Sharma, and S. S. Bhasin, "The effect of ferrule presence and type of dowel on fracture resistance of endodontically treated teeth restored with metal-ceramic crowns," *Journal of Conservative Dentistry*, vol. 17, no. 2, pp. 183–187, 2014.

[25] N. Z. Baba and C. J. Goodacre, "Restoration of endodontically treated teeth: contemporary concepts and future perspectives," *Endodontic Topics*, vol. 31, no. 1, pp. 68–83, 2014.

[26] C. C. H. Ng, H. B. Dumbrigue, M. I. Al-Bayat, J. A. Griggs, and C. W. Wakefield, "Influence of remaining coronal tooth structure location on the fracture resistance of restored endodontically treated anterior teeth," *Journal of Prosthetic Dentistry*, vol. 95, no. 4, pp. 290–296, 2006.

[27] M. Naumann, A. Preuss, and M. Rosentritt, "Effect of incomplete crown ferrules on load capacity of endodontically treated maxillary incisors restored with fiber posts, composite build-ups, and all-ceramic crowns: an in vitro evaluation after chewing simulation," *Acta Odontologica Scandinavica*, vol. 64, no. 1, pp. 31–36, 2006.

[28] P. L. B. Tan, S. A. Aquilino, D. G. Gratton et al., "In vitro fracture resistance of endodontically treated central incisors with varying ferrule heights and configurations," *The Journal of Prosthetic Dentistry*, vol. 93, no. 4, pp. 331–336, 2005.

[29] J. A. Sorensen and M. J. Engelman, "Ferrule design and fracture resistance of endodontically treated teeth," *The Journal of Prosthetic Dentistry*, vol. 63, no. 5, pp. 529–536, 1990.

[30] A. Jotkowitz and N. Samet, "Rethinking ferrule—a new approach to an old dilemma," *British Dental Journal*, vol. 209, no. 1, pp. 25–33, 2010.

[31] G. Maroulakos, W. W. Nagy, and E. D. Kontogiorgos, "Fracture resistance of compromised endodontically treated teeth restored with bonded post and cores: an in vitro study," *The Journal of Prosthetic Dentistry*, vol. 114, no. 3, pp. 390–397, 2015.

[32] L. Zhou and Q. Wang, "Comparison of fracture resistance between cast posts and fiber posts: a meta-analysis of literature," *Journal of Endodontics*, vol. 39, no. 1, pp. 11–15, 2013.

[33] B. Dejak and A. Młotkowski, "The influence of ferrule effect and length of cast and FRC posts on the stresses in anterior teeth," *Dental Materials*, vol. 29, no. 9, pp. e227–e237, 2013.

[34] J. Hegde, R. Ramakrishna, K. Bashetty, S. Srirekha, L. Lekha, and C. Champa, "An in vitro evaluation of fracture strength of endodontically treated teeth with simulated flared root

canals restored with different post and core systems," *Journal of Conservative Dentistry*, vol. 15, no. 3, pp. 223–227, 2012.

[35] A. Bacchi, M. B. Fernandes dos Santos, M. J. Pimentel, C. R. Caetano, M. A. C. Sinhoreti, and R. L. X. Consani, "Influence of post-thickness and material on the fracture strength of teeth with reduced coronal structure," *Journal of Conservative Dentistry*, vol. 16, no. 2, pp. 139–143, 2013.

[36] J. R. Pereira, A. Lins Do Valle, F. K. Shiratori, J. S. Ghizoni, and E. A. Bonfante, "The effect of post material on the characteristic strength of fatigued endodontically treated teeth," *Journal of Prosthetic Dentistry*, vol. 112, no. 5, pp. 1225–1230, 2014.

[37] D. Sendhilnathan and S. Nayar, "The effect of post-core and ferrule on the fracture resistance of endodontically treated maxillary central incisors," *Indian Journal of Dental Research*, vol. 19, no. 1, pp. 17–21, 2008.

[38] R. R. Barcellos, D. P. D. Correia, A. P. Farina, M. F. Mesquita, C. C. R. Ferraz, and D. Cecchin, "Fracture resistance of endodontically treated teeth restored with intra-radicular post: the effects of post system and dentine thickness," *Journal of Biomechanics*, vol. 46, no. 15, pp. 2572–2577, 2013.

[39] M. Raedel, C. Fiedler, S. Jacoby, and K. W. Boening, "Survival of teeth treated with cast post and cores: a retrospective analysis over an observation period of up to 19.5 years," *Journal of Prosthetic Dentistry*, vol. 114, no. 1, article 1655, pp. 40–45, 2015.

[40] S. M. L. B. Camarinha, L. C. Pardini, L. D. F. R. Garcia, S. Consani, and F. D. C. P. Pires-de-Souza, "Cast metal core adaptation using two impression materials and intracanal techniques," *Brazilian Journal of Oral Sciences*, vol. 8, no. 3, pp. 128–131, 2009.

[41] L. W. Stockton, "Factors affecting retention of post systems: a literature review," *Journal of Prosthetic Dentistry*, vol. 81, no. 4, pp. 380–385, 1999.

[42] H. O'Kray, T. S. Marshall, and T. M. Braun, "Supplementing retention through crown/preparation modification: an in vitro study," *Journal of Prosthetic Dentistry*, vol. 107, no. 3, pp. 186–190, 2012.

[43] L. H. A. Raposo, G. R. Silva, P. C. F. Santos-Filho et al., "Effect of anti-rotation devices on biomechanical behaviour of teeth restored with cast post-and-cores," *International Endodontic Journal*, vol. 43, no. 8, pp. 681–691, 2010.

[44] A. Gopi, R. K. Dhiman, and D. Kumar, "A simple antirotational mechanism in a posterior two piece post and core," *Medical Journal Armed Forces India*, vol. 71, supplement 2, pp. S601–S604, 2015.

[45] H. Cho, K. X. Michalakis, Y. Kim, and H. Hirayama, "Impact of interproximal groove placement and remaining coronal tooth structure on the fracture resistance of endodontically treated maxillary anterior teeth," *Journal of Prosthodontics*, vol. 18, no. 1, pp. 43–48, 2009.

[46] A. Kutesa-Mutebi and Y. I. Osman, "Effect of the ferrule on fracture resistance of teeth restored with prefabricated posts and composite cores," *African Health Sciences*, vol. 4, no. 2, pp. 131–135, 2004.

[47] I. Tacir and Z. Polat, "The effect of ferrule on the fracture resistance of teeth restored with cast dowel system," *Biotechnology and Biotechnological Equipment*, vol. 20, no. 3, pp. 157–161, 2006.

[48] "The glossary of prosthodontic terms," *The Journal of Prosthetic Dentistry*, vol. 94, no. 1, pp. 10–92, 2005.

[49] R. W. Loney, W. E. Kotowicz, and G. C. McDowell, "Three-dimensional photoelastic stress analysis of the ferrule effect in cast post and cores," *The Journal of Prosthetic Dentistry*, vol. 63, no. 5, pp. 506–512, 1990.

[50] M. Nayak, K. Prasada, and D. Shetty, "Fracture resistance of endodontically treated teeth restored with custom cast post core using non uniform and uniform ferrule length luted with two different cements: in vitro study," *Indian Endodontology*, vol. 22, no. 1, pp. 78–86, 2010.

[51] S. Goyal, P. V. Shyamala, R. Miglani, and L. Narayanan, "Metal collars—are they serving any purpose?" *Journal of Conservative Dentistry*, vol. 10, no. 1, pp. 14–18, 2007.

[52] N. R. Da Silva, L. H. A. Raposo, A. Versluis, A. J. Fernandes-Neto, and C. J. Soares, "The effect of post, core, crown type, and ferrule presence on the biomechanical behavior of endodontically treated bovine anterior teeth," *Journal of Prosthetic Dentistry*, vol. 104, no. 5, pp. 306–317, 2010.

[53] M. G. Roscoe, P. Y. Noritomi, V. R. Novais, and C. J. Soares, "Influence of alveolar bone loss, post type, and ferrule presence on the biomechanical behavior of endodontically treated maxillary canines: strain measurement and stress distribution," *Journal of Prosthetic Dentistry*, vol. 110, no. 2, pp. 116–126, 2013.

[54] A. M. E. Marchionatti, V. F. Wandscher, J. Broch et al., "Influence of periodontal ligament simulation on bond strength and fracture resistance of roots restored with fiber posts," *Journal of Applied Oral Science*, vol. 22, no. 5, pp. 450–458, 2014.

[55] A. R. Giovani, L. P. Vansan, M. D. de Sousa Neto, and S. M. Paulino, "In vitro fracture resistance of glass-fiber and cast metal posts with different lengths," *Journal of Prosthetic Dentistry*, vol. 101, no. 3, pp. 183–188, 2009.

[56] R. Del Castillo, C. Ercoli, G. N. Graser, R. H. Tallents, and M. E. Moss, "Effect of ring liner and casting ring temperature on the dimension of cast posts," *Journal of Prosthetic Dentistry*, vol. 84, no. 1, pp. 32–37, 2000.

[57] P. A. Hansen, "Predictable casting for dimensional shrinkage of fast-cast post-and-cores," *Operative Dentistry*, vol. 39, no. 4, pp. 367–373, 2014.

[58] D. F. Pascoe, "Analysis of the geometry of finishing lines for full crown restorations," *The Journal of Prosthetic Dentistry*, vol. 40, no. 2, pp. 157–162, 1978.

[59] R. J. Hoard, A. A. Caputo, R. M. Contino, and M. E. Koenig, "Intracoronal pressure during crown cementation," *The Journal of Prosthetic Dentistry*, vol. 40, no. 5, pp. 520–525, 1978.

[60] K. Dreyer and Jørgensen, "The relationship between retention and convergence angle in cemented veneer crowns," *Acta Odontologica Scandinavica*, vol. 13, no. 1, pp. 35–40, 1955.

[61] M. R. Dimashkieh, E. H. Davies, and J. A. von Fraunhofer, "Measurement of the cement film thickness beneath full crown restorations," *British Dental Journal*, vol. 137, no. 7, pp. 281–284, 1974.

[62] P. Aditya, V. N. V. Madhav, S. V. Bhide, and A. Aditya, "Marginal discrepancy as affected by selective placement of die-spacer: an in vitro study," *Journal of Indian Prosthodontist Society*, vol. 12, no. 3, pp. 143–148, 2012.

[63] W. B. Eames, S. J. O'Neal, J. Monteiro, C. Miller, J. D. Roan Jr., and K. S. Cohen, "Techniques to improve the seating of castings," *The Journal of the American Dental Association*, vol. 96, no. 3, pp. 432–437, 1978.

[64] R. Grajower, Y. Zuberi, and I. Lewinstein, "Improving the fit of crowns with die spacers," *The Journal of Prosthetic Dentistry*, vol. 61, no. 5, pp. 555–563, 1989.

[65] R. Pilo, H. S. Cardash, H. Baharav, and M. Helft, "Incomplete seating of cemented crowns: a literature review," *The Journal of Prosthetic Dentistry*, vol. 59, no. 4, pp. 429–433, 1988.

[66] A. Ishikiriama, J. de Freitas Oliveira, D. F. Vieira, and J. Mondelli, "Influence of some factors on the fit of cemented crowns," *The Journal of Prosthetic Dentistry*, vol. 45, no. 4, pp. 400–404, 1981.

[67] J. R. Strub, O. Pontius, and S. Koutayas, "Survival rate and fracture strength of incisors restored with different post and core systems after exposure in the artificial mouth," *Journal of Oral Rehabilitation*, vol. 28, no. 2, pp. 120–124, 2001.

[68] P. Milot and R. S. Stein, "Root fracture in endodontically treated teeth related to post selection and crown design," *The Journal of Prosthetic Dentistry*, vol. 68, no. 3, pp. 428–435, 1992.

[69] P. Gateau, M. Sabek, and B. Dailey, "Fatigue testing and microscopic evaluation of post and core restorations under artificial crowns," *The Journal of Prosthetic Dentistry*, vol. 82, no. 3, pp. 341–347, 1999.

[70] A. G. Gegauff, "Effect of crown lengthening and ferrule placement on static load failure of cemented cast post-cores and crowns," *Journal of Prosthetic Dentistry*, vol. 84, no. 2, pp. 169–179, 2000.

[71] L. Shamseddine, R. Eid, F. Homsy, and H. Elhusseini, "Effect of tapering internal coronal walls on fracture resistance of anterior teeth treated with cast post and core: in vitro study," *Journal of Dental Biomechanics*, vol. 5, 2014.

10

Developmental Immunotoxicity, Perinatal Programming, and Noncommunicable Diseases: Focus on Human Studies

Rodney R. Dietert

Department of Microbiology and Immunology, College of Veterinary Medicine, Cornell University, North Tower Road, Ithaca, NY 14853, USA

Correspondence should be addressed to Rodney R. Dietert; rrd1@cornell.edu

Academic Editor: Gernot Zissel

Developmental immunotoxicity (DIT) is a term given to encompass the environmentally induced disruption of normal immune development resulting in adverse outcomes. A myriad of chemical, physical, and psychological factors can all contribute to DIT. As a core component of the developmental origins of adult disease, DIT is interlinked with three important concepts surrounding health risks across a lifetime: (1) the Barker Hypothesis, which connects prenatal development to later-life diseases, (2) the hygiene hypothesis, which connects newborns and infants to risk of later-life diseases and, (3) fetal programming and epigenetic alterations, which may exert effects both in later life and across future generations. This review of DIT considers: (1) the history and context of DIT research, (2) the fundamental features of DIT, (3) the emerging role of DIT in risk of noncommunicable diseases (NCDs) and (4) the range of risk factors that have been investigated through human research. The emphasis on the human DIT-related literature is significant since most prior reviews of DIT have largely focused on animal research and considerations of specific categories of risk factors (e.g., heavy metals). Risk factors considered in this review include air pollution, aluminum, antibiotics, arsenic, bisphenol A, ethanol, lead (Pb), maternal smoking and environmental tobacco smoke, paracetamol (acetaminophen), pesticides, polychlorinated biphenyls, and polyfluorinated compounds.

1. Introduction

Early-life environmental insults affecting the developing immune system can have significant health ramifications not only for the exposed offspring but also potentially extending to additional generations. Developmental immunotoxicity (DIT) appears to play a significant role in the current global epidemic of non-communicable diseases (NCDs) [1, 2]. This review of DIT begins with the history of DIT placed in the context of the area of immunology known as immunotoxicology and charts the emergence of recent concepts concerning early developmental programming as it impacts later-life health. It also describes the current state of the science for DIT and the likely applications of DIT assessment as it may impact both human health and environmental protection. In particular, the paper discusses (1) the history of DIT research, (2) the role of critical windows of vulnerability for the developing immune system, (3) frequent outcomes of DIT, (4) consideration of the microbiome in DIT, (5) the role of prenatal epigenetic alterations in immunotoxicity, and (6) the

connection between DIT, elevated risk of comorbid chronic diseases, and current epidemic of NCDs.

2. History of DIT Research

2.1. Emergence within Immunotoxicology. Immunotoxicology, the study of the adverse impact of environmental conditions (e.g., exposure to food, drugs, chemicals, microbial agents, and physical and psychosocial factors) on the immune system, began to gain recognition during the 1970s and early 1980s [3] with the initial focus on use of surrogates for host resistance in animal models [4, 5] and concern about environmentally induced immunosuppression [6]. The search for assays and parameters that were predictive of chemical- or drug-induced immunotoxicity centered on measures that could replace then cumbersome and costly host challenges with infectious agents or transplantable cancer cells. Not surprisingly loss of immune protection (i.e., immunosuppression) and increased susceptibility to infections and/or cancer were a driving concern. This also coincided with the era in which the HIV-induced immunosuppression associated with AIDS was an increasing human health challenge [7, 8]. A coordinated effort to identify the best predictor of immunotoxicity resulted in the development of the tier system of assays providing a strategy of immunotoxicity testing [9] and the concept that a limited combination of immune measures could be effective for identifying immunotoxic chemicals [10, 11]. In addition to the identification of chemicals that could produce immunosuppression in humans [12], the detection of chemicals with sensitizing potential was an early systematic concern within immunotoxicology [13, 14].

The examination of adverse insults to the developing immune system, a subsection of immunotoxicology known as developmental immunotoxicity (DIT), was among the first research initiatives within immunotoxicology. As early as the 1970s, animal studies revealed the persistent nature of immune problems resulting from early-life insult. Studies involving drugs [15, 16], heavy metals [17, 18], pesticides [19], mold toxins [20–22], and polycyclic aromatic hydrocarbons [23] suggested that the developmental periods of immune system formation, dissemination, and acquired host defense capacities represent developmental windows that need to be research and public safety priorities. Yet, developmental studies represented only one of several aspects of immunotoxicological research and the term "developmental immunotoxicity" was not prevalent in the literature until the mid-1990s [24, 25].

DIT did not achieve a priority position for research and safety evaluation within immunotoxicology until approximately the late 1990s–early 2000s. Among the important events were a workshop on childhood health risks coordinated by the March of Dimes and EPA [26–28], the publication of a seminar text on compiling DIT research [29], and the increasing recognition of fetal programming of later-life health and disease [30–32]. Basic features of developmental immunotoxicity (DIT) have emerged during decades of research. These features are shown as follow

DIT

  (i) is directly linked with immune dysfunction and increased risk of NCDs,

  (ii) stems from critical developmental windows of immune vulnerability restricted to the young,

  (iii) can happen at lower exposure levels than usually produce adult-exposure immunotoxicity,

  (iv) often involves a broader spectrum of adverse immune outcome versus adult-exposure immunotoxicity,

  (v) usually produces more persistent effects than those following adult exposure,

  (vi) can lead to latent dysfunction that may be masked until it is triggered by a later-life event,

  (vii) often manifests as immune dysfunctional imbalances (suppression of some immune responses along with the inappropriate enhancement of others),

  (viii) may produce different sex-based outcomes,

  (ix) is not routinely assessed in most required safety testing protocols to date,

  (x) can occur via several different biological pathways (e.g., impaired immune maturation, epigenetic alteration, and immune-microbiome disruption).

The DIT literature is sufficiently extensive to permit fundamental characterizations. This information is derived from [1, 27, 33–40].

2.2. DIT and the Barker Hypothesis. The impetus for a greater focus on DIT was aided by the findings of Barker and colleagues that maternal undernutrition during prenatal development could increase the risk of cardiovascular disease (CVD) in the offspring [41–43]. This led to what has been termed the "Barker Hypothesis" [44]. Originally, the linkage between fetal environment-adult disease was focused solely on maternal nutrition and CVD (including both coronary heart disease and hypertension) as an example linking early developmental conditions and fetal programming to later-life adult disease. But it became clear that the same relationship could exist for many other adult chronic diseases and conditions (e.g., renal disease and type 2 diabetes, in adult offspring that were also affected by the fetal nutritional environment) [45, 46].

2.3. DIT and Developmental Origins of Adult Health and Disease (DOHaD). As the net was cast beyond just maternal-fetal nutritional status to include a wide array of environmental conditions and factors, the concept of developmental origins of health and disease (DOHaD) emerged [47, 48] to connect critical windows of development with specific childhood and adult health risks. Immune damage, dysfunction, and/or imbalances are now known to persist long after either toxicant levels of chemical exposures return to normal or physical-psychosocial stressors have been removed [33, 34]. In fact, part of the challenge in deciphering pathways resulting in DIT and fetal programming of adverse immune status is that evidence of prior problematic exposure conditions may remain largely hidden. For this reason, DIT testing usually requires careful consideration about exposure windows and immunological assessment tools [35, 36, 49]. The opportunity to examine the different functional responses of the immune system in response to various challenges has emerged as a key component of safety assessment [35, 50, 51].

3. Fundamental Features of DIT

3.1. Heightened Sensitivity of the Developing Immune System. One of the hallmarks of the developing immune system is that it exhibits an increased sensitivity for most environmentally induced toxicity compared with the fully matured immune system of the adult. Additionally, DIT often occurs at exposure doses that are below those producing other developmental effects [52–55]. Luebke et al. [33] reviewed the evidence of comparative age-based sensitivity for five of the most extensively studied drugs and environmental chemicals: diethylstilbestrol (DES), diazepam (DZP), lead (Pb), 2,3,7,8-tetrachlorodibenzo-p-dioxin (TCDD), and tributyltin oxide (TBO). They concluded that early development appears to be a time of increased sensitivity to xenobiotics and risk of adverse immune outcomes that are likely to persist into later life.

This increased risk of developmental immune insult compared with that of the adult has been seen across broad categories of drugs and chemicals as well as among different dietary and physical/psychological factors [1, 29, 37]. This differential, age-based sensitivity can take different forms, which are reviewed in detail in Dietert and Piepenbrink [38]. In many cases, the lowest dose required to produce immune disruption is several fold to several magnitudes lower in early life than in the adult [33]. Additionally, a broader array of immune parameters are likely to be affected following exposure of the nonadult versus the adult [54, 56]. Prenatal and early postnatal exposures are more likely to produce persistent adverse immune outcomes [57–60].

3.2. Critical Developmental Windows. The identification and consideration of both systemic and tissue-oriented developmental vulnerabilities for the immune system have undergone progressive evolution since the original series of immune "critical windows" emerged from a national workshop [27, 28]. As was illustrated in Dietert [1], for most key developmental steps of immune maturation, multiple environmental disruptors have been identified. The effect of inhibition or delay of a critical developmental step can increase the risk of multiple later-life diseases. For example, key processes of T cell selection in the thymus can be affected by maternal exposure to certain heavy metals, plasticizers, dioxins, polycyclic chlorinated biphenyls, tobacco smoke, and certain drugs. Not surprisingly, the adverse health outcomes that have been associated with environmental targeting of thymus-directed processes are largely restricted to prenatal development and cover virtually every category of disease including cancer as well as autoimmune and allergic diseases and childhood vaccine failures [1].

Each immune developmental window has its own unique vulnerabilities that are best detected via age-relevant safety screening [38]. For example, Bunn et al. [61] demonstrated that while Pb was immunotoxic across all windows of prenatal developmental, later gestational maternal exposures were more likely to result in profound T helper 2- (Th2-) favored functional skewing in the juvenile rat.

Application of the critical windows concept for enhanced immune-associated disease prevention has been explored by Jenmalm and Duchén [62]. These authors stressed that dietary interventions capable of aiding prevention of allergy are most likely to be effective if directed toward specific prenatal, perinatal, and early postnatal developmental windows [62].

4. Frequent Outcomes of DIT and Risk of Noncommunicable Diseases (NCDs)

One of the outcomes of the recent human studies on DIT and fetal programming of immune-based disease is an increasing realization that these processes are major contributors to the ongoing epidemic of noncommunicable diseases (NCDs) (most of which are chronic diseases). NCDs are the major cause of death globally and include cardiovascular disease as well as cancer [63]. What has become clear is that the vast majority of NCDs cannot be maintained in the absence of misregulated (usually unresolving) inflammation [39, 64, 65]. This means that improper immune homeostasis in tissues is likely to be required for NCD onset and/or maintenance. Human studies supported by animal model research have established the importance of the prenatal and early postnatal environment for maturation of innate immune cells in concert with formation of the microbiome in mucosal tissues and other sites (e.g., skin).

One of the impediments to recognizing this DIT-NCD linkage is that historic examination of immunotoxicity often focused on changes in primary and secondary immune organs. However, the majority of immune cells actually reside outside of these organs in mucosal and other tissues such as the gut, brain, skin, liver, endocrine, reproductive, urogenital, and cardiovascular systems. It is these tissues that are most often involved with NCDs, and the status of these resident immune cells is often at issue relative to tissue pathology. A shift in focus in immune evaluation to consider the impact of DIT and later-life status of cells such as skin dendritic cells, microglia, Kupffer cells, and immune cells of the BALT and GALT should provide a clearer picture of the cause-effect relationship between DIT and certain NCDs [66]. Table 1 provides examples of environmental factors and conditions that are thought to contribute to later-life human disease via DIT and immune dysfunction. NCDs represent the majority of examples shown in Table 1.

The significance of the prevention of DIT as a strategy to reduce the prevalence of NCDs has been strengthened with the awareness that NCDs exist as tightly intertwined patterns of comorbid risks. This paradigm of tightly interlinked chronic diseases and conditions was described in a series of papers illustrating the health risk trajectories that exist when children are diagnosed with a number of different immune-/inflammatory-driven conditions: asthma, recurrent infections, schizophrenia, autoimmune thyroiditis, celiac disease, inflammatory disease, and psoriasis [2, 34, 67, 68]. Cancer is one of the common outcomes in the tissue receiving the primary inflammatory insult [40]. Even end-stage conditions such as chronic kidney disease and frailty form part of these interlinked patterns of chronic diseases and conditions [39, 69].

As an example, one interconnected pattern of comorbidity exists among a triad of autoimmune conditions: type 1 diabetes, celiac disease, and autoimmune thyroiditis. Children diagnosed with type 1 diabetes have a predictably greater risk for developing celiac disease and/or autoimmune thyroiditis [70, 71]. While the mechanism remains to be elucidated, childhood asthma, obesity, and sleep disorders are similarly interlinked in a triad [72, 73]. Tanaka et al. [74] and Anders et al. [75] have pointed out that clinical depression is a largely immune driven, inflammatory-based condition that is another comorbid outcome intrinsically connected to many different NCDs/chronic diseases.

TABLE 1: DIT and increased risk of human disease*.

Disease, disorder, or susceptibility state	Suggested early-life immune-modulating risk factor	Reference(s)
Acute myeloid leukemia	Benzene	[173]
Allergic sensitization	Polychlorinated biphenyls	[170]
Asthma	Maternal paracetamol use	[155]
Atherosclerosis	Maternal hypercholesterolemia	[174]
Atopic dermatitis	Maternal smoking	[175]
Allergic rhinitis	Antibiotics in infancy	[176]
Autism spectrum disorders	Maternal immune activation	[177]
Bipolar disorder	Gestational influenza	[178]
Cardiovascular disease	Childhood abuse	[179]
Celiac disease	Elective cesarean delivery	[180]
Crohn's disease	Maternal smoking	[181]
Chronic obstructive pulmonary disease	Smoke from biomass fuels	[182]
Depression	Childhood trauma	[183]
Endometriosis	Environmental tobacco smoke	[184]
Hypertension	Pesticides (DDT)	[185]
Insulin resistance	Maternal diet	[186]
Lack of protection against diphtheria and tetanus following childhood vaccination	Perfluorinated pollutants	[171]
Multiple sclerosis	Vitamin D insufficiency	[187]
Myalgic encephalomyelitis (Chronic fatigue syndrome)	Childhood trauma	[188, 189]
Narcolepsy (specific subpopulation)	H1N1 flu vaccination	[190, 191]
Obesity/overweight risk	Cesarean delivery	[192]
Otitis media	Maternal smoking/ETS	[193–195]
Parkinson's disease	Pesticides	[164, 196]
Preeclampsia	Traffic-related air pollution	[197]
Psoriasis	Environmental tobacco smoke	[198]
Respiratory infections	Polychlorinated biphenyls	[199, 200]
Rheumatoid arthritis	Maternal smoking	[201]
Schizophrenia	Prenatal immune activation	[202, 203]
Sudden infant death syndrome	Maternal smoking and alcohol consumption	[133]
Type 1 diabetes	Lack of or short-duration breastfeeding	[204]
Ulcerative colitis	Urban living	[205]

*This table includes both noncommunicable and communicable diseases and conditions. Environmental risk factors are provided to illustrate an example and are not intended to be an exhaustive listing. The focus is on human studies and data.

The ramification of these comorbid disease interconnections is that there is increased value in avoiding fetal programming that results in childhood-onset, immune dysfunction-based NCDs. These implications led four immunotoxicologists to call for required DIT testing of chemicals and drugs as a step to better protect children from the risk of NCDs [2].

5. Human Studies Involving DIT: Alphabetical List of Risk Factors

Most prior reviews of DIT have focused largely on animal research. This section examines the wide range of risk factors for DIT that has been evaluated among human populations. Evidence supporting the occurrence of DIT among human populations has been obtained from both exposed populations as well as via epidemiological studies. The risk factors are presented alphabetically rather than being grouped into different categories (e.g., chemicals, drugs, physical, and psychological factors).

In many of these studies antibody titers against either a common virus or childhood vaccinations have been used as a biomarker of DIT. While limited as an overall immune measure, there are significant benefits to this approach: (1) serum antibody levels are easily determined, (2) a majority of children will have been vaccinated according to a predictable and standard schedule, and (3) the microbial infection or vaccine challenge of the child's immune system will enable a detection of potential dysfunction in an actively responding immune system and, based on animal data, these are among the most sensitive parameters for measuring DIT. Other studies reach beyond vaccination data to examine associations between exposure/environmental conditions and immune-based chronic diseases during childhood. Among the most commonly used are asthma, allergic rhinitis, atopic dermatitis, type 1 diabetes, celiac disease, and inflammatory bowel disease. Only a portion of these disease-association studies has overt human immune function associated with them. For the remainder, there has been a tendency to rely more on linking DIT immune function animal data with information on human immune disease-associations.

5.1. Air Pollution. Ambient air pollution including specific components (e.g., polycyclic aromatic hydrocarbons, particulate matter) has been implicated in respiratory and cardiovascular diseases via improperly controlled inflammation. Nadeau et al. [76] examined groups of asthmatic and nonasthmatic children in Fresno, CA, for pollutant exposure, T regulatory (Treg) cell activity (that would help to control Th2 mediated asthma symptoms), and DNA methylation. The researchers found that increased exposure to ambient air pollutants was associated with increased methylation of CpG islands at the Foxp3 locus as well as reduced Foxp3 expression [76]. They also reported reduced numbers of Fox3p+ Treg cells and reduced Treg activity particularly among the asthmatic children. The authors concluded that increased air pollution exposure in children is associated with increased asthma morbidity via epigenetic alterations and a possible immune mechanism [76].

Kerkhof et al. [77] found evidence in children that traffic-related air pollution (e.g., particulate matter (PM) 2.5, 10, soot, and nitrogen dioxide) increased the prevalence of doctor-diagnosed asthma by year 8 particularly among children with specific variant alleles for the toll-like receptor (TLR) genes 2 and 4. The investigators suggested that their results are consistent with the suspected involvement of innate immune response in the linkage between exposure to traffic pollution and risk of childhood asthma [77].

Calderón-Garcidueñas et al. [78] compared immune markers in asymptomatic children from two different city areas (Southwest Mexico City versus Polotitlán, Mexico as a control city) with vastly different burdens of urban air pollution. They found that children exposed to the severe air pollution had immune dysregulation with reduced levels of IFN-γ and natural killer cells with evidence of elevated systemic inflammation (elevated C-reactive protein and prostaglandin E metabolites).

Indoor air pollution, beyond that of environmental tobacco smoke, which is discussed in a later section, has also been associated with human DIT. Herberth et al. [79] studied the effects of home renovation (e.g., painting, flooring, and new furniture) on inflammatory biomarker profiles of six-year-old children. Significant increases in serum IL-8 and macrophage chemotactic protein 1 (MCP-1) were associated with home renovation activities. Installation of new wall-to-wall carpet gave the strongest single activity association with these markers.

5.2. Aluminum.

Aluminum exposure during prenatal and childhood development can occur via a variety of routes including via food, certain drugs (aluminum-containing antacids), drinking water, and air [80] including some parenteral nutrition products [81]. The immune system appears to be a sensitive target for aluminum [82]. However, a prevalent opportunity for repeated exposure is alum (aluminum oxyhydroxide)-containing vaccines. Alum is an adjuvant designed to promote a protective immune response, which may include a component of local inflammation (via specific cytokine release). One of the concerns with aluminum is the potential to sometimes induce inappropriate inflammation involving innate immune cells such as macrophages. In some individuals, such as those carrying HLA-DRB1*01, there appears to be an elevated risk of persistent macrophagic myofasciitis [83, 84], and this link has been proposed as one route to autoimmune/inflammatory syndrome induced by adjuvants (ASIA) [85].

There is evidence to suggest that febrile responses in children following alum-containing vaccination may represent an inflammation-driven hyperresponse that occurs in a subset of children, possibly those possessing certain cytokine gene alleles [86]. A proposed mechanistic basis for alum-induction of DIT in a subpopulation of children was discussed by Terhune and Deth [87]. These authors suggested that the Th2 biasing and inflammasome activating effects of aluminum may present a problem for children carrying genetic variants of certain cytokine genes (e.g., IL-4, IL-13, IL-33, and IL-18). In some subpopulations of children,

aluminum adjuvants might enhance the production of nontarget directed IgE thereby elevating the risk of allergy and atopy [87]. Other investigators have suggested that alum may play a role in the induction of Crohn's disease in genetically susceptible individuals [88].

5.3. Antibiotics.

Antibiotic use in early life has been associated with an elevated risk of immune-based diseases such as childhood asthma. Raciborski et al. [89] found that antibiotic use during the first three years of life was associated with a significantly elevated risk of asthma by 6–8 years of age among 1461 children in Warszawa, Poland. The highest association was found between infants who completed three courses of antibiotic within the first year of life and later childhood asthma (OR = 5.59, 95% CI: 2.6–12.01) [89]. Not all authors agree on this association. Heintze and Petersen [90] argue that various forms of bias weaken the literature on perinatal antibiotic use and risk of childhood asthma. However, the impact of repeated antibiotic use on the microbiome during immune development provides a potential mechanistic basis for DIT, Th2 skewing, and misregulated inflammation [91].

Extensive antibiotic use is of particular concern when viewed in the context of the hygiene hypothesis or the recently-described "Completed Self" model (i.e., where unimpeded comaturation of the development immune system and infant microbiome is critical) [91] (see Figure 1). Under the "Completed Self" paradigm, successful development of a balanced, well-regulated immune system needs comaturation with a complete microbiome in the infant. The developing immune system receives important signals from the commensal microbes and eventually matures to perceive self as a combination of the mammalian cells and commensal microbes. The successful merger of the infant's mammalian and microbial components into the fully formed human-microbial superorganism may well represent the single most important step distinguishing later-life health from disease. As a result, any prenatal or postnatal environmental exposure that interferes with timely and effective self-completion is a significant health risk [91]. This new immunological view of what constitutes a fully completed infant could impact risk-benefit considerations for antibiotic administration in early life.

5.4. Arsenic.

Arsenic is found in both inorganic and organic forms. Most of the environmental health concerns have focused on the inorganic forms of arsenic (e.g., arsenite or arsenate) with exposure occurring primarily via ingestion of contaminated food and water and secondarily via inhalation. Some forms of arsenic (e.g., arsenic trioxide) have been used in the treatment of leukemias. The topic of arsenic-induced immunotoxicity was recently reviewed by Dangleben et al. [92]. These authors stressed the increased vulnerability of infants and children to arsenic-induced immune dysfunction and the potential for early-life exposures to produce later-life health problems.

Studies of exposed human populations also suggest that arsenic is a major concern for DIT, and several studies have examined children in Mexico and Bangladesh among

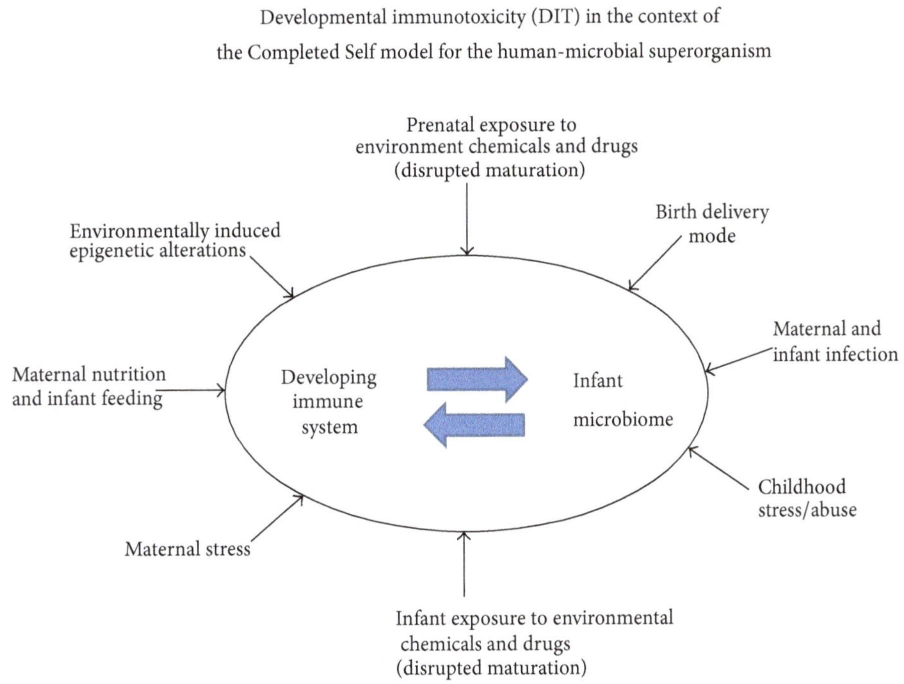

Developmental immunotoxicity (DIT) in the context of
the Completed Self model for the human-microbial superorganism

FIGURE 1: This figure depicts a model following the "Completed Self" paradigm [91] in which the immune system and infant microbiome need to comature without interference or disruption to reduce later-life health risks. The categories of environmental risk factors reported to cause prenatal and/or postnatal disruption are illustrated.

highly exposed populations. Soto-Peña et al., [93] found that children in Mexico (6–10 years old) with arsenic exposure primarily from drinking water (evaluated based on urinary levels) had peripheral blood mononuclear cells (PBMs) that were shifted in ex vivo stimulated function (proliferation and cytokine secretion). Rocha-Amador et al. [94] found that children in Mexico living in an area with high exposure to arsenic via drinking water had increased apoptosis among PBMs compared with those from an area with lower exposure levels. In a study of Bangladeshi children where a significant exposure to arsenic can occur via drinking water, Ahmed et al. [95] found that prenatal exposure to arsenic interfered with thymic function affecting T cell development. The proposed route of insult was via oxidative damage and possible misregulation of apoptosis. The same investigators demonstrated that prenatal exposure to arsenic was associated with increased placental inflammation increasing oxidative stress and altering both T cell and cytokine profiles in cord blood [96].

This suggests that, at physiologically-relevant exposures, arsenic-induced DIT can manifest almost immediately during fetal development. This is consistent with the findings of arsenic-exposed children in Mexico where increased arsenic levels were associated with increased basal nitric oxide production by monocytes and increased superoxide anion produced by activated monocytes [97]. Taken together these studies suggest that a proinflammatory state is part of the profile of arsenic-induced human DIT. Lower resistance to certain infectious diseases has been associated with early-life exposure to arsenic. In a prospective population-based cohort study, 1,552 Bangladeshi infants were examined for both lower respiratory tract and diarrhea-associated infections and compared versus maternal arsenic levels during the pregnancy (measured at two time points via urine) [98]. Rahman et al. [98] found that the highest quadril of maternal arsenic exposure versus the lowest had a significantly elevated risk of both forms of mucosal tissue infections. Lower respiratory tract infections had a 69% increased relative risk for infants of high arsenic exposed mothers adjusted relative risk (RR = 1.69; 95% confidence interval (CI), 1.36–2.09), whereas there was a 20% increased risk of diarrheal-associated infections (RR = 1.20; 95% CI, 1.01–1.43) among the same groups.

5.5. Bisphenol A. Bisphenol A (BPA) is used in a variety of food and beverage containers. Most human chemical exposure occurs via food and beverages although exposure via air, dust, and water is also possible. Sources of BPA include food storage containers, water bottles, baby bottles, and polycarbonate tableware. BPA has received significant immune system evaluation in recent years although the majority of studies, to date, have been performed in rodents.

Rogers et al. [99] recently reviewed the immunotoxicologic profile of BPA suggesting that it (1) increases Th2 polarization of dendritic cells, (2) alters macrophage inflammatory cytokine production and metabolism but with different dose-dependent effects, (3) decreases T regulatory cells, (4) alters the relative proportions of immunoglobulin (Ig) producing cells, and (5) polarizes CD4+ T helper (Th) cells although the direction of polarization (e.g., Th1 versus Th2) has differed among studies.

Human studies for BPA and DIT are comparatively limited to date. In a National Health and Nutrition Examination Survey (NHANES) study, children and teens less than 18 years of age exhibited an inverse correlation of BPA exposure (urinary levels of BPA) with antibody levels against cytomegalovirus [100]. Kim et al. [101] examined the genomic alteration patterns of Egyptian prepubescent girls (ages 10–13) relative to both genome-wide methylation and methylation of genes previously identified as sensitive to BPA exposure. Among those genes prominently modified were those involved with immune response and autoimmune thyroid disease. Taken together, the animal and human studies suggest that early-life exposure to problematic doses of BPA produces altered gene expression related to immune function and inflammatory responses. However, more research is needed to define the boundaries of these alterations and the impact on various immune-related diseases in later life.

5.6. Cesarean Section. Cesarean section (CS) can be a medical necessity in some circumstances. However, the increased prevalence of elective CS (versus vaginal delivery (VD)) has created a public health concern [102]. CS has been reported to alter the course of immune development by producing Th skewing, innate immune dysfunction, and an increased likelihood of exacerbated inflammatory responses (reviewed in [103–105]). There are a minimum of four possible factors with Cesarean delivery that may contribute to subsequent DIT: (1) failure to properly seed the newborn's mucosal tissues with microbiota from the maternal vaginal tract, (2) the prophylactic use of antibiotics, (3) other drug administration connected with the Cesarean operation, and (4) the contrasting placental immune-stress-hormonal environment between the two delivery modes.

In the first category, birth delivery mode can significantly affect the microbiota and the subsequent immune-microbiome interactions. In a Canadian study, Azad et al. [106] found that infants delivered by elective Caesarean were much lower in the bacterial diversity and richness of their microbiome. In the fourth category from above, the immune physiology of vaginal delivery (versus CS) appears to create a strikingly different environment for the full-term fetus. A cross-sectional study of 375 women in The Netherlands compared spontaneous, term VDs versus elective CSs for signs of intrauterine inflammation. Houben et al. [107] found that measures of placental inflammation and amniotic fluid proinflammatory cytokines (IL-6, TNF-α, and IL-8) were significantly elevated with VD versus CS. The investigators suggested that increased sterile inflammation during labor and VD delivery may play a critical role in normal parturition and facilitate subsequent maturational processes (e.g., immune and airway maturation) in the newborn [107].

CS has been associated with altered levels of immune cell populations, cytokines, and chemokines in neonates leading Cho and Norman [105] to suggest that it should not be recommended except where there is a clear medical

indication or a benefit over risk estimate including long-term consideration for the infant child. For example, CS has been found to skew the infant immune profiles toward a Th2 biased capacity [108]. Innate immune maturational markers are also affected. Elective CS without labor was found to be associated with reduced surface expression of two different toll-like receptors (TLRs): TLR2 and TLR4. In contrast, labor and vaginal delivery appears to upregulate these TLRs to adult levels [109]. Because these TLRs are important in innate immunity, the authors suggest that labor is an important component of ongoing immune maturation [109]. The concentrations of the chemokine, RANTES (CCL5), a chemokine important in recruiting immune cells to inflammatory sites, were found to be lower in neonates from CS than VD [110]. In a prospective study of full-term deliveries, Malamitsi-Puchner et al. [111] found that VD neonates had elevated levels of both soluble IL-2 receptor and TNF-α compared with CS delivered babies. Taken together, these studies suggest that neonatal immune profiles, including early inflammatory interactions, are locked into a less mature, more-fetal-like state following CS versus VD deliveries. Not surprisingly, this appears to have consequences relative to risk of childhood chronic diseases.

CS with the outcome of low bacterial diversity in the infant is reported to increase the risk of several immune-based diseases emerging in children including asthma [112, 113], atopic dermatitis [114], celiac disease [115], and type 1 diabetes [116, 117]. A meta-analysis of 23 studies on CS and asthma estimated that the increased risk associated with this birth delivery mode was estimated at 20% [118]. Of note is the observation that specific subpopulations may be at an increased risk for the disease-promoting aspects of CS. For example, Magnus et al. [119] found that the association between CS and childhood asthma (at 3 years of age) was strongest among children of nonatopic mothers.

5.7. Childhood Abuse. In children who experience abuse, the developing immune system appears to become wired for dysfunctional responses. In the Nurses' Health Study II, Bertone-Johnson [120] found that women reporting moderate to severe childhood or adolescent abuse had significantly elevated levels of two inflammatory markers CRP and IL-6 as adults. The authors argued that early-life stress may program the immune system for dysregulation and that subsequent immune dysregulation elevates the risk of certain chronic diseases. Slopen et al. [121] make a similar link between childhood adverse experiences, misregulated inflammation, and risk of cardiovascular disease.

5.8. Diethylstilbestrol. While human immunological studies on diethylstilbestrol (DES) are limited compared with other health-related studies, there are reports suggesting that prenatally-exposed offspring are at a higher risk of immune-based disease. Overall DES daughters exposed in utero self-reported an increased risk of all immune-based diseases (infections, allergies, and autoimmune conditions). Within specific categories, the women experienced more infectious diseases than non-DES exposed daughters [122]. In a separate study, Strohsnitter et al. [123] examined the incidence of selected autoimmune conditions among DES daughters. They found no overall increase in disease associations for rheumatoid arthritis (RA), systemic lupus erythematosus (SLE), optic neuritis (ON), or idiopathic thrombocytopenic purpura (ITP). However, there was a significant increase in the onset of RA by 45 years of age in the DES-exposed versus nonexposed groups [123].

5.9. Ethanol.

There are substantial data from animals suggesting that developmental exposure to alcohol produces DIT [55, 124] and can elevate the risk of non-communicable diseases possibly via inflammatory processes [125]. Maternal consumption of alcohol during pregnancy can produce immune-related adverse outcomes in the offspring. In fact, later gestation appears to be particularly sensitive to the effect of ethanol [126]. Among the reported long-term effects was interference with the immune response to influenza virus challenge in mice [127].

Remarkably, human studies are limited for low-level ethanol intake and DIT-related outcomes. Most studies following children exposed in utero to alcohol have focused on growth and behavioral outcomes [128, 129]. Carson et al. [130] utilized the COPSAC prospective birth cohort comprising 411 children born to asthmatic mothers. The children were considered full term and lacked congenital abnormality, systemic illness, or history of mechanical ventilation or lower airway infection. For this study group, the risk of offspring atopic dermatitis was reported to be significantly elevated for any maternal alcohol consumption during pregnancy (HR 1.44, 95% CI 1.05–1.99, $P = 0.024$) even after exclusion of effects of maternal smoking or atopic dermatitis [130].

Two studies reported negative results for maternal alcohol intake and childhood asthma. Yuan et al. [131] examined the incidence of hospitalization for asthma to age 12 among children from 10,440 singleton full-term births in Denmark between the years 1984 and 1987. The authors reported no significant associations between alcohol and no alcohol consumption (HR 0.95; 95% CI 0.70–1.29) including different doses of alcohol as well as binge drinking. In a second study, Shaheen et al. [132] examined maternal alcohol consumption during pregnancy relative to risk of childhood atopic disease (asthma and hayfever) measured at seven years of age within the Avon Longitudinal Study of Parents and Children (ALSPAC). They found no elevated risk for late gestational alcohol consumption with asthma or hayfever and no difference among mothers carrying different alleles for the alcohol dehydrogenase gene [132].

A case-controlled study in Ireland with infants born in 1994–2001 examined factors that are potentially involved with sudden infant death syndrome (SIDS) [133]. McDonnell Naughton et al. [133] reported that mothers of infants with SIDS were more likely to have consumed alcohol during pregnancy than controls (HR 3.59, 95% CI 1.40–9.20).

5.10. Lead (Pb).

A cadre of heavy metals has been examined for DIT and associated health risks in both children and adults. Among the most consistent observations with lead (Pb) are elevated risk of oxidative damage and a skewing toward Th2-driven responses with elevated levels of IgE. As an indicator of Pb's ability to produce misregulated inflammation, Pineda-Zavaleta et al. [134] found the macrophages isolated from Pb-exposed children stimulated in vitro with lipopolysaccharide overproduced superoxide anion. Karmaus et al. [135] reported that Pb exposure was associated with elevated IgE in children. Li et al. [136] reported a negative correlation between circulating CD4+T cells and blood lead levels. Lutz et al. [137] found that combined exposure to Pb and environmental tobacco smoke was strongly associated with elevated serum IgE levels in children. The human data are consistent with the animal studies suggesting that Th skewing, increased oxidative stress and tissue damage, and misregulated inflammation are among the adverse immune outcomes following developmental exposure to Pb [138].

5.11. Maternal Smoking and Environmental Tobacco Smoke.

There are several suggested developmental risk factors for asthma. Among these, maternal smoking during pregnancy and exposure of the infant to environmental tobacco smoke (ETS) were identified by Selgrade et al. [139] as having the most convincing body of evidence connecting environmental exposure to DIT and risk of childhood asthma. Additionally, Prescott [140] identified early life exposure to tobacco smoke producing altered immune function as being an important contributor to risk of allergic diseases. Among the pathways proposed to be involved is the capacity of maternal smoking to alter TLR-mediated responses in infant innate immune cells [140]. Noakes et al. [141] suggest that smoking induced TLR alterations will affect not only the developing immune system but also the "hygiene hypothesis" effects of immune-microbiome interactions in the newborn. The capacity of DIT to disrupt integrity of the immune-microbiome (the Completed Self model) is depicted in Figure 1.

Wilson et al. [142] reported that exposure of children to secondhand smoke produced significant changes in cytokine levels particularly reducing the level of IFN-γ. As previously mentioned in the section on Pb, Lutz et al. [137] reported an interaction of environmental risk factors in which Pb-exposed children also exposed to ETS had elevated IgE and IL-4 levels and altered T cell populations. Similar results were obtained by Tebow et al. [143] for exposure covering both prenatal and postnatal periods. These researchers found that parental smoking was associated with a disrupted balance of IFN-γ to IL-4 among children of smokers. While IL-4 levels were unchanged in the comparison of children with parental smokers versus non-smokers, reduced IFN-γ was associated with parental smoking and a dose response relationship appeared to exist. Therefore, the balance of IFN-γ to IL-4 was shifted toward the latter.

Elevated risk of allergic diseases is not the only immune-based concern with early-life exposure to tobacco smoke. Kum-Nji et al. [144] reviewed the literature regarding ETS and childhood infection and concluded that there is no longer a doubt about this association. Supporting evidence has been seen using childhood vaccination. In an examination of 200 infants with a history of parental allergy, Baynam et al. [145]

found that, among children with parents who smoked, infants carrying a variant of the IL-4 receptor gene (the IL-4Ralpha 551 QR/QQ genotype) exhibited significantly altered immune responses. These included reduced IgG responses, reductions in certain T cell responses (e.g., those associated with IFN-γ production), and altered innate immune (defective TLR-driven) responses upon vaccination with tetanus toxoid. These studies suggest that early-life exposure to smoking causes immune dysbiosis (targeted inappropriately exaggerated responses as well as suppression) that includes both an elevated risk of certain allergic diseases as well as potentially impaired responses to childhood vaccination. In keeping with many other DIT studies involving other risk factors, it also suggests that some human subpopulations are likely to have enhanced vulnerability for smoking-related DIT.

Disrupted immune maturation is not the only pathway through which maternal smoking and ETS appear to affect later-life immune function. Wilhelm-Benartzi [146] found that childhood ETS exposure produced epigenetic marks in genes associated with both immune function and immune signaling.

5.12. Paracetamol. Prenatal and early infant exposure to paracetamol (acetaminophen) has been associated with an increased risk of a variety of wheeze-associated disorders in the child including asthma. In the case of prenatal exposure, a study from Denmark examined 197,060 singletons born in northern Denmark in 1996–2008 [147]. Paracetamol exposure during any trimester of the pregnancy resulted in an adjusted odds ratio of 1.35 (95% confidence interval: 1.17–1.57) for risk of asthma by the end of 2009 [131]. For infant exposure, Gonzalez-Barcala et al. [148] studied 20, 000 children in Galicia, Spain, and reported that paracetamol use during the first year of life led to a significant increased risk of asthma in 6-7-year-old children (odds ratio (OR) 2.04 (1.79–2.31)). Henderson and Shaheen [149] recently reviewed the epidemiological data regarding prenatal and infant exposure to paracetamol and an increased risk of childhood asthma. They argue that the evidence is sufficiently strong as to be compelling for this association but also point out that mechanistic causation remains a significant data gap.

One of the potential confounding factors is prevalence of infections and the use of antibiotics, which may coincide with administration of paracetamol [150]. Heintze and Petersen [90] argued that failure to distinguish among the confounding effects of these two factors would significantly weaken the proposed associations. However, Muc et al. [151] performed a cross-sectional study of 1063 primary school children in Portugal in which they partitioned the factors of paracetamol in early childhood and antibiotic administration relative to risk of asthma. Paracetamol use and antibiotic administration were independently found to increase the risk in children of current asthma (at the time of evaluation) as well as ever having asthma. Because frequency of paracetamol use was connected to increased allergic symptoms, the researchers suggested that dose-dependent associations may be present among the data [151]. Not all studies have reported positive associations for paracetamol and asthma. However, based on

an understanding of the pathways through which paracetamol is likely to affect offspring immune status and childhood health, Thiele et al. [152] called for a reconsideration of safety and dosage recommendation during pregnancy.

For potential infant use, McBride [153] argued that risk data combined with the likelihood of glutathione depletion by paracetamol in the airways suggested that children at risk for asthma should avoid the use of paracetamol. Selgrade et al. [139] pointed out that accompanying animal data have been generally lacking in DIT models of the human paracetamol-asthma linkage. However, these authors also point to the overall importance of oxidative stress and inflammation as likely routes for xenobiotic-induced, DIT-related asthma. This would be consistent with findings of several research groups.

Evidence from several studies suggests that disruption of effective oxygen species regulation is a likely route to the elevated risk. Kang et al. [154] reported that postnatal pediatric use of paracetamol was more likely to produce asthma among children carrying specific genetic alleles associated with control of oxidative inflammation (*NAT2*, *Nrf2*, and *GSTP1*). Shaheen et al. [155] examined the effect of specific maternal alleles for nuclear erythroid 2 p45-related factor 2 (*Nrf2*) and glutathione S-transferase (GST) polymorphisms within data from the Avon Longitudinal Study of Parents and Children. They found that maternal *Nrf2* allelic differences had an effect on early gestation exposure to paracetamol and childhood asthma, while the presence of the *GSTT1* allele was important in late gestational exposure to paracetamol [155]. Taken together, these studies suggest that subpopulation differences are likely to exist for the relative risks of association between prenatal exposure to paracetamol and childhood-onset asthma.

5.13. Pesticides. Pesticides fall into several different chemical categories (e.g., organophosphate, organochlorine, and pyrethroids). However, humans are likely to be exposed to pesticide mixtures rather than to a single pesticide, and mixtures may result in unanticipated interactions among the pesticides at the molecular level [156]. Human exposure to certain pesticides at sufficient doses has been known to produce a variety of effects on physiological systems with some outcomes potentially linked to their endocrine disrupting activity [157] and altered oxidative stress [158]. In particular, most of the human findings primarily concern early life exposure and childhood neurodevelopmental impairment. In a prospective longitudinal study conducted in the French West Indies, Boucher et al. [159] reported that exposure to the organochlorine pesticide, chlordecone, was associated with impaired neurodevelopment in 18-month-old infants. The effects were seen in boys but not girls.

Three epidemiological studies are significant in pointing to similar conclusions regarding prenatal pesticide exposure and later childhood neurodeficits. In the Columbia University study, Rauh et al. [160] found an inverse association between Working Memory Index and Full-Scale IQ in inner-city children at age seven and the level of prenatal exposure to chlorpyrifos, an organophosphate pesticide. In a Mount Sinai Children's Environmental Health Study, Engel et al. [161]

reported that prenatal exposure to organophosphate pesticides was negatively associated with cognitive function by 12 months of age but also continuing later into childhood. In a multi-institutional California study among predominately Latino farmworker families, Bouchard et al. [162] reported that prenatal exposure to organophosphate pesticides was associated with reduced intellectual development at age seven.

Among pesticides, the exposure risks not only involve childhood-onset conditions but also later-life-appearing diseases (e.g., neurodegenerative). Zhou et al. [163] found that early-life exposure of mice to paraquat led to a later silencing in the gene (PINK1) responsible for producing a neuroprotective peptide. At the same time these pesticides activated the brain's innate immune cell resident microglia populations to generate excessive oxidative damage among neurons [164]. The reduced neuroprotection coupled with the increased risk of immune-mediated oxidative damage shifts the equilibrium of the aging brain toward neurodegeneration.

There is a suggestion that pesticide exposure may affect the risk of immune-driven NCDs. In the U.S. Agricultural Health Study, Hoppin et al. [165] found that exposure to pesticides elevated the risk for atopic (but not nonatopic) asthma among farm women. In fact the exposure to pesticides nullified the beneficial effect of growing up on a farm relative to risk of asthma. In this study, a total of 7 of 16 insecticides, 2 of 11 herbicides, and 1 of 4 fungicides were associated with an elevated risk of atopic asthma while permethrin use was the only pesticide associated with an increased risk of nonatopic asthma [165]. The study design [165] did not permit a comparison of differential developmental sensitivities and the potential role of pesticide-induced DIT in risk of asthma. However, the apparent nullification of immune-microbiome protection against asthma (i.e., hygiene hypothesis) raises intriguing questions.

Corsini et al. [166] recently reviewed the literature on pesticides and immunotoxicity. Based on human studies, these investigators concluded that the potential role of pesticides in immunotoxicity is unclear at present. They pointed out the serious limitations of most of the available studies including problems in accessing exposure levels and quite divergent approaches to assessment. The researchers called for better studies that would include pre- and postexposure information and be designed with appropriately matched controls. Beyond the weaknesses discussed by Corsini et al. [166], other weaknesses include a general lack of data regarding early developmental exposures and information regarding potential hypervulnerability for pesticide-induced DIT among human subpopulations.

5.14. Polychlorinated Biphenyls. Polychlorinated biphenyls (PCBs) are in a category of persistent organic pollutants (POPs) that can present human health challenges long after release into the environment. Stølevik et al. [167] examined the effects of exposure to PCBs and dioxin among Norwegian mother-child pairs and potential immune effects. They found that exposure to PCBs and dioxins was associated with increased incidence of respiratory infections and reduced antibody response against one (measles) of several childhood vaccinations. This is consistent with the findings of Heilmann et al. [168, 169] who studied perinatal PCB exposure and immune outcomes among children of the Faroe Islands. These researchers reported reduced antibody titers up to age seven to common childhood vaccinations following largely maternal diet-based perinatal exposure to PCBs. For the strongest associations, these investigators found that a doubling of serum PCB concentrations resulted in an approximately 20% reduction in antibody levels. Approximately 28% of the Faroe Islands children were found to be effectively unprotected against the childhood preventable diseases based on the extent of antibody suppression [168, 169].

Significantly for risk of NCDs, Grandjean et al. [170] found that prenatal and lactational exposure of Faroe Island children to marine pollutants including PCBs increased the risk of allergic sensitization. These findings are consistent with the apparent capacity of PCBs to produce disruption of immune homeostasis with effects including not only immunosuppression but also inappropriately enhanced and misdirected immune responses.

5.15. Polyfluorinated and Perfluorinated Compounds. The impact of developmental exposure to perfluorooctane sulfonic acid (PFOS) and perfluorooctanoic acid (PFOA) was examined in a prospective cohort birth study in the Faroe Islands [171]. The researchers found that a twofold increase in the levels of PFOS and PFOA at age five resulted in a several-fold increased likelihood of being unprotected against preventable childhood illnesses at age seven. In this case, lack of protection was defined as being below a protective level of antibodies against diphtheria and tetanus [171]. These findings have potentially stark implications for the health protection of children. In fact, the investigators determined that if benchmark dose (BMD) was calculated for the various polyfluorinated compounds using antibody levels as the driver and these were converted to safety limits for PFCs, the current limits may be several hundredfold too high [172].

6. Conclusions

DIT and fetal programming are emerging as significant contributors not only to later-life immune dysfunction and misregulated inflammation but also to increased risk of NCDs and particularly chronic diseases. Given the present epidemic of NCDs, the interrelated comorbidities that exist among a myriad of chronic diseases, and the role of NCDs as the greatest cause of death worldwide, better preventative strategies are needed.

Animal model research of DIT dates back several decades and helped to establish the fundamental characteristics surrounding early-life immune vulnerability for later-life disease. Recently, human DIT-related data have shown the relevance of the animal model information concerning dose sensitivity, subpopulation vulnerability, and health ramifications. While data gaps still exist for some categories of environmental risk factors (e.g., bisphenol A, certain pesticides), the way forward seems clear.

Better identification of DIT risk and improved protection of age-, sex-, and genotype-based hypervulnerable subpopulations are needed. This may well require a different approach to safety testing. With the potential for epigenetic alterations to be produced in utero and inheritance of altered immune- and inflammation-related gene expression across generations, it is apparent that efforts to reduce the prevalence of NCDs need to focus on early life. Reducing the prevalence of DIT is an important first step in comprehensive efforts to reduce the prevalence and global impact of NCDs.

Abbreviations

ALSPAC:	Avon Longitudinal Study of Parents and Children
Alum:	Aluminum oxyhydroxide
BMD:	Benchmark dose
CI:	Confidence interval
COPSAC:	Copenhagen Prospective Study on Asthma in Childhood
CRP:	C-Reactive protein
CS:	Cesarean section
CVD:	Cardiovascular disease
DES:	Diethylstilbestrol
DIT:	Developmental immunotoxicity
DOHaD:	Developmental origins of health and disease
DZP:	Diazepam
HLA:	Human leukocyte antigen
Ig:	Immunoglobulin
IgE:	Immunoglobulin E
IFN-γ:	Interferon-gamma
Il-4:	Interleukin-4
IL-6:	Interleukin-6
IL-8:	Interleukin-8
NHANES:	National Health and Nutrition Examination Survey
NCDs:	Noncommunicable diseases
Pb:	Lead
PFOA:	Perfluorooctanoic acid
PFOS:	Perfluorooctane sulfonic acid
POPs:	Persistent organic pollutants
RR:	Relative risk
Th:	T helper
Th2:	T helper 2
TBT:	Tributyltin oxide
TCDD:	2,3,7,8-Tetrachlorodibenzo-p-dioxin
TLR:	Toll-like receptor
TNF-α:	Tumor necrosis factor-alpha
VD:	Vaginal delivery.

Conflict of Interests

The author declares that he has no conflict of interests regarding the publication of this paper.

Acknowledgment

The author thanks Janice Dietert, Performance Plus Consulting, for her editorial suggestions.

References

[1] R. R. Dietert, "Developmental immunotoxicology: focus on health risks," *Chemical Research in Toxicology*, vol. 22, no. 1, pp. 17–23, 2009.

[2] R. R. Dietert, J. C. DeWitt, D. R. Germolec, and J. T. Zelikoff, "Breaking patterns of environmentally influenced disease for health risk reduction: Immune perspectives," *Environmental Health Perspectives*, vol. 118, no. 8, pp. 1091–1099, 2010.

[3] R. V. House and M. J. Selgrade, "A quarter-century of immunotoxicology: looking back, looking forward," *Toxicological Sciences*, vol. 118, no. 1, pp. 1–3, 2010.

[4] J. H. Dean, M. I. Luster, and G. A. Boorman, "Methods and approaches for assessing immunotoxicity: an overview," *Environmental Health Perspectives*, vol. 43, pp. 27–29, 1982.

[5] M. K. Selgrade, M. J. Daniels, G. R. Burleson, L. D. Lauer, and J. H. Dean, "Effects of 7,12-dimethylbenz[a]anthracene, benzo[a]pyrene and cyclosporin A on murine cytomegalovirus infection: studies of resistance mechanisms," *International Journal of Immunopharmacology*, vol. 10, no. 7, pp. 811–818, 1988.

[6] J. G. Vos, "Immune suppression as related to toxicology," *Journal of Immunotoxicology*, vol. 4, pp. 175–200, 2007.

[7] D. J. Barrett, "Characterization of the acquired immune deficiency syndrome at the cellular and molecular level," *Molecular and Cellular Biochemistry*, vol. 63, no. 1, pp. 3–11, 1984.

[8] H. C. Lane and A. S. Fauci, "Immunologic abnormalities in the acquired immunodeficiency syndrome," *Annual Review of Immunology*, vol. 3, pp. 477–500, 1985.

[9] M. I. Luster, C. Portier, D. G. Pait, and D. R. Germolec, "The use of animal tests in risk assessment for immunotoxicology," *Toxicology in Vitro*, vol. 8, no. 5, pp. 945–950, 1994.

[10] M. I. Luster, C. Portier, D. G. Pait et al., "Risk assessment in immunotoxicology. I. Sensitivity and predictability of immune tests," *Fundamental and Applied Toxicology*, vol. 18, no. 2, pp. 200–210, 1992.

[11] M. I. Luster, C. Portier, D. G. Pait et al., "Risk assessment in immunotoxicology. II. Relationships between immune and host resistance tests," *Fundamental and Applied Toxicology*, vol. 21, no. 1, pp. 71–82, 1993.

[12] J. G. Vos and H. Van Loveren, "Experimental studies on immunosuppression: how do they predict for man?" *Toxicology*, vol. 129, no. 1, pp. 13–26, 1998.

[13] D. A. Basketter, E. Selbie, E. W. Scholes, D. Lees, I. Kimber, and P. A. Botham, "Results with OECD recommend positive control sensitizers in the maximization, Buehler and local lymph node assays," *Food and Chemical Toxicology*, vol. 31, no. 1, pp. 63–67, 1993.

[14] D. A. Basketter, J. N. Bremmer, M. E. Kammuller et al., "The identification of chemicals with sensitizing or immunosuppressive properties in routine toxicology," *Food and Chemical Toxicology*, vol. 32, no. 3, pp. 289–296, 1994.

[15] M. I. Luster, R. E. Faith, and J. A. McLachlan, "Alterations of the antibody response following in utero exposure to diethylstilbestrol," *Bulletin of Environmental Contamination and Toxicology*, vol. 20, no. 4, pp. 433–437, 1978.

[16] M. I. Luster, R. E. Faith, J. A. McLachlan, and G. C. Clark, "Effect of in utero exposure to diethylstilbestrol on the immune response in mice," *Toxicology and Applied Pharmacology*, vol. 47, no. 2, pp. 279–285, 1979.

[17] M. I. Luster, R. E. Faith, and C. A. Kimmel, "Depression of humoral immunity in rats following chronic developmental lead exposure," *Journal of Environmental Pathology and Toxicology*, vol. 1, no. 4, pp. 397–402, 1978.

[18] R. E. Faith, M. I. Luster, and C. A. Kimmel, "Effect of chronic developmental lead exposure on cell-mediated immune functions," *Clinical and Experimental Immunology*, vol. 35, no. 3, pp. 413–420, 1979.

[19] J. M. Spyker-Cranmer, J. B. Barnett, D. L. Avery, and M. F. Cranmer, "Immunoteratology of chlordane: cell-mediated and humoral immune responses in adult mice exposed in utero," *Toxicology and Applied Pharmacology*, vol. 62, no. 3, pp. 402–408, 1982.

[20] V. Jagadeesan, C. Rukmini, M. Vijayaraghavan, and P. G. Tulpule, "Immune studies with T-2 toxin: effect of feeding and withdrawal in monkeys," *Food and Chemical Toxicology*, vol. 20, no. 1, pp. 83–87, 1982.

[21] R. R. Dietert, S. E. Bloom, M. A. Qureshi, and U. C. Nanna, "Hematological toxicology following embryonic exposure to aflatoxin-B1," *Proceedings of the Society for Experimental Biology and Medicine*, vol. 173, no. 4, pp. 481–485, 1983.

[22] R. R. Dietert, M. A. Qureshi, U. C. Nanna, and S. E. Bloom, "Embryonic exposure to aflatoxin-B1: mutagenicity and influence on development and immunity," *Environmental Mutagenesis*, vol. 7, no. 5, pp. 715–725, 1985.

[23] P. Urso and N. Gengozian, "Depressed humoral immunity and increased tumor incidence in mice following in utero exposure to benzo[a]pyrene," *Journal of Toxicology and Environmental Health*, vol. 6, no. 3, pp. 569–576, 1980.

[24] M. Schlumpf, E. E. Bütikofer, A. A. Schreiber, R. Parmar, H. R. Ramseier, and W. Lichtensteiger, "Delayed developmental immunotoxicity of prenatal benzodiazepines," *Toxicology in Vitro*, vol. 8, no. 5, pp. 1061–1065, 1994.

[25] S. D. Holladay and B. J. Smith, "Alterations in murine fetal thymus and liver hematopoietic cell populations following developmental exposure to 7,12- dimethylbenz[a]anthracene," *Environmental Research*, vol. 68, no. 2, pp. 106–113, 1995.

[26] S. G. Selevan, C. A. Kimmel, and P. Mendola, "Identifying critical windows of exposure for children's health," *Environmental Health Perspectives*, vol. 108, no. 3, pp. 451–455, 2000.

[27] S. D. Holladay and R. J. Smialowicz, "Development of the murine and human immune system: differential effects of immunotoxicants depend on time of exposure," *Environmental Health Perspectives*, vol. 108, 3, pp. 463–473, 2000.

[28] R. R. Dietert, R. A. Etzel, D. Chen et al., "Workshop to identify critical windows of exposure for children's health: immune and respiratory systems work group summary," *Environmental Health Perspectives*, vol. 108, no. 3, pp. 483–490, 2000.

[29] S. D. Holladay, *Developmental Immunotoxicology*, CRC Press, Boca Raton, Fla, USA, 2004.

[30] S. Langley-Evans, "Fetal programming of immune function and respiratory disease," *Clinical and Experimental Allergy*, vol. 27, no. 12, pp. 1377–1379, 1997.

[31] A. M. V. Ward and D. I. W. Phillips, "Fetal programming of stress responses," *Stress*, vol. 4, no. 4, pp. 263–271, 2001.

[32] D. J. P. Barker, "The developmental origins of insulin resistance," *Hormone Research*, vol. 64, no. 3, pp. 2–7, 2005.

[33] R. W. Luebke, D. H. Chen, R. Dietert, Y. Yang, M. King, and M. I. Luster, "The comparative immunotoxicity of five selected compounds following developmental or adult exposure," *Journal of Toxicology and Environmental Health B*, vol. 9, no. 1, pp. 1–26, 2006.

[34] J. C. Dewitt, M. M. Peden-Adams, D. E. Keil, and R. R. Dietert, "Current status of developmental immunotoxicity: early-life patterns and testing," *Toxicologic Pathology*, vol. 40, no. 2, pp. 230–236, 2012.

[35] R. R. Dietert and M. P. Holsapple, "Methodologies for developmental immunotoxicity (DIT) testing," *Methods*, vol. 41, no. 1, pp. 123–131, 2007.

[36] M. Collinge, L. A. Burns-Naas, G. J. Chellman et al., "Developmental immunotoxicity (DIT) testing of pharmaceuticals: current practices, state of the science, knowledge gaps, and recommendations," *Journal of Immunotoxicology*, vol. 9, no. 2, pp. 210–230, 2012.

[37] A. H. Piersma, E. C. Tonk, S. L. Makris, K. M. Crofton, R. R. Dietert, and H. van Loveren, "Juvenile toxicity testing protocols for chemicals," *Reproductive Toxicology*, vol. 34, pp. 482–486, 2012.

[38] R. R. Dietert and M. S. Piepenbrink, "Perinatal immunotoxicity: why adult exposure assessment fails to predict risk," *Environmental Health Perspectives*, vol. 114, no. 4, pp. 477–483, 2006.

[39] R. R. Dietert, J. C. DeWitt, and R. W. Luebke, "Reducing the prevalence of immune-based chronic dsisease," in *Immunotoxicity, Immune Dysfunction, and Chronic Disease*, R. R. Dietert and R. W. Dietert, Eds., pp. 419–440, Humana, New York, NY, USA, 2012.

[40] R. R. Dietert, "Role of developmental immunotoxicity and immune dysfunction in chronic disease and cancer," *Reproductive Toxicology*, vol. 31, no. 3, pp. 319–326, 2011.

[41] D. J. P. Barker, P. D. Winter, C. Osmond, B. Margetts, and S. J. Simmonds, "Weight in infancy and death from ischaemic heart disease," *The Lancet*, vol. 2, no. 8663, pp. 577–580, 1989.

[42] D. J. P. Barker, A. R. Bull, C. Osmond, and S. J. Simmonds, "Fetal and placental size and risk of hypertension in adult life," *British Medical Journal*, vol. 301, no. 6746, pp. 259–262, 1990.

[43] D. J. Barker, "The intrauterine environment and adult cardiovascular disease," *Ciba Foundation Symposium*, vol. 156, pp. 3–10, 1991.

[44] N. Paneth and M. Susser, "Early origin of coronary heart disease (the "Barker hypothesis"). Hypotheses, no matter how intriguing, need rigorous attempts at refutation," *British Medical Journal*, vol. 310, no. 6977, pp. 411–412, 1995.

[45] H. Wendy E, M. Rees, E. Kile, J. D. Mathews, and Z. Wang, "A new dimension to the Barker hypothesis: low birthweight and susceptibility to renal disease," *Kidney International*, vol. 56, no. 3, pp. 1072–1077, 1999.

[46] M. J. Holness, M. L. Langdown, and M. C. Sugden, "Early-life programming of susceptibility to dysregulation of glucose metabolism and the development of type 2 diabetes mellitus," *Biochemical Journal*, vol. 349, no. 3, pp. 657–665, 2000.

[47] S. Darney, B. Fowler, P. Grandjean, J. Heindel, D. Mattison, and W. Slikker Jr., "Prenatal Programming and Toxicity II (PPTOX II): role of environmental stressors in the developmental origins of disease," *Reproductive Toxicology*, vol. 31, no. 3, p. 271, 2011.

[48] R. Barouki, P. D. Gluckman, P. Grandjean, M. Hanson, and J. J. Heindel, "Developmental origins of non-communicable disease: implications for research and public health," *Environmental Health*, vol. 11, p. 42, 2012.

[49] J. C. DeWitt, M. M. Peden-Adams, D. E. Keil, and R. R. Dietert, "Developmental immunotoxicity (DIT): assays for evaluating effects of exogenous agents on development of the immune system," in *Current Protocols in Toxicology*, chapter 18, p. 15, 2012.

[50] G. R. Burleson and F. G. Burleson, "Testing human biologicals in animal host resistance models," *Journal of Immunotoxicology*, vol. 5, no. 1, pp. 23–31, 2008.

[51] M. Collinge, M. Thorn, V. Peachee, and K. White Jr., "Validation of a Candida albicans delayed-type hypersensitivity (DTH) model in female juvenile rats for use in immunotoxicity assessments," *Journal of Immunotoxicology*, vol. 10, no. 4, pp. 341–348, 2013.

[52] E. C. M. Tonk, D. M. G. de Groot, A. H. Penninks et al., "Developmental immunotoxicity of methylmercury: the relative sensitivity of developmental and immune parameters," *Toxicological Sciences*, vol. 117, no. 2, pp. 325–335, 2010.

[53] E. C. M. Tonk, A. Verhoef, L. J. J. de la Fonteyne et al., "Developmental immunotoxicity in male rats after juvenile exposure to di-n-octyltin dichloride (DOTC)," *Reproductive Toxicology*, vol. 32, no. 3, pp. 341–348, 2011.

[54] E. C. M. Tonk, A. Verhoef, E. R. Gremmer, H. van Loveren, and A. H. Piersma, "Relative sensitivity of developmental and immune parameters in juvenile versus adult male rats after exposure to di(2-ethylhexyl) phthalate," *Toxicology and Applied Pharmacology*, vol. 260, no. 1, pp. 48–57, 2012.

[55] E. C. Tonk, A. Verhoef, E. R. Gremmer, H. van Loveren, and A. H. Piersma, "Developmental immunotoxicity in male rats after juvenile exposure to ethanol," *Toxicology*, vol. 309, pp. 91–99, 2013.

[56] R. R. Dietert, J.-E. Lee, J. Olsen, K. Fitch, and J. A. Marsh, "Developmental immunotoxicity of dexamethasone: comparison of fetal versus adult exposures," *Toxicology*, vol. 194, no. 1-2, pp. 163–176, 2003.

[57] B. C. Gehrs, M. M. Riddle, W. C. Williams, and R. J. Smialowicz, "Alterations in the developing immune system of the F344 rat after perinatal exposure to 2, 3, 7, 8-tetrachlorodibenzo-p-dioxin: II. Effects on the pup and the adult," *Toxicology*, vol. 122, pp. 229–240, 1997.

[58] T. E. Miller, K. A. Golemboski, R. S. Ha, T. Bunn, F. S. Sanders, and R. R. Dietert, "Developmental exposure to lead causes persistent immunotoxicity in Fischer 344 rats," *Toxicological Sciences*, vol. 42, no. 2, pp. 129–135, 1998.

[59] D. B. Walker, W. C. Williams, C. B. Copeland, and R. J. Smialowicz, "Persistent suppression of contact hypersensitivity, and altered T-cell parameters in F344 rats exposed perinatally to 2,3,7,8-tetrachlorodibenzo-p- dioxin (TCDD)," *Toxicology*, vol. 197, no. 1, pp. 57–66, 2004.

[60] I. Hussain, M. S. Piepenbrink, K. J. Fitch, J. A. Marsh, and R. R. Dietert, "Developmental immunotoxicity of cyclosporin-A in rats: age-associated differential effects," *Toxicology*, vol. 206, no. 2, pp. 273–284, 2005.

[61] T. L. Bunn, P. J. Parsons, E. Kao, and R. R. Dietert, "Exposure to lead during critical windows of embryonic development: differential immunotoxic outcome based on stage of exposure and gender," *Toxicological Sciences*, vol. 64, no. 1, pp. 57–66, 2001.

[62] M. C. Jenmalm and K. Duchén, "Timing of allergy-preventive and immunomodulatory dietary interventions—are prenatal, perinatal or postnatal strategies optimal?" *Clinical and Experimental Allergy*, vol. 43, pp. 273–278, 2013.

[63] D. E. Bloom, E. T. Cafiero, E. Jané-Llopis et al., *The Global Economic Burden of Noncommunicable Diseases*, World Economic Forum, Geneva, Switzerland, 2011.

[64] R. R. Dietert, "Misregulated inflammation as an outcome of early-life exposure to endocrine-disrupting chemicals," *Reviews in Environmental Health*, vol. 27, pp. 117–131, 2012.

[65] S. L. Prescott, "Early-life environmental determinants of allergic diseases and the wider pandemic of inflammatory noncommunicable diseases," *Journal of Allergy and Clinical Immunology*, vol. 131, pp. 23–30, 2013.

[66] R. R. Dietert and R. W. Dietert, Eds., *Immunotoxicity, Immune Dysfunction, and Chronic Disease*, Humana, New York, NY, USA, 2012.

[67] R. R. Dietert and J. T. Zelikoff, "Pediatric immune dysfunction and health risks following early-life immune insult," *Current Pediatric Reviews*, vol. 5, no. 1, pp. 36–51, 2009.

[68] R. R. Dietert and J. T. Zelikoff, "Identifying patterns of immune-related disease: use in disease prevention and management," *World Journal of Pediatrics*, vol. 6, no. 2, pp. 111–118, 2010.

[69] R. R. Dietert, "Immune system disorders," in *Aging and Vulnerability to Environmental Chemicals: Age-Related Disorders and Their Origins in Environmental Exposures*, B. Weiss, Ed., Royal Society of Chemistry, London, UK, 2012.

[70] A. Pham-Short, K. C. Donaghue, G. Ambler, A. K. Chan, and M. E. Craig, "Coeliac disease in Type 1 diabetes from 1990 to 2009: higher incidence in young children after longer diabetes duration," *Diabetic Medicine*, vol. 29, pp. e286–e289, 2012.

[71] D. Greco, M. Pisciotta, F. Gambina, and F. Maggio., "Graves' disease in subjects with type 1 diabetes mellitus: a prevalence study in western Sicily (Italy)," *Primary Care Diabetes*, vol. 5, no. 4, pp. 241–244, 2011.

[72] C. Papoutsakis, K. N. Priftis, M. Drakouli et al., "Childhood overweight/obesity and asthma: is there a link? A systematic review of recent epidemiologic evidence," *Journal of the Academy of Nutrition and Dietetics*, vol. 113, pp. 77–105, 2013.

[73] H. Lazaratou, A. Soldatou, and D. Dikeos, "Medical comorbidity of sleep disorders in children and adolescents," *Current Opinion in Psychiatry*, vol. 25, pp. 391–397, 2012.

[74] M. Tanaka, S. Anders, and D. K. Kinney, "Environment, the immune system, and depression: an integrative review and discussion of the infection-defense hypothesis," in *Immunotoxicity, Immune Dysfunction, and Chronic Disease*, R. R. Dietert and R. W. Dietert, Eds., Humana, New York, NY, USA, 2012.

[75] S. Anders, M. Tanaka, and D. K. Kinney, "Depression as an evolutionary strategy for defense against infection," *Brain, Behavior, and Immunity*, vol. 31, pp. 9–22, 2013.

[76] K. Nadeau, C. McDonald-Hyman, E. M. Noth et al., "Ambient air pollution impairs regulatory T-cell function in asthma," *Journal of Allergy and Clinical Immunology*, vol. 126, no. 4, pp. 845.e10–852.e10, 2010.

[77] M. Kerkhof, D. S. Postma, B. Brunekreef et al., "Toll-like receptor 2 and 4 genes influence susceptibility to adverse effects of traffic-related air pollution on childhood asthma," *Thorax*, vol. 65, no. 8, pp. 690–697, 2010.

[78] L. Calderón-Garcidueñas, M. Macías-Parra, H. J. Hoffmann et al., "Immunotoxicity and environment: immunodysregulation and systemic inflammation in children," *Toxicological Pathology*, vol. 37, pp. 161–169, 2009.

[79] G. Herberth, R. Gubelt, S. Röder et al., "Increase of inflammatory markers after indoor renovation activities: The LISA Birth Cohort Study," *Pediatric Allergy and Immunology*, vol. 20, no. 6, pp. 563–570, 2009.

[80] D. Krewski, R. A. Yokel, E. Nieboer et al., "Human health risk assessment for aluminium, aluminium oxide, and aluminium hydroxide," *Journal of Toxicology and Environmental Health B*, vol. 10, no. 1, pp. 1–269, 2007.

[81] R. L. Poole, K. P. Pieroni, S. Gaskari, T. Dixon, and J. A. Kerner, "Aluminum exposure in neonatal patients using the least contaminated parenteral nutrition solution products," *Nutrients*, vol. 4, pp. 1566–1574, 2012.

[82] Y. Z. Zhu, D. W. Liu, Z. Y. Liu, and Y. F. Li, "Impact of aluminum exposure on the immune system: a mini review," *Environmental Toxicology and Pharmacology*, vol. 35, pp. 82–87, 2013.

[83] E. Israeli, N. Agmon-Levin, M. Blank, and Y. Shoenfeld, "Macrophagic myofaciitis a vaccine (alum) autoimmune-related disease," *Clinical Reviews in Allergy and Immunology*, vol. 41, no. 2, pp. 163–168, 2011.

[84] R. K. Gherardi and F. J. Authier, "Macrophagic myofasciitis: characterization and pathophysiology," *Lupus*, vol. 21, no. 2, pp. 184–189, 2012.

[85] O. Vera-Lastra, G. Medina, P. Cruz-Dominguez Mdel, L. J. Jara, and Y. Shoenfeld, "Autoimmune/inflammatory syndrome induced by adjuvants (Shoenfeld's syndrome): clinical and immunological spectrum," *Expert Reviews in Clinical Immunology*, vol. 9, pp. 361–373, 2013.

[86] T. Nakayama, Y. Kashiwagi, H. Kawashima, T. Kumagai, K. J. Ishii, and T. Ihara, "Alum-adjuvanted H5N1 whole virion inactivated vaccine (WIV) enhanced inflammatory cytokine productions," *Vaccine*, vol. 30, pp. 3885–3890, 2012.

[87] T. D. Terhune and R. C. Deth, "How aluminum adjuvants could promote and enhance non-target IgE synthesis in a genetically-vulnerable sub-population," *Journal of Immunotoxicology*, vol. 10, pp. 210–222, 2013.

[88] A. Lerner, "Aluminum as an adjuvant in Crohn's disease induction," *Lupus*, vol. 21, no. 2, pp. 231–238, 2012.

[89] F. Raciborski, A. Tomaszewska, J. Komorowski et al., "The relationship between antibiotic therapy in early childhood and the symptoms of allergy in children aged 6–8 years—the questionnaire study results," *International Journal of Occupational Medicine and Environmental Health*, vol. 25, pp. 470–480, 2012.

[90] K. Heintze and K. U. Petersen, "The case of drug causation of childhood asthma: antibiotics and paracetamol," *European Journal of Clinical Pharmacology*, vol. 69, pp. 1197–1209, 2013.

[91] R. R. Dietert and J. M. Dietert, "The completed self: an immunological view of the human-microbiome superorganism and risk of chronic diseases," *Entropy*, vol. 14, pp. 2036–2065, 2012.

[92] N. L. Dangleben, C. F. Skibola, and M. T. Smith, "Arsenic immunotoxicity: a review," *Environmental Health*, vol. 12, p. 73, 2013.

[93] G. A. Soto-Peña, A. L. Luna, L. Acosta-Saavedra et al., "Assessment of lymphocyte subpopulations and cytokine secretion in children exposed to arsenic," *FASEB Journal*, vol. 20, no. 6, pp. 779–781, 2006.

[94] D. O. Rocha-Amador, J. Calderón, L. Carrizales, R. Costilla-Salazar, and I. N. Pérez-Maldonado, "Apoptosis of peripheral blood mononuclear cells in children exposed to arsenic and fluoride," *Environmental Toxicology and Pharmacology*, vol. 32, no. 3, pp. 399–405, 2011.

[95] S. Ahmed, K. B. Ahsan, M. Kippler et al., "In utero arsenic exposure is associated with impaired thymic function in newborns possibly via oxidative stress and apoptosis," *Toxicological Sciences*, vol. 129, pp. 305–314, 2012.

[96] S. Ahmed, S. M.-E. Khoda, R. S. Rekha et al., "Arsenic-associated oxidative stress, inflammation, and immune disruption in human placenta and cord blood," *Environmental Health Perspectives*, vol. 119, no. 2, pp. 258–264, 2011.

[97] A. L. Luna, L. C. Acosta-Saavedra, L. Lopez-Carrillo et al., "Arsenic alters monocyte superoxide anion and nitric oxide production in environmentally exposed children," *Toxicology and Applied Pharmacology*, vol. 245, no. 2, pp. 244–251, 2010.

[98] A. Rahman, M. Vahter, E.-C. Ekström, and L.-Å. Persson, "Arsenic exposure in pregnancy increases the risk of lower respiratory tract infection and diarrhea during infancy in Bangladesh," *Environmental Health Perspectives*, vol. 119, no. 5, pp. 719–724, 2011.

[99] J. A. Rogers, L. Metz, and V. W. Yong, "Review: endocrine disrupting chemicals and immune responses: a focus on bisphenol-A and its potential mechanisms," *Molecular Immunology*, vol. 53, pp. 421–430, 2013.

[100] E. M. Rees Clayton, M. Todd, J. B. Dowd, and A. E. Aiello, "The impact of bisphenol A and triclosan on immune parameters in the U.S. population, NHANES 2003–2006," *Environmental Health Perspectives*, vol. 119, no. 3, pp. 390–396, 2011.

[101] J. H. Kim, L. S. Rozek, A. S. Soliman et al., "Bisphenol A-associated epigenomic changes in prepubescent girls: a cross-sectional study in Gharbiah, Egypt," *Environmental Health*, vol. 12, p. 33, 2013.

[102] J. Unterscheider, M. McMenamin, and F. Cullinane, "Rising rates of caesarean deliveries at full cervical dilatation: a concerning trend," *European Journal of Obstetrics Gynecology and Reproductive Biology*, vol. 157, no. 2, pp. 141–144, 2011.

[103] J. Neu and J. Rushing, "Cesarean Versus Vaginal Delivery: long-term infant outcomes and the Hygiene Hypothesis," *Clinics in Perinatology*, vol. 38, no. 2, pp. 321–331, 2011.

[104] R. R. Dietert, "Natural childbirth and breastfeeding as preventive measures of immune-microbiome dysbiosis and misregulated inflammation," *Journal of Ancient Diseases & Preventive Remedies*, vol. 1, p. 103, 2013.

[105] C. E. Cho and M. Norman, "Cesarean section and development of the immune system in the offspring," *American Journal of Obstetrics and Gynecology*, vol. 208, pp. 249–254, 2013.

[106] M. B. Azad, T. Konya, H. Maughan et al., "Gut microbiota of healthy Canadian infants: profiles by mode of delivery and infant diet at 4 months," *Canadian Medical Association Journal*, vol. 19, pp. 385–394, 2013.

[107] M. L. Houben, P. G. J. Nikkels, G. M. van Bleek et al., "The association between intrauterine inflammation and spontaneous vaginal delivery at term: A Cross-Sectional Study," *PLoS ONE*, vol. 4, no. 8, article e6572, 2009.

[108] V. C. Romero, E. C. Somers, V. Stolberg et al., "Developmental programming for allergy: a secondary analysis of the Mothers, Omega-3, and Mental Health Study," *American Journal of Obstetrics & Gynecology*, vol. 208, pp. 316.e1–316.e6, 2013.

[109] C.-M. Shen, S.-C. Lin, D.-M. Niu, and Y. R. Kou, "Labour increases the surface expression of two toll-like receptors in the cord blood monocytes of healthy term newborns," *Acta Paediatrica, International Journal of Paediatrics*, vol. 98, no. 6, pp. 959–962, 2009.

[110] B. Królak-Olejnik and I. Olejnik, "Late-preterm cesarean delivery and chemokines concentration in the umbilical cord blood of neonates," *Journal of Maternal-Fetal and Neonatal Medicine*, vol. 25, pp. 1810–1813, 2012.

[111] A. Malamitsi-Puchner, E. Protonotariou, T. Boutsikou, E. Makrakis, A. Sarandakou, and G. Creatsas, "The influence of

the mode of delivery on circulating cytokine concentrations in the perinatal period," *Early Human Development*, vol. 81, no. 4, pp. 387–392, 2005.

[112] C. Roduit, S. Scholtens, J. C. De Jongste et al., "Asthma at 8 years of age in children born by caesarean section," *Thorax*, vol. 64, no. 2, pp. 107–113, 2009.

[113] M. B. Azad and A. L. Kozyrskyj, "Perinatal programming of asthma: the role of gut microbiota," *Clinical and Developmental Immunology*, vol. 2012, Article ID 932072, 9 pages, 2012.

[114] T. R. Abrahamsson, H. E. Jakobsson, A. F. Andersson, B. Björkstén, L. Engstrand, and M. C. Jenmalm, "Low diversity of the gut microbiota in infants with atopic eczema," *Journal of Allergy and Clinical Immunology*, vol. 129, no. 2, pp. 434–440, 2012.

[115] E. Decker, M. Hornef, and S. Stockinger, "Cesarean delivery is associated with celiac disease but not inflammatory bowel disease in children," *Gut Microbes*, vol. 2, no. 2, pp. 91–98, 2011.

[116] J. Phillips, N. Gill, K. Sikdar, S. Penney, and L. A. Newhook, "History of cesarean section associated with childhood onset of T1DM in Newfoundland and Labrador, Canada," *Journal of Environmental and Public Health*, vol. 2012, Article ID 635097, 6 pages, 2012.

[117] E. Bonifacio, K. Warncke, C. Winkler, M. Wallner, and A.-G. Ziegler, "Cesarean section and interferon-induced helicase gene polymorphisms combine to increase childhood type 1 diabetes risk," *Diabetes*, vol. 60, no. 12, pp. 3300–3306, 2011.

[118] S. Thavagnanam, J. Fleming, A. Bromley, M. D. Shields, and C. R. Cardwell, "A meta-analysis of the association between Caesarean section and childhood asthma," *Clinical and Experimental Allergy*, vol. 38, no. 4, pp. 629–633, 2008.

[119] M. C. Magnus, S. E. Håberg, H. Stigum et al., "Delivery by Cesarean section and early childhood respiratory symptoms and disorders: the Norwegian mother and child cohort study," *American Journal of Epidemiology*, vol. 174, no. 11, pp. 1275–1285, 2011.

[120] E. R. Bertone-Johnson, B. W. Whitcomb, S. A. Missmer, E. W. Karlson, and J. W. Rich-Edwards, "Inflammation and early-life abuse in women," *American Journal of Preventive Medicine*, vol. 43, pp. 611–620, 2012.

[121] N. Slopen, K. C. Koenen, and L. D. Kubzansky, "Childhood adversity and immune and inflammatory biomarkers associated with cardiovascular risk in youth: a systematic review," *Brain, Behavior, and Immunity*, vol. 26, no. 2, pp. 239–250, 2012.

[122] A. J. J. M. Vingerhoets, J. Assies, K. Goodkin, G. L. Van Heck, and M. H. Bekker, "Prenatal diethylstilbestrol exposure and self-reported immune-related diseases," *European Journal of Obstetrics Gynecology and Reproductive Biology*, vol. 77, no. 2, pp. 205–209, 1998.

[123] W. C. Strohsnitter, K. L. Noller, R. Troisi et al., "Autoimmune disease incidence among women prenatally exposed to diethylstilbestrol," *Journal of Rheumatology*, vol. 37, no. 10, pp. 2167–2173, 2010.

[124] E. C. Tonk, D. M. de Groot, A. P. Wolterbeek et al., "Developmental immunotoxicity of ethanol in an extended one-generation reproductive toxicity study," *Archives of Toxicology*, vol. 87, no. 2, pp. 323–335, 2013.

[125] X. Zhang, N. Lan, P. Bach et al., "Prenatal alcohol exposure alters the course and severity of adjuvant-induced arthritis in female rats," *Brain, Behavior, and Immunity*, vol. 26, no. 3, pp. 439–450, 2012.

[126] X.-D. Ping, F. L. Harris, L. A. S. Brown, and T. W. Gauthier, "In vivo dysfunction of the term alveolar macrophage after in utero ethanol exposure," *Alcoholism*, vol. 31, no. 2, pp. 308–316, 2007.

[127] J. McGill, D. K. Meyerholz, M. Edsen-Moore et al., "Fetal exposure to ethanol has long-term effects on the severity of influenza virus infections," *Journal of Immunology*, vol. 182, no. 12, pp. 7803–7808, 2009.

[128] S. J. Kelly, N. Day, and A. P. Streissguth, "Effects of prenatal alcohol exposure on social behavior in humans and other species," *Neurotoxicology and Teratology*, vol. 22, no. 2, pp. 143–149, 2000.

[129] N. L. Day, A. Helsel, K. Sonon, and L. Goldschmidt, "The association between prenatal alcohol exposure and behavior at 22 years of age," *Alcoholism: Clinical and Experimental Research*, vol. 37, pp. 1171–1178, 2013.

[130] C. G. Carson, L. B. Halkjaer, S. M. Jensen, and H. Bisgaard, "Alcohol intake in pregnancy increases the child's risk of atopic dermatitis. The COPSAC prospective birth cohort study of a high risk population," *PLoS One*, vol. 7, article e42710, 2012.

[131] W. Yuan, H. T. Sørensen, O. Basso, and J. Olsen, "Prenatal maternal alcohol consumption and hospitalization with asthma in childhood: A Population-Based Follow-up Study," *Alcoholism*, vol. 28, no. 5, pp. 765–768, 2004.

[132] S. O. Shaheen, C. Rutterford, L. Zuccolo et al., "Prenatal alcohol exposure and childhood atopic disease: a Mendelian randomization approach," *Journal of Allergy and Clinical Immunology*, 2013.

[133] M. McDonnell Naughton, C. McGarvey, M. O. Regan, and T. Matthews, "Maternal smoking and alcohol consumption during pregnancy as risk factors for sudden infant death," *Irish Medical Journal*, vol. 105, no. 4, pp. 105–108, 2012.

[134] A. P. Pineda-Zavaleta, G. García-Vargas, V. H. Borja-Aburto et al., "Nitric oxide and superoxide anion production in monocytes from children exposed to arsenic and lead in region Lagunera, Mexico," *Toxicology and Applied Pharmacology*, vol. 198, no. 3, pp. 283–290, 2004.

[135] W. Karmaus, K. R. Brooks, T. Nebe, J. Witten, N. Obi-Osius, and H. Kruse, "Immune function biomarkers in children exposed to lead and organochlorine compounds: A Cross-Sectional Study," *Environmental Health*, vol. 4, no. 1, article 5, 2005.

[136] S. Li, Z. Zhengyan, L. I. Rong, and C. Hanyun, "Decrease of CD4+ T-lymphocytes in children exposed to environmental lead," *Biological Trace Element Research*, vol. 105, no. 1–3, pp. 19–25, 2005.

[137] P. M. Lutz, E. A. Kelty, T. D. Brown, T. J. Wilson, G. Brock, and R. E. Neal, "Environmental cigarette smoke exposure modulates IgE levels of Pb-exposed children," *Toxicology*, vol. 291, no. 1–3, pp. 43–50, 2012.

[138] C. A. Leifer and R. R. Dietert, "Early life environment and developmental immunotoxicity in inflammatory dysfunction and disease," *Toxicological and Environmental Chemistry*, vol. 93, no. 7, pp. 1463–1485, 2011.

[139] M. K. Selgrade, R. B. Blain, K. M. Fedak, and M. A. Cawley, "Potential risk of asthma associated with in utero exposure to xenobiotics," *Birth Defects Research C*, vol. 99, pp. 1–13, 2013.

[140] S. L. Prescott, "Effects of early cigarette smoke exposure on early immune development and respiratory disease," *Paediatric Respiratory Reviews*, vol. 9, no. 1, pp. 3–10, 2008.

[141] P. S. Noakes, J. Hale, R. Thomas, C. Lane, S. G. Devadason, and S. L. Prescott, "Maternal smoking is associated with impaired neonatal toll-like-receptor-mediated immune responses," *European Respiratory Journal*, vol. 28, no. 4, pp. 721–729, 2006.

[142] K. M. Wilson, S. C. Wesgate, J. Pier et al., "Secondhand smoke exposure and serum cytokine levels in healthy children," *Cytokine*, vol. 60, pp. 34–37, 2012.

[143] G. Tebow, D. L. Sherrill, I. C. Lohman et al., "Effects of parental smoking on interferon γ production in children," *Pediatrics*, vol. 121, no. 6, pp. e1563–e1569, 2008.

[144] P. Kum-Nji, L. Meloy, and H. G. Herrod, "Environmental tobacco smoke exposure: prevalence and mechanisms of causation of infections in children," *Pediatrics*, vol. 117, no. 5, pp. 1745–1754, 2006.

[145] G. Baynam, S.-K. Khoo, J. Rowe et al., "Parental smoking impairs vaccine responses in children with atopic genotypes," *Journal of Allergy and Clinical Immunology*, vol. 119, no. 2, pp. 366–374, 2007.

[146] C. S. Wilhelm-Benartzi, B. C. Christensen, D. C. Koestler et al., "Association of secondhand smoke exposures with DNA methylation in bladder carcinomas," *Cancer Causes and Control*, vol. 22, no. 8, pp. 1205–1213, 2011.

[147] A. B. T. Andersen, D. K. Farkas, F. Mehnert, V. Ehrenstein, and R. Erichsen, "Use of prescription paracetamol during pregnancy and risk of asthma in children: a population-based Danish cohort study," *Clinical Epidemiology*, vol. 4, no. 1, pp. 33–40, 2012.

[148] F. J. Gonzalez-Barcala, S. Pertega, T. P. Castro et al., "Exposure to paracetamol and asthma symptoms," *European Journal of Public Health*, vol. 23, pp. 706–710, 2013.

[149] A. J. Henderson and S. O. Shaheen, "Acetaminophen and asthma," *Paediatric Respiratory Reviews*, vol. 14, pp. 9–15, 2013.

[150] A. R. Scialli, R. Ang, J. Breitmeyer, and M. A. Royal, "Childhood asthma and use during pregnancy of acetaminophen: a critical review," *Reproductive Toxicology*, vol. 30, no. 4, pp. 508–519, 2010.

[151] M. Muc, C. Padez, and A. M. Pinto, "Exposure to paracetamol and antibiotics in early life and elevated risk of asthma in childhood," *Advances in Experimental Medicine and Biology*, vol. 788, pp. 393–400, 2013.

[152] K. Thiele, T. Kessler, P. Arck, A. Erhardt, and G. Tiegs, "Acetaminophen and pregnancy: short- and long-term consequences for mother and child," *Journal of Reproductive Immunology*, vol. 97, pp. 128–139, 2013.

[153] J. T. McBride, "The association of acetaminophen and asthma prevalence and severity," *Pediatrics*, vol. 128, no. 6, pp. 1181–1185, 2011.

[154] S. H. Kang, Y. H. Jung, H. Y. Kim et al., "Effect of paracetamol use on the modification of the development of asthma by reactive oxygen species genes," *Annuals of Allergy, Asthma & Immunology*, vol. 110, pp. 364–369, 2013.

[155] S. O. Shaheen, R. B. Newson, S. M. Ring, M. J. Rose-Zerilli, J. W. Holloway, and A. J. Henderson, "Prenatal and infant acetaminophen exposure, antioxidant gene polymorphisms, and childhood asthma," *Journal of Allergy and Clinical Immunology*, vol. 126, no. 6, pp. 1141–1148, 2010.

[156] A. F. Hernández, T. Parrón, A. M. Tsatsakis, M. Requena, R. Alarcón, and O. López-Guarnido, "Toxic effects of pesticide mixtures at a molecular level: their relevance to human health," *Toxicology*, vol. 307, pp. 136–145, 2013.

[157] L. S. Kjeldsen, M. Ghisari, and E. C. Bonefeld-Jørgensen, "Currently used pesticides and their mixtures affect the function of sex hormone receptors and aromatase enzyme activity," *Toxicology and Applied Pharmacology*, vol. 272, no. 2, pp. 453–464, 2013.

[158] N. Bonvallot, M. Tremblay-Franco, C. Chevrier et al., "Metabolomics tools for describing complex pesticide exposure in pregnant women in brittany (france)," *PLoS One*, vol. 21, article e64433, 2013.

[159] S. Boucher, M. N. Simard, G. Muckle et al., "Exposure to an organochlorine pesticide (chlordecone) and development of 18-month-old infants," *Neurotoxicology*, vol. 35, pp. 162–168, 2013.

[160] V. Rauh, S. Arunajadai, M. Horton et al., "Seven-year neurodevelopmental scores and prenatal exposure to chlorpyrifos, a common agricultural pesticide," *Environmental Health Perspectives*, vol. 119, no. 8, pp. 1196–1201, 2011.

[161] S. M. Engel, J. Wetmur, J. Chen et al., "Prenatal exposure to organophosphates, paraoxonase 1, and cognitive development in childhood," *Environmental Health Perspectives*, vol. 119, no. 8, pp. 1182–1188, 2011.

[162] M. F. Bouchard, J. Chevrier, K. G. Harley et al., "Prenatal exposure to organophosphate pesticides and IQ in 7-year-old children," *Environmental Health Perspectives*, vol. 119, no. 8, pp. 1189–1195, 2011.

[163] H. Zhou, C. Huang, J. Tong, and X.-G. Xia, "Early exposure to paraquat sensitizes dopaminergic neurons to subsequent silencing of PINK1 gene expression in mice," *International Journal of Biological Sciences*, vol. 7, no. 8, pp. 1180–1187, 2011.

[164] T. Taetzsch and M. L. Block, "Pesticides, microglial NOX2, and Parkinson's disease," *Journal of Biochemical and Molecular Toxicology*, vol. 27, pp. 137–149, 2013.

[165] J. A. Hoppin, D. M. Umbach, S. J. London et al., "Pesticides and atopic and nonatopic asthma among farm women in the agricultural health study," *American Journal of Respiratory and Critical Care Medicine*, vol. 177, no. 1, pp. 11–18, 2008.

[166] E. Corsini, M. Sokooti, C. L. Galli, A. Moretto, and C. Colosiom, "Pesticide induced immunotoxicity in humans: a comprehensive review of the existing evidence," *Toxicology*, vol. 307, pp. 123–135, 2013.

[167] S. B. Stølevik, U. C. Nygaard, E. Namork et al., "Prenatal exposure to polychlorinated biphenyls and dioxins from the maternal diet may be associated with immunosuppressive effects that persist into early childhood," *Food and Chemical Toxicology*, vol. 51, pp. 165–172, 2013.

[168] C. Heilmann, P. Grandjean, P. Weihe, F. Nielsen, and E. Budtz-Jørgensen, "Reduced antibody responses to vaccinations in children exposed to polychlorinated biphenyls," *PLoS Medicine*, vol. 3, no. 8, article e311, 2006.

[169] C. Heilmann, E. Budtz-Jørgensen, F. Nielsen, B. Heinzow, P. Weihe, and P. Grandjean, "Serum concentrations of antibodies against vaccine toxoids in children exposed perinatally to immunotoxicants," *Environmental Health Perspectives*, vol. 118, no. 10, pp. 1434–1438, 2010.

[170] P. Grandjean, L. K. Poulsen, C. Heilmann, U. Steuerwald, and P. Weihe, "Allergy and sensitization during childhood associated with prenatal and lactational exposure to marine pollutants," *Environmental Health Perspectives*, vol. 118, no. 10, pp. 1429–1433, 2010.

[171] P. Grandjean, E. W. Andersen, E. Budtz-Jørgensen et al., "Serum vaccine antibody concentrations in children exposed to perfluorinated compounds," *Journal of the American Medical Association*, vol. 307, no. 4, pp. 391–397, 2012.

[172] P. Grandjean and E. Budtz-Jørgensen, "Immunotoxicity of perfluorinated alkylates: calculation of benchmark doses based on serum concentrations in children," *Environmental Health*, vol. 12, p. 35, 2013.

[173] M. Vinceti, K. J. Rothman, C. M. Crespi et al., "Leukemia risk in children exposed to benzene and PM10 from vehicular traffic: a case-control study in an Italian population," *European Journal of Epidemiology*, vol. 27, pp. 781–790, 2012.

[174] W. Palinski, T. Yamashita, S. Freigang, and C. Napoli, "Developmental programming: maternal hypercholesterolemia and immunity influence susceptibility to atherosclerosis," *Nutrition Reviews*, vol. 65, no. 12, pp. S182–S187, 2007.

[175] D. Hinz, M. Bauer, S. Röder et al., "Cord blood Tregs with stable FOXP3 expression are influenced by prenatal environment and associated with atopic dermatitis at the age of one year," *Allergy*, vol. 67, no. 3, pp. 380–389, 2012.

[176] W. K. Kim, J. W. Kwon, J. H. Seo et al., "Interaction between IL13 genotype and environmental factors in the risk for allergic rhinitis in Korean children," *Journal of Allergy and Clinical Immunology*, vol. 130, pp. 421–426, 2012.

[177] B. Gesundheit, J. P. Rosenzweig, D. Naor et al., "Immunological and autoimmune considerations of Autism Spectrum Disorders," *Journal Autoimmunity*, vol. 44, pp. 1–7, 2013.

[178] R. Parboosing, Y. Ba, L. Shen, C. A. Schaefer, and A. S. Brown, "Gestational influenza and bipolar disorder in adult offspring," *Journal of the American Medical Association Psychatry*, vol. 70, no. 7, pp. 677–685, 2013.

[179] G. M. Hosang, S. L. Johnson, J. Kiecolt-Glaser et al., "Gender specific association of child abuse and adult cardiovascular disease in a sample of patients with basal cell carcinoma," *Child Abuse & Neglect*, vol. 37, pp. 374–379, 2013.

[180] K. Mårild, O. Stephansson, S. Montgomery, J. A. Murray, and J. F. Ludvigsson, "Pregnancy outcome and risk of celiac disease in offspring: a nationwide case-control study," *Gastroenterology*, vol. 142, no. 1, pp. 39–45, 2012.

[181] S. E. Roberts, C. J. Wotton, J. G. Williams, M. Griffith, and M. J. Goldacre, "Perinatal and early life risk factors for inflammatory bowel disease," *World Journal of Gastroenterology*, vol. 17, no. 6, pp. 743–749, 2011.

[182] R. Kodgule and S. Salvi, "Exposure to biomass smoke as a cause for airway disease in women and children," *Current Opinion in Allergy and Clinical Immunology*, vol. 12, no. 1, pp. 82–90, 2012.

[183] S. Lu, H. Peng, L. Wang et al., "Elevated specific peripheral cytokines found in major depressive disorder patients with childhood trauma exposure: a cytokine antibody array analysis," *Comprehensive Psychiatry*, vol. 54, no. 7, pp. 953–961, 2013.

[184] M. Kvaskoff, A. Bijon, F. Clavel-Chapelon, S. Mesrine, and M. C. Boutron-Ruault, "Childhood and adolescent exposures and the risk of endometriosis," *Epidemiology*, vol. 24, pp. 261–269, 2013.

[185] M. La Merrill, P. M. Cirillo, M. B. Terry, N. Y. Krigbaum, J. D. Flom, and B. A. Cohn, "Prenatal exposure to the pesticide DDT and hypertension diagnosed in women before age 50: A Longitudinal Birth Cohort Study," *Environmental Health Perspective*, vol. 121, pp. 594–599, 2013.

[186] J. A. Thompson and T. R. H. Regnault, "In utero origins of adult insulin resistance and vascular dysfunction," *Seminars in Reproductive Medicine*, vol. 29, no. 3, pp. 211–224, 2011.

[187] M. W. Koch, L. M. Metz, S. M. Agrawal, and V. W. Yong, "Environmental factors and their regulation of immunity in multiple sclerosis," *Journal of Neurological Sciences*, vol. 324, pp. 10–16, 2013.

[188] M. Maes, F. N. M. Twisk, M. Kubera, and K. Ringel, "Evidence for inflammation and activation of cell-mediated immunity in Myalgic Encephalomyelitis/Chronic Fatigue Syndrome (ME/CFS): increased interleukin-1, tumor necrosis factor-α,

PMN-elastase, lysozyme and neopterin," *Journal of Affective Disorders*, vol. 136, no. 3, pp. 933–939, 2012.

[189] S. Kempke, P. Luyten, S. Claes et al., "The prevalence and impact of early childhood trauma in Chronic Fatigue Syndrome," *Journal of Psychiatric Research*, vol. 47, pp. 664–669, 2013.

[190] A. Szakács, N. Darin, and T. Hallböök, "Increased childhood incidence of narcolepsy in western Sweden after H1N1 influenza vaccination," *Neurology*, vol. 80, pp. 1315–1321, 2013.

[191] L. Wijnans, C. Lecomte, and C. de Vries, "The incidence of narcolepsy in Europe: before, during, and after the influenza A(H1N1)pdm09 pandemic and vaccination campaigns," *Vaccine*, vol. 31, pp. 1246–1254, 2013.

[192] H. Li, R. Ye, L. Pei, A. Ren, X. Zheng, and J. Liu, "Caesarean delivery, caesarean delivery on maternal request and childhood overweight: a Chinese birth cohort study of 181–380 children," *Pediatric Obesity*, 2013.

[193] R. G. Jense, A. Koch, P. Homøe, and Bjerregaard, "Tobacco smoke increases the risk of otitis media among Greenlandic Inuit children while exposure to organochlorines remain insignificant," *Environment International*, vol. 54, pp. 112–118, 2013.

[194] Z. Csákányi, A. Czinner, J. Spangler, T. Rogers, and G. Katona, "Relationship of environmental tobacco smoke to otitis media (OM) in children," *International Journal of Pediatric Otorhinolaryngology*, vol. 76, pp. 989–993, 2012.

[195] O. C. Erdivanli, Z. O. Coskun, K. C. Kazikdas, and M. Demirci, "Prevalence of otitis media with effusion among Primary School Children in Eastern Black Sea, in Turkey and the effect of smoking in the development of otitis media with effusion," *Indian Journal of Otolaryngology and Head and Neck Surgery*, vol. 64, no. 1, pp. 17–21, 2012.

[196] Y. H. Yuan, J. D. Sun, M. M. Wu, J. F. Hu, S. Y. Peng, and N. H. Chen, "Rotenone could activate microglia through NFκB associated pathway," *Neurochemical Research*, vol. 38, pp. 1553–1560, 2013.

[197] G. Pereira, F. Haggar, A. W. Shand, C. Bower, A. Cook, and N. Nassar, "Association between pre-eclampsia and locally derived traffic-related air pollution: A Retrospective Cohort Study," *Journal of Epidemiology and Community Health*, vol. 67, pp. 147–152, 2013.

[198] M. G. Ozden, N. S. Tekin, M. A. Gürer et al., "Environmental risk factors in pediatric psoriasis: A Multicenter Case-Control Study," *Pediatric Dermatology*, vol. 28, pp. 306–312, 2011.

[199] A. Glynn, A. Thuvander, M. Aune et al., "Immune cell counts and risks of respiratory infections among infants exposed pre- and postnatally to organochlorine compounds: A Prospective Study," *Environmental Health: A Global Access Science Source*, vol. 7, article 62, 2008.

[200] S. B. Stølevik, U. C. Nygaard, E. Namork et al., "Prenatal exposure to polychlorinated biphenyls and dioxins is associated with increased risk of wheeze and infections in infants," *Food and Chemical Toxicology*, vol. 49, no. 8, pp. 1843–1848, 2011.

[201] J. J. K. Jaakkola and M. Gissler, "Maternal smoking in pregnancy as a determinant of rheumatoid arthritis and other inflammatory polyarthropathies during the first 7 years of life," *International Journal of Epidemiology*, vol. 34, no. 3, pp. 664–671, 2005.

[202] M. A. Burt, Y. C. Tse, P. Boksa, and T. P. Wong, "Prenatal immune activation interacts with stress and corticosterone exposure later in life to modulate N-methyl-d-aspartate receptor synaptic function and plasticity," *International Journal of Neuropsychopharmacology*, vol. 3, pp. 1–14, 2013.

[203] N. Yoshimi, F. Futamura, and K. Hashimoto, "Prenatal immune activation and subsequent peripubertal stress as a new model of schizophrenia," *Expert Reviews in Neurotherapy*, vol. 13, pp. 747–750, 2013.

[204] E. Patelarou, C. Girvalaki, H. Brokalaki, A. Patelarou, Z. Androulaki, and C. Vardavas, "Current evidence on the associations of breastfeeding, infant formula, and cow's milk introduction with type 1 diabetes mellitus: a systematic review," *Nutrition Reviews*, vol. 70, pp. 509–519, 2012.

[205] P. López-Serrano, J. L. Pérez-Calle, M. T. Pérez-Fernández, J. M. Fernández-Font, D. Boixeda de Miguel, and C. M. Fernández-Rodríguez, "Environmental risk factors in inflammatory bowel diseases. Investigating the hygiene hypothesis: A Spanish Case-Control Study," *Scandinavian Journal Gastroenterology*, vol. 45, pp. 1464–1471, 2010.

11

Transplantation of Encapsulated Pancreatic Islets as a Treatment for Patients with Type 1 Diabetes Mellitus

Meirigeng Qi[1,2]

[1] *Division of Transplantation/Department of Surgery, University of Illinois at Chicago, IL 60612, USA*
[2] *Department of Diabetes and Metabolic Diseases Research, Beckman Research Institute of the City of Hope, 1500 E. Duarte Road, Duarte, CA 91010, USA*

Correspondence should be addressed to Meirigeng Qi; mqi@coh.org

Academic Editor: Stefano La Rosa

Encapsulation of pancreatic islets has been proposed and investigated for over three decades to improve islet transplantation outcomes and to eliminate the side effects of immunosuppressive medications. Of the numerous encapsulation systems developed in the past, microencapsulation have been studied most extensively so far. A wide variety of materials has been tested for microencapsulation in various animal models (including nonhuman primates or NHPs) and some materials were shown to induce immunoprotection to islet grafts without the need for chronic immunosuppression. Despite the initial success of microcapsules in NHP models, the combined use of islet transplantation (allograft) and microencapsulation has not yet been successful in clinical trials. This review consists of three sections: introduction to islet transplantation, transplantation of encapsulated pancreatic islets as a treatment for patients with type 1 diabetes mellitus (T1DM), and present challenges and future perspectives.

1. Introduction

1.1. Type 1 Diabetes and Its Treatment. Type 1 diabetes mellitus (T1DM), also known as insulin-dependent diabetes mellitus, is an autoimmune disease that causes a progressive destruction of the insulin-producing pancreatic β cells [1, 2]. As a result, patients require exogenous insulin to maintain normal blood glucose levels. In patients with T1DM, long-term hyperglycemia often causes complications such as nephropathy, neuropathy, and retinopathy. According to a report from the American Diabetes Association (ADA), there are nearly three million children and adults living with T1DM in the USA and millions of others affected worldwide [3]. Management of T1DM and other associated complications is burdensome to both individuals and to society as a whole.

Insulin injection is a common method to directly control blood glucose levels. However, intensive insulin therapy can induce more frequent episodes of hypoglycemic symptoms in certain populations of patients with T1DM [4, 5].

Whole pancreas transplantation, which has been conducted since 1966, is a therapeutic way of stopping the progression of diabetic complications without increasing the incidence of hypoglycemic events [6–10]. The Graft survival rate has been well maintained post-surgery, with a survival rate of 76% after one year and 62% after three years. Long-term normoglycemia under insulin independence has been achieved with a 5-year graft survival rate of 50–70% [11]. Unfortunately, this procedure, which is usually performed simultaneously with kidney transplantation, involves complicated surgical procedures and consequential complications. Major complications include graft thrombosis, graft pancreatitis, pancreatic fistulae, and pseudocyst formation [12].

Islet transplantation is considered as an improved way to cure T1DM in comparison with insulin injection and whole pancreas transplantation. Absence of insulin in patients with T1DM forces them to use exogenous insulin to maintain normal blood glucose, which can delay or prevent health complications. Theoretically, exogenous insulin can replace

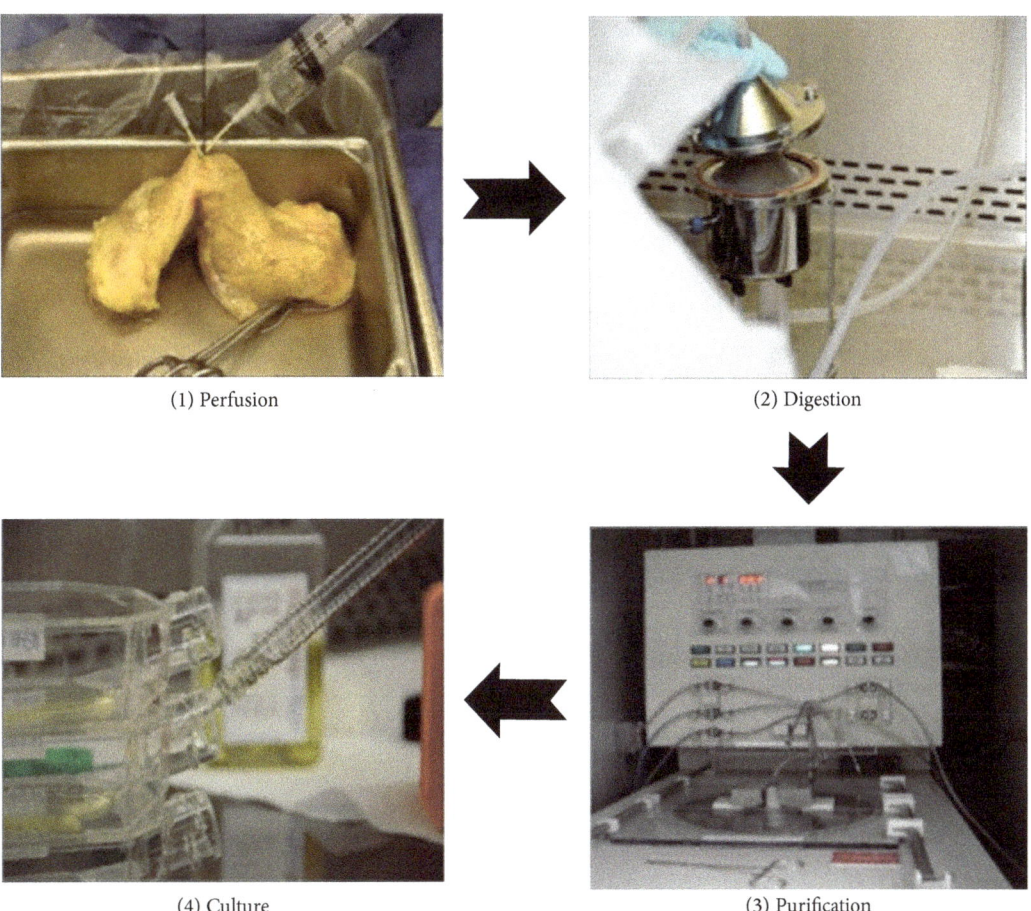

(1) Perfusion

(2) Digestion

(4) Culture

(3) Purification

FIGURE 1: Human islet isolation procedure. (1) Pancreas perfused with enzymatic solution; (2) pancreatic tissue digested in Ricordi isolation chamber; (3) digested tissue purified in COBE 2991 cell separator; (4) purified islets cultured at 37°C/5% CO_2.

β cells in islets, but practically, the insulin injection cannot maintain stable blood glucose levels. Pancreatic islet transplantation is a procedure to selectively transplant the endocrine part of a whole pancreas (about 2% of the pancreas mass). In comparison with whole pancreas transplantation, islet transplantation can be conducted via a minimally invasive approach and is associated with minimal or no complications. The islets can be infused via a catheter that has percutaneous portal venous access [13]. Therefore, this procedure can be applied to a wider range of recipients. More importantly, the islet transplantation can provide glycemic control without exogenous insulin and risks of hypoglycemia. The first experimental islet transplantation was conducted in a rodent model in 1972; several years after this a whole pancreas transplantation was initiated in a human patient [14]. Generally speaking, clinical allogeneic islet transplantation involves four chronological steps: procurement of donor pancreas, isolation of pancreatic islets (Figure 1 and Table 1), assessment of isolated islets (Table 2), and transplantation of harvested islets and patient followup.

Although islet transplantation has been widely accepted in recent years, the protocol has not obtained a license and is not accepted as a standard clinical treatment. Currently, many islet transplantation centers are planning or initiating license applications for clinical allogeneic islet transplantation.

1.2. Limitation of Islet Transplantation and Initiation of Encapsulation. Although the field of islet transplantation has progressed rapidly, the long-term success of allogeneic islet transplantation remains questionable. Patients from the original Edmonton trial had an insulin-independence rate of approximately 10% at five years after transplantation [20]. This rate, based on a recent study, is as high as 50%, but the combination of an optimized immunosuppressive regimen and a sophisticated transplant center is required [21]. As discussed elsewhere, the reasons for long-term graft loss can be summarized into the two following categories.

(i) Immunosuppression Associated Factors. Islet recipients must take immunosuppressive medications to prevent allogeneic rejections. Any imperfect immunosuppressive protocol can lead to graft loss. But after long-term usage, even the optimized medications can be toxic to the transplanted islets directly or cause dysfunction of other organs [20]. In addition to the damage allogeneic rejection can cause to the

TABLE 1: Enzyme types used for human islet isolation.

Enzyme types	Manufacture	Concentration	Digestion time (min)
Sigma type V collagenase	Sigma	1 g/350 mL	14
BM Type P collagenase	Boehringer-Mannheim	0.7 g/350 mL	25
Liberase HI	Roche Applied Science	0.5 g/350 mL	16
Liberase MTF C/T, GMP grade	Roche Applied Science		19
Collagenase		0.5 g/350 mL	
Thermolysin		0.015 g/350 mL	
Collagenase NB 1 (premium and GMP)	SERVA Electrophoresis GmbH		14
Collagenase		1600–2286 PZ units/350 mL	
Neutral Protease		200–286 DMC units/350 mL	
VitaCyte C1 collagenase	VitaCyte		20
CIzyme collagenase HA		15–18 units/g tissue	
CIzyme thermolysin		1.25 DMC units/g tissue	

MTF: mammalian tissue free.
GMP: good manufacturing practice.
DMC: dimethylcasein.

TABLE 2: Product-Release Test for islets before transplantation.

Test	Test method	Criteria
Purity	DTZ staining is used for islet identity, which is visualized by qualified personnel	≥30%
Viability	Fluorescent dye (FDA and PI) staining is used for islet viability, which is determined by qualified personnel	≥70%
Islet yield	DTZ staining is used for islet identity and islet number is counted by qualified personnel	First transplant: ≥5,000 IEQ/kg RBW Second transplant: ≥10,000 IEQ/kg RBW
Transplant tissue volume	Centrifuge and measure packed cell volume in conical tube	≤10 mL
Microbiological test	Gram stain on 100 μL smear with microscopic examination by qualified personnel	No intact organism observed
Endotoxin content	QCL-1000 Chromogenic LAL Test Kit, Cat number 50-647U, (BioWhittaker, Inc.)	≤5 EU/kg body weight of the potential recipient
Glucose static incubation	*In vitro* insulin release in 1.6 mM and 16.7 mM glucose. Expressed by SI	≥1.5

DTZ: dithizone.
FDA: fluorescein diacetate, for live cells.
PI: propidium iodide, for dead cells.
RBW: recipient body weight.
SI: stimulation index.

transplanted islets, recurrence of autoimmune attacks on the transplanted islets has also drawn investigator's attention. Histological studies have shown that islet transplantation triggers recurrent autoimmune effects that can cause β-cell destruction [22, 23]. Another study has revealed that the presence of pretransplant autoreactivity could lead to strengthened autoimmune reactions targeting β cells [24].

(ii) Nonimmunosuppressive Associated Factors. Nonimmunosuppresive factors including insufficient islet mass and poor islet quality can cause the dysfunction of islets in the long term. Islets are transplanted through the portal system and engraft in the liver; this can cause islet graft loss by (1) instant blood-mediated inflammatory reaction (IBMIR) [24]; (2) hypoxia-related islet cell death [25]. It has been reported that approximately 60% of pancreatic islets are destroyed due

to IBMIR after intraportal transplantation [26]. This reaction leads to the disruption of islets due to the activation of complement and coagulation systems [27, 28]. Tissue factor together with monocyte chemoattractant protein (MCP-1) and other inflammatory mediators cause the activation of coagulation and complement system. Poor clinical outcomes of islet transplantation are often associated with increased intensity of IBMIR [29]. In terms of hypoxia-related islet loss, the devascularization caused during the isolation, as well as the implantation of the islets into low oxygen tension within the liver, directly damages the islet cells [25]. The indirect cause of islet loss can be considered as the result of the activation of innate immune system by the hypoxia environment itself. Consequently, the release of inflammatory cytokines, such as tumor necrosis factor-α (TNF-α), interferon-γ (IFN-γ), and interleukin-1β (IL-1β), damages the islet graft [30].

With the above-mentioned limitations, the field of islet transplantation has been trying to find an alternative strategy to minimize the limitations for both donors and patients. Specifically, two avenues of research are being investigated. First, to find a possible method to decrease islet loss or provide an unlimited source of islet cells for transplantation. Second, to find an alternative approach to avoid the use of immunosuppressive medications. Immunoisolation of pancreatic islets, also known as encapsulation, not only allows for transplantation of cells without immunosuppression but also increases the chance of using cells from a nonhuman origin.

2. Transplantation of Encapsulated Pancreatic Islets as a Treatment for Patients with T1MD

2.1. Overview of Encapsulation. Cell encapsulation technology is based on the concept of immunoisolation, which was originally presented by Prehn et al. from as early as 1954. Prehn et al. used a type of immunoisolation instrument called the diffusion chamber device [31]. In that study, the diffusion chamber device was used to prevent the homograft from provoking an immune reaction in the host. Later on this technology was used to protect transplanted cells, known as "artificial cells" [32–36]. Since islet cells can be isolated and transplanted successfully, the encapsulation technology was soon applied in the field of islet transplantation. Many types of encapsulation technologies have been investigated over the last three decades in different animals such as mice [37], rats [38], dogs [39, 40], and monkeys [41, 42]. These studies demonstrate the feasibility of restoring normoglycemia by implanting allo- and xenografts without immunosuppression. Furthermore, the studies reveal the inconsistency of transplantation outcomes due to differences in encapsulation strategy and in animal models. The studies also suggest that long-term graft survival might depend on enriched and consistent blood supply to the grafts. In the light of the experiences accumulated from the large amount of transplant studies performed in different animal models, scientists and clinicians attempted a trial involving encapsulated allogeneic islet transplantation in patients with T1DM [15, 17, 18, 43]. The following sections describe the encapsulation technologies, characterize insulin release from encapsulated islets, depict immunology and biocompatibility factors of the devices, outline the approach of local/short-term immunomodulation, report the trials of clinical encapsulated islet transplantation, and discuss alternative cell sources for encapsulation.

2.2. Cell Encapsulation Technology. Encapsulation technology provides the means for islet cell survival in the absence of immunosuppressive drugs. The principle of encapsulation is that transplanted cells are contained within an artificial compartment separated from the immune system by a semipermeable membrane. The capsule should protect the cells from potential damage caused by antibodies, complement proteins, and immune cells. Therefore, the capsule is often referred to as an "immunoisolation device." As well as the protective mechanism provided by the capsules, islet

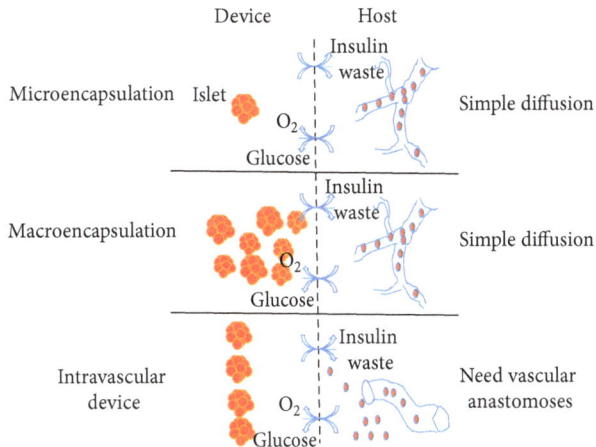

FIGURE 2: Schematic representation of immunoisolation device or bioartificial pancreas. They can be commonly separated into two categories, intravascular and extravascular devices. The latter can further be divided into macroencapsulation and microencapsulation devices. Intravascular and extravascular classifications are based on whether or not it is connected directly to the blood circulation. The macroencapsulation and microencapsulation classifications depend on whether it contains one or more islets in the device.

cells within the capsules can also release insulin to control blood glucose levels, since this membrane enables small molecules to diffuse in (glucose, oxygen, and nutrients) and out (metabolic wastes). Thus, the encapsulation system is also regarded as a "bioartificial pancreas." The immunoisolation device or bioartificial pancreas can be commonly separated into two categories, intravascular and extravascular devices. The latter can further be divided into macroencapsulation and microencapsulation devices (Figure 2). Intravascular and extravascular classifications are based on whether or not it is connected directly to the blood circulation. The macroencapsulation and microencapsulation classifications depend on whether it contains one or more islets in the device.

2.2.1. Intravascular Device. The intravascular device is designed to have a small chamber directly connected to the host's vascular system [44, 45]. Since the device is closely located to the blood supply, oxygen and nutrition diffuse into the device rapidly. The main biomaterial is the intravascular device is composed of copolymer polyacrylonitrile-polyvinyl chloride (PAN-PVC), which is similar to the material used in extravascular devices [46]. This kind of encapsulation system was initially used with autologous islet transplantation in the rodent model and normoglycemia was achieved for three months [47]. Furthermore, autologous islets in this device normalized the blood glucose in the monkey model. Although the modified versions of intravascular devices have been tested in allogeneic and xenogeneic transplant models [48, 49], such an encapsulation system has never been developed to the clinical level. The major concern that hampers the clinical application of the device is the development of thrombosis, which requires intensive anticoagulation treatment.

2.2.2. Extravascular Device. The extravascular device is fabricated based on the principle of planar or tubular diffusion chambers. This type of device does not need anastomosis when it is implanted into the host and has an advantage over the intravascular device in terms of clinical application. The process of producing the extravascular device is called encapsulation.

The main advantage of macroencapsulation is the ease of implantation and the retrieval of the device. They may be implanted in the peritoneal cavity and in subcutaneous sites [50, 51]. On the other hand, one disadvantage of macroencapsulation that makes the device less applicable is the difficulty in the diffusion of nutrients and oxygen through the device, which tends to harm islets [45]. It has been reported that a tubular device made by copolymer PAN-PVC dramatically reduced adhesion and fibrosis, which has been observed in earlier studies. A set of encapsulated allogeneic islet transplantations in patients with T1DM was conducted using the more biocompatible tubular devices. The result showed that 2 weeks of graft survival was achieved without using any immunosuppressive medications [16]. However, this type of device was weak structurally and ruptured easily during implantation. Furthermore, the large number of islets required in the device leads the islets to clump together and undergo central necrosis. To overcome the drawback of the weak structure, different types of macroencapsulation systems have been proposed in the past [52–55]. A sheet type immunoisolation device made of alginate was reported by Storrs from Islet Sheet Medical [56]. This type of macroencapsulation device can be retrieved intact, which is an additional advantage in terms of clinical safety. Moreover, retrievability of the device allows for the quantitative assessment of islet viability and function. To overcome the problem of hypoxia and central necrosis of the implanted islets, a vascularization-enhanced macroencapsulation device was produced by TheraCyte [57]. This device is suitable for subcutaneous implantation and greatly beneficiated patients with T1DM. TheraCyte reported that islets encapsulated in such device survived for an extended period of time in a xenotransplanted animal model [58]. Most recently, another study using this device revealed that islet allografts were protected in immunized recipients [59].

The main advantages of the microencapsulation system over macroencapsulation are its stable mechanical structure, large surface area-to-volume ratio, and improved diffusion profile. Due to the flexible and adjustable characteristics, the microcapsules are mostly fabricated from hydrogels. Over the past 30 years, hydrogels including alginate [60], poly(hydroxyethyl methacrylate-methyl methacrylate), agarose [61], acrylonitrile copolymers, chitosan [62], and polyethylene glycol (PEG) [63] have been frequently used for microencapsulation. To date, the most preferable material for microencapsulation is alginate. The principle of making microcapsules is based on the envelopment of individual islets in a droplet, which is transformed into a rigid capsule by gelification (in the case of alginate beads) followed by polycation coating (in the case of multiple-layered microcapsules).

Alginate, a collective term for a family of polysaccharides synthesized by seaweed and bacteria, is used in a wide range of foods, pharmaceutical products, and other applications [64]. In molecular terms, alginates are binary linear polysaccharides composed of two monomers, α-L-guluronic (G) and β-D-mannuronic (M) acid, which form M blocks, G blocks, and blocks of alternating sequence (MG) [65]. In nature, alginates are found to exhibit great variations in composition and arrangement of the two monomers in a polymer chain. Blocks of repeating G units (G blocks) form cavities that bind divalent cations, which cross-link G blocks of other alginate chains [66]. This in turn allows for the formation of gels as capsules. Hence, G block sequences are required for the alginate to form a strong gel with divalent ions such as Ca^{2+}, Ba^{2+}, and Sr^{2+}. A strong correlation therefore exists between the sequential structure and functional properties of alginates.

To increase the stability and to reduce the permeability of alginate gel beads, a polycation layer is traditionally added to the alginate gel core [67–70]. However, the successful use of alginate-polycation capsules as carriers for insulin producing cells *in vivo* has been hampered by the capsule's lack of biocompatibility as well as their mechanical instability. These disadvantages have made controlled insulin release and immunoprotection of islets difficult to achieve. The major obstacle for stability is swelling, causing an increase in pore size and ultimately breakage. This is caused by the loss of calcium from the calcium-alginate gel by, for example, phosphate and citrate, which can bind calcium, and nongelling ions such as sodium that over time will exchange some of the calcium in the gel [71].

2.3. Insulin Release Kinetics of Encapsulated Islets. Pancreatic β cells, which constitute 65–80% of the total cells in an islet, play a fundamental role in controlling metabolism through insulin secretion. Insulin release from β cells is controlled by the β cell's electrical activity, metabolic events, and ion signaling. These sets of intricate actions display the complex kinetic profile of biphasic and pulsatile responses to real-time changes in glucose levels [72, 73]. Insulin secretion is a complex and dynamic process. Glucose catabolism generates ATP through the mitochondrial Tricarboxylic Acid Cycle (TCA cycle), which consequently closes ATP-sensitive K^+ (K_{ATP}) channels, initiates plasma membrane depolarization, and increases Ca^{2+} concentration, through the rapid influx of Ca^{2+} via voltage-dependent calcium channels (VDCCs). This glucose-stimulated increase in Ca^{2+} concentration triggers the fusion of insulin granules with the cell membrane and the exocytosis of insulin, C-peptide, and proinsulin [74–77] (Figure 3(a)). Alternate pathways for insulin secretion, independent from K_{ATP} and Ca^{2+} concentrations, have been described [78, 79]. However, the K_{ATP} and Ca^{2+} concentration-mediated pathway remains the primary mechanism of glucose-stimulated insulin secretion. The normal response of β cells to glucose stimulation is the biphasic secretion process. The first phase corresponds to a transient and clear increase in the secretion rate. This is followed by a sharp decrease to the lowest secretion rate and a constantly flat or gradually increasing second phase that lasts as long as glucose stimulation is applied (Figure 3(b)). The

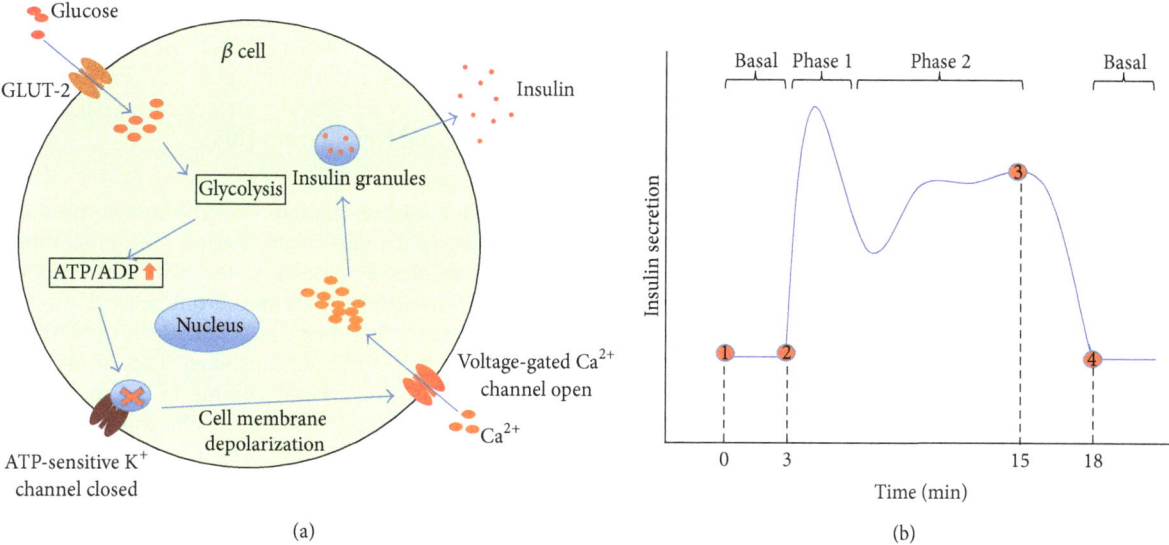

FIGURE 3: Diagram of insulin secretion from pancreatic β cells. (a) Cellular representation of an insulin-release process; (b) Graphical display of the biphasic insulin secretion.

secretion profiles, which are influenced by the environmental stimuli and controlled by the intrinsic characteristics of β cells, are thought to be important for insulin effects; however, the underlying mechanism of such dynamics has not been fully revealed [80, 81].

In physiological conditions, because of the rich blood supply to the pancreas, the β cells in islets detect hyperglycemia and release insulin rapidly to maintain glucose homeostasis. The transplanted naked islets lose direct connections to blood vessels, so diffusion is the only method for glucose and insulin to transport between the body and the islets. Regarding the transplanted encapsulated islets, the situation is presumably worse because molecules have to diffuse through the capsules. Therefore, it is of the upmost importance to understand the kinetics of insulin release from encapsulated islets.

The first known article regarding the kinetics of insulin release from encapsulated islets was published in 1988 by a research group from France. In this study glucose stimulated insulin release from islets, which were encapsulated in two different sized alginate-polylysine microcapsules (350 μm and 650 μm), were compared. The results showed that upon high glucose stimulation, the smaller microcapsules released a significantly higher amount of insulin compared to the larger microcapsules. However, the amount of insulin secreted from the smaller encapsulated islets was seven times less than that from naked islets [82]. In a recent study from 2009, the insulin release profile from encapsulated mouse insulinoma 6 (MIN6) cells was compared to that from nonencapsulated MIN6 cells. The kinetics of insulin release was more sluggish and the insulin release rate was lower in the encapsulated cells compared to the nonencapsulated cells [83]. Apparently, from the previously discussed studies, encapsulated islets or cells tend to show reduced insulin secretion when compared to nonencapsulated islets or cells. An interesting conclusion drawn from the combination of

this study [83] and another study [84] is that the slowed insulin release was due to a delayed uptake of glucose through the semipermeable membrane, but not primarily due to a slowed release of insulin from the encapsulated islets. The aforementioned studies, therefore, imply that the challenge of optimizing the microencapsulation system is not only to make capsules of a reduced size, but also to adjust the permeability properties of the capsule pores in order to allow for the ease of diffusion of glucose molecules.

Recently, a microfluidic perifusion system has been introduced and developed in our research group. This system was designed to more precisely measure multiple key parameters that directly control β-cell insulin secretion and viability, such as mitochondrial electrical potentials, calcium influx, and insulin kinetics [85–87]. Most recently, this technology has been applied to evaluate microencapsulated islets. Our group has also developed a novel microfluidic-based cellular array capable of trapping individual microencapsulated islets in hydrodynamic traps. Using this device, we demonstrated high trapping efficacy for microencapsulated islets (~99%), with minimal physical stress on the cells (data not shown). The unique integration of an atmospheric component has also allowed the device to study impacts of hypoxia on microencapsulated islets.

2.4. Immunology and Biocompatibility. Immunology studies the host's defense mechanisms against invasion of foreign organisms, either living or non-living. The immune response is often divided into two categories, innate and acquired immune reaction. The innate immune response is nonspecific and exists in all individuals. It does not distinguish between different organisms and acts rapidly upon the exposure of foreign invaders. The innate immune reaction typically initiates with cellular mediators such as macrophages and neutrophils. The acquired immune reaction is specific and not actively present in all individuals. This specific immune response requires the recognition of a specific antigen by lymphocytes including T and B cells.

Biomaterials are not firmly considered as organisms [88]; however, implantation of biomaterials in a host triggers an immune reaction, which involves many components of the immune system. Biocompatibility is commonly defined as the ability of a biomaterial or other medical device to perform its function properly in a specific application with an appropriate response in the host [89, 90]. As indicated by Williams DF, "biocompatibility refers to the ability of a biomaterial to perform its desired function with respect to a medical therapy, without eliciting any undesirable local or systemic effects in the recipients or beneficiary of that therapy, but generating the most appropriate beneficial cellular or tissue response in that specific situation, and optimizing the clinically relevant performance of that therapy" [89]. The immunoisolation device is not constructed solely by material for the main structure and it also contains islet cells. Therefore, in order for the device to be biocompatible, the bioartificial pancreas must carry out its proper function and it must not harm the host. For an immunoisolation device, biocompatibility has been referred to as the degree of fibrosis after implantation into the host. Recently work has focused on the implantation of microcapsules in larger animals, primarily NHPs, to evaluate the biocompatibility of the microcapsules for clinical islet transplantation.

2.4.1. Implantation of Empty Microcapsules.
The purpose of immunoisolation is to avoid immune rejection from the host. However, the device itself can trigger inflammatory reactions and different immune reactions. All biomaterials elicit an immune response from the host; known as the foreign body reaction. The foreign body reaction is considered as a nonspecific immune response and the reaction occurs as soon as the foreign materials are introduced to the host. The mechanisms and processes of the foreign body reaction are described extensively in several articles [91–94]. Generally speaking, the full process of the foreign body reaction can be described chronologically in the following order.

(i) Surgical procedure introduces an injury. This triggers the initial inflammatory reaction to the biomaterials starting with the formation of a provisional matrix [95, 96].

(ii) Proteins from blood and interstitial fluids are in direct contact and attach to the biomaterials. These proteins trigger the activation of the coagulation system, the complement proteins, and the platelets [97–99].

(iii) As a result of the activation of inflammatory mediators, wound healing regulators, and other types of immune cell reactions, fibrotic tissue will form over the foreign materials. The main inflammatory and wound healing mediators involved in this fibrotic formation are TNF-α [100], IFN-γ [101], IL-6 [102], IL-8 [102], MCP-1 [102], macrophage inflammatory protein (MIP)-1β [102], IL-4 [100], IL-13 [103], IL-10

[100, 104, 105], transforming growth factor (TGF)-β [106], and platelet derived growth factor (PDGF) [107]. The main immune cells associated with fibrosis formation are: monocytes, macrophages, dendritic cells, and lymphocytes [108].

As noted earlier, alginate is the most commonly used material for islet microencapsulation. The biocompatibility of microcapsules has been tested with the implantation of empty microcapsules in numerous animal models. The peritoneal cavity has been selected as an optimal site for *in vivo* analysis of microencapsulated islet implantation, as this site can harbor a large volume of microcapsules [14]. Furthermore, this site is easily accessible during implantation and is relatively safe. It has been reported previously that empty microcapsules, composed of purified alginate, do not elicit any significant foreign body reaction after implantation into the peritoneal cavity of rodents [109, 110]. However, implantation of empty microcapsules into the portal vein of pigs provoke extensive pericapsular cellular overgrowth [111]. This result indicates that portal vein microcapsule transplantation is incompatible with the current alginate composition.

2.4.2. Implantation of Microcapsules Containing Allogeneic Islets.
The evaluation of the function of microencapsulated islets in large animals is a necessary transit point between scientific studies in rodents and its clinical application for humans. Allotransplantation in large animals has been performed to mimic clinical islet transplantation. Soon-Shiong et al. initially reported the long-term reversal of diabetes in dogs using microencapsulated islet allografts [112]. In this study, encapsulated canine islets, using alginate-PLL microcapsules, were transplanted into the peritoneal cavity at a dose of 15,000–20,000 IEQ/kg. Two years graft survival was achieved in recipients that received a single encapsulated islet transplant with a month of anti-inflammatory medication. Recently, allografts in alginate-PLL microcapsules were tested in the absence of antirejection medications in pigs but large-scale studies were not documented [113, 114]. In 2008, Wang et al. published work on the normalization of blood glucose levels in dogs for up to 214 days with a single transplantation of microencapsulated allogeneic islets without immunosuppressive medication [39]. In this study, an encapsulation system consisting of alginate, $CaCl_2$, PMCG, cellulose sulfate (CS), and PLL was first introduced in this animal model. The amount of islets used in this study was 20,000–90,000 IEQ/kg, which is significantly higher than that in similar previous studies [112]. This study implies that more islets are needed to normalize blood glucose levels if immunosuppressive medications are not administrated after transplantation. Although the NHP is considered as an optimal allotransplantation model, little is published in terms of microencapsulated islet transplantation. In our previous study, we conducted allogeneic islet transplantations in baboons using the modified PMCG microcapsules. Two diabetic baboons were transplanted with an average of 16,475 IEQ/kg encapsulated islets (2-3 transplants) and

neither baboon achieved normoglycemia after transplantation. Evenly distributed microcapsules were observed in the peritoneal cavity. Retrieved microcapsules at 4 weeks posttransplant were intact and free of cellular overgrowth around the microcapsules.

In summary, a great amount of encapsulated islets are required to normalize blood glucose levels in large animals.

2.4.3. Implantation of Microcapsules Containing Xenogeneic Tissue.

Due to the shortage of donor tissues for patients with T1DM, xenotransplantation has drawn the attention of research facilities. Most xenotransplantation uses microencapsulated porcine islets as donor tissue. Sun et al. found that microencapsulated porcine islets transplanted into spontaneously diabetic cynomolgus monkeys survived for 120–800 days with no immunosuppression [115]. Other groups have tested their encapsulated porcine islets in nondiabetic monkeys [41, 42]. It is notable that all of these transplanted porcine islets were encapsulated in alginate-polycation based microcapsules, which is a microcapsule with less antibody permeability.

In our previous study, human islets encapsulated in Ca^{2+}/Ba^{2+}-alginate microbeads were transplanted into the peritoneal cavity of a diabetic baboon at a dose of 36,000 IEQ/kg. After transplantation, decreased blood glucose and positive C-peptide production were observed up to 2 weeks. Adhesion and clumping of the microcapsules were observed during laparotomy at day 76 posttransplant. Microcapsules that were retrieved at this point presented with fibrotic overgrowth. Xenogeneic tissue can trigger a stronger immune mediated rejection compared to allogeneic tissue, which may explain islet graft dysfunction in this study. Antibody responses against the encapsulated islets were found 20–35 days posttransplant. Similar results were observed in the transplantation of microencapsulated human islets into the peritoneal cavity of diabetic cynomolgus monkey (unpublished data).

It has been reported that transplantation of macroencapsulated pig islets can reverse diabetes in primates for 6 months without immunosuppression [116]. Most recently, Veriter et al. have reported the result of subcutaneous transplantation of macroencapsuled pig islets coencapsulated with mesenchymal stem cells. In this study, a significant correction of glycated hemoglobin was achieved in diabetic primate model [117].

2.5. Local or Short-Term Immunomodulation.

As mentioned earlier, a variety of natural and synthetic polymers have been used in islet encapsulation. However, inconsistency and poor long-term results have been a major limitation for clinical application. The graft failure is usually initiated by several factors including poor biocompatibility of the implanted materials, hypoxic conditions for islets inside of the capsules, and incomplete immunoprotection [118–120]. Thus, local or short-term immunomodulation and a nonsystematic immunosuppressive treatment have been investigated to improve the encapsulated islet transplant outcomes.

Biocompatibility of capsules is crucial for the long-term survival of the islet graft. It was demonstrated that a 10-day immunosuppressive medication regimen significantly reduced the fibrotic overgrowth around the intraportally implanted empty microcapsules [121]. Our group also tested the beneficial effects of 2-week long T-cell directed immunosuppressive medication and anti-inflammatory agents (TNF-α blocker) on the biocompatibility of Ca^{2+}/Ba^{2+}-alginate microbeads in cynomolgus monkeys. The results showed that the medications could only prevent fibrotic overgrowth on the surface of the implanted empty microbeads for as long as the medications were administered. This suggests that the extended use of immunosuppressants may have to be administrated to make the Ca^{2+}/Ba^{2+}-alginate microbeads biocompatible, which diminishes the goal of the encapsulation strategy (unpublished data).

Incomplete immunoprotection is mainly caused by the uncontrollable passage of proinflammatory cytokines and other immunoreactive molecules with low molecular weights, such as IL-1β (17.5 KD) and TNF-α (51 KD) through the biopolymer membrane [30, 122, 123].

Therefore, strategies to block those cytokines have been studied in recent years to improve the graft survival after encapsulated islet transplantation. In a recent study, a peptide inhibitor for the cell surface IL-1 receptor (IL-1R) was conjugated to the hydrogel for capsules to block the interaction between the immobilized cells and the cytokines [124]. In another strategy, Sertoli cells were used in co-encapsulation with islets cells. These cells are located in the convoluted seminiferous tubules of testes and have been shown to inhibit T-and B-cell proliferation and IL-2 production [125]. Cotransplantation of islets with Sertoli cells was shown to have varying protective effects on graft survival in allo-[126], concordant (rat to mouse) and discordant (fish to mouse) xeno- [127, 128], and autoimmune [129] transplant models. It was published that the Sertoli cells improve the functional performance of alginate-PLL microencapsulated islets in xenotransplant models (rat-mouse) [130]. However, this approach has not advanced significantly enough to be used in clinical trials.

2.6. Encapsulated Islet Transplantation in Patients with T1DM.

Table 3 lists the clinical trials of encapsulated islets transplanted in patients with T1DM. Soon-Shiong et al. reported a successful human encapsulated islet transplant in a diabetic patient who was receiving immunosuppression for a functioning kidney graft [15]. In the study, a total of 15,000 IEQ/kg alginate-PLL encapsulated islets were implanted intraperitoneally. Insulin independence was demonstrated for 9 months after the procedure, with tight glycemic control noted.

Scharp et al. subcutaneously implanted a PAN-PVC macroencapsulation device containing allogeneic islets into 9 patients [16]. The results concluded that macroencapsulated human islets could survive at the subcutaneous site and that semipermeable membranes can be designed to protect against both allogeneic immune responses and the autoimmune reactions of patients with T1DM.

TABLE 3: Encapsulated islet transplantation in patients with T1DM.

Investigator or company	Type of encapsulation	Islet source (patient number)	Immunosuppression	Transplant site
Soon-Shiong et al. [15]	A-PLL microcapsule	Allogeneic (1)	Yes, after kidney transplantation	Peritoneal cavity
Scharp et al. [16]	PAN-PVC diffusion chamber	Allogeneic (9)	No	Subcutaneous site
Calafiore et al. [17]	A-PLO microcapsule	Allogeneic (4)	No	Peritoneal cavity
Tuch et al. [18]	Ba^{2+}-alginate microbeads	Allogeneic (4)	No	Peritoneal cavity
Amcyte, Inc.	A-PLL microcapsule	Allogeneic (12 intended)	No	Peritoneal cavity
Novocell, Inc. (ViaCyte, Inc.)	PEG conformal coating	Allogeneic (12 intended)	No	Peritoneal cavity
Living Cell Technologies (LCT)	A-PLO microcapsule	Porcine insulin-producing cells (DIABECEL)	No	Peritoneal cavity
Jacobs-Tulleneers-Thevissen et al. [19]	Ca^{2+}/Ba^{2+}-alginate microbeads	Allogeneic (1)	No	Peritoneal cavity
Sernova Corp.	Macroencapsulation Cell Pouch System	Allogeneic (under preparation)	NR	Subcutaneous site

A-PLL: alginate-polylysine-alginate microcapsule.
PAN-PVC: polyacrylonitrile-polyvinyl chloride.
A-PLO: alginate-polyornitine-alginate microcapsule.
NR: not reported.
PEG: poly(ethylene glycol).

Calafiore et al. transplanted alginate-PLO microcapsulated islets in a human clinical trial without immunosuppression. In 2006, the results of the first two patients were published and both patients showed increased C-peptide serum levels, as a measure of islet graft function. Several weeks after transplantation, these two patients presented with an ephemeral incline in exogenous insulin consumption [17]. In 2011, the same group published the results of encapsulated islet transplantation in 4 patients, which included the follow-up results of the initial two patients reported in 2006 and two other patients transplanted afterwards [131]. So far, the results from 4 patients have been reported. In all cases the group observed no side effects of the grafting procedure, nor any evidence of immune sensitization. All patients exhibited a lower intake of exogenous insulin, approximately half of the pretransplantation consumption levels.

Tuch et al. transplanted allogeneic islets encapsulated in Ba^{2+}-alginate microbeads into four diabetic patients without immunosuppression. C-peptide was present on day one after transplantation, but disappeared within a period of one to four weeks. In a recipient of multiple islet infusions, C-peptide was detected at 6 weeks after the third infusion and remained detectable for 30 months. Neither insulin requirement nor glycemic control were altered in any of the patients [18].

From 2005 to 2006, two companies, Amcyte, Inc., and Novocell, Inc. announced clinical trials involving encapsulated islet transplantation in patients with T1DM. Amcyte, Inc. planned to conduct clinical trials in twelve patients using islets encapsulated in alginate-PLL microcapsules. These microcapsules were further embedded into a macrocapsule for implantation. Another company, Novocell, Inc. (current name ViaCyte, Inc.), initiated phase 1/2 clinical trials of PEG-encapsulated islet allograft implantation in patients with T1DM. Twelve patients were enrolled in this clinical trial. However, this particular study was terminated. Currently, there is limited information available regarding these two clinical trials.

Xenotransplantation has attracted much attention in the field of islet transplantation. In the light of such consideration, transplantation of microencapsulated xenogeneic islets, especially porcine islets, has commenced in patients with T1DM. In 1996, Living Cell Technologies (LCT), a company based in New Zealand, initiated a clinical trial involving encapsulated porcine islet transplantation. In this trial, porcine islets were encapsulated in alginate-PLO microcapsules and implanted into the peritoneal cavity of patients without immunosuppression. Nine and a half years after transplantation, laparotomy of one of the patients showed the presence of microcapsules in the peritoneal cavity, some of which still contained live pig islet cells. However, the majority of cells appeared to be necrotic [132]. As of now, the company reported in their website that a total of 14 patients with T1DM were enrolled in the phase 1/2 clinical trial of DIABECEL conducted in New Zealand and Russia [43]. The first four patients received approximately 10,000 IEQ/kg encapsulated islets and showed an average reduction of 76% in episodes of clinically significant hypoglycemia unawareness after 30–52 weeks of followup. Four patients from each of the second and third groups received 15,000 and 20,000 IEQ/kg of encapsulated islets respectively and the followup of these particular patients is ongoing. The last two patients have received a dose at 5,000 IEQ/kg and were enrolled to construct the dose ranging data needed to determine a target product profile for phase 3 clinical trials. Based on the most recent newsletter from the website, a registration study has been launched in 2013 for phase 2b/3 clinical trials, in which 30 patients were enrolled. The LCT product, DIABECEL, is expected to be commercially available in 2016 [43].

Most recently, Jacobs-Tulleneers-Thevissen et al. published work on transplantation of Ca^{2+}/Ba^{2+}-alginate microbeads containing allogeneic islets in a patient [19]. The alginate microbeads were harvested 3 months after transplantation and were conglomerated in the peritoneal cavity. In another report, Sernova Corp announced a commercial product of the macroencapsulation device called the Cell Pouch System. This device can be subcutaneously implanted. The device has a unique ability of releasing antirejection drugs locally. The Cell Pouch System is currently preparing for clinical trials [133].

2.7. Alternative to Allogeneic Islets from Deceased Donors for Clinical Encapsulated Islet Transplantation. As mentioned before, in the ongoing clinical islet transplantation protocols, the donor pool cannot provide enough islets to treat all potential patients. Therefore, different cell sources have been investigated to overcome this problem, including xenogeneic pig islets [134–136], genetically engineered insulin-producing cells [137], and insulin-producing cells differentiated from stem cells [138–140]. Since these cell types are potential alternative cell sources for clinical islet transplantation, they are also being considered for clinical encapsulated islet transplantation. However, to date only encapsulated porcine islets have been tested in patients with T1DM [43]. The encapsulation of other cell types has only been tested in experimental animal models to investigate the features of growth, differentiation, and maturation [37, 141, 142].

3. The Present and Future

At present, there is a large amount of islet encapsulation-related research in progress around the world trying to eliminate the use of immunosuppressants in patients with T1DM. This research is largely uncoordinated and a well-documented systematic analysis of the various capsule types has not been completed. The correlation between NHPs and human subjects in biocompatibility of device and function of transplanted islets is poorly demonstrated. Despite the numerous clinical trials conducted by academic institutes and biotechnological companies, encapsulated islet transplantation has not been perfected [17–19, 43, 131]. With regard to the mixed set of results, there are three main factors limiting the progression of microencapsulated islet transplantation towards clinical application. First, the variability of raw materials in the manufacturing process has impeded the development of a reliable microencapsulation system.

Second, current biocompatibility testing relies heavily on *in vivo* rodent models, which does not strongly support patients with T1DM. Finally, there is a significant inconsistency in results observed among individual laboratories even with the use of similar biomaterials and experimental approaches.

Taking all these obstacles into account, the development of a centralized *in vitro* and *in vivo* testing center in the future would allow for a more comprehensive, consistent, and species-specific examination of biocompatibility for the encapsulation system. A collaborative consortium may need to be organized, which should lead to the standardization in material selections, techniques, animal models, and procedures. Under active collaboration between research facilities, the end goal of providing islet encapsulation as a viable cure for patients with T1DM without immunosuppressant would be achievable.

Conflict of Interests

The author declares that there is no conflict of interests.

Acknowledgments

This study was conducted as part of the Chicago Diabetes Project (CDP), an international collaboration, to find a functional cure for diabetes. The author would like to thank the CDP for financial support, as well as CDP members, Dr. Igor Lacik and Dr. Berit L. Strand, for sharing their knowledge of islet encapsulation. The author especially thanks Dr. Jose Oberholzer and Dr. Yong Wang for supervising the paper and Dr. James McGarrigle for reviewing and editing the paper.

References

[1] S. Sakaguchi, N. Sakaguchi, M. Asano, M. Itoh, and M. Toda, "Immunologic self-tolerance maintained by activated T cells expressing IL- 2 receptor α-chains (CD25): breakdown of a single mechanism of self- tolerance causes various autoimmune diseases," *Journal of Immunology*, vol. 155, no. 3, pp. 1151–1164, 1995.

[2] S. Sakaguchi, "Naturally arising CD4+ regulatory T cells for immunologic self-tolerance and negative control of immune responses," *Annual Review of Immunology*, vol. 22, pp. 531–562, 2004.

[3] American Diabetes Association, http://www.diabetes.org.

[4] "The effect of intensive treatment of diabetes on the development and progression of long-term complications in insulin-dependent diabetes mellitus. The Diabetes Control and Complications Trial Research Group," *The New England Journal of Medicine*, vol. 329, pp. 977–986, 1993.

[5] E. F. M. Wijdicks, R. H. Wiesner, and R. A. F. Krom, "Neurotoxicity in liver transplant recipients with cyclosporine immunosuppression," *Neurology*, vol. 45, no. 11, pp. 1962–1964, 1995.

[6] A. C. Gruessner and D. E. R. Sutherland, "Pancreas transplant outcomes for United States (US) cases as reported to the United Network for Organ Sharing (UNOS) and the International Pancreas Transplant Registry (IPTR)," *Clinical Transplants*, pp. 45–56, 2008.

[7] A. C. Gruessner and D. E. R. Sutherland, "Pancreas transplant outcomes for United States (US) and non-US cases as reported to the United Network for Organ Sharing (UNOS) and the International Prancreas Transplant Registry (IPTR) as of June 2004," *Clinical Transplantation*, vol. 19, no. 4, pp. 433–455, 2005.

[8] M. Mora Porta, M. J. Ricart, R. Casamitjana et al., "Pancreas and kidney transplantation: long-term endocrine function," *Clinical Transplantation*, vol. 24, no. 6, pp. E236–E240, 2010.

[9] N. Demartines, M. Schiesser, and P. Clavien, "An evidence-based analysis of simultaneous pancreas-kidney and pancreas transplantation alone," *American Journal of Transplantation*, vol. 5, no. 11, pp. 2688–2697, 2005.

[10] C. Jahansouz, S. C. Kumer, M. Ellenbogen, and K. L. Brayman, "Evolution of β-cell replacement therapy in diabetes mellitus: pancreas transplantation," *Diabetes Technology and Therapeutics*, vol. 13, no. 3, pp. 395–418, 2011.

[11] D. J. Cohen, L. St. Martin, L. L. Christensen, R. D. Bloom, and R. S. Sung, "Kidney and pancreas transplantation in the United States, 1995-2004," *American Journal of Transplantation*, vol. 6, no. 5, pp. 1153–1169, 2006.

[12] P. R. Johnson and K. E. Jones, "Pancreatic islet transplantation," *Seminars in Pediatric Surgery*, vol. 21, pp. 272–280, 2012.

[13] R. C. Gaba, R. Garcia-Roca, and J. Oberholzer, "Pancreatic islet cell transplantation: an update for interventional radiologists," *Journal of Vascular and Interventional Radiology*, vol. 23, no. 5, pp. 583–594, 2012.

[14] W. F. Ballinger and P. E. Lacy, "Transplantation of intact pancreatic islets in rats," *Surgery*, vol. 72, no. 2, pp. 175–186, 1972.

[15] P. Soon-Shiong, R. E. Heintz, N. Merideth et al., "Insulin independence in a type 1 diabetic patient after encapsulated islet transplantation," *The Lancet*, vol. 343, no. 8903, pp. 950–951, 1994.

[16] D. W. Scharp, C. J. Swanson, B. J. Olack et al., "Protection of encapsulated human islets implanted without immunosuppression in patients with type I or type II diabetes and in nondiabetic control subjects," *Diabetes*, vol. 43, no. 9, pp. 1167–1170, 1994.

[17] R. Calafiore, G. Basta, G. Luca et al., "Microencapsulated pancreatic islet allografts into nonimmunosuppressed patients with type 1 diabetes," *Diabetes Care*, vol. 29, no. 1, pp. 137–138, 2006.

[18] B. E. Tuch, G. W. Keogh, L. J. Williams et al., "Safety and viability of microencapsulated human islets transplanted into diabetic humans," *Diabetes Care*, vol. 32, no. 10, pp. 1887–1889, 2009.

[19] D. Jacobs-Tulleneers-Thevissen, M. Chintinne, Z. Ling et al., "Sustained function ofalginate-encapsulated human islet cell implants in the peritoneal cavity of mice leading to a pilot study in a type 1 diabetic patient," *Diabetologia*, vol. 56, pp. 1605–1614, 2013.

[20] E. A. Ryan, B. W. Paty, P. A. Senior et al., "Five-year follow-up after clinical islet transplantation," *Diabetes*, vol. 54, no. 7, pp. 2060–2069, 2005.

[21] M. D. Bellin, F. B. Barton, A. Heitman et al., "Potent induction immunotherapy promotes long-term insulin independence after islet transplantation in type 1 diabetes," *American Journal of Transplantation*, vol. 12, pp. 1576–1583, 2012.

[22] A. A. Rossini, "Autoimmune diabetes and the circle of tolerance," *Diabetes*, vol. 53, no. 2, pp. 267–275, 2004.

[23] G. Worcester Human Islet Transplantation, "Autoimmunity after islet-cell allotransplantation," *The New England Journal of Medicine*, vol. 355, pp. 1397–1399, 2006.

[24] R. Hilbrands, V. A. L. Huurman, P. Gillard et al., "Differences in baseline lymphocyte counts and autoreactivity are associated with differences in outcome of islet cell transplantation in type 1 diabetic patients," *Diabetes*, vol. 58, no. 10, pp. 2267–2276, 2009.

[25] P. Carlsson, F. Palm, A. Andersson, and P. Liss, "Markedly decreased oxygen tension in transplanted rat pancreatic islets irrespective of the implantation site," *Diabetes*, vol. 50, no. 3, pp. 489–495, 2001.

[26] N. R. Barshes, S. Wyllie, and J. A. Goss, "Inflammation-mediated dysfunction and apoptosis in pancreatic islet transplantation: implications for intrahepatic grafts," *Journal of Leukocyte Biology*, vol. 77, no. 5, pp. 587–597, 2005.

[27] W. Bennet, B. Sundberg, C. Groth et al., "Incompatibility between human blood and isolated islets of langerhans: a finding with implications for clinical intraportal islet transplantation?" *Diabetes*, vol. 48, no. 10, pp. 1907–1914, 1999.

[28] L. Özmen, K. N. Ekdahl, G. Elgue, R. Larsson, O. Korsgren, and B. Nilsson, "Inhibition of thrombin abrogates the instant blood-mediated inflammatory reaction triggered by isolated human islets: possible application of the thrombin inhibitor Melagatran in clinical islet transplantation," *Diabetes*, vol. 51, no. 6, pp. 1779–1784, 2002.

[29] H. Johansson, A. Lukinius, L. Moberg et al., "Tissue factor produced by the endocrine cells of the islets of langerhans is associated with a negative outcome of clinical islet transplantation," *Diabetes*, vol. 54, no. 6, pp. 1755–1762, 2005.

[30] A. Rabinovitch and W. L. Suarez-Pinzon, "Cytokines and their roles in pancreatic islet β-cell destruction and insulin-dependent diabetes mellitus," *Biochemical Pharmacology*, vol. 55, no. 8, pp. 1139–1149, 1998.

[31] R. T. Prehn, J. M. Weaver, and G. H. Algire, "The diffusion-chamber technique applied to a study of the nature of homograft resistance," *Journal of the National Cancer Institute*, vol. 15, no. 3, pp. 509–517, 1954.

[32] J. Koo and T. M. S. Chang, "Secretion of erythropoietin from microencapsulated rat kidney cells: preliminary results," *International Journal of Artificial Organs*, vol. 16, no. 7, pp. 557–560, 1993.

[33] T. M. S. Chang, "Semipermeable microcapsules," *Science*, vol. 146, no. 3643, pp. 524–525, 1964.

[34] D. A. Cieslinski and H. D. Humes, "Tissue engineering of a bioartificial kidney," *Biotechnology and Bioengineering*, vol. 43, no. 7, pp. 678–681, 1994.

[35] H. Wong and T. M. S. Chang, "Bioartificial liver: implanted artificial cells microencapsulated living hepatocytes increases survival of liver failure rats," *International Journal of Artificial Organs*, vol. 9, no. 5, pp. 335–336, 1986.

[36] P. Aebischer, M. Goddard, A. P. Signore, and R. L. Timpson, "Functional recovery in hemiparkinsonian primates transplanted with polymer-encapsulated PC12 cells," *Experimental Neurology*, vol. 126, no. 2, pp. 151–158, 1994.

[37] J. L. Foster, G. Williams, L. J. Williams, and B. E. Tuch, "Differentiation of transplanted microencapsulated fetal pancreatic cells," *Transplantation*, vol. 83, no. 11, pp. 1440–1448, 2007.

[38] T. Meyer, B. Höcht, and K. Ulrichs, "Xenogeneic islet transplantation of microencapsulated porcine islets for therapy of type I diabetes: long-term normoglycemia in STZ-diabetic rats without immunosuppression," *Pediatric Surgery International*, vol. 24, no. 12, pp. 1375–1378, 2008.

[39] T. Wang, J. Adcock, W. Kühtreiber et al., "Successful allotransplantation of encapsulated islets in pancreatectomized canines

for diabetic management without the use of immunosuppression," *Transplantation*, vol. 85, no. 3, pp. 331–337, 2008.

[40] A. G. Abalovich, M. C. Bacqué, D. Grana, and J. Milei, "Pig pancreatic islet transplantation into spontaneously diabetic dogs," *Transplantation Proceedings*, vol. 41, no. 1, pp. 328–330, 2009.

[41] D. Dufrane, R. Goebbels, A. Saliez, Y. Guiot, and P. Gianello, "Six-month survival of microencapsulated pig islets and alginate biocompatibility in primates: proof of concept," *Transplantation*, vol. 81, no. 9, pp. 1345–1353, 2006.

[42] R. B. Elliott, L. Escobar, R. Calafiore et al., "Transplantation of micro- and macroencapsulated piglet islets into mice and monkeys," *Transplantation Proceedings*, vol. 37, no. 1, pp. 466–469, 2005.

[43] Living Cell Technologies. DIABECELL, http://www.lctglobal.com/Products-and-Services/Diabecell.

[44] R. P. Lanza, J. L. Hayes, and W. L. Chick, "Encapsulated cell technology," *Nature Biotechnology*, vol. 14, no. 9, pp. 1107–1111, 1996.

[45] D. W. Scharp, N. S. Mason, and R. E. Sparks, "Islet immunoisolation: the use of hybrid artificial organs to prevent islet tissue rejection," *World Journal of Surgery*, vol. 8, no. 2, pp. 221–229, 1984.

[46] C. K. Colton and E. S. Avgoustiniatos, "Bioengineering in development of the hybrid artificial pancreas," *Journal of Biomechanical Engineering*, vol. 113, no. 2, pp. 152–170, 1991.

[47] W. L. Chick, A. A. Like, and V. Lauris, "Beta cell culture on synthetic capillaries: an artificial endocrine pancreas," *Science*, vol. 187, no. 4179, pp. 847–849, 1975.

[48] T. Maki, J. P. A. Lodge, M. Carretta et al., "Treatment of severe diabetes mellitus for more than one year using a vascularized hybrid artificial pancreas," *Transplantation*, vol. 55, no. 4, pp. 713–718, 1993.

[49] T. Maki, I. Otsu, J. J. O'Neil et al., "Treatment of diabetes by xenogeneic islets without immunosuppression: use of a vascularized bioartificial pancreas," *Diabetes*, vol. 45, no. 3, pp. 342–347, 1996.

[50] K. Tatarkiewicz, J. Hollister-Lock, R. R. Quickel, C. K. Colton, S. Bonner-Weir, and G. C. Weir, "Reversal of hyperglycemia in mice after subcutaneous transplantation of macroencapsulated islets," *Transplantation*, vol. 67, no. 5, pp. 665–671, 1999.

[51] W. Wang, Y. Gu, H. Hori et al., "Subcutaneous transplantation of macroencapsulated porcine pancreatic endocrine cells normalizes hyperglycemia in diabetic mice," *Transplantation*, vol. 76, no. 2, pp. 290–296, 2003.

[52] T. Aung, M. Kogire, K. Inoue et al., "Insulin release from a bioartificial pancreas using a mesh reinforced polyvinyl alcohol hydrogel tube: an in vitro study," *ASAIO Journal*, vol. 39, no. 2, pp. 93–96, 1993.

[53] T. Aung, K. Inoue, M. Kogire et al., "Comparison of various gels for immobilization of islets in bioartificial pancreas using a mesh-reinforced polyvinyl alcohol hydrogel tube," *Transplantation Proceedings*, vol. 27, no. 1, pp. 619–621, 1995.

[54] H. Hayashi, K. Inoue, T. Aung et al., "Long survival of xenografted bioartificial pancreas with a mesh-reinforced polyvinyl alcohol hydrogel bag employing a B-cell line (MIN6)," *Transplantation Proceedings*, vol. 28, no. 3, pp. 1428–1429, 1996.

[55] M. Qi, Y. Gu, N. Sakata et al., "PVA hydrogel sheet macroencapsulation for the bioartificial pancreas," *Biomaterials*, vol. 25, no. 27, pp. 5885–5892, 2004.

[56] R. Storrs, R. Dorian, S. R. King, J. Lakey, and H. Rilo, "Preclinical development of the Islet Sheet," *Annals of the New York Academy of Sciences*, vol. 944, pp. 252–266, 2001.

[57] TheraCyte, http://www.theracyte.com/TheTechnology.htm.

[58] A. K. Sörenby, M. Kumagai-Braesch, A. Sharma, K. R. Hultenby, A. M. Wernerson, and A. B. Tibell, "Preimplantation of an immunoprotective device can lower the curative dose of islets to that of free islet transplantation-studies in a rodent model," *Transplantation*, vol. 86, no. 2, pp. 364–366, 2008.

[59] M. Kumagai-Braesch, S. Jacobson, H. Mori et al., "The TheraCyte device protects against islet allograft rejection in immunized hosts," *Cell Transplantation*, vol. 22, pp. 1137–1146, 2013.

[60] P. de Vos, M. M. Faas, B. Strand, and R. Calafiore, "Alginate-based microcapsules for immunoisolation of pancreatic islets," *Biomaterials*, vol. 27, no. 32, pp. 5603–5617, 2006.

[61] H. Iwata, H. Amemiya, T. Matsuda, H. Takano, R. Hayashi, and T. Akutsu, "Evaluation of microencapsulated islets in agarose gel as bioartificial pancreas by studies of hormone secretion in culture and by xenotransplantation," *Diabetes*, vol. 38, supplement 1, pp. 224–225, 1989.

[62] B. A. Zielinski and P. Aebischer, "Chitosan as a matrix for mammalian cell encapsulation," *Biomaterials*, vol. 15, no. 13, pp. 1049–1056, 1994.

[63] G. M. Cruise, O. D. Hegre, F. V. Lamberti et al., "In vitro and in vivo performance of porcine islets encapsulated in interfacially photopolymerized poly(ethylene glycol) diacrylate membranes," *Cell Transplantation*, vol. 8, no. 3, pp. 293–306, 1999.

[64] O. Smidsrød and G. Skjåk-Bræk, "Alginate as immobilization matrix for cells," *Trends in Biotechnology*, vol. 8, pp. 71–78, 1990.

[65] A. Haug, B. Larsen, and O. Smidsrød, "A study of the constitution of alginic acid by partial hydrolysis," *Acta Chemica Scandinavica*, vol. 20, pp. 183–190, 1966.

[66] G. T. Grant, E. R. Morris, and D. A. Rees, "Biological interactions between polysaccharides and divalent cations: the egg box model," *FEBS Letters*, vol. 32, no. 1, pp. 195–198, 1973.

[67] G. M. R. Vandenbossche, M. E. Bracke, C. A. Cuvelier, H. E. Bortier, M. M. Mareel, and J.-P. Remon, "Host reaction against alginate-polylysine microcapsules containing living cells," *Journal of Pharmacy and Pharmacology*, vol. 45, no. 2, pp. 121–125, 1993.

[68] B. Thu, P. Bruheim, T. Espevik, O. Smidsrød, P. Soon-Shiong, and G. Skjåk-Bræk, "Alginate polycation microcapsules: i. Interaction between alginate and polycation," *Biomaterials*, vol. 17, no. 10, pp. 1031–1040, 1996.

[69] B. Thu, P. Bruheim, T. Espevik, O. Smidsrød, P. Soon-Shiong, and G. Skjåk-Bræk, "Alginate polycation microcapsules: iI. Some functional properties," *Biomaterials*, vol. 17, no. 11, pp. 1069–1079, 1996.

[70] B. Kulseng, B. Thu, T. Espevik, and G. Skjåk-Bræk, "Alginate polylysine microcapsules as immune barrier: permeability of cytokines and immunoglobulins over the capsule membrane," *Cell Transplantation*, vol. 6, no. 4, pp. 387–394, 1997.

[71] B. Thu, *Alginate polycation microcapsules: a study of some molecular and functional properties relevant to their use as bioartificial pancreas [thesis]*, NTNU, Trondheim, Norway, 1996.

[72] D. S. Luciani, S. Misler, and K. S. Polonsky, "Ca^{2+} controls slow $NAD(P)H$ oscillations in glucose-stimulated mouse pancreatic islets," *Journal of Physiology*, vol. 572, no. 2, pp. 379–392, 2006.

[73] N. Pørksen, M. Hollingdal, C. Juhl, P. Butler, J. D. Veldhuis, and O. Schmitz, "Pulsatile insulin secretion: detection, regulation,

and role in diabetes," *Diabetes*, vol. 51, supplement 1, pp. S245–S254, 2002.

[74] C. Warnotte, P. Gilon, M. Nenquin, and J. Henquin, "Mechanisms of the stimulation of insulin release by saturated fatty acids: a study of palmitate effects in mouse β-cells," *Diabetes*, vol. 43, no. 5, pp. 703–711, 1994.

[75] J. C. Henquin, W. Schmeer, M. Nenquin, and H. P. Meissner, "Effects of a calcium channel agonist on the electrical, ionic and secretory events in mouse pancreatic B-cells," *Biochemical and Biophysical Research Communications*, vol. 131, no. 2, pp. 980–986, 1985.

[76] A. P. Babenko, L. Aguilar-Bryan, and J. Bryan, "A view of SUR/K(IR)6.X, k(atp) channels," *Annual Review of Physiology*, vol. 60, pp. 667–687, 1998.

[77] M. W. Roe, J. F. Worley III, Y. Tokuyama et al., "NIDDM is associated with loss of pancreatic β-cell L-type Ca^{2+} channel activity," *American Journal of Physiology—Endocrinology and Metabolism*, vol. 270, no. 1, pp. E133–E140, 1996.

[78] M. Gembal, P. Gilon, and J.-C. Henquin, "Evidence that glucose can control insulin release independently from its action on ATP-sensitive K^+ channels in mouse B cells," *The Journal of Clinical Investigation*, vol. 89, no. 4, pp. 1288–1295, 1992.

[79] S. G. Straub and G. W. G. Sharp, "Glucose-stimulated signaling pathways in biphasic insulin secretion," *Diabetes/Metabolism Research and Reviews*, vol. 18, no. 6, pp. 451–463, 2002.

[80] J. Henquin, M. Nenquin, P. Stiernet, and B. Ahren, "In vivo and in vitro glucose-induced biphasic insulin secretion in the mouse: pattern and role of cytoplasmic Ca^{2+} and amplification signals in β-cells," *Diabetes*, vol. 55, no. 2, pp. 441–451, 2006.

[81] M. Komjati, P. Bratusch-Marrain, and W. Waldhausl, "Superior efficacy of pulsatile versus continuous hormone exposure on hepatic glucose production in vitro," *Endocrinology*, vol. 118, no. 1, pp. 312–319, 1986.

[82] D. Chicheportiche and G. Reach, "In vitro kinetics of insulin release by microencapsulated rat islets: effect of the size of the microcapsules," *Diabetologia*, vol. 31, no. 1, pp. 54–57, 1988.

[83] R. Barrientos, S. Baltrusch, S. Sigrist, G. Legeay, A. Belcourt, and S. Lenzen, "Kinetics of insulin secretion from MIN6 pseudoislets after encapsulation in a prototype device of a bioartificial pancreas," *Hormone and Metabolic Research*, vol. 41, no. 1, pp. 5–9, 2009.

[84] S. Baltrusch and S. Lenzen, "Novel insights into the regulation of the bound and diffusible glucokinase in MIN6 β-cells," *Diabetes*, vol. 56, no. 5, pp. 1305–1315, 2007.

[85] J. S. Mohammed, Y. Wang, T. A. Harvat, J. Oberholzer, and D. T. Eddington, "Microfluidic device for multimodal characterization of pancreatic islets," *Lab on a Chip*, vol. 9, no. 1, pp. 97–106, 2009.

[86] A. F. Adewola, D. Lee, T. Harvat et al., "Microfluidic perifusion and imaging device for multi-parametric islet function assessment," *Biomedical Microdevices*, vol. 12, no. 3, pp. 409–417, 2010.

[87] D. Lee, Y. Wang, J. E. Mendoza-Elias et al., "Dual microfluidic perifusion networks for concurrent islet perifusion and optical imaging," *Biomedical Microdevices*, vol. 14, no. 1, pp. 7–16, 2012.

[88] A. Remes and D. F. Williams, "Immune response in biocompatibility," *Biomaterials*, vol. 13, no. 11, pp. 731–743, 1992.

[89] D. F. Williams, "On the mechanisms of biocompatibility," *Biomaterials*, vol. 29, no. 20, pp. 2941–2953, 2008.

[90] Z. Lifeng, H. Yan, Y. Dayun et al., "The underlying biological mechanisms of biocompatibility differences between bare and TiN-coated NiTi alloys," *Biomedical Materials*, vol. 6, no. 2, Article ID 025012, 2011.

[91] D. L. Coleman, R. N. King, and J. D. Andrade, "The foreign body reaction: a chronic inflammatory response," *Journal of Biomedical Materials Research*, vol. 8, no. 5, pp. 199–211, 1974.

[92] J. M. Anderson, A. Rodriguez, and D. T. Chang, "Foreign body reaction to biomaterials," *Seminars in Immunology*, vol. 20, no. 2, pp. 86–100, 2008.

[93] M. J. A. van Luyn, J. A. Plantinga, L. A. Brouwer, I. M. S. L. Khouw, L. F. M. H. de Leij, and P. B. van Wachem, "Repetitive subcutaneous implantation of different types of (biodegradable) biomaterials alters the foreign body reaction," *Biomaterials*, vol. 22, no. 11, pp. 1385–1391, 2001.

[94] B. C. Jham, N. G. Nikitakis, M. A. Scheper, J. C. Papadimitriou, B. A. Levy, and H. Rivera, "Granulomatous foreign-body reaction involving oral and perioral tissues after injection of biomaterials: a series of 7 cases and review of the literature," *Journal of Oral and Maxillofacial Surgery*, vol. 67, no. 2, pp. 280–285, 2009.

[95] J. M. Anderson, "Inflammatory response to implants," *ASAIO Transactions*, vol. 34, no. 2, pp. 101–107, 1988.

[96] A. Rosengren, L. M. Bjursten, and N. Danielsen, "Analysis of the inflammatory response to titanium and PTFE implants in soft tissue by macrophage phenotype quantification," *Journal of Materials Science*, vol. 9, no. 7, pp. 415–420, 1998.

[97] C. J. Wilson, R. E. Clegg, D. I. Leavesley, and M. J. Pearcy, "Mediation of biomaterial-cell interactions by adsorbed proteins: a review," *Tissue Engineering*, vol. 11, no. 1-2, pp. 1–18, 2005.

[98] M. B. Gorbet and M. V. Sefton, "Biomaterial-associated thrombosis: roles of coagulation factors, complement, platelets and leukocytes," *Biomaterials*, vol. 25, no. 26, pp. 5681–5703, 2004.

[99] B. G. Keselowsky, A. W. Bridges, K. L. Burns et al., "Role of plasma fibronectin in the foreign body response to biomaterials," *Biomaterials*, vol. 28, no. 25, pp. 3626–3631, 2007.

[100] D. M. Mosser and J. P. Edwards, "Exploring the full spectrum of macrophage activation," *Nature Reviews Immunology*, vol. 8, no. 12, pp. 958–969, 2008.

[101] I. M. Khouw, P. B. van Wachem, R. J. van der Worp, T. K. van den Berg, L. F. de Leij, and M. J. van Luyn, "Systemic anti-IFN-gamma treatment and role of macrophage subsets in the foreign body reaction to dermal sheep collagen in rats," *Journal of Biomedical Materials Research*, vol. 49, pp. 297–304, 2000.

[102] J. A. Jones, D. T. Chang, H. Meyerson et al., "Proteomic analysis and quantification of cytokines and chemokines from biomaterial surface-adherent macrophages and foreign body giant cells," *Journal of Biomedical Materials Research A*, vol. 83, no. 3, pp. 585–596, 2007.

[103] A. K. McNally and J. M. Anderson, "Macrophage fusion and multinucleated giant cells of inflammation," *Advances in Experimental Medicine and Biology*, vol. 713, pp. 97–111, 2011.

[104] D. M. Mosser, "The many faces of macrophage activation," *Journal of Leukocyte Biology*, vol. 73, no. 2, pp. 209–212, 2003.

[105] S. M. van Putten, M. Wübben, W. E. Hennink, M. J. A. van Luyn, and M. C. Harmsen, "The downmodulation of the foreign body reaction by cytomegalovirus encoded interleukin-10," *Biomaterials*, vol. 30, no. 5, pp. 730–735, 2009.

[106] P. Falk, E. Angenete, M. Bergstrom, and M. L. Ivarsson, "TGF-beta1 promotes transition of mesothelial cells into fibroblast phenotype in response to peritoneal injury in a cell culture model," *International Journal of Surgery*, vol. 11, no. 9, pp. 977–982, 2013.

[107] J. Donovan, X. Shiwen, J. Norman, and D. Abraham, "Platelet-derived growth factor alpha and beta receptors have overlapping

functional activities towards fibroblasts," *Fibrogenesis & Tissue Repair*, vol. 6, article 10, 2013.

[108] S. Yamashiro, H. Kamohara, J. Wang, D. Yang, W. Gong, and T. Yoshimura, "Phenotypic and functional change of cytokine-activated neutrophils: inflammatory neutrophils are heterogeneous and enhance adaptive immune responses," *Journal of Leukocyte Biology*, vol. 69, no. 5, pp. 698–704, 2001.

[109] P. de Vos, C. G. van Hoogmoed, J. van Zanten, S. Netter, J. H. Strubbe, and H. J. Busscher, "Long-term biocompatibility, chemistry, and function of microencapsulated pancreatic islets," *Biomaterials*, vol. 24, no. 2, pp. 305–312, 2003.

[110] M. Qi, I. Lacik, G. Kollárikováet al., "A recommended laparoscopic procedure for implantation of microcapsules in the peritoneal cavity of non-human primates," *Journal of Surgical Research*, vol. 168, no. 1, pp. e17–e123, 2011.

[111] C. Toso, J. Oberholzer, I. Ceausoglu et al., "Intra-portal injection of 400-μm microcapsules in a large-animal model," *Transplant International*, vol. 16, no. 6, pp. 405–410, 2003.

[112] P. Soon-Shiong, E. Feldman, R. Nelson et al., "Long-term reversal of diabetes by the injection of immunoprotected islets," *Proceedings of the National Academy of Sciences of the United States of America*, vol. 90, no. 12, pp. 5843–5847, 1993.

[113] R. Calafiore, G. Basta, G. Luca et al., "Transplantation of allogeneic/xenogeneic pancreatic islets containing coherent microcapsules in adult pigs," *Transplantation Proceedings*, vol. 30, no. 2, pp. 482–483, 1998.

[114] R. Calafiore, G. Basta, G. Luca et al., "Transplantation of pancreatic islets contained in minimal volume microcapsules in diabetic high mammalians," *Annals of the New York Academy of Sciences*, vol. 875, pp. 219–232, 1999.

[115] Y. Sun, X. Ma, D. Zhou, I. Vacek, and A. M. Sun, "Normalization of diabetes in spontaneously diabetic cynomologus monkeys by xenografts of microencapsulated porcine islets without immunosuppression," *The Journal of Clinical Investigation*, vol. 98, no. 6, pp. 1417–1422, 1996.

[116] D. Dufrane, R. Goebbels, and P. Gianello, "Alginate macroencapsulation of pig islets allows correction of streptozotocin-induced diabetes in primates up to 6 months without immunosuppression," *Transplantation*, vol. 90, no. 10, pp. 1054–1062, 2010.

[117] S. Veriter, P. Gianello, Y. Igarashi et al., "Improvement of subcutaneous bioartificial pancreas vascularization and function by co-encapsulation of pig islets and mesenchymal stem cells in primates," *Cell Transplantation*, 2013.

[118] S. K. Tam, J. Dusseault, S. Polizu, M. Ménard, J. Hallé, and L. Yahia, "Impact of residual contamination on the biofunctional properties of purified alginates used for cell encapsulation," *Biomaterials*, vol. 27, no. 8, pp. 1296–1305, 2006.

[119] M. Figliuzzi, T. Plati, R. Cornolti et al., "Biocompatibility and function of microencapsulated pancreatic islets," *Acta Biomaterialia*, vol. 2, no. 2, pp. 221–227, 2006.

[120] P. de Vos, B. de Haan, and R. van Schilfgaarde, "Effect of the alginate composition on the biocompatibility of alginate-polylysine microcapsules," *Biomaterials*, vol. 18, no. 3, pp. 273–278, 1997.

[121] Z. Mathe, P. Bucher, D. Bosco et al., "Short-term immunosuppression reduces fibrotic cellular infiltration around Barium-M-alginate microbeads injected intraportally," *Transplantation Proceedings*, vol. 36, no. 4, pp. 1199–1200, 2004.

[122] M. de Groot, T. A. Schuurs, and R. van Schilfgaarde, "Causes of limited survival of microencapsulated pancreatic islet grafts," *Journal of Surgical Research*, vol. 121, no. 1, pp. 141–150, 2004.

[123] J. Y. Jang, D. Y. Lee, S. J. Park, and Y. Byun, "Immune reactions of lymphocytes and macrophages against PEG-grafted pancreatic islets," *Biomaterials*, vol. 25, no. 17, pp. 3663–3669, 2004.

[124] J. Su, B. Hu, W. L. Lowe Jr., D. B. Kaufman, and P. B. Messersmith, "Anti-inflammatory peptide-functionalized hydrogels for insulin-secreting cell encapsulation," *Biomaterials*, vol. 31, no. 2, pp. 308–314, 2010.

[125] R. Charles, L. Lu, S. Qian, and J. J. Fung, "Stromal cell-based immunotherapy in transplantation," *Immunotherapy*, vol. 3, no. 12, pp. 1471–1485, 2011.

[126] G. S. Korbutt, J. F. Elliott, and R. V. Rajotte, "Cotransplantation of allogeneic islets with allogeneic testicular cell aggregates allows long-term graft survival without systemic immunosuppression," *Diabetes*, vol. 46, no. 2, pp. 317–322, 1997.

[127] J. M. Dufour, R. V. Rajotte, T. Kin, and G. S. Korbutt, "Immunoprotection of rat islet xenografts by cotransplantation with Sertoli cells and a single injection of antilymphocyte serum," *Transplantation*, vol. 75, no. 9, pp. 1594–1596, 2003.

[128] H. Yang and J. R. Wright Jr., "Co-encapsulation of sertoli enriched testicular cell fractions further prolongs fish-to-mouse islet xenograft survival," *Transplantation*, vol. 67, no. 6, pp. 815–820, 1999.

[129] G. S. Korbutt, W. L. Suarez-Pinzon, R. F. Power, R. V. Rajotte, and A. Rabinovitch, "Testicular Sertoli cells exert both protective and destructive effects on syngeneic islet grafts in non-obese diabetic mice," *Diabetologia*, vol. 43, no. 4, pp. 474–480, 2000.

[130] G. Luca, R. Calafiore, G. Basta et al., "Improved function of rat islets upon co-microencapsulation with Sertoli's cells in alginate/poly-L-ornithine," *AAPS PharmSciTech*, vol. 2, no. 3, p. E15, 2001.

[131] G. Basta, P. Montanucci, G. Luca et al., "Long-term metabolic and immunological follow-up of nonimmunosuppressed patients with type 1 diabetes treated with microencapsulated islet allografts: four cases," *Diabetes care*, vol. 34, no. 11, pp. 2406–2409, 2011.

[132] R. B. Elliott, L. Escobar, P. L. J. Tan, M. Muzina, S. Zwain, and C. Buchanan, "Live encapsulated porcine islets from a type 1 diabetic patient 9.5 yr after xenotransplantation," *Xenotransplantation*, vol. 14, no. 2, pp. 157–161, 2007.

[133] Cell Pouch System, http://www.sernova.com.

[134] C. G. Groth, "Transplantation of porcine fetal pancreas to diabetic patients," *The Lancet*, vol. 345, no. 8951, p. 735, 1995.

[135] C. G. Groth, O. Korsgren, A. Tibell et al., "Transplantation of porcine fetal pancreas to diabetic patients," *The Lancet*, vol. 344, no. 8934, pp. 1402–1404, 1994.

[136] R. A. Valdés-González, L. M. Dorantes, G. N. Garibay et al., "Xenotransplantation of porcine neonatal islets of Langerhans and Sertoli cells: a 4-year study," *European Journal of Endocrinology*, vol. 153, no. 3, pp. 419–427, 2005.

[137] A. T. Cheung, B. Dayanandan, J. T. Lewis et al., "Glucose-dependent insulin release from genetically engineered K cells," *Science*, vol. 290, no. 5498, pp. 1959–1962, 2000.

[138] B. Bose, S. P. Shenoy, S. Konda, and P. Wangikar, "Human embryonic stem cell differentiation into insulin secreting beta-cells for diabetes," *Cell Biology International*, vol. 36, pp. 1013–1020, 2012.

[139] K. R. Prabakar, J. Dominguez-Bendala, R. D. Molano et al., "Generation of glucose-responsive, insulin-producing cells from human umbilical cord blood-derived mesenchymal stem cells," *Cell Transplantation*, vol. 21, pp. 1321–1339, 2012.

[140] C. L. Basford, K. J. Prentice, A. B. Hardy et al., "The functional and molecular characterisation of human embryonic stem cell-derived insulin-positive cells compared with adult pancreatic beta cells," *Diabetologia*, vol. 55, no. 2, pp. 358–371, 2012.

[141] B. E. Tuch, T. C. Hughes, and M. D. M. Evans, "Encapsulated pancreatic progenitors derived from human embryonic stem cells as a therapy for insulin-dependent diabetes," *Diabetes/Metabolism Research and Reviews*, vol. 27, no. 8, pp. 928–932, 2011.

[142] S. K. Dean, Y. Yulyana, G. Williams, K. S. Sidhu, and B. E. Tuch, "Differentiation of encapsulated embryonic stem cells after transplantation," *Transplantation*, vol. 82, no. 9, pp. 1175–1184, 2006.

12

Blatchford Score Is Superior to AIMS65 Score in Predicting the Need for Clinical Interventions in Elderly Patients with Nonvariceal Upper Gastrointestinal Bleed

Khalid Abusaada, Fnu Asad-ur-Rahman, Vladimir Pech, Umair Majeed, Shengchuan Dai, Xiang Zhu, and Sally A. Litherland

Florida Hospital Internal Medicine Program, Florida Hospital, 601 Rollins Street, Orlando, FL 32803, USA

Correspondence should be addressed to Khalid Abusaada; khalid.abusaada.md@flhosp.org

Academic Editor: Spilios Manolakopoulos

Background. Blatchford and AIMS65 scores were developed to risk stratify patients with upper gastrointestinal bleed (UGIB). We sought to assess the performance of Blatchford and AIMS65 scores in predicting outcomes in elderly patients with nonvariceal UGIB. *Methods.* A retrospective cohort study of elderly patients (over 65 years of age) with nonvariceal UGIB admitted to a tertiary care center. Primary outcome was a combined outcome of in-hospital mortality, need for any therapeutic endoscopic, radiologic, or surgical intervention, rebleeding within 30 days, or blood transfusion. Secondary outcome was a combined outcome of in-hospital mortality or need for an intervention to control the bleed. *Results.* 164 patients were included. The primary outcome occurred in 119 (72.5%) patients. The secondary outcome occurred in 12 patients (7.2%). Blatchford score was superior to AIMS65 score in predicting the primary outcome (area under the receiver-operator curve (AUROC) 0.84 versus 0.68, resp., $p < 0.001$). Both scores performed poorly in predicting the secondary outcome (AUROC 0.56 versus 0.52, resp., $p = 0.18$). *Conclusions.* Blatchford score could be useful in predicting the need for hospital based interventions in elderly patients with nonvariceal UGIB. Blatchford and AIMS65 scores are poor predictors of the need for a therapeutic intervention to control bleeding.

1. Introduction

Upper gastrointestinal bleeding (UGIB) is a frequent presenting symptom in the elderly. The elderly, defined as individuals 65 years of age or older, form a population that has a high percentage of multiple comorbidities with related polypharmacy, including the concomitant use of antiplatelet treatments, which puts them at higher risk for gastrointestinal bleed and for clinical decompensation under the stress caused by acute bleeding [1].

The most common cause of nonvariceal UGIB in elderly patients is peptic ulcer disease and gastritis/esophagitis [2–6]. In-hospital mortality from UGIB in elderly patients in previous reports ranged between 0 and 8.4% [1–3, 7]. However, the studies that reported the higher mortality rates included variceal bleed [1, 3, 7].

Despite being a common presenting symptom, there is little information in the literature to guide physicians on the management of nonvariceal UGIB in the elderly.

Blatchford score was developed to predict a composite outcome of inpatient mortality, in-hospital rebleeding, endoscopic or surgical intervention, and need for blood transfusion in the general population presenting with UGIB [8]. Blatchford score was proposed as a tool to triage patients with UGIB to outpatient versus inpatient treatment [9–11].

Recently, the AIMS65 score was derived from a large database of UGIB patients to predict mortality [12]. Comparison of the two scores had conflicting results in the general population [13, 14]. In addition, the performance of Blatchford and AIMS65 scores in elderly patients has not been validated.

In this study we sought to compare the performance of Blatchford and AIMS65 scoring systems in predicting clinically meaningful outcomes and the need for an intervention to control the bleeding in elderly patients with nonvariceal upper GIB.

2. Methods

This is a retrospective cohort study. All research reviews were conducted under protocols approved by the local Institutional Review Board (IRBNet# 519910) and all data were collected and analyzed in a HIPAA compliant manner to ensure patient privacy and data integrity.

The study was conducted in a large tertiary care center. Patients over the age of 65 years admitted to our institution between 2009 and 2011 with a diagnosis of GIB from any source were identified using International Classification of Disease Ninth Edition (ICD9) codes. After the identification of patients with a diagnosis of GIB, charts were reviewed and data was extracted by trained internal medicine residents. All reviewers received training on data extraction and a database was created to standardize the process. Patients with known liver cirrhosis, presentation with acute liver failure, or history of variceal bleed were excluded. Patients also were excluded if GIB was not the presenting symptom to the emergency department (ED).

For each patient included in the study, the following data were collected through manual chart review: age, sex, medical history, albumin level, international normalized ratio, blood urea nitrogen, hemoglobin, systolic blood pressure on admission, pulse, changes in mental state including syncope and dizziness, presence of melena, associated comorbidities and medication use, findings on colonoscopy and esophagogastroduodenoscopy (EGD), other procedures, and pathology reports.

The scores of interest were Blatchford score and AIMS65 score. Each of these scores was calculated using information available at time of presentation to ED.

The Blatchford score was calculated from eight clinical or laboratory variables as defined by Blatchford et al. [8]. AIMS65 score was calculated from five clinical and laboratory variables as described by Saltzman et al. [12] (Table 1). Altered mental status in AIMS65 score was defined as a change in baseline mental or neurologic state documented by the ED physician or admitting physician at time of admission including dizziness, syncope, and presyncope.

Upper GIB bleed was defined as presentation with hematemesis or other UGIB symptoms with source of bleeding in the upper GI tract identified by endoscopy or other imaging studies such as a bleeding scan or angiography.

The primary outcome was a composite endpoint of inpatient mortality, readmission within 30 days for rebleed, need for blood transfusion, or need for any endoscopic, radiologic, or surgical intervention. The secondary outcome was a combined outcome of in-hospital mortality or need for an intervention to control the source of bleeding.

TABLE 1: Blatchford score and AIMS65 score.

Risk factor	Score
Blatchford score	
Blood urea (mmol/L)	
≥6.5 <8.0	2
≥8.0 <10.0	3
≥10.0 ≤25.0	4
>25	6
Hemoglobin (g/dL) for men	
≥12.0 <13.0	1
≥10.0 <12.0	3
<10.0	6
Hemoglobin (g/dL) for women	
≥10.0 < 12.0	1
<10.0	6
Systolic blood pressure (mm Hg)	
100–109	1
90–99	2
<90	3
Other factors	
Pulse ≥ 100 (per min)	1
Melena	1
Syncope on presentation	2
Liver disease	2
Heart failure	2
AIMS65 score	
Albumin < 3.0 mg/dL	1
Age > 65	1
Altered mental status	1
Systolic blood pressure (mm Hg) < 90 mm Hg	1
INR > 1.5	1

INR, international normalized ratio.

3. Statistical Analysis

Baseline characteristics and outcomes were summarized by frequency tabulation and means with standard deviations as appropriate. Discriminative ability of the scoring systems for predicting outcomes was evaluated by receiver-operator characteristic curve analysis.

The area under the receiver-operating characteristic curve (AUROC) was calculated and compared for both scores using the DeLong test [15]. A cutoff point was selected according to the maximal sum of the sensitivity and the specificity for each score. Patients were considered to be in the low risk group for each score if they fell below the cutoff point or in the high risk group if they were at or above the cutoff point. Estimates of sensitivity, specificity, and positive and negative predictive values were calculated for each score. Comparison between low and high risk groups for each score was performed using the chi score test and Fisher's exact test as appropriate. All statistical comparisons were 2 tailed, with p value < 0.05 considered statistically significant. The data analysis was performed by using STATA, version 13.0 (StataCorp, College Station, TX).

TABLE 2: Patient characteristics and outcomes.

Characteristics	Number (%)
Baseline characteristics	
Age, mean (SD)	78.8 (0.54)
Gender (male)	75 (47%)
PPI at home	76 (46%)
NSAIDs at home	25 (15.2%)
Charlson comorbidity index, mean (SD)	5.79 (2.4)
Presentation	
Hematochezia	23 (14%)
Melena	95 (58%)
Hematemesis	53 (32%)
Unstable comorbidity on admission	13 (9.2%)
Source of bleeding	
Peptic ulcer disease	45 (27%)
Gastritis	75 (45%)
Duodenitis	8 (5%)
Esophagitis	44 (27%)
Neoplasm	1 (0.6%)
Normal endoscopy	5 (3%)
Mallory Weiss tear	1 (0.6%)
Arteriovenous malformation	7 (4%)
Ulcerated gastric polyp	3 (2%)
No endoscopy	9 (5%)
Management and outcomes	
Upper endoscopy only	100 (60%)
Colonoscopy only	2 (1.2%)
Upper endoscopy and colonoscopy	54 (33%)
No endoscopic procedure	8 (5%)
In-hospital mortality	1 (0.6%)
Intervention to control bleeding source	9 (5.5%)
Need for a nonurgent intervention to treat findings on endoscopic procedure	2 (1.2%)
Readmission in 30 days for rebleeding	33 (20.5%)
Received blood transfusion	105 (64%)

PPI: proton pump inhibitor, NSAIDs: nonsteroidal anti-inflammatory drugs, and SD: standard deviation.

4. Results

One hundred and sixty-four (164) patients were included in the study based on inclusion and exclusion criteria. Demographic and clinical characteristics, treatments, and outcomes are shown in Table 2. No endoscopic investigations were done on 5% of the patients because either the patient declined the procedure or the treating physician decided against the procedure for clinical reasons.

In-hospital mortality was 0.63% (1 patient). This patient died from a sigmoid colon perforation after colonoscopy. Most of the patients (92.8%) in our cohort did not need a therapeutic endoscopic, surgical, or radiologic intervention. In these patients the bleeding stopped spontaneously with supportive and conservative management.

An intervention to control the bleeding source was performed in 9 patients (5.5%). Two patients (1.2%) needed a nonurgent intervention (Schatzki's ring dilatation and pancreatic cancer diagnosis with subsequent referral for palliative measures).

The composite outcome of in-hospital mortality, need for any intervention, readmission in 30 days for GIB, and need for blood transfusion occurred in 119 patients (72.5%); most of the outcome was driven by need for blood transfusion, which was required in 105 (64% of patients).

When comparing AUROC for predicting the primary composite outcome of in-hospital mortality, need for any intervention, readmission for rebleed within 30 days, or need for blood transfusion, Blatchford score (0.80 95% CI 0.71–0.88) was superior to AIMS65 score (0.68 95% CI 0.60–0.77) ($p = 0.02$) (Figure 1).

A Blatchford score more than or equal to 1 was able to identify 99% of high risk patients; however, only 3 patients (1.85% of the patients) had a score of 0. A Blatchford score more than or equal to 2 identified 97.5 of the high risk patients. Using a Blatchford score more than or equal to 2 as a cutoff resulted in 14 (8.5%) patients being classified as low risk. No patients in this group died or required an intervention; however, three patients received blood transfusion. This resulted in a sensitivity of 97.5% and specificity of 24.4% when a Blatchford score more than or equal to 2 is counted as high risk (Table 3). The primary outcome occurred in 77% of patients in the high risk group and in 21% in the low risk group ($p < 0.001$).

Blatchford score and AIMS65 scores did not perform well in predicting the secondary outcome of in-hospital mortality or need for an intervention to control the bleeding [AUROC 0.56 (95% CI 0.34–0.70) versus 0.52 (95% CI 0.37–0.67)] for Blatchford and AIMS65 scores, respectively ($p = 0.97$) (Figure 2). Blatchford score more than or equal to 2 had 100% sensitivity and 100% negative predictive value for in-hospital mortality or need for an urgent intervention; however the specificity and the positive predictive value were very low (9 and 6.6%, resp.) (Table 4).

5. Discussion

The study evaluated the performance of Blatchford and AIMS65 scores in elderly patients presenting with nonvariceal upper GIB.

The low mortality rate in our cohort is within the range of mortality rates in elderly patients with nonvariceal upper GIB reported in prior studies [1–3, 7]. Prior studies on nonvariceal upper GIB in the general population had wide variation in mortality which is believed to be related to the definition of upper GIB and the populations studied [16]. We chose to define UGIB based on endoscopic findings rather than using presenting symptoms if other than hematemesis. In patients with GIB who do not present with hematemesis, an upper GI source is identified in only 30–74% of patients [17, 18]. In patients with hematochezia, it is estimated that about 10% have an upper source of bleeding identified [19, 20]. This makes the use of symptoms to define UGIB unreliable.

TABLE 3: Performance of the scores in predicting the combined outcome of inpatient mortality, need for any intervention, readmission for rebleed within 30 days, and need for blood transfusion.

Score	Sensitivity %	Specificity %	PPV %	NPV %	AUROC (95% CI)
Blatchford score ≥2	97.5	25	79	81	0.80 (0.71–0.89)
AIMS65 score ≥2	68	64	83	43	0.68 (0.60–0.77)

PPV: positive predictive value. NPV: negative predictive value. AUROC: area under receiver-operator curve.

TABLE 4: Performance of the scores in predicting inpatient mortality or need for an urgent intervention to control bleeding.

Score	Sensitivity %	Specificity %	PPV %	NPV %	AUROC (95% CI)
Blatchford score ≥2	100	9	6.6	100	0.56 (0.34–0.70)
AIMS65 score ≥2	70	41.5	6	92.7	0.52 (0.36–0.67)

PPV: positive predictive value. NPV: negative predictive value. AUROC: area under receiver-operator curve.

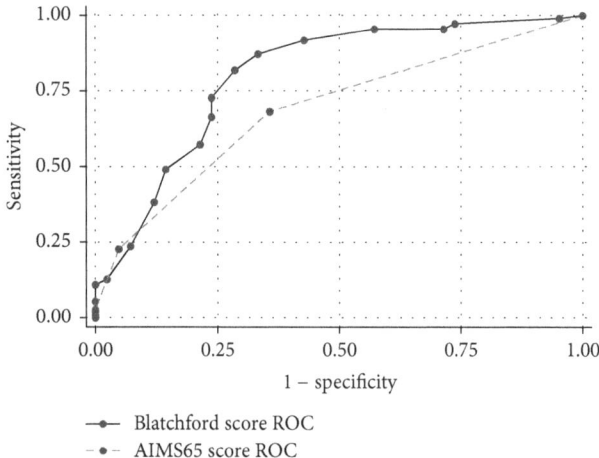

FIGURE 1: Area under receiver-operating characteristic (ROC) curve for Blatchford score and AIMS65 score in predicting composite outcome of in-hospital mortality, need for any intervention, readmission for rebleed within 30 days, or need for blood transfusion.

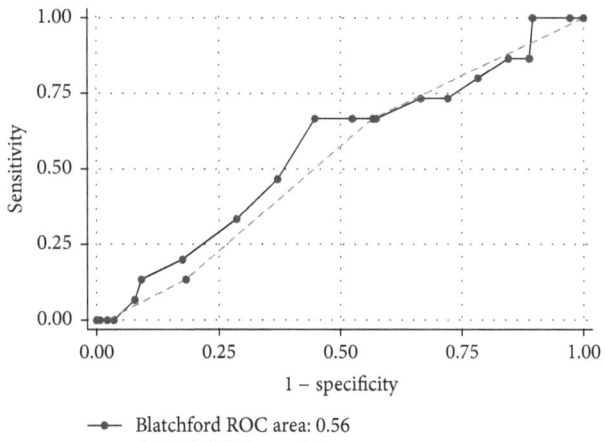

FIGURE 2: Area under receiver-operating characteristic (ROC) curve for Blatchford score and AIMS65 score in predicting the combined outcome of in-hospital mortality or need for urgent intervention to control bleeding.

The need for an intervention to control bleeding in our cohort of elderly patient was also low (5.5%). This is much lower than rates of endoscopic interventions in prior studies of UGIB in the general population which ranged from 21 to 56% [21–25]. The low intervention and mortality rates in our study could be explained at least in part with the lower incidence of PUD in our population (27%) compared to other studies in which PUD represented 22–56% of the sample as well as exclusion of variceal bleeding. It has been suggested that the incidence of PUD in UGIB is exaggerated in studies of UGIB outcomes and it represents only about 20–30% of causes which is consistent with our findings [26]. This is likely related to differences in population and inclusion criteria used as some studies included variceal bleed [21–23] and patients who developed bleeding while hospitalized [22–24] and excluded patients who did not undergo endoscopy in the first 24 h of presentation [21, 24] and relied on clinical rather than endoscopic criteria to define upper GIB [21–23, 27]. For example, Pang et al. included only patients with UGIB who underwent an inpatient endoscopy within 24 hours in Hong Kong [21]. They had an intervention rate of 27% and a PUD incidence of 50%. 71% of the interventions were related to PUD and 15% were related to variceal bleed [21]. On the other hand, the multicenter study by Laursen et al. in Europe reported a PUD incidence of 31%, variceal bleed of 7%, and an intervention rate of 19% [27]. In addition, the lower rates of intervention could also be related to the older age of the population itself. Wang et al. reported an intervention rate of 9% in older adults (>60 years) with UGIB [25]. Our results are consistent with other studies in the elderly which reported that esophagitis [4] and gastritis [5] are the most common cause of nonvariceal GIB in older patients and are in line with other studies of the etiology of upper GIB in the elderly [6]. We believe that the population in our study is representative of the elderly population in the community.

Blatchford score was originally developed to predict similar outcomes in the general population presenting to the ED with an upper GIB. Stanley et al. [9] showed that outpatient management of patients with upper GIB with a Blatchford score of 0 is safe [9]. It has also been suggested that a threshold of Blatchford score more than or equal to 2 could be used as a decision cutoff for hospital admission in upper GIB [10, 11].

In our cohort of elderly patients only 1.8% of the patients had a Blatchford score of 0. This is largely due to increased prevalence of comorbidities and anemia in this population. A Blatchford score more than or equal to 2 identified 97.7 of the high risk patients. Blatchford score more than or equal to 2 has a high sensitivity for the combined outcome of in-hospital mortality, need for any intervention, and need for blood transfusion and readmission for rebleed in elderly patients with GIB. Even though the specificity of the test is very low using this cutoff, using Blatchford score more than or equal to 2 as a criterion for admission has the potential to reduce admissions for GIB by 8% in elderly patients. Although 3 patients (19%) in the low risk category required blood transfusion, none of them died or required an intervention to control the bleed and a Blatchford score more than or equal to 2 was able to identify 97.7% of the high risk patients. This high sensitivity and low specificity were pointed out by others [28] and are consistent with results of previous studies on the performance of Blatchford score in upper GIB in the general population [9–11].

AIMS65 score performed poorly in our cohort of elderly patients in predicting the need for admission. Our population was different from that whose AIMS65 score was originally derived and validated [12, 14]. We think that its reliance on age and albumin as factors in the score contributed to the poor performance in elderly patients with no advanced liver disease like ours.

Most elderly patients in our study stopped bleeding with supportive care only without the need for an intervention to control the bleed. However, both Blatchford and AIMS65 scores performed poorly in predicting the combined outcome of in-hospital mortality or the need for an intervention to control bleeding. A Blatchford score more than or equal to 2 has a very low specificity resulting in a low AUROC of 0.57 in predicting this outcome. Therefore, both Blatchford and AIMS65 scores have no clinical use in predicting which patients would benefit from an urgent intervention. However, Blatchford score more than or equal to 2 has 100% sensitivity for the secondary outcome. Therefore, a low score excludes the need for an intervention and a Blatchford score more than or equal to 2 can be used as a triaging tool to identify low risk patients who can be treated in the outpatient setting.

Limitations. The study is limited by the retrospective design of the study which may have compromised the data validity; however, the study was conducted using a structured protocol and training for data abstraction to limit bias. The study was conducted in a single institution which potentially could limit the generalizability of its results. In addition, 5% of the patients did not undergo endoscopic procedure; thus, the etiology of the bleed was uncertain; however, the outcomes of interest were available for those patients and exclusion of these patients could result in a selection bias. Furthermore, our results apply only to elderly patients with nonvariceal UGIB as patients with known liver disease or acute hepatic failure were excluded.

6. Conclusion

Nonvariceal UGIB in most elderly patients ceases spontaneously with supportive care without the need for an invasive intervention. Blatchford score is useful in predicting the need for hospital based interventions such as blood transfusion in elderly patient with nonvariceal UGIB and can serve as a triaging tool to identify low risk patients who can be treated as outpatients. However, it has low specificity and it should not be relied upon to predict the need for a therapeutic intervention. AIMS65 score is of no use to predict outcomes in elderly patients with UGIB. Further work is needed to develop better predictors of the need for an urgent intervention to control the bleed.

Additional Points

Institutional Review Board Approval. All research reviews were conducted under protocols approved by the local Institutional Review Board (IRB) and all data were collected and analyzed in accordance with the ethical standards as laid down in the 1964 Declaration of Helsinki and its later amendments or comparable ethical standards.

Competing Interests

The authors have no conflict of interests to declare.

Acknowledgments

The authors would like to acknowledge Dr. Debby Sentana, Dr. Fnu Vikram, and Dr. Jinendra Satiya for their help with the study.

References

[1] P. Charatcharoenwitthaya, N. Pausawasdi, N. Laosanguaneak, J. Bubthamala, T. Tanwandee, and S. Leelakusolvong, "Characteristics and outcomes of acute upper gastrointestinal bleeding after therapeutic endoscopy in the elderly," *World Journal of Gastroenterology*, vol. 17, no. 32, pp. 3724–3732, 2011.

[2] D. C. Brown, J. S. Collins, and A. H. Love, "Outcome and benefits of upper gastrointestinal endoscopy in the elderly," *The Ulster Medical Journal*, vol. 58, no. 2, pp. 177–181, 1989.

[3] A. A. Alkhatib, F. A. Elkhatib, A. Maldonado, S. M. Abubakr, and D. G. Adler, "Acute upper gastrointestinal bleeding in elderly people: presentations, endoscopic findings, and outcomes," *Journal of the American Geriatrics Society*, vol. 58, no. 1, pp. 182–185, 2010.

[4] J. Zimmerman, V. Shohat, E. Tsvang, R. Arnon, R. Safadi, and D. Wengrower, "Esophagitis is a major cause of upper gastrointestinal hemorrhage in the elderly," *Scandinavian Journal of Gastroenterology*, vol. 32, no. 9, pp. 906–909, 1997.

[5] S. H. Tariq, N. Zia, M. L. Omran et al., "Gastritis is the most common cause of gastrointestinal bleeding in older persons," *Journal of the American Geriatrics Society*, vol. 48, article S53, 2000.

[6] S. H. Tariq and G. Mekhjian, "Gastrointestinal bleeding in older adults," *Clinics in Geriatric Medicine*, vol. 23, no. 4, pp. 769–784, 2007.

[7] W. N. Segal and J. P. Cello, "Hemorrhage in the upper gastrointestinal tract in the older patient," *The American Journal of Gastroenterology*, vol. 92, no. 1, pp. 42–46, 1997.

[8] O. Blatchford, W. Murray, and M. Blatchford, "A risk score to predict need for treatment for upper-gastrointestinal hemorrhage," *The Lancet*, vol. 356, pp. 1318–1321, 2000.

[9] A. J. Stanley, D. Ashley, H. R. Dalton et al., "Outpatient management of patients with low-risk upper-gastrointestinal haemorrhage: multicentre validation and prospective evaluation," *The Lancet*, vol. 373, no. 9657, pp. 42–47, 2009.

[10] I. R. Le Jeune, A. L. Gordon, D. Farrugia, R. Manwani, I. N. Guha, and M. W. James, "Safe discharge of patients with low-risk upper gastrointestinal bleeding (UGIB): can the use of Glasgow-Blatchford Bleeding Score be extended?" *Acute Medicine*, vol. 10, no. 4, pp. 176–181, 2011.

[11] J. M. Recio-Ramírez, M. D. P. Sánchez-Sánchez, J. A. Peña-Ojeda et al., "The predictive capacity of the Glasgow-Blatchford score for the risk stratification of upper gastrointestinal bleeding in an emergency department," *Revista Española de Enfermedades Digestivas*, vol. 107, no. 5, pp. 262–267, 2015.

[12] J. R. Saltzman, Y. P. Tabak, B. H. Hyett, X. Sun, A. C. Travis, and R. S. Johannes, "A simple risk score accurately predicts in-hospital mortality, length of stay, and cost in acute upper GI bleeding," *Gastrointestinal Endoscopy*, vol. 74, no. 6, pp. 1215–1224, 2011.

[13] E. Yaka, S. Yilmaz, N. O. Dogan, and M. Pekdemir, "Comparison of the glasgow-blatchford and AIMS65 scoring systems for risk stratification in upper gastrointestinal bleeding in the emergency department," *Academic Emergency Medicine*, vol. 22, no. 1, pp. 23–30, 2015.

[14] B. H. Hyett, M. S. Abougergi, J. P. Charpentier et al., "The AIMS65 score compared with the Glasgow-Blatchford score in predicting outcomes in upper GI bleeding," *Gastrointestinal Endoscopy*, vol. 77, no. 4, pp. 551–557, 2013.

[15] E. R. DeLong, D. M. DeLong, and D. L. Clarke-Pearson, "Comparing the areas under two or more correlated receiver operating characteristic curves: a nonparametric approach," *Biometrics*, vol. 44, no. 3, pp. 837–845, 1988.

[16] V. Jairath, M. Martel, R. F. A. Logan, and A. N. Barkun, "Why do mortality rates for nonvariceal upper gastrointestinal bleeding differ around the world? A systematic review of cohort studies," *Canadian Journal of Gastroenterology*, vol. 26, no. 8, pp. 537–543, 2012.

[17] M. D. Witting, L. Magder, A. E. Heins, A. Mattu, C. A. Granja, and M. Baumgarten, "ED predictors of upper gastrointestinal tract bleeding in patients without hematemesis," *The American Journal of Emergency Medicine*, vol. 24, no. 3, pp. 280–285, 2006.

[18] N. Palamidessi, R. Sinert, L. Falzon, and S. Zehtabchi, "Nasogastric aspiration and lavage in emergency department patients with hematochezia or melena without hematemesis," *Academic Emergency Medicine*, vol. 17, no. 2, pp. 126–132, 2010.

[19] S. E. Byers, C. R. Chudnofsky, B. Sorondo, P. Dominici, and S. J. Parrillo, "Incidence of occult upper gastrointestinal bleeding in patients presenting to the ED with hematochezia," *The American Journal of Emergency Medicine*, vol. 25, no. 3, pp. 340–344, 2007.

[20] D. M. Jensen and G. A. Machicado, "Diagnosis and treatment of severe hematochezia. The role of urgent colonoscopy after purge," *Gastroenterology*, vol. 95, no. 6, pp. 1569–1574, 1988.

[21] S. H. Pang, J. Y. L. Ching, J. Y. W. Lau, J. J. Y. Sung, D. Y. Graham, and F. K. L. Chan, "Comparing the Blatchford and pre-endoscopic Rockall score in predicting the need for endoscopic therapy in patients with upper GI hemorrhage," *Gastrointestinal Endoscopy*, vol. 71, no. 7, pp. 1134–1140, 2010.

[22] S. B. Laursen, J. M. Hansen, and O. B. Schaffalitzky de Muckadell, "The glasgow blatchford score is the most accurate assessment of patients with upper gastrointestinal hemorrhage," *Clinical Gastroenterology and Hepatology*, vol. 10, no. 10, pp. 1130–1135, 2012.

[23] R. V. Bryant, P. Kuo, K. Williamson et al., "Performance of the Glasgow-Blatchford score in predicting clinical outcomes and intervention in hospitalized patients with upper GI bleeding," *Gastrointestinal Endoscopy*, vol. 78, no. 4, pp. 576–583, 2013.

[24] B. J. Kim, M. K. Park, S. Kim et al., "Comparison of scoring systems for the prediction of outcomes in patients with nonvariceal upper gastrointestinal bleeding: a prospective study," *Digestive Diseases and Sciences*, vol. 54, no. 11, pp. 2523–2529, 2009.

[25] C.-Y. Wang, J. Qin, J. Wang, C.-Y. Sun, T. Cao, and D.-D. Zhu, "Rockall score in predicting outcomes of elderly patients with acute upper gastrointestinal bleeding," *World Journal of Gastroenterology*, vol. 19, no. 22, pp. 3466–3472, 2013.

[26] S. Boonpongmanee, D. E. Fleischer, J. C. Pezzullo et al., "The frequency of peptic ulcer as a cause of upper-GI bleeding is exaggerated," *Gastrointestinal Endoscopy*, vol. 59, no. 7, pp. 788–794, 2004.

[27] S. B. Laursen, H. R. Dalton, I. A. Murray et al., "Performance of new thresholds of the Glasgow Blatchford score in managing patients with upper gastrointestinal bleeding," *Clinical Gastroenterology and Hepatology*, vol. 13, no. 1, pp. 115–121.e2, 2015.

[28] S. Ahn, K. S. Lim, Y.-S. Lee, and J.-L. Lee, "Blatchford score is a useful tool for predicting the need for intervention in cancer patients with upper gastrointestinal bleeding," *Journal of Gastroenterology and Hepatology*, vol. 28, no. 8, pp. 1288–1294, 2013.

13

Mathematical Modelling and Tuberculosis: Advances in Diagnostics and Novel Therapies

Alice Zwerling, Sourya Shrestha, and David W. Dowdy

Johns Hopkins Bloomberg School of Public Health, Baltimore, MD 21205, USA

Correspondence should be addressed to Alice Zwerling; azwerli1@jhu.edu

Academic Editor: Aliya Naheed

As novel diagnostics, therapies, and algorithms are developed to improve case finding, diagnosis, and clinical management of patients with TB, policymakers must make difficult decisions and choose among multiple new technologies while operating under heavy resource constrained settings. Mathematical modelling can provide helpful insight by describing the types of interventions likely to maximize impact on the population level and highlighting those gaps in our current knowledge that are most important for making such assessments. This review discusses the major contributions of TB transmission models in general, namely, the ability to improve our understanding of the epidemiology of TB. We focus particularly on those elements that are important to appropriately understand the role of TB diagnosis and treatment (i.e., what elements of better diagnosis or treatment are likely to have greatest population-level impact) and yet remain poorly understood at present. It is essential for modellers, decision-makers, and epidemiologists alike to recognize these outstanding gaps in knowledge and understand their potential influence on model projections that may guide critical policy choices (e.g., investment and scale-up decisions).

1. Introduction

Recent decades have seen renewed interest in tuberculosis (TB) research, notably in areas of diagnostic test development and novel treatment regimens for TB and multidrug resistant TB (MDR-TB) [1–3]. New advances bring great potential to reduce TB burden and mortality, but resources remain highly constrained in most TB endemic settings. Mathematical modelling can serve to estimate the impact of various interventions on outcomes of interest; they can provide helpful insight by describing the types of interventions likely to maximize impact on the population level and highlighting those gaps in our current knowledge that are most important for making such assessments [4–8]. While the term "mathematical modelling" is used to describe a variety of techniques, this review will focus on transmission models designed to assess or understand the population-level (epidemiological) impact of TB control interventions.

The compartmental model, in which a population is divided into subpopulations or "compartments" on the basis of such characteristics as TB status, has historically been the most common form of TB mathematical model. Although other types of models, such as agent-based and network models, have been used to model specific transmission dynamics of TB [9–11], they are in general less frequently used in TB transmission models, where we are modeling airborne transmission of a chronic infection, compared to other infectious disease systems. In this outlook, we focus on compartmental models, which have been influential in modeling transmission dynamics of numerous infectious diseases, including droplet-borne respiratory diseases (e.g., influenza), sexually transmitted infections, and vector-borne diseases [12, 13]. The prototypical "SIR" model divides the population into susceptible (S), infected (I), and recovered (R) compartments, and transmission dynamics are described using rates of flow between these compartments. Given the complexities of TB pathology and the presence of a potentially long latency, compartmental models of TB are typically modified reflecting TB pathology, relevant context, and the research question of interest. Figure 1 depicts a simplified compartmental model for TB transmission, in which the population is subdivided into compartments of individuals who have never been infected with TB, those who have been

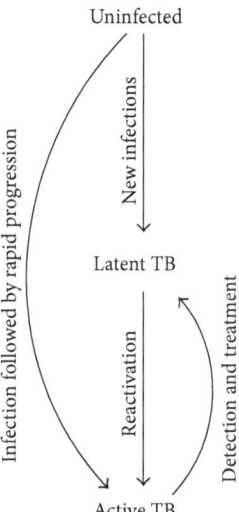

FIGURE 1: A simple epidemiological model of TB. Uninfected individuals that are exposed to TB can become infected with TB, which can result in either a long-standing infection that is asymptomatic and noninfectious (latent TB) or progress at some point ("reactivation") to a condition that is infectious and generally symptomatic (active TB). Detection and effective treatment can cure active TB. For simplicity, some other important features of natural history of TB are not shown here (but are generally included in compartmental models of TB), including reinfection, spontaneous resolution ("self-cure"), and mortality.

infected but are not currently infectious (latent TB), and those who are actively infectious and symptomatic. By evaluating the rates at which people flow from one compartment to another under different scenarios, such models can provide insight about not only the direct effects of those interventions on those who receive them, but also the indirect effects that occur through a reduction in transmission to the population as a whole.

Here, we use the compartmental model as a tool to highlight a major contribution of TB transmission models in general, namely, the ability to improve our understanding of the epidemiology of TB. We focus particularly on those elements that are important to appropriately understand the role of TB diagnosis and treatment (i.e., what elements of better diagnosis or treatment are likely to have greatest population-level impact) and yet remain poorly understood at present. It is essential for modellers, decision-makers, and epidemiologists alike to recognize these outstanding gaps in knowledge and understand their potential influence on model projections that may guide critical policy choices (e.g., investment and scale-up decisions). Only through such shared understanding can epidemiologists direct data collection efforts at the highest-yield targets, decision-makers understand both the value and limitations of model-based projections, and modelers seek to refine their tools in response to emerging data and policy needs.

2. Modelling Transmission

2.1. Infectiousness over Time. A key advantage of transmission models is that they incorporate the process of infection; in other words, interventions that lead to faster diagnosis of TB also benefit the population by reducing transmission [14]. However, the process of transmission is also an area of great uncertainty in TB. A commonly used measure to describe infectiousness is the effective reproductive ratio (R_e), which represents the average number of secondary cases arising from a primary case of active TB in a population with its existing level of immunity. Notably, R_e depend on both the process of generating infectious particles and social mixing or contact patterns within the host population.

The impact of a given diagnostic intervention on TB transmission will depend on its effect on R_e, as it is deployed in the population. Our ability to estimate the number of effective secondary cases produced by each index case and how a diagnostic intervention may reduce this number is therefore critical. However, accurately assessing the reproductive ratio for TB, much less the effect of a diagnostic intervention on that ratio, requires a better understanding of the context in which TB transmission occurs. Unfortunately, we currently lack a tool that can reliably detect recent TB transmission or infection: tests for latent TB infection do not differentiate between recent and remote infection, and tests for active TB likewise do not differentiate the timing of initial transmission leading to infectiousness [15, 16]. Unlike acute infections (e.g., influenza, measles, and diarrheal illness), the time from infection to disease in TB can be as short as a few months, or as long as decades. Even animal models are limited in this regard; with the exception of nonhuman primates, animal models including mice, guinea pigs, and rabbits do not approximate the human latent TB infection phase [17], and there is no animal model for human social interactions.

The effective reproductive ratio for TB in different populations depends on three processes: the generation of infectious particles, contact between infectious individuals and other members of society, and susceptibility of the host population [7]. The clinical course of TB infection and disease comprises a spectrum that is dynamic over time and varies between and within individuals [18] and includes elements of infectiousness, symptom burden, and changing social interactions (e.g., staying home when sick) that are all poorly understood. Better data to inform these dynamic processes would help to improve our estimates of the impact expected from different TB diagnostic interventions, and mathematical models can highlight which data elements are most critical [19].

2.2. Generation of Infectious Particles. As TB is an airborne disease, generation of infectious particles ("droplet nuclei") is essential to transmission [20]. This process depends on both the infectious agent (e.g., ability to survive in small particles and to infect lung alveolar epithelium when inhaled) and the host (e.g., generation of particles sufficiently small to remain airborne and that contain infectious organisms). The presence of visible *M. tuberculosis* bacilli on microscopic examination of sputum (sputum smear status) is a correlate of

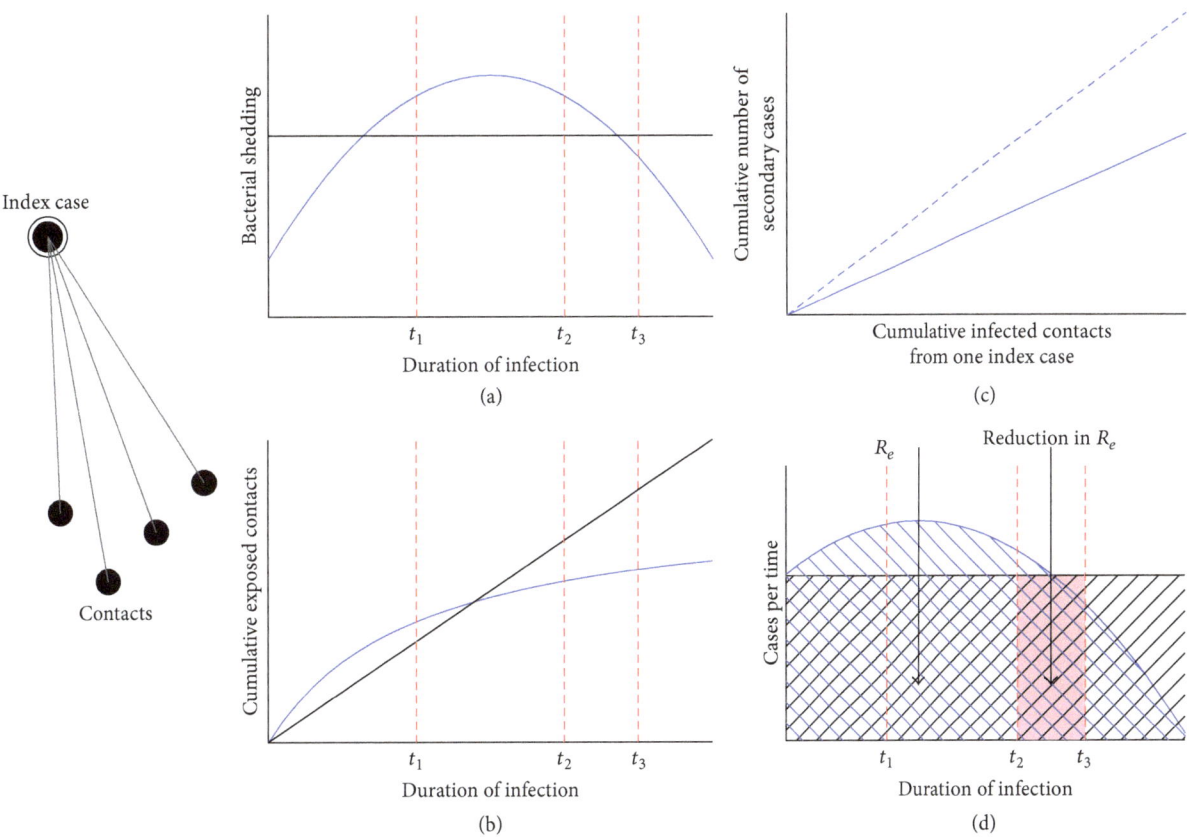

FIGURE 2: (a) The rate of bacterial shedding over the duration of infection may be a constant function (black line) or change over time (blue line). (b) The cumulative number of contacts exposed to TB over the duration of infection may increase linearly over time (black line) or may plateau as contact pool becomes saturated or patient is too ill to circulate in the community. The potential impact of a novel intervention may depend on this assumption; given a linear increase, earlier intervention (t_1) would be likely preferred. While given the second curve with only a small increase and plateau, the impact between intervening at t_1 and t_2 might not be as great; therefore other factors including cost-effectiveness may come into play. (c) The cumulative number of secondary cases resulting from one index case in relation to the number of cumulative infected contacts: there are factors associated with bacterial virulence and host susceptibility that impact the rate of progression from infection to disease. This rate may be steeper among immunosuppressed contacts, for example, (dotted line) compared with immunocompetent contact (solid line). (d) The effective reproductive number (R_e) is the number of secondary cases generated over a given time period. Bacterial shedding, contact mixing pattern, and bacterial and host susceptibility all contribute to the overall rate of secondary cases generated over time; depending on what assumptions are made these rates could be thought to stay constant over time or vary, perhaps tapering off over the duration of infection. By reducing the time to diagnosis and treatment initiation we hope to reduce the number of secondary cases but the amount of impact depends on assumptions around the shape of the curve over time. The hashed area represents the secondary cases generated from one index case while the shaded area represents the potential reduction in secondary cases given an intervention at t_2. Figure adapted with permission from Dowdy et al. [7].

infectiousness, but individuals with smear-negative TB may still contribute a substantial proportion of TB transmission on the population level [21]. This has important implications for diagnosis, which traditionally rests on sputum smear microscopy as an integral part of the diagnostic algorithm. For novel diagnostic tests to have important impact on TB epidemiology, they must improve upon sputum smear, in terms of its ability to identify those cases that contribute to community transmission. Whole genome sequencing is now frequently used in high-income countries to identify transmission clusters and super-spreaders [22–25], but these evaluations occur post hoc and only in lower-burden or research settings. Understanding how other diagnostic interventions are likely to alter the total number of infectious particles generated by a single representative individual with

active TB may help to understand the likely impact of those interventions on the population level.

Within the context of diagnostic interventions, it becomes important to understand how both the generation of infectious TB particles and the rate of contact with susceptible individuals change over time with the evolving TB disease course (Figures 2(a) and 2(b)). Assumptions relating to these processes have important implications for the potential impact of diagnostic interventions [7]. For example, if diagnostics are deployed in such a way that most infectious contacts have already occurred by the time new diagnostic tests can be accessed, the impact of those novel tests on TB incidence will be limited—even if the tests are perfectly sensitive and specific. Similarly, if diagnostic tests are implemented without the infrastructure necessary to link people who test positive to appropriate treatment, the infectious course will remain unaltered. Specifically, Dowdy et al. used a model that included subclinical TB disease phase and found that ignoring the possibility of infectiousness prior to seeking care resulted in models that could overestimate the impact of passive diagnostic testing (i.e., testing that relies on symptomatic presentation by patients) by 50% or more [7]. This model demonstrated that active case detection of prevalent cases in the community is likely to have greater impact on the duration of infectiousness, and thus on TB incidence, than passive diagnosis. It also showed that estimates of the relative impact of different diagnostic strategies depend critically on improving our understanding of when in the disease process TB transmission occurs.

2.3. Contact between Infectious Individuals and Other Members of Society. Generation of an infectious particle will only cause transmission of TB if that particle contacts the lung epithelium of another individual. Such contact depends on social mixing patterns between people with active TB and other members of society. For example, if an index case only has extended exposure to household contacts, close friends and family there may be a point in time where the cumulative number of infected contacts reaches a plateau, with no or very few new contacts exposed (Figure 2(b)). In such a scenario, increasing levels of bacterial shedding from the index case may not result in more infections if the pool of susceptible contacts has reached saturation. Similarly, low levels of bacterial shedding during early onset of the disease, even prior to the patient recognizing any symptoms, may account for a significant proportion of transmission events if the duration of that period is long and characterized by more frequent airborne contacts (e.g., if people continue to work and interact with society during that time). Like the ability to generate infectious particles, the trajectory of social contact is likely to vary between individuals and across settings, and the point in that trajectory at which diagnostic interventions are deployed will determine the population-level impact of those interventions. Many models assume the simplest case (constant rate of contact over time), but the number of susceptible contacts most likely declines over time unless index cases are hospitalized, imprisoned, or otherwise introduced into a new population. This phenomenon likely decreases the potential impact of passive diagnostic testing, as most transmission events may occur early in the disease course. Kasaie et al. [10] employed agent based models to explore scenarios where transmission was dominated by either community or household transmission and the potential impact of household based contact tracing. The authors found that 75–95% of household infections would have occurred prior to the diagnosis of the focal case in the household, and, hence, household contact tracing by itself was unlikely to be transformative in terms of TB epidemiology. Better understanding the degree to which contact rate changes over time may be essential for better estimating the impact of novel diagnostic tests for TB.

2.4. Susceptibility of the Host Population. A third important determinant of the rate of TB transmission over time, and

thus of the impact of diagnostic testing, is the susceptibility of the host population to developing active TB after a potentially infectious contact. This concept of susceptibility therefore encompasses both susceptibility to infection and susceptibility to progression if infection occurs. While not necessarily intrinsic to host susceptibility, bacterial strain virulence also plays an important role [26, 27]. Further determinants of TB susceptibility, including HIV, older age, diabetes, smoking, and malnutrition, have been described in the literature; however, the degree to which these determinants of susceptibility overlap with potential transmission events is only now becoming understood [28]. In settings where many infectious contacts occur with individuals of higher susceptibility profiles, R_e will be substantially higher than if those contacts occur with less susceptible people, as depicted in Figure 2(c). Indeed, one of the major reasons for the dramatic declines in TB incidence seen throughout much of the Western world is likely a reduction in the susceptibility profile of the population, while the TB rise in Africa is driven by the HIV epidemic [29].

2.5. Sensitivity and Uncertainty Analyses. Transmission modelling results are often accompanied by sensitivity and uncertainty analyses, which can achieve two important goals. First, some parameters used in the model can contain large uncertainty or variability in the estimates, arising from either the dearth of high quality data or the variability of estimates derived from different sources. Uncertainty analyses help give readers perspective on how uncertainty in model inputs might translate into uncertainty in model results. Second, sensitivity analyses of the model input parameters can provide critical information on which model parameters have the most influence on model results. Typical sensitivity analyses include one-way and multivariate sensitivity analyses. In one-way sensitivity analysis, one observes changes in the model outcome as a result of change in a single focal parameter, holding other parameters constant. In contrast, in a multivariate sensitivity analysis, one varies all or most of the model parameters over selected ranges and computes the model outcomes. By analyzing the correlation between the model outcome and a given parameter, one can assess the role of the parameter in the outcome [30]. Sensitivity and uncertainty analyses also do not address uncertainties arising from uncertainty or variability in the model structure.

3. The Role of Modeling: TB Diagnostics

3.1. Background. The field of TB diagnostics has seen major growth in the last decade, and many novel technologies are now available for use, with even more in the pipeline. Arguably the greatest technological breakthrough in TB control over the past decade has been a new diagnostic test: Xpert MTB/RIF, a molecular test for TB and rifampin resistance capable of providing results in two hours with minimal human resource requirement [31]. Important questions are now arising as policymakers must consider implementing rapidly expanding options for TB diagnostics, while drawing on limited budgets.

Mathematical modeling can help policymakers understand the potential population-level impact and cost-effectiveness associated with implementing novel diagnostic tests. Importantly, models can consider a wide variety of settings, populations, and diagnostic algorithms to help inform the "right diagnostic approach for the right setting"—in other words, helping us to understand what population characteristics will lead to different approaches having greater or less impact. Whereas decision-makers often express an interest in models that will project the future under different implementation scenarios, understanding the factors that drive the impact of different diagnostic approaches is often a more important long-term goal—and models are uniquely positioned to provide this kind of insight.

Lin et al. have conducted modelling studies to estimate the potential impact of new diagnostic tools using detailed models of the diagnostic pathway and integrating operational and dynamic transmission models [32, 33]. This work compared the reduction in incidence, prevalence, and mortality of pulmonary TB achieved by new diagnostic tools against a baseline case of sputum smear microscopy. They demonstrated the importance of including operational context and the diagnostic pathway in models evaluating novel diagnostics; for example, the epidemiologic impact of a new more accurate tool was greatest in settings where access to tuberculosis care was good but existing diagnostic strategies have poor sensitivity and was less dependent on its relative performance. These models can be informative both for guiding decisions around novel tools and the impact of alternative diagnostic pathways; however useful projections rely on capturing the relevant structure of the transmission dynamics and diagnostic pathway at work.

Matching the appropriate diagnostic test and algorithm to a given setting is an important task but one that requires understanding of interactions between population epidemiology, test characteristics, operational considerations (e.g., feasibility of scale-up), and resource requirements. Depending on the interventions being considered, different assumptions may be required—such as those relating to test accuracy (e.g., sensitivity and specificity), use (e.g., diagnostic algorithm and purpose of the test), underlying population, and costs. Improved understanding of which assumptions are most critical to specific decisions regarding TB diagnostics can help the TB control community direct data-gathering efforts and make more informed decisions in the future.

3.2. Summary: Infectiousness over Time and Implications for Models of Diagnostic Interventions. Figure 2(d) depicts the rate of transmissions that will ultimately lead to a secondary case of infectious TB, over the disease course of an index case. Upon contact with a diagnostic intervention (t_2) that results in treatment that would otherwise be delayed (t_3), the shaded area between those two times and under the curve represents the reduction in R_e achieved. This figure demonstrates that the potential impact of diagnostic interventions depends on not only their accuracy but also how early in the disease course they can be deployed and the shape of the "transmission curve" before versus after contact with the diagnostic intervention. Understanding this shape is

key to the development of accurate models of TB diagnostics and incorporates the elements discussed above: generation of infectious particles, contact, and susceptibility. The duration between t_2 and t_3 likewise depends on characteristics of the health system and patients' interactions with that system [32, 33]. The potential impact of novel diagnostics can be attenuated not only by flaws in the test, but also by delays in care seeking, diagnosis, and treatment (i.e., longer time to t_2 in Figure 2(d)).

In summary, although active case finding is a stated goal, at present we must still rely on symptomatic presentation by patients for most TB diagnoses to occur. Mathematical models can help decision-makers understand the potential impact of novel TB diagnostic tests, but they also highlight the key data gaps that prevent us from being able to make more accurate, evidence-based projections. Those data gaps include insufficient knowledge about the trajectories of infectiousness, mixing, and population susceptibility over time, including how those trajectories are influenced by the pathogen, host, and health system. If we are to understand the population-level impact of novel TB diagnostics, the next wave of epidemiological data gathering must address these deficiencies in our current understanding.

4. The Role of Modeling: TB Drugs and Drug Resistance

4.1. Background. For the first time in many decades [34] new first-line drug regimens are being considered for treatment of TB. Some of these regimens make repurposed use of existing drug compounds (e.g., fluoroquinolones) and others use novel compounds (e.g., PA-824) [35–37]. The possibility of new first-line drug regimens for TB offers an opportunity to further investigate the dynamics of TB drug resistance, which will be a key consideration in the roll-out of any such regimen. Existing second-line regimens require prolonged, costly, uncomfortable treatment (often 24 months with up to 8 months of daily injections) with a much greater risk of side effects including neuropsychiatric effects, loss of hearing, and kidney failure [38–40]. Since such regimens are very challenging to complete, it is essential to limit our dependence on such regimen from a population perspective. However, transmission of resistance can spur a vicious cycle: as resistant strains of TB become more prevalent, they spread more rapidly, in turn increasing the transmission burden of drug resistant TB. Mathematical models can help guide decision-making and elucidate key knowledge gaps in this complex arena [41–46]. In the context of resistance to new first-line drug regimens, the role of modeling is particularly important for two different reasons.

First, drug resistance is a multifactorial process, and the emergence of drug resistance in a population setting depends on several underlying factors [47]. As with diagnostic considerations above, these include factors intrinsic to the pathogen, including genetic barriers to drug resistance [48–52]; factors related to contact/transmission, including TB prevalence (i.e., transmission burden) and treatment success [48]; and factors related to host susceptibility, including HIV prevalence [53].

While we have developed a rudimentary understanding of some of these factors, models can help to demonstrate where more comprehensive data are necessary to understand the likely dynamics of TB drug resistance under pressure from new drugs and new regimens.

Second, novel regimens are, by definition, implemented in settings that have no data as to how the regimen will affect TB dynamics on the population level. In such data-free situations, models are essential for making "first-pass" projections and for informing which data are the most essential to collect. Mathematical models can shape our understanding by extrapolating relevant information from existing epidemics (e.g., of MDR-TB). Such understanding can form a basis for well-informed, targeted policies for appropriate deployment of new regimens, augmentation of those regimens with drug susceptibility testing (DST), and ongoing collection of epidemiological data.

4.2. A Simple Model of Drug Resistance in TB. In the absence of detailed data, a reasonable approach to understand the emergence and transmission dynamics of drug resistance is to construct simplified transmission models of drug resistant TB. One such simplified model might subdivide TB strains into two categories: those that are sensitive to a hypothetical first-line TB drug regimen (DS-TB) and those that are resistant (DR-TB) [46, 54, 55]. This is illustrated schematically in Figure 3. In this framework, resistance is acquired during treatment via de novo mutations and propagated via ongoing transmission thereafter. In comparison to the model shown in Figure 1, the model in Figure 3 now consists of two arms, representing transmission cycles of DS-TB and DR-TB. This framework allows for exploration of different aspects of DR-TB including the relative fitness of DS-TB and DR-TB, relative treatment success, and acquisition of resistance during treatment. These characterizations can be informed by data from existing experience with other resistant strains (e.g., MDR-TB) and expanded to consider additional illustrative scenarios.

4.3. Reproductive Fitness of Drug Resistant TB. Analogous to the effective reproductive ratio R_e discussed above, we can develop a similar concept of $R_{e,\text{dr}}$ as applied to drug resistant strains. This quantity is the average number of secondary DR-TB infections resulting from a single primary DR-TB infection, in the presence of an existing DS-TB epidemic. This effective reproductive ratio can serve as a theoretical basis of the reproductive fitness of the resistant strains—resistant strains with $R_{e,\text{dr}}$ of 1 have comparable potential as DS-TB to spread throughout the population, whereas those with $R_{e,\text{dr}} < 1$ have less potential to spread, and those with $R_{e,\text{dr}} > 1$ have the potential, given sufficient time, to replace DS-TB in the population.

The relationship between key drivers of drug resistance and $R_{e,\text{dr}}$ can inform the relative importance of each factor in influencing the long-term emergence of DR-TB. One revealing insight afforded by this exercise is that the rate of acquisition of drug resistance does not affect the effective reproductive ratio. This implies that transmission of DR-TB is much more important than the acquisition of resistance

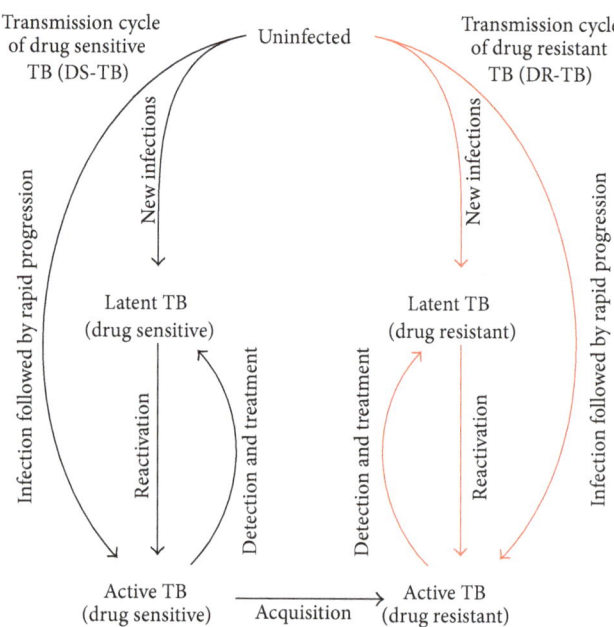

FIGURE 3: A simple epidemiological model of drug resistant (DR-)TB. This model divides the transmission cycle of TB into two arms: transmission of DS-TB and DR-TB (which is shown in red). For simplicity and comparability, the transmission cycle of DR-TB is structurally similar to DS-TB. The difference between DS-TB and DR-TB can be characterized by difference in rates of transition between different compartments. (E.g., if the transmission fitness of DR-TB is less than that of DS-TB, the rates of new infections of DR-TB are lower compared to DS-TB.) The acquisition of drug resistance during treatment resulting from de novo mutations is a primary way in which drug resistance enters the population. Subsequently, drug resistance can spread via transmission events. Increasing the rate at which DR-TB is successfully diagnosed and treated (e.g., through drug susceptibility testing and regimen modification) can be modeled as an increase in the flow from compartment "Active DR-TB" back to "Latent DR-TB" (or, in an alternative formulation, back to uninfected).

during treatment in terms of affecting long-term trajectories of DR-TB after scale-up of a new first-line regimen. Just as the product of transmission rate (cases per time) and the effective duration of infection make up the effective reproductive ratio R_e (see Figure 2), the relative transmission rate and relative duration of infectiousness of DR-TB versus DS-TB determine $R_{e,\text{dr}}$ relative to $R_{e,\text{ds}}$, as shown in Figure 4(a).

4.4. The Trajectories of DR-TB after Launch of a New First-Line Drug Regimen. Trajectories of the prevalence of DR-TB produced by simulating this model can further elucidate the role of these different drivers of TB drug resistance over time. During the first years following regimen introduction (first 5 years after the launch of new first-line drug regimen), acquisition during treatment is a more important determinant of DR-TB at the population level than is transmission, whereas transmission becomes more important in later years. This shift reflects the changing balance between a constant risk of acquisition per treatment episode and a transmission risk that is proportional to an expanding pool of prevalent DR-TB.

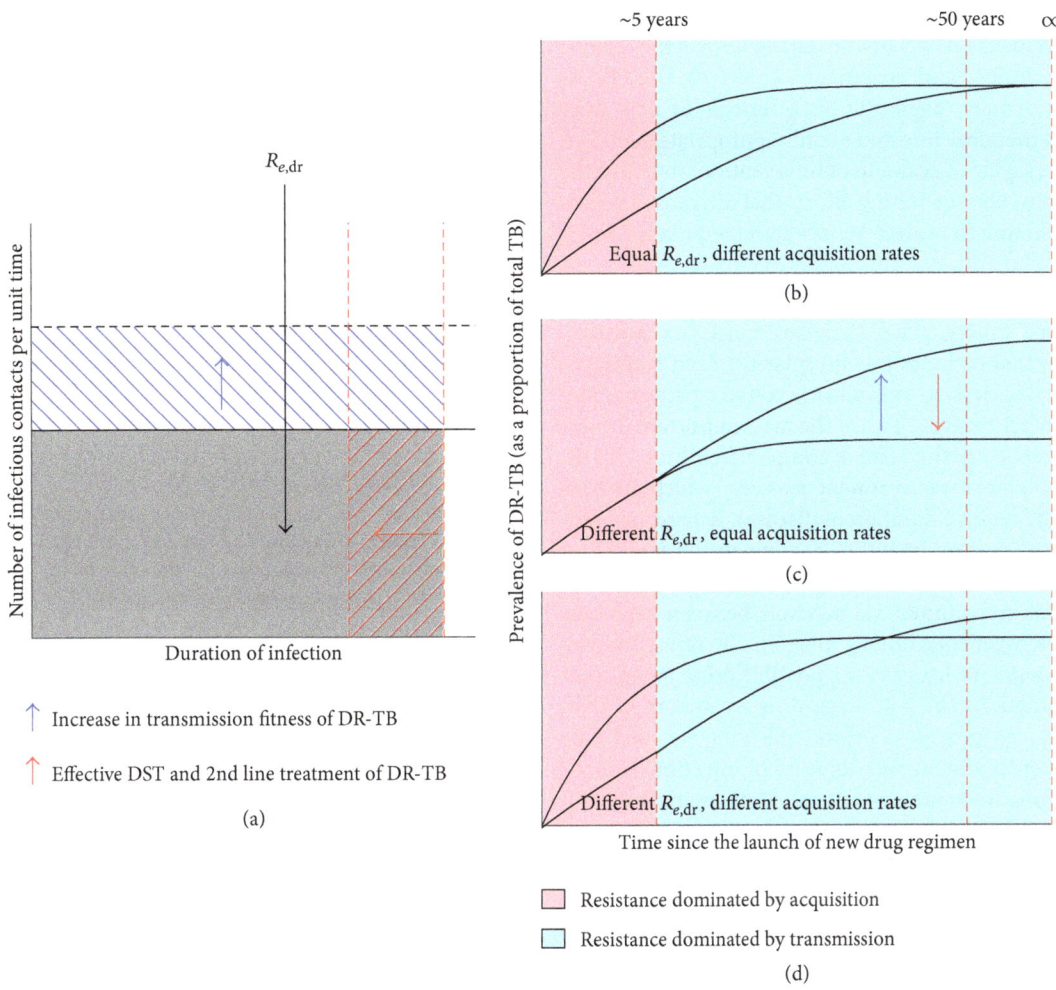

FIGURE 4: Proliferation of drug resistance following the launch of new first-line drug regimen. (a) The effective reproductive ratio of DR-TB ($R_{e,dr}$) is the expected number of secondary cases of active, resistant TB resulting from a single case of DR-TB (shown as the grey shaded area). An increase in the relative transmission fitness of DR-TB (e.g., due to compensatory mutations; shown by the blue arrow) increases $R_{e,dr}$ (shown by the blue hatched area). Shortening the average duration of DR-TB infections (e.g., by deployment of DST, and effective second-line treatment; shown by the red arrow) decreases $R_{e,dr}$ (shown by the red hatched area). However, the rate of acquisition of drug resistance (e.g., due to de novo mutations against drugs in the treatment regimen) does not factor in the calculation of $R_{e,dr}$ (b, c, and d). The trajectories of the prevalence of DR-TB just following the launch of a hypothetical new drug regimen are affected by both the acquisition rates and the $R_{e,dr}$ of DR-TB, but their effects will be more pronounced at different time periods. Acquisition-driven drug resistance is expected to be more frequent in the first 5 years (pink area), while transmission-driven TB relatively later (blue area). (b) For two hypothetical DR-TB strains with similar $R_{e,dr}$, but different acquisition rates, we may observe difference in their prevalence in the short term, but over time they are expected to result in similar levels of resistance. (c) In contrast, for strains with similar acquisition rates, but different $R_{e,dr}$, we may not observe significant difference in their prevalence in the short term, but the levels of drug resistance can diverge significantly. Factors that affect $R_{e,dr}$ will affect the trajectories of DR-TB prevalence—for example, deployment of DST that achieve reduction in average duration of infection (red arrow) can reduce prevalence of DR-TB over longer term. (d) DR-TB strain with larger acquisition rate and smaller $R_{e,dr}$ is expected to be more prevalent over the short term compared to a strain with lower acquisition rate and higher $R_{e,dr}$, but the prevalence of DR-TB is flipped between two hypothetical strains over longer term. Hence, short term prevalence of DR-TB alone may not be a reliable predictor of the prevalence over longer term. Figures are only illustrative and not drawn to scale.

4.5. Consequences of Public Health Interventions.

The method by which new drug regimens are rolled out, and in particular the role of concomitant drug susceptibility testing, will ultimately shape the trajectory of DR-TB prevalence over time. In particular, the effect of various implementation strategies on the effective duration of DR-TB (i.e., shortening that duration by speeding the process of diagnosis and initiation of appropriate treatment) will be critical. Individuals with active DR-TB that remain undetected or untreated will fuel drug resistance through ongoing transmission. Early detection of drug resistance via drug susceptibility testing (DST) and rapid initiation of effective therapy will be key to controlling this spread. Surveillance data on the prevalence of DR-TB during the first few years after the launch of new first line regimens will reflect acquisition rather than transmission burden and therefore may not be indicative of longer term trajectories. It is therefore important to collect not only surveillance data, but also data to inform the relative transmission fitness and treatment success of DR-TB. As with models of new diagnostic tests, models of new drug regimens can therefore inform not only appropriate decision-making with respect to scale-up of interventions, but also the epidemiological data-gathering efforts that are most likely to enhance our ability to project impact at the population level.

4.6. Summary: Models of Drug Resistance under New First-Line Regimens. Emergence of drug resistance is a multifactorial process that includes the interplay between pathogens (e.g., genetic barriers to resistance), contact patterns, and duration of infectiousness. Two of the most important drivers of drug resistance are the relative competitive fitness of DR-strains and the relative treatment success (which in turn determines the relative duration of disease). Regarding competitive fitness, lab experiments (e.g., competition assay) may provide basic insight, but fitness in the lab may not correlate with fitness as transmitted via aerosols between host systems with heterogeneous mixing [56, 57], different pathogen characteristics [58–60], and in the possible presence of compensatory mutations [61, 62]. Regarding treatment success, program data can provide a helpful start, but detailed data on relapse after treatment and duration of infectiousness for those failing treatment are also critical. Mathematical models again play an important role in understanding the system of DR-TB, deploying appropriate interventions (e.g., DST), and driving the collection of key epidemiological data.

5. Conclusions

Mathematical models continue to provide valuable insight into potential impact and cost-effectiveness of strategies to improve both diagnosis and treatment of TB. While often expected to provide projections of alternative futures, their greater contribution may lie in informing decisions as to the best path given existing data, providing better understanding of the key drivers of impact, and informing more relevant data collection efforts in the future. In both of the systems described here (diagnostics and drug regimens), host, pathogen, and health system factors combine to drive infectiousness, mixing patterns, and population susceptibility. Models can demonstrate how the interplay between these elements drives TB epidemiology under the influence of novel interventions; one important way of achieving this aim is by describing interventions' effects on the effective reproductive ratio R_e. Future efforts to control TB will benefit from increased collaboration between epidemiologists, decision-makers, and modellers. Models of TB diagnostics and novel drug regimens represent two realms in which such discussions are starting to take place.

Conflict of Interests

The authors declare that there is no conflict of interests regarding the publication of this paper.

Authors' Contribution

Alice Zwerling and Sourya Shrestha contributed equally to the conception and writing of this paper.

References

[1] R. McNerney, M. Maeurer, I. Abubakar et al., "Tuberculosis diagnostics and biomarkers: needs, challenges, recent advances, and opportunities," *Journal of Infectious Diseases*, vol. 205, supplement 2, pp. S147–S158, 2012.

[2] C. C. Boehme, S. Saacks, and R. J. O'Brien, "The changing landscape of diagnostic services for tuberculosis," *Seminars in Respiratory and Critical Care Medicine*, vol. 34, no. 1, pp. 17–31, 2013.

[3] TB Alliance, *Confronting TB: What It Takes, Global Report 2008*, TB Alliance, New York, NY, USA, 2008.

[4] A. Y. Sun, M. Pai, H. Salje, S. Satyanarayana, S. Deo, and D. W. Dowdy, "Modeling the impact of alternative strategies for rapid molecular diagnosis of tuberculosis in Southeast Asia," *The American Journal of Epidemiology*, vol. 178, no. 12, pp. 1740–1749, 2013.

[5] M. O. Fofana, G. M. Knight, G. B. Gomez, R. G. White, and D. W. Dowdy, "Population-level impact of shorter-course regimens for tuberculosis: a model-based analysis," *PLoS ONE*, vol. 9, no. 5, Article ID e96389, 2014.

[6] D. W. Dowdy, I. Lotia, A. S. Azman, J. Creswell, S. Sahu, and A. J. Khan, "Population-level impact of active tuberculosis case finding in an Asian megacity," *PLoS ONE*, vol. 8, no. 10, Article ID e77517, 2013.

[7] D. W. Dowdy, S. Basu, and J. R. Andrews, "Is passive diagnosis enough? The impact of subclinical disease on diagnostic strategies for tuberculosis," *American Journal of Respiratory and Critical Care Medicine*, vol. 187, no. 5, pp. 543–551, 2013.

[8] C. M. Denkinger, M. Pai, and D. W. Dowdy, "Do we need to detect isoniazid resistance in addition to rifampicin resistance in diagnostic tests for tuberculosis?" *PLoS ONE*, vol. 9, no. 1, Article ID e84197, 2014.

[9] T. Cohen, C. Colijn, B. Finklea, and M. Murray, "Exogenous re-infection and the dynamics of tuberculosis epidemics: local effects in a network model of transmission," *Journal of the Royal Society Interface*, vol. 4, no. 14, pp. 523–531, 2007.

[10] P. Kasaie, J. R. Andrews, W. D. Kelton, and D. W. Dowdy, "Timing of tuberculosis transmission and the impact of household contact tracing: an agent-based simulation model," *The American Journal of Respiratory and Critical Care Medicine*, vol. 189, no. 7, pp. 845–852, 2014.

[11] M. Murray, "Determinants of cluster distribution in the molecular epidemiology of tuberculosis," *Proceedings of the National Academy of Sciences of the United States of America*, vol. 99, no. 3, pp. 1538–1543, 2002.

[12] R. Anderson, R. May, and B. Anderson, *Infectious Diseases of Humans: Dynamics and Control*, Oxford Science Publications, 1991.

[13] M. J. Keeling and P. Rohani, *Modeling Infectious Diseases in Humans and Animals*, Princeton University Press, Princeton, NJ, USA, 2007.

[14] N. A. Menzies, T. Cohen, H.-H. Lin, M. Murray, and J. A. Salomon, "Population health impact and cost-effectiveness of tuberculosis diagnosis with Xpert MTB/RIF: a dynamic simulation and economic evaluation," *PLoS Medicine*, vol. 9, no. 11, Article ID e1001347, 2012.

[15] M. Pai, C. M. Denkinger, S. V. Kik et al., "Gamma interferon release assays for detection of *Mycobacterium tuberculosis* infection," *Clinical Microbiology Reviews*, vol. 27, no. 1, pp. 3–20, 2014.

[16] S. D. Lawn, "Diagnosis of pulmonary tuberculosis," *Current Opinion in Pulmonary Medicine*, vol. 19, no. 3, pp. 280–288, 2013.

[17] A. S. Dharmadhikari and E. A. Nardell, "What animal models teach humans about tuberculosis," *American Journal of Respiratory Cell and Molecular Biology*, vol. 39, no. 5, pp. 503–508, 2008.

[18] G. Delogu and D. Goletti, "The spectrum of tuberculosis infection: new perspectives in the era of biologics," *Journal of Rheumatology*, vol. 41, no. 91, pp. 11–16, 2014.

[19] D. Dowdy, C. Dye, and T. Cohen, "Data needs for evidence-based decisions: a tuberculosis modeler's 'wish list'," *International Journal of Tuberculosis and Lung Disease*, vol. 17, no. 7, pp. 866–877, 2013.

[20] E. A. Nardell, "Catching droplet nuclei: toward a better understanding of tuberculosis transmission," *American Journal of Respiratory and Critical Care Medicine*, vol. 169, no. 5, pp. 553–554, 2004.

[21] A. Tostmann, S. V. Kik, N. A. Kalisvaart et al., "Tuberculosis transmission by patients with smear-negative pulmonary tuberculosis in a large cohort in the Netherlands," *Clinical Infectious Diseases*, vol. 47, no. 9, pp. 1135–1142, 2008.

[22] J. M. Bryant, S. R. Harris, J. Parkhill et al., "Whole-genome sequencing to establish relapse or re-infection with *Mycobacterium tuberculosis*: a retrospective observational study," *The Lancet Respiratory Medicine*, vol. 1, no. 10, pp. 786–792, 2013.

[23] J. M. Bryant, D. M. Grogono, D. Greaves et al., "Whole-genome sequencing to identify transmission of *Mycobacterium abscessus* between patients with cystic fibrosis: a retrospective cohort study," *The Lancet*, vol. 381, no. 9877, pp. 1551–1560, 2013.

[24] T. M. Walker, C. L. C. Ip, R. H. Harrell et al., "Whole-genome sequencing to delineate *Mycobacterium tuberculosis* outbreaks: a retrospective observational study," *The Lancet Infectious Diseases*, vol. 13, no. 2, pp. 137–146, 2013.

[25] A. Roetzer, R. Diel, T. A. Kohl et al., "Whole genome sequencing versus traditional genotyping for investigation of a *Mycobacterium tuberculosis* outbreak: a longitudinal molecular epidemiological study," *PLoS Medicine*, vol. 10, no. 2, Article ID e1001387, 2013.

[26] M. Beisiegel, H.-J. Mollenkopf, K. Hahnke et al., "Combination of host susceptibility and *Mycobacterium tuberculosis* virulence define gene expression profile in the host," *European Journal of Immunology*, vol. 39, no. 12, pp. 3369–3384, 2009.

[27] M. Beisiegel, M. Kursar, M. Koch et al., "Combination of host susceptibility and virulence of mycobacterium tuberculosis determines dual role of nitric oxide in the protection and control of inflammation," *Journal of Infectious Diseases*, vol. 199, no. 8, pp. 1222–1232, 2009.

[28] P. D. O. Davies and J. M. Grange, "Factors affecting susceptibility and resistance to tuberculosis," *Thorax*, vol. 56, supplement 2, pp. ii23–ii29, 2001.

[29] E. L. Corbett, C. J. Watt, N. Walker et al., "The growing burden of tuberculosis: global trends and interactions with the HIV epidemic," *Archives of Internal Medicine*, vol. 163, no. 9, pp. 1009–1021, 2003.

[30] M. A. Sanchez and S. M. Blower, "Uncertainty and sensitivity analysis of the basic reproductive rate: tuberculosis as an example," *American Journal of Epidemiology*, vol. 145, no. 12, pp. 1127–1137, 1997.

[31] C. C. Boehme, P. Nabeta, D. Hillemann et al., "Rapid molecular detection of tuberculosis and rifampin resistance," *The New England Journal of Medicine*, vol. 363, no. 11, pp. 1005–1015, 2010.

[32] H.-H. Lin, I. Langley, R. Mwenda et al., "A modelling framework to support the selection and implementation of new tuberculosis diagnostic tools," *International Journal of Tuberculosis and Lung Disease*, vol. 15, no. 8, pp. 996–1004, 2011.

[33] H.-H. Lin, D. Dowdy, C. Dye, M. Murray, and T. Cohen, "The impact of new tuberculosis diagnostics on transmission: why context matters," *Bulletin of the World Health Organization*, vol. 90, pp. 739–747, 2012.

[34] S. Keshavjee and P. E. Farmer, "Tuberculosis, drug resistance, and the history of modern medicine," *The New England Journal of Medicine*, vol. 367, no. 10, pp. 931–936, 2012.

[35] C. Lienhardt, M. Raviglione, M. Spigelman et al., "New drugs for the treatment of tuberculosis: needs, challenges, promise, and prospects for the future," *Journal of Infectious Diseases*, vol. 205, supplement 2, pp. S241–S249, 2012.

[36] World Health Organization (WHO), *STOP TB: Working Group on New TB Drugs Pipeline of TB Drugs*, World Health Organization (WHO), Geneva, Switzerland, 2014, http://www.newtbdrugs.org/pipeline.php.

[37] K. E. Dooley, E. L. Nuermberger, and A. H. Diacon, "Pipeline of drugs for related diseases: tuberculosis," *Current Opinion in HIV and AIDS*, vol. 8, no. 6, pp. 579–585, 2013.

[38] E. W. Orenstein, S. Basu, N. S. Shah et al., "Treatment outcomes among patients with multidrug-resistant tuberculosis: systematic review and meta-analysis," *The Lancet Infectious Diseases*, vol. 9, no. 3, pp. 153–161, 2009.

[39] J. S. Mukherjee, M. L. Rich, A. R. Socci et al., "Programmes and principles in treatment of multidrug-resistant tuberculosis," *The Lancet*, vol. 363, no. 9407, pp. 474–481, 2004.

[40] N. R. Gandhi, P. Nunn, K. Dheda et al., "Multidrug-resistant and extensively drug-resistant tuberculosis: a threat to global control of tuberculosis," *The Lancet*, vol. 375, no. 9728, pp. 1830–1843, 2010.

[41] M. Lipsitch and B. R. Levin, "Population dynamics of tuberculosis treatment: mathematical models of the roles of non-compliance and bacterial heterogeneity in the evolution of drug resistance," *International Journal of Tuberculosis and Lung Disease*, vol. 2, no. 3, pp. 187–199, 1998.

[42] B. R. Levin, M. Lipsitch, V. Perrot et al., "The population genetics of antibiotic resistance," *Clinical Infectious Diseases*, vol. 24, supplement 1, pp. S9–S16, 1997.

[43] C. Dye, B. G. Williams, M. A. Espinal, and M. C. Raviglione, "Erasing the world's slow stain: strategies to beat multidrug-resistant tuberculosis," *Science*, vol. 295, no. 5562, pp. 2042–2046, 2002.

[44] C. Dye and M. A. Espinal, "Will tuberculosis become resistant to all antibiotics?" *Proceedings of the Royal Society B: Biological Sciences*, vol. 268, no. 1462, pp. 45–52, 2001.

[45] T. Cohen, C. Dye, C. Colijn, B. Williams, and M. Murray, "Mathematical models of the epidemiology and control of drug-resistant TB," *Expert Review of Respiratory Medicine*, vol. 3, no. 1, pp. 67–79, 2009.

[46] S. M. Blower, P. M. Small, and P. C. Hopewell, "Control strategies for tuberculosis epidemics: new models for old problems," *Science*, vol. 273, no. 5274, pp. 497–500, 1996.

[47] B. Müller, S. Borrell, G. Rose, and S. Gagneux, "The heterogeneous evolution of multidrug-resistant *Mycobacterium tuberculosis*," *Trends in Genetics*, vol. 29, no. 3, pp. 160–169, 2013.

[48] M. Zignol, W. van Gemert, D. Falzon et al., "Surveillance of anti-tuberculosis drug resistance in the world: an updated analysis, 2007–2010," *Bulletin of the World Health Organization*, vol. 90, no. 2, pp. 111D–119D, 2012.

[49] J. G. Pasipanodya and T. Gumbo, "A new evolutionary and pharmacokinetic-pharmacodynamic scenario for rapid emergence of resistance to single and multiple anti-tuberculosis drugs," *Current Opinion in Pharmacology*, vol. 11, no. 5, pp. 457–463, 2011.

[50] D. Laurenzo and S. A. Mousa, "Mechanisms of drug resistance in *Mycobacterium tuberculosis* and current status of rapid molecular diagnostic testing," *Acta Tropica*, vol. 119, no. 1, pp. 5–10, 2011.

[51] M. Coscolla and S. Gagneux, "Does *M. tuberculosis* genomic diversity explain disease diversity?" *Drug Discovery Today: Disease Mechanisms*, vol. 7, no. 1, pp. e43–e59, 2010.

[52] S. Borrell and S. Gagneux, "Strain diversity, epistasis and the evolution of drug resistance in *Mycobacterium tuberculosis*," *Clinical Microbiology and Infection*, vol. 17, no. 6, pp. 815–820, 2011.

[53] N. R. Gandhi, A. Moll, A. W. Sturm et al., "Extensively drug-resistant tuberculosis as a cause of death in patients co-infected with tuberculosis and HIV in a rural area of South Africa," *The Lancet*, vol. 368, no. 9547, pp. 1575–1580, 2006.

[54] S. M. Blower, A. R. McLean, T. C. Porco et al., "The intrinsic transmission dynamics of tuberculosis epidemics," *Nature Medicine*, vol. 1, no. 8, pp. 815–821, 1995.

[55] S. Shrestha, G. M. Knight, M. Fofana et al., "Drivers and trajectories of resistance to new first-line drug regimens for tuberculosis," *Open Forum Infectious Diseases*, vol. 1, 2014.

[56] R. J. F. Ypma, H. K. Altes, D. van Soolingen, J. Wallinga, and W. M. van Ballegooijen, "A sign of superspreading in tuberculosis: highly skewed distribution of genotypic cluster sizes," *Epidemiology*, vol. 24, no. 3, pp. 395–400, 2013.

[57] J. L. Gardy, J. C. Johnston, S. J. H. Sui et al., "Whole-genome sequencing and social-network analysis of a tuberculosis outbreak," *The New England Journal of Medicine*, vol. 364, no. 8, pp. 730–739, 2011.

[58] C. Colijn, T. Cohen, and M. Murray, "Latent coinfection and the maintenance of strain diversity," *Bulletin of Mathematical Biology*, vol. 71, no. 1, pp. 247–263, 2009.

[59] T. Cohen, P. D. van Helden, D. Wilson et al., "Mixed-strain *Mycobacterium tuberculosis* infections and the implications for tuberculosis treatment and control," *Clinical Microbiology Reviews*, vol. 25, no. 4, pp. 708–719, 2012.

[60] T. Cohen and M. Murray, "Modeling epidemics of multidrug-resistant *M. tuberculosis* of heterogeneous fitness," *Nature Medicine*, vol. 10, no. 10, pp. 1117–1121, 2004.

[61] B. R. Levin, V. Perrot, and N. Walker, "Compensatory mutations, antibiotic resistance and the population genetics of adaptive evolution in bacteria," *Genetics*, vol. 154, no. 3, pp. 985–997, 2000.

[62] G. Brandis, M. Wrande, L. Liljas, and D. Hughes, "Fitness-compensatory mutations in rifampicin-resistant RNA polymerase," *Molecular Microbiology*, vol. 85, no. 1, pp. 142–151, 2012.

14

Ensuring Confidentiality of Geocoded Health Data: Assessing Geographic Masking Strategies for Individual-Level Data

Paul A. Zandbergen

Department of Geography, University of New Mexico, Albuquerque, NM 87131, USA

Correspondence should be addressed to Paul A. Zandbergen; zandberg@unm.edu

Academic Editor: Ada Youk

Public health datasets increasingly use geographic identifiers such as an individual's address. Geocoding these addresses often provides new insights since it becomes possible to examine spatial patterns and associations. Address information is typically considered confidential and is therefore not released or shared with others. Publishing maps with the locations of individuals, however, may also breach confidentiality since addresses and associated identities can be discovered through reverse geocoding. One commonly used technique to protect confidentiality when releasing individual-level geocoded data is geographic masking. This typically consists of applying a certain amount of random perturbation in a systematic manner to reduce the risk of reidentification. A number of geographic masking techniques have been developed as well as methods to quantify the risk of reidentification associated with a particular masking method. This paper presents a review of the current state-of-the-art in geographic masking, summarizing the various methods and their strengths and weaknesses. Despite recent progress, no universally accepted or endorsed geographic masking technique has emerged. Researchers on the other hand are publishing maps using geographic masking of confidential locations. Any researcher publishing such maps is advised to become familiar with the different masking techniques available and their associated reidentification risks.

1. Introduction

The widespread availability of powerful geocoding tools in commercial Geographic Information System (GIS) software and the interest in spatial analysis at the individual level have made mapping residential addresses of individuals a widely employed technique in public health research [1–6]. Spatial analysis and mapping of georeferenced, individual-level health data can help identify important geographical patterns [1, 2, 7, 8]. However, given the need and/or legal requirement to preserve the confidentiality of microdata, the possibilities of undertaking geographical analysis on certain types of individual-level data are often limited [9, 10]. As a result of restrictions on access to confidential data, important information may remain inaccessible.

Releasing locations of individuals in digital or paper format presents reidentifications risk since these locations can be reverse geocoded to find the addresses and identities associated with those locations. Geographic masking techniques have been developed to reduce the risk of reidentification.

The present review describes the background for sharing and individual-level data, the use of geocoding and reverse geocoding of health-related datasets, and the effectiveness of geographic masking techniques to preserve confidentiality.

2. Individual-Level Data and Geocoding

Datasets collected as part of public health research often contain confidential information. This may include the individual's name, gender, age, race, ethnicity, income, and other socioeconomic characteristics, as well as the specific health-related conditions of interest in the particular study. The collection of this type of individual information for research purposes falls under human subjects' research. This type of data cannot be released publicly since this would violate the confidentiality clauses of human subjects' research [11]. Typically, when researchers publish their results, only aggregate data on the entire sample or specific subsamples can be released.

Increasingly, the individual-level information collected as part of health-related research contains geographic identifiers. This can be relatively coarse in the form of the local jurisdiction (city or municipality) or postal code or much finer grained in the form of the exact street address. Some data collection protocols may also include the collection of coordinates using GPS units in the field. These geographic identifiers add value to the research in a number of different ways. First, if limited demographic and socioeconomic variables are available on the study subjects, their location can provide proxy variables. For example, it is very common to associate the study subjects with the demographic characteristics of the census enumeration unit they are located in. Second, the location of study subjects can provide insight into other variables which may be related to health outcomes. Examples include the time it takes to travel to the nearest health facility of interest, the distance to pollution sources, or the air/water/soil quality at their residential location.

Street addresses represent the most commonly used geographic identifiers for individual level data. Address information can be converted into locations on a map using a process known as geocoding [1, 12]. Geocoding can be accomplished using desktop GIS software or online mapping services. Automated geocoding methods can convert large address databases very quickly.

Geocoding is not error-free. Typically, a certain number of records do not geocode due to incomplete or incorrect information. Geocoded locations may also not be accurate due to incorrect reference information or errors in the geocoding process [1]. These errors, however, are relatively well understood and have received substantial attention in the literature [1, 13–20]. The datasets used for geocoding as well as the geocoding techniques themselves are also gradually improving [21, 22].

A review of articles published in recent volumes of some of the leading public health research journals reveals that geocoding is very widely used. In addition, several new health journals have emerged with a clear emphasis on the spatial dimensions of health, such as the *International Journal of Health Geographics* and *Spatial and Spatio-temporal Epidemiology*. This confirms that geocoding has become firmly established as an analytical tool in public health research [6].

3. Reverse Geocoding

The widespread use of geocoding not only presents unprecedented opportunities for analysis, for example, [23–25]; it also presents challenges to preserving the confidentiality of public health datasets [2, 6, 26]. In short, the release of geographic information at the individual level can breach confidentiality. For example, publishing the street address of an individual makes it possible to look up the associated name(s) in directories and property databases. Publishing a location as coordinates (e.g., latitude/longitude) means that these can be plotted on a map and then associated with an address. Publishing a map in paper or digital form also means that the locations can be associated with an address.

Figure 1 illustrates an example where a published coordinate is published on a map to identify a specific residence.

These techniques are collectively referred to as "reverse geocoding" [27–34]. Formally, reverse geocoding consists of determining the street address associated with a published location in paper or digital format. Reverse geocoding can lead to reidentification because the street address can then be associated with one or several individuals using common directories. Conceptually, reverse geocoding is like putting regular address geocoding in reverse, as illustrated in Figure 2.

Reidentification of individual addresses using reverse geocoding has been shown to be relatively easy and accurate. For example, [29] created a hypothetical map of geocoded patient addresses and were able to correctly identify 79% of the addresses using manual reverse geocoding techniques in GIS. The same authors employed a similar approach using semiautomated reverse geocoding based on image analysis and were able to correctly identify 26% of the addresses [35]. In another example, following Hurricane Katrina, a local newspaper published a map of mortality locations. Using a combination of GIS methods and field work, researchers were able to correctly identify the original residence for most of the locations in the published map [36]. More recently, a study of crime incidents in Vienna, Austria, determined the accuracy of reverse geocoding for several online mapping services [28]. Findings indicate that 68% of probable victims could be identified by name using online reverse geocoding and online address and telephone directories.

Current trends towards spatial data of greater detail and the availability of free online reverse geocoding tools increase the risk of reidentification [1]. For example, online geocoding services such as Google Maps and Microsoft's Bing Maps provide very accurate building-level geocoding and reverse geocoding as part of their (free) online mapping services. This has made accurate and relatively sophisticated "map-hacking" tools available to anybody with an internet connection and modest computer skills. The leading GIS software platform, ArcGIS by Esri, has also added a Reverse Geocoding tool to its standard set of data processing and analysis tools. This has further established reverse geocoding as a robust and standard GIS tool.

4. Benefits and Risks of Data Sharing

When trying to determine if and how locational information on individuals can be released, the following considerations need to balanced: (1) the need to protect confidentiality—this is part of an individual's right to privacy and most often a condition in the collection of the original data, (2) the desire to preserve the original pattern in the locations—this reflects the interest in trying to obtain useful information by utilizing individual level spatial data instead of aggregated data, (3) the usefulness of sharing data for the benefit of researchers and the benefit of the public at large. These considerations are conflicting in the sense that confidentiality is protected by maximizing changes to individual locations, while preserving the original pattern is accomplished by minimizing changes.

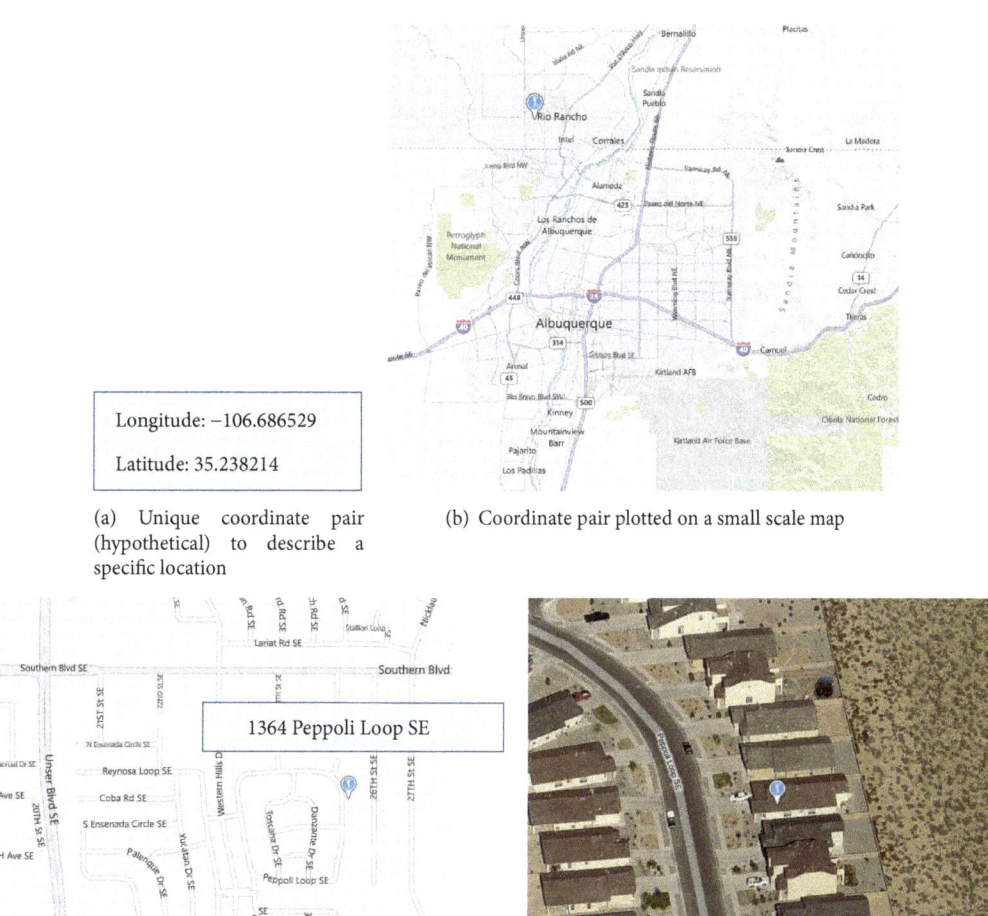

(a) Unique coordinate pair (hypothetical) to describe a specific location

Longitude: −106.686529

Latitude: 35.238214

(b) Coordinate pair plotted on a small scale map

(c) Coordinate pair plotted on a large scale map

1364 Peppoli Loop SE

(d) Oblique aerial imagery of the location

FIGURE 1: Disclosure of confidential information by publishing coordinates. Figure 1(a) shows an example of a hypothetical set of coordinates. Plotting these on a small scale map (b) provides an approximate location (i.e., Rio Rancho). Zooming in using a large scale map (c) provides a very exact location, which can be used to identify the street address associated with the set of coordinates (e.g., 1364 Peppoli Loop SE). Aerial imagery (d) can be used to confirm the specific residence.

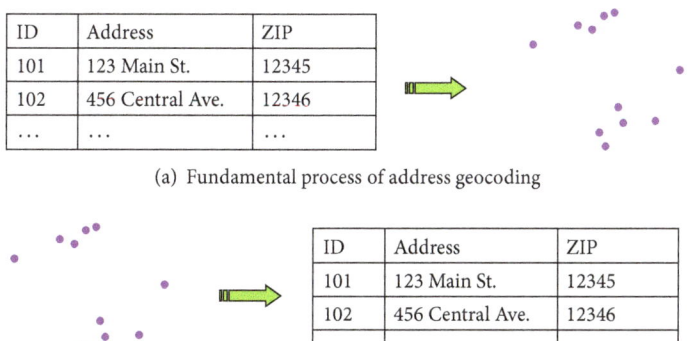

ID	Address	ZIP
101	123 Main St.	12345
102	456 Central Ave.	12346
...	...	...

(a) Fundamental process of address geocoding

ID	Address	ZIP
101	123 Main St.	12345
102	456 Central Ave.	12346
...	...	...

(b) Fundamental process of reverse address geocoding

FIGURE 2: Geocoding and reverse geocoding. Geocoding (a) is the process of assigning locations (i.e., coordinates) to address information. A tabular dataset of addresses becomes a map. Reverse geocoding (b) literally puts this in reverse and converts mapped locations to addresses. Errors in the geocoding and reverse geocoding process may result in mismatched address information; that is, the addresses obtained using reverse geocoding may not be identical to those used in the original geocoding.

The objective of any confidentiality protection method is to find a balance between reducing the risk for reidentification and preserving the properties of the original data.

These challenges in trying to balance the need for confidentiality with the potential benefits from providing researchers and others access to georeferenced individual health data have been widely recognized. For example, the National Research Council published a report in 2007 called "Putting People on the Map: Protecting Confidentiality with Linked Social-Spatial Data" [37]. The Panel on Confidentiality Issues Arising from the Integration of Remotely Sensed and Self-Identifying Data concluded that:

> "Recent research on technical approaches for reducing the risk of identification and breach of confidentiality has demonstrated promise for future success. At this time, however, no known technical strategy or combination of technical strategies for managing linked spatial-social data adequately resolves conflicts among the objectives of data linkage, open access, data quality, and confidentiality protection across datasets and data uses [37]."

The present review documents some of the progress that has been made since the publication of this report and other studies with a similar message [38, 39]. Specifically, the review summarizes the state-of-the-art of geographic masking as one of the "technical approaches" referred to in the NRC report.

5. Confidentiality Protection Strategies

The simplest and most rigorous way to protect the confidentiality of study subjects is to simply not share any of the individual-level data collected as part of the research. For many datasets, this may be the best default option unless convincing arguments are available to release the data in some manner. One of the most practical and convincing arguments is that making data available has become a requirement of many funding agencies [40, 41].

One possible solution is to provide very restricted access to the individual-level data. This is the approach adopted by most cancer registries [10]. Individual-level cancer data records are collected and organized by cancer registries. Access to the individual records is restricted to researchers whose protocols have met the requirements of human subjects' review. Researchers are often restricted as to where they can use the data (sometimes on-site only) and what they are allowed to publish in terms of detailed results. This type of restricted access gives researchers the opportunity to work with the original, individual records, but subsequent releases of the data are strictly controlled. These detailed and institutionalized protocols are not very common for other types of health-related datasets.

Another commonly used solution is to release the data in spatially aggregated form [9]. This is analogous to reporting summary data in tabular form for selected subsets of the original data. For individual-level geocoded data, aggregation is typically accomplished by combining individual locations within a meaningful spatial unit. This could consist of local or regional jurisdictions, such as cities, counties, or census enumeration units. Figure 3 illustrates the basic process for spatial aggregation. To preserve confidentiality, only the aggregated dataset is published or shared.

For many applications, however, the release of spatially aggregated data is much less useful compared to having access to the individual locations [26]. Many spatial analytical techniques, such as general point-pattern analysis and cluster detection, are much less powerful or simply not possible using aggregated data.

Finally, an alternative solution is to modify the data in such a way that the risk for reidentification is greatly reduced without aggregating the data to coarser units of analysis. This includes altering the original locations in some systematic manner, also referred to as geographic masking.

6. Ensuring Confidentiality Using Geographic Masking

Geographic masking is the process of altering the coordinates of point location data to limit the risk of reidentification upon release of the data. In effect, the purpose of geographic masking is to make it much more difficult to accurately reverse geocode the released data. Figure 4 illustrates the general concept of geographic masking.

The term geographic masking was first described in some detail in 1999 [26]. The term was introduced as an extension of masking techniques for nonspatial microdata [42, 43]. While geographic masking is the most widely accepted term, other terms have also been used, including "geomasking" [44–47], "jittering" [48, 49], and "dithering" [50]. The original description of geographic masking methods [26] included several different types of masking, including (1) affine transformations, which accomplish displacement using translations, changes in scale, and rotation, and (2) random perturbation, which accomplish displacement by adding a certain amount of random noise to the coordinates. The transformation approach has not been widely adopted, mostly because the new coordinates no longer have the same real-world context. For example, once a rotation or translation has been applied to a set of locations, it no longer makes sense to overlay these coordinates on top of other spatial data layers. As a result, geographic masking has become largely synonymous with applying random perturbation to coordinates.

Geographic masking is actively being used by public health researchers that use individual-level data. A number of studies were identified that met the following two conditions: (1) the article included a map with geocoded locations of individual-level health information and (2) specific mention was made that the geocoded locations were modified in some way for reasons of confidentiality (even if the term "geographic masking" was not used explicitly). The following section reviews the nature of these maps and the details reported on the geographic masking methods employed.

A study in Cape Code published maps with the location of residential addresses of patients diagnosed with cancer [48]. The geographic masking approach was described as

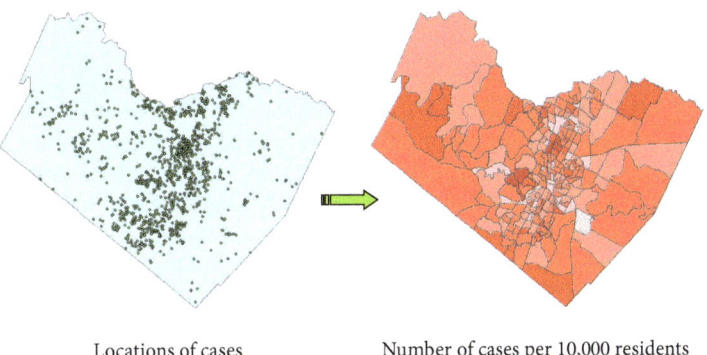

Locations of cases   Number of cases per 10,000 residents

FIGURE 3: Spatial aggregation of individual cases using census enumeration units. Individual geocoded locations (left) are aggregated using census tracts (right). The count of the number of cases per census tract is used to determine relevant population-weighted indices, such as the number of cases per 10,000 residents. Determining incidence or disease rates, as opposed to raw counts, is one of the primary reasons for aggregation. As a secondary benefit, spatial aggregation greatly reduced the reidentification risk.

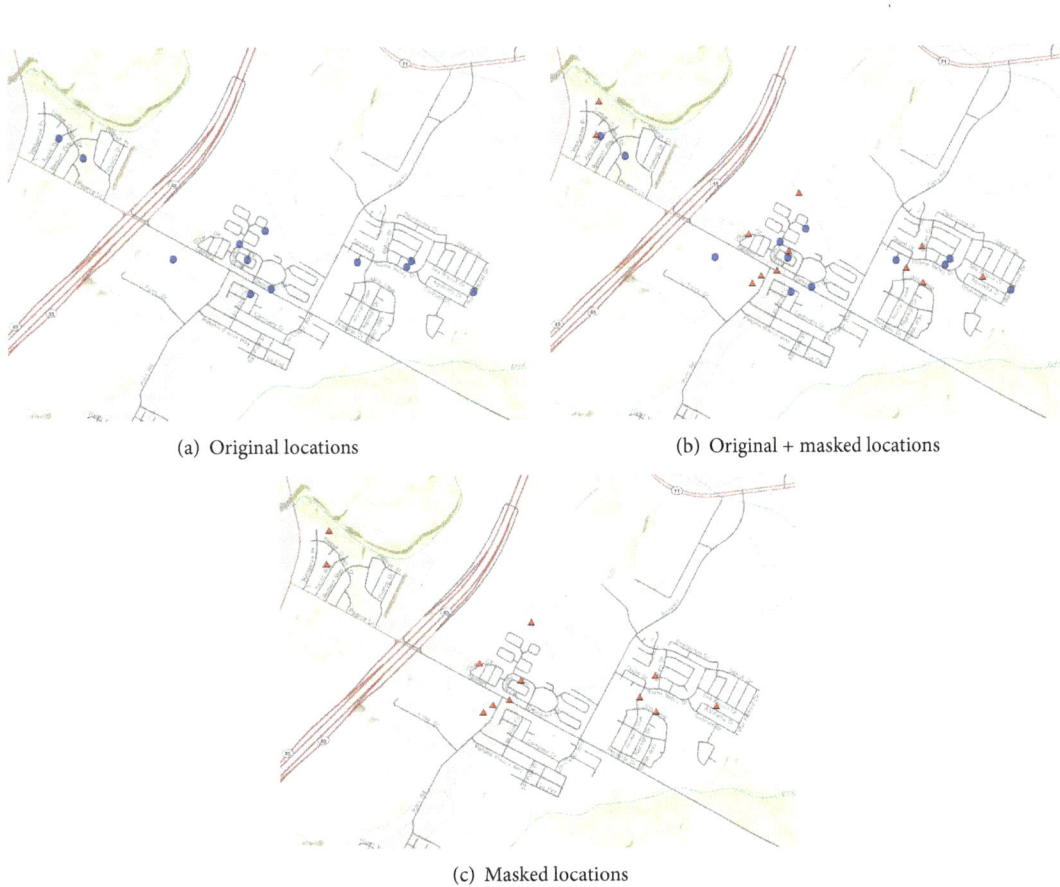

(a) Original locations   (b) Original + masked locations

(c) Masked locations

FIGURE 4: Conceptual illustration of geographic masking. A set of original locations (a) is created using address geocoding or field data collection using GPS. These locations correspond very closely to the residences of interest, although a certain amount of error might be present. For each location, a masked representation is created (b) by displacing the original location using one of several algorithms. Most algorithms include a certain degree of randomness in the displacement. The original locations are removed from the dataset, resulting in a set of masked locations (c) for publication and distribution purposes. The set of masked locations has the same number of observations as the set of original locations.

"for confidentiality reasons, the points have been jittered [48]." A study in Churchill County, NV (USA), published maps with the location of residential address of childhood leukemia cases [51]. The geographic masking approach was described as "locations are enlarged and "jittered" to maintain confidentiality [51]." A study in England published maps of the locations of farms where bovine tuberculosis was found [52]. The geographic masking approach was described as "the map shows the location of each farm, jittered randomly within a circular disc of radius 5 km to preserve confidentiality [52]." A study in North Carolina published maps with the locations of the residential addresses of children screened for blood lead [24]. The geographic masking approach was described as "for publicly displayed maps... we randomly moved the actual location of the child within a fixed radial buffer, a technique known as jittering [24]." A study in Minnesota published maps with the locations of the residential addresses of persons diagnosed with cancer [53]. The geographic masking approach was described as "... plots the residential locations in this data, where we have added a random "jitter" to each in order to protect the confidentiality of the patients (and explaining why some of the cases appear to lie outside of the spatial domain) [53]." A study in Massachusetts (USA) published maps with the locations of the residential addresses of infants born to mothers living near a known PCB-contaminated Superfund site [54]. The geographic masking approach was described as "residence locations are jittered with 1% random noise to protect the confidentiality of participants [54]." A study in Perth, Western Australia (USA), published maps with the locations of the residential addresses of children who visited the emergency room with a principal diagnosis of asthma [54, 55]. The geographic masking approach was described as "case and control cases have been jittered [55]."

While these examples do not represent a comprehensive survey of all the published studies that employ geographic masking, they illustrate a number of characteristics. First, the term "jittering" is widely used instead of "geographic masking." Although jittering is generally used to suggest some type of random perturbation, the examples vary in their use of the term. Second, a number of examples provide specifics on the nature of the geographic masking method, such as "jittered randomly within a circular disc of radius 5 km [52]" or "jittered with 1% random noise to protect confidentiality of participants [54]." Several other examples, however, simply state that locations have been altered without any further description.

7. Different Approaches to Geographic Masking

A number of different geographic masking techniques have been developed over the years. All of these include some degree of randomization in order to reduce the risk of reidentification. Figure 5 provides a visual representation of each of these methods.

(1) Random Direction and Fixed Radius. Masked points are placed on a random location on a circle around the original location. Masked points are not placed inside the circle itself.

(2) Random Perturbation within a Circle. Masked locations are placed anywhere within a circular area around the original location. Since every location within the circle is equally likely, masked locations are more likely to be placed at larger distances compared to small distances. A variation on this technique is the use of random direction and random radius. In this technique, masked points are displaced using a vector with random direction and random radius. The radius is constrained by a maximum value. This effectively results in a circular area where masked locations can be placed, but the masked locations are as likely to be at large distances compared to small distances. These two techniques therefore only differ slightly in the probability of how close masked locations are placed to the original locations.

(3) Gaussian Displacement. The direction of displacement is random, but the distance follows a Gaussian distribution. The dispersion of the distribution can be varied based on other parameters of interest, such as local population density.

(4) Donut Masking. This technique is similar to random displacement within a circle, but a smaller internal circle is utilized within which displacement is not allowed. In effect, this sets a minimum and maximum level for the displacement. Masked locations are placed anywhere within the allowable area. A slightly different approach to donut masking is the use of a random direction and two random radii: one for maximum and one for minimum displacement. These two techniques only differ slightly in the probability of how close masked locations are placed to the original locations. Both approaches enforce a minimum amount of displacement.

(5) Bimodal Gaussian Displacement. This is a variation on the Gaussian masking technique, employing a bimodal Gaussian distribution for the random distance function. In effect, this approximates donut masking, but with a less uniform probability of placement.

While these methods are presented here as separate methods, several are slightly revised versions of each other. For example, donut masking and bimodal Gaussian displacement are very similar in terms of the general area where masked locations are placed relative to the original locations.

These five techniques have been described to varying degrees in the literature. Random direction and fixed radius have been used by [56]. Random perturbation within a circle has been studied by [26, 50, 56, 57]. Gaussian displacement has been studied by [57, 58]. Donut masking was originally proposed by [59] and has been studied in a number of more recent studies [44, 46, 47, 60]. Bimodal Gaussian displacement has been studied by [61]. These studies specifically focus on the development or testing of one or more masking methods. The earlier review of applications of geographic masking to real-world datasets has indicated

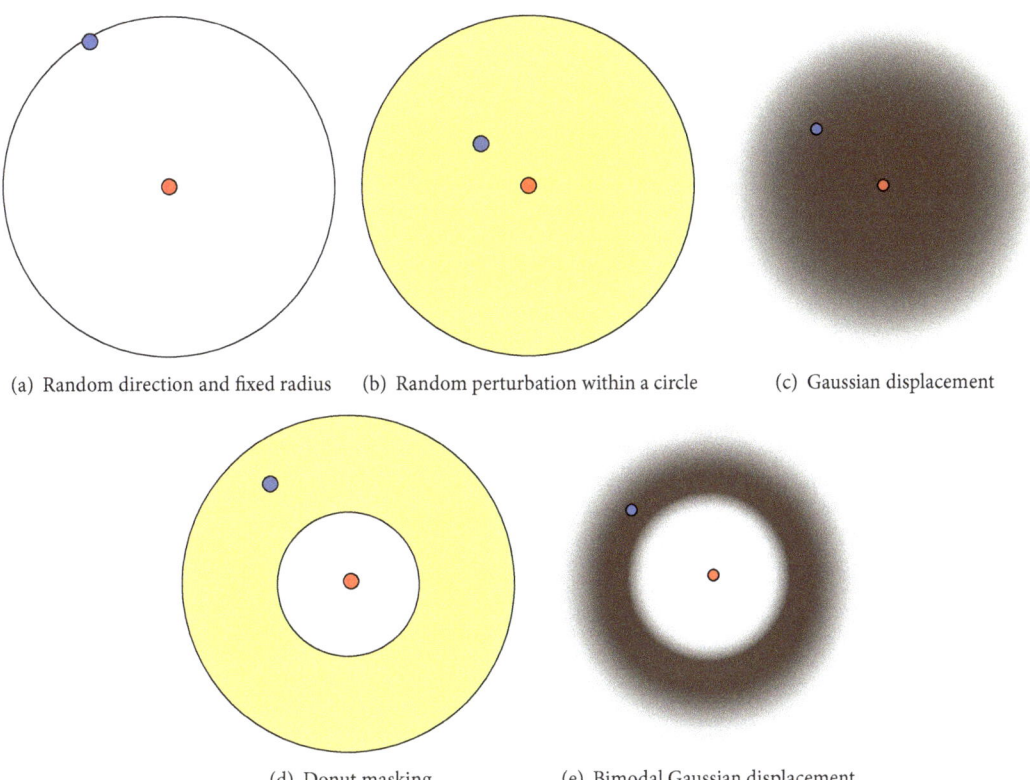

(a) Random direction and fixed radius   (b) Random perturbation within a circle   (c) Gaussian displacement

(d) Donut masking   (e) Bimodal Gaussian displacement

FIGURE 5: Graphical representation of common geographic masking techniques. The red dot indicates the original location and the blue dot one of the many possible masked locations.

that some studies do not mention the specific technique by name. Among those studies that do provide a description of the technique, the random perturbation is by far the most widely used. This suggests that the slightly more sophisticated methods that have received attention in the literature of geographic masking have so far not been adopted.

A number of other techniques have been mentioned in the literature, such as moving each location to the midpoint of the nearest street segment or to the nearest street intersection [62]. Technically speaking, however, these techniques are microspatial aggregation methods since several original locations may end up at the same "masked" location. While these methods warrant attention as an alternative to other methods of spatial aggregation, they have received very limited attention in the literature.

Determining the amount of displacement necessary to achieve confidentiality has been addressed by several of the studies on geographic masking [56], but no universal guidelines have emerged. However, it is widely agreed upon that the amount of displacement should be inversely proportional to the local population density [26, 47, 56, 58, 61]. For example, consider a residence in a rural area with a very low population density. It is quite possible that there are no other residences within 100 meters of this residence. A displacement of 100 meters would therefore not be very effective in reducing the reidentification disk. By contrast, a residence in a very densely populated urban area may be likely to have numerous other residences within 100 meters, and a displacement of 100

meters may be more than sufficient to substantially lower the reidentification risk. All masking techniques described above include at least one parameter that controls the overall magnitude of displacement, for example, the radius corresponding to the maximum displacement or the standard deviation for techniques employing a normal distribution. This parameter should be scaled inversely proportional to local population density (expressed as people per unit area). Instead of using the population density of census enumeration areas, several studies have proposed using the local density of residential addresses as a more reliable way to adjust the magnitude of displacement [44, 47, 63].

One variation on geographic masking is the use of additional spatial filters to ensure masked locations fall within predefined areas of interest. For example, displacement could be limited to a physical land base by excluding surface water bodies (e.g., oceans, bays, rivers, and lakes) to ensure that no masked locations appear in areas which are obviously uninhabited. Another potential use of such filters is to ensure masked locations stay within the same enumeration units (e.g., census block group, postal code) as the original location. The use of such additional spatial filters is illustrated in Figure 6.

While conceptually relatively simple, no studies on geographic masking have specifically addressed the use of such additional spatial filters. It is therefore not known, for example, to what extent their use increases the risk for reidentification.

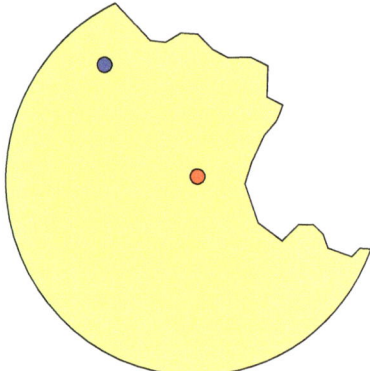

FIGURE 6: Example of geographic masking technique (i.e., random placement within a circle) using an additional spatial filter to constrain displacement. The red dot represents the original location; the yellow area represents all possible locations for the masked location; and the blue dot represents one possible masked location selected randomly. This filter can be used to avoid placement in areas where logically no population resides (such as water bodies or parks) or to limit displacement to a particular enumeration unit (such as the same census tract or postal code).

8. Effectiveness of Geographic Masking in Preserving Confidentiality

One critical aspect in evaluating the effectiveness of geographic masking is to determine how the masking algorithm has reduced the risk of reidentification. In other words, what is the probability of discovery of the masked dataset? This is critical for finding the much-desired balance between protecting confidentiality and maintaining data utility.

Many early studies on geographic masking essentially postulated that a "substantial" displacement of the original point location would suffice to preserve confidentiality [56, 64]. More recently, determining the nature or magnitude of displacement required to effectively accomplish this has started to receive more attention [44, 46, 61, 65].

Several approaches have been developed to determine the degree of confidentiality provided by specific geographic masking techniques. The most widely embraced approach that has started to receive interest in recent years employs the concept of "spatial k-anonymity." This extends the concept of "k-anonymity," which provides a quantitative estimate of the probability of discovery for tabular data [66–70]. Traditional k-anonymity implies that data for a particular individual will only be released if there is a minimum of $k-1$ individuals with the same combination of characteristics. When a particular value for k is determined, data tables can be empirically examined to ensure that the expectation for k-anonymity is met.

The concept of k-anonymity is best illustrated with an example, adapted from [66] and shown in Figure 7. Consider a set of health-related records with personal identifiers such as name, birthdate, sex, ethnicity, street address, and ZIP code, in addition to health-related data such as diagnosis, treatment, and insurance. To protect confidentiality, individual identifiers need to be removed from the data prior to

release, including name and address. While this may appear to be sufficient to protect confidentiality, consider a second set of records consisting of publicly available voting records. In many jurisdictions these records include the individual's name, birthdate, sex, street address, and ZIP code, in addition to voting-related data such as party affiliation and the nature of participation in the last election. The voting records can be used to reidentify the individuals in the anonymized health records. In this particular example, the combination of ZIP code, birthdate, and gender in most cases will uniquely identify a single individual. The value for k would be 1, which is of course unacceptable. A possible solution is to replace the exact birthdate with the birth year, although in some cases this may not be sufficient. For an actual set of data files, empirical values for k can be determined to see the effects of specific anonymization techniques on the risk of reidentification.

The k-anonymity concept can be expanded to include geographic identifiers. Spatial k-anonymity is an emerging concept that has started to receive some attention for testing and comparing geographic masking techniques [65, 71, 72]. Similar to k-anonymity for nonspatial data, spatial k-anonymity provides a quantitative estimate of the probability of discovery, but now considers reverse geocoding instead of database record linkage as the primary mechanism for reidentification.

Spatial k-anonymity has been applied fairly extensively to the protection of privacy in location-based services [71, 73–75]. In the context of individual residential locations, however, spatial k-anonymity has not been well developed. In general, determining an estimate for spatial k-anonymity for residential locations relies on a comparison between the amount of displacement of a location introduced by masking and the density of the local population of interest. A relatively large displacement in an area of high population density would provide a high degree of spatial k-anonymity. One proposed approach to implement this logic is referred to as the "nth nearest neighbor number" method, that is, the number of potential residential locations which are in closer proximity to the masked location than the original location [44, 47, 63]. This approach employs the empirically observed distribution of actual residential locations. The nth nearest neighbor values can be used to provide an empirical estimate of spatial k-anonymity, similar to the example of database record linkage discussed previously. One shortcoming of this approach is that it relies upon the availability of high resolution residential address points or buildings. A variation on this approach has been developed using population density for census enumeration areas instead of the distribution of actual residential locations [61]. While there have been few studies using spatial k-anonymity to examine the reidentification risk associated with masked datasets, in a typical setting larger displacements have been shown to result in the highest values for spatial k-anonymity [44, 47, 61], as expected.

Given the nature of geographic masking, any type or amount of displacement or perturbation of the original locations will still allow for the theoretical possibility that the masked location is in relatively close proximity to the "true"

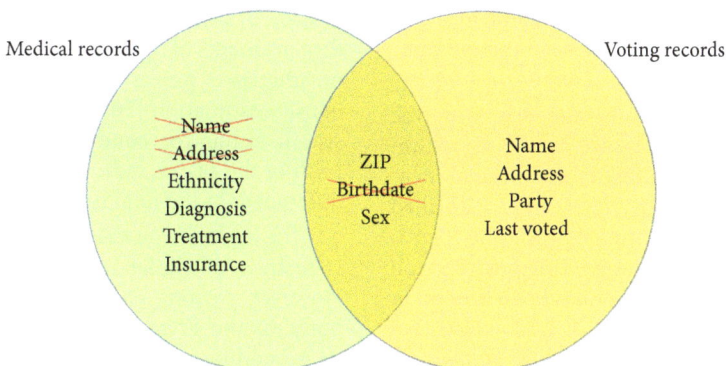

FIGURE 7: Illustration of the k-anonymity concept using record linkage. Medical records contain a number of different fields which are removed to protect confidentiality, including name and address. When combined with voting records, however, it becomes possible to uniquely identify individuals in the medical records by combining fields for ZIP code, birthday, and sex. The k-anonymity provided by the released data is unacceptably low. By removing the field for birthdate (or replacing it with birth year), the k-anonymity is substantially increased and may reach acceptable levels. The concept of k-anonymity provides a quantitative measure of confidentiality protection. More specifically, it is a number that can be calculated for each subset of the data. For the example of medical record and voting records, values for k-anonymity can be calculated prior to release for all combination of ZIP code and sex or any other field of interest. Adapted from [66].

location. However, the actual distance is not as important as the probability of discovery, which is more effectively characterized by an analysis based on spatial k-anonymity. Therefore, if a location is displaced by a substantial distance, but the spatial k-anonymity value is still very low, the probability of discovery is still substantial. This could be the case in a low density rural area where even a substantial displacement may not provide adequate protection of confidentiality.

A standard for confidentiality protection when publishing individual-level locations does not exist at the present time. However, as a general guideline for researchers, such a standard could be based on achieving a high level of spatial k-anonymity. The basic question for research into geographic masking techniques should therefore be which geographic masking parameters are necessary to obtain high values for spatial k-anonymity? More specifically, which geographic masking parameters are necessary to provide a specified minimum level of k-anonymity for a given dataset? The use of quantifiable measure of the probability of discovery in the form of an index for spatial k-anonymity greatly facilitates this line of reasoning. For example, for a specific case-study of emergency department visits in the area of Boston, MA (USA), an average displacement of 0.25 km was found to result in a spatial k-anonymity value of 20 or higher for 99% of the original locations [61].

There has been surprisingly little research comparing the effectiveness of different geographic masking techniques. Most studies have examined only a single method in the context of a specific scenario. Despite this lack of comparative studies, there appears to be general agreement that donut masking and bimodal Gaussian displacement are preferred over other techniques since they enforce a minimum amount of displacement. Random perturbation within a circle and simple Gaussian displacement may result in masked locations which are very close to the original locations. For simple Gaussian displacement these nearby locations are in fact the most likely. This is undesirable since it presents a high risk of reidentification through reverse geocoding. While this argument is supported by logic, few studies have provided empirical analysis to demonstrate these potential advantages [46]. The lack of comparative analysis of masking techniques provides a clear indication for desirable future research directions.

9. Multiple Releases of Masked Data and Disclosure of Masking Methods

Confidentiality may be breached by releasing multiple versions of the same masked datasets [57]. For example, an agency responsible for releasing location information may rerun the geographic masking algorithm with every request for a particular dataset to ensure that each release is unique. If such multiple releases were made available, these could be combined to aid in the reidentification of the original locations. Multiple releases at least in theory make it possible to reverse engineer the masking algorithm used to create the masked datasets. Therefore, even if the masking algorithm itself is not released, multiple releases of the data may present an increased reidentification risk.

Different masking techniques will vary in their robustness to this form of reidentification. However, most techniques in their basic form are symmetrical (i.e., displacement direction is random and displacement distance does not depend on direction). As a result, the average location of a large number of masked locations will start to approximate the original location. Additional perturbation may be introduced if separate masked locations are in close proximity to each other and can therefore not be distinguished in multiple versions of the masked data sets. Even in this scenario, however, averaged locations of multiple locations in multiple masked datasets will provide insights into the masking methods, which in itself will lead to increased disclosure risk. While this effect has been recognized in the literature on geographic masking [57, 58], very limited empirical testing has been carried out.

One additional aspect to consider is the release of the specific geographic masking technique together with the masked dataset. Conceivably, knowledge of the algorithm provides additional knowledge to identify the original location. Similar to the way geocoded locations can be identified using reverse geocoding, masked locations could be identified using "reverse geographic masking." This has received some attention in the literature [57], but has been limited in terms of datasets and masking methods. It is expected that different masking techniques will vary in their robustness to this form of reidentification. For example, the random direction and fixed radius method are not expected to be very robust in this regard.

10. Effects of Masking on Spatial-Analytic Methods

Typically the most compelling reason to release individual-level health datasets in some form is that they provide more useful information than the summarized or spatially aggregated versions of the same data. Many types of analysis are only possible using the individual points. It is therefore critical to determine to what extent the properties of these datasets are preserved by geographic masking. If geographic masking results in a point pattern whose properties do not closely resemble those of the original point locations, then the individual-level dataset is of much lower analytical value.

Research on the effects of geographic masking on the spatial-analytic properties of a set of location is essential in order to determine whether masking technique strike a meaningful balance between the protection of confidentiality and the ability to derive relevant spatial relationships. What follows is a summary of the studies to date on this subject. A study in Franklin County, Ohio, Kwan et al. [56] used the residential addresses of 541 deaths due to lung cancer to examine the effects of two different masking techniques: random direction with a fixed radius and random placement within a circle, using different radii for both methods. Effects of masking were determined by using kernel density estimation and the cross K-function. Findings indicated a consistent tradeoff between the amount of perturbation and the accuracy of the analytical results [56]. A study using artificial clusters of point locations masked using bimodal Gaussian displacement examined the robustness of cluster detection using SaTScan [61]. Results showed a gradual decrease in cluster detection sensitivity and specificity with an increase in the average displacement distance. A study on household travel surveys employed donut masking for a set of selected households and examined the influence of masking on measures of the build environment [60]. Results showed a gradual reduction in the utility of these measures with larger displacement distances. A study on the location of burglaries determined the effect of masking on measures of spatial point patterns (Nearest Neighbor Index) and on measures of clustering after spatial aggregation (Moran's I) [47]. Results

indicated very minor effects of geographic masking for displacements of up to 250 m. A study using masked versions of simulated points determined the robustness of kernel density estimation [50] and found a strong influence of the search radius (or bandwidth). Displacements greater than 1/5th of the search radius were found to result in substantial differences in the final results.

The literature on the effects of geographic masking on the robustness of spatial-analytic technique is relatively limited. However, lessons can be learned from the much larger body of the literature on the effects of positional errors in geocoding on spatial analyses [1, 13–16, 18, 20, 76–82]. While geographic masking is not a type of geocoding error, the net effect on spatial analysis is very similar: locations are displaced in a systematic manner and this introduces a certain amount of error in the spatial analytic procedures using these locations as input. The primary difference is that the displacements in geographic masking falls within a very specific range and often follows a uniform or normal distribution, while positional errors in geocoding follow a log-normal distribution [16, 83]. This means that a set of locations obtained using geocoding typically contains a large proportion of locations with a relatively small error (up to 100 meters or thereabouts) and a much smaller but not insignificant proportion of locations with a much larger error (up to several hundred meters or even kilometers). Despite this difference, the geocoding literature provides some useful insights into the effects of location displacement on the outcome of spatial analysis. In general, this research suggests that the effects are highly dependent on the type of analysis method and the specific scale of the analysis. For example, research on kernel density analysis suggests that the robustness of results is highly dependent on the search radius employed in constructing the kernel [15] with very small values for the radius producing very unreliable results. Similarly, concordance with census enumeration units is dependent on the typical size of the polygons being used, with smaller units resulting in larger errors in the analysis [15, 84].

While most studies have examined the effect of geographic masking using very specific spatial-analytical procedures, other less technical approaches have also been used. For example, [62, 64] have used human study subjects to identify the effect of masking techniques on the visual impact of point patterns.

11. Alternatives to Masking

Geographic masking methods have been under development for over 10 years. Despite the development of several different masking techniques, there is no general consensus on which technique is most suited for a particular task. Based on the progress in developing and testing masking techniques, it is unclear whether advances in geographic masking will lead to the widespread adoption and recommendation of a particular set of techniques. It is therefore worthwhile to consider what alternatives are available. These alternatives fall into a number of categories.

One approach to more traditional geographic masking is the use of more complex spatial manipulations of the data. Proposed approaches include spatial smoothing [85], multiple imputation [86], and linear programming [65]. While these methods manipulate the original locations using spatial analytic methods, they do not fall under what are commonly referred to as geographic masking techniques.

A more radical alternative to geographic masking is the use of synthetic data. In this approach, a dataset is created which has properties that are very similar to that of the original data, but the identities of all individuals have been modified. This approach has been successfully developed for tabular datasets [87].

Software agents present another alternative. In this approach, software is used to provide controlled access to original individual data records without releasing identifiable details [88]. Analysis results are returned based on the individual records. This approach does not suffer from the limitations presented by releasing spatially aggregated data. There is a concern that certain properties of the original data could be inferred from the analysis results, but in general the risk of reidentification is much lower compared to the release of individual-level masked datasets [88]. While very promising in concept, the use of software agents to handle confidential health datasets is not very widespread, in part, because of the challenges related to establishing the secure computer infrastructure to implement the approach.

Yet another alternative is to employ flexible aggregation methods which are much finer than traditional census units, but which do not reveal exact individual locations [89]. Such flexible aggregation methods provide an easily quantifiable measure for the risk of reidentification, while at the same time minimizing the degree of aggregation to limit the decrease in the utility of the data.

While a number of alternatives to geographic masking have emerged, there have been no comparative studies to examine the relative strengths of various approaches for a specific application. As a result, there is currently no clear guidance on when geographic masking method should be employed and when alternatives should be considered.

12. Conclusions

The growing body of knowledge on geographic masking indicates that it is possible to provide a quantitative estimate of the degree of confidentiality provided by a specific masking technique for a given study area. It is also possible to quantitatively determine the effects of geographic masking on the robustness of specific analytic techniques. This suggests that finding a balance between confidentiality protection and data utility is technically possible for a given scenario. Despite this recent progress, at the present time there is no universally accepted or endorsed geographic masking method. Research and funding agencies do not provide any guidance on what masking methods to use or how to use them.

This gap can likely be attributed to a number of factors. First, while awareness of confidentiality concerns is high, spatial literacy among most health researchers is not. Geocoding and basic spatial analysis techniques have become widely used in public health research, but topics such as reverse geocoding, geographic masking, and spatial k-anonymity have not yet become part of the vocabulary of mainstream public health research. Second, the number of studies on geographic masking is still relatively small and the research community has not presented a very strong case for a particular set of methods that would be effective for a range of different scenarios. Third and perhaps most important, it is not clear that geographic masking presents the best alternative among several approaches to protect confidentiality while providing controlled access to individual-level data for analysis and surveillance purposes. While geographic masking clearly holds promise, it is limited in what can be accomplished technically and alternative approaches may prove more effective at achieving the same general goals for specific applications.

This suggests a number of different avenues for future research. First, research on geographic masking is clearly in its early stages, and more work is needed to compare existing approaches and to develop new ones. Second, technical guidelines are needed on the use of geographic masking. While decisions on if and how to release georeferenced individual-level health data are obviously not based on technical criteria alone, a better understanding of the possibilities and limitations of geographic masking should contribute to more informed decisions. Third, several alternatives to geographic masking have been developed and research is needed to compare the strengths and weaknesses of these approaches relative to more established masking techniques.

Researchers on the other hand are publishing maps using geographic masking of confidential locations, in the absence of clear guidelines on how to best accomplish this. Any researcher publishing such maps is advised to become very familiar with the different techniques available and their associated reidentification risks.

Conflict of Interests

The author declares that there is no conflict of interests regarding the publication of this paper.

Acknowledgments

Research reported in this paper was supported by the National Institute of Environmental Health Sciences of the National Institutes of Health under Award no. 1R21ES019666-01. The content is solely the responsibility of the authors and does not necessarily represent the official views of the National Institutes of Health.

References

[1] P. A. Zandbergen, "Geocoding quality and implications for spatial analysis," *Geography Compass*, vol. 3, no. 2, pp. 647–680, 2009.

[2] G. Rushton, M. P. Armstrong, J. Gittler et al., *Geocoding Health Data: The Use of Geographic Codes in Cancer Prevention and Control, Research and Practice*, CRC Press, 2010.

[3] N. Krieger, J. T. Chen, P. D. Waterman, M.-J. Soobader, S. V. Subramanian, and R. Carson, "Geocoding and monitoring of US socioeconomic inequalities in mortality and cancer incidence: does the choice of area-based measure and geographic level matter? The public health disparities geocoding project," *American Journal of Epidemiology*, vol. 156, no. 5, pp. 471–482, 2002.

[4] T. Abe and D. Stinchcomb, "Geocoding practices in cancer registries," in *Geocoding Health Data*, pp. 111–125, CRC Press, 2010.

[5] N. Krieger, "Place, space, and health: GIS and epidemiology," *Epidemiology*, vol. 14, no. 4, pp. 384–385, 2003.

[6] J. M. Bissette, J. A. Stover, L. M. Newman, P. C. Delcher, K. T. Bernstein, and L. Matthews, "Assessment of geographic information systems and data confidentiality guidelines in STD programs," *Public Health Reports*, vol. 124, supplement 2, p. 58, 2009.

[7] D. B. Richardson, N. D. Volkow, M.-P. Kwan, R. M. Kaplan, M. F. Goodchild, and R. T. Croyle, "Medicine. Spatial turn in health research," *Science*, vol. 339, no. 6126, pp. 1390–1392, 2013.

[8] A. Gemmill, R. B. Gunier, A. Bradman, B. Eskenazi, and K. G. Harley, "Residential proximity to methyl bromide use and birth outcomes in an agricultural population in california," *Environmental Health Perspectives*, vol. 121, no. 6, pp. 737–743, 2013.

[9] N. H. Fefferman, E. A. O'Neil, and E. N. Naumova, "Confidentiality and confidence: is data aggregation a means to achieve both?" *Journal of Public Health Policy*, vol. 26, no. 4, pp. 430–449, 2005.

[10] G. Rushton, M. P. Armstrong, J. Gittler et al., "Geocoding in cancer research: a review," *The American Journal of Preventive Medicine*, vol. 30, no. 2, pp. S16–S24, 2006.

[11] J. P. Reiter and S. K. Kinney, "Sharing confidential data for research purposes: a primer," *Epidemiology*, vol. 22, no. 5, pp. 632–635, 2011.

[12] D. W. Goldberg, J. P. Wilson, and C. A. Knoblock, "From text to geographic coordinates: the current state of geocoding," *URISA Journal*, vol. 19, no. 1, pp. 33–46, 2007.

[13] P. A. Zandbergen, "Influence of geocoding quality on environmental exposure assessment of children living near high traffic roads," *BMC Public Health*, vol. 7, article 37, 2007.

[14] P. A. Zandbergen and J. W. Green, "Error and bias in determining exposure potential of children at school locations using proximity-based GIS techniques," *Environmental Health Perspectives*, vol. 115, no. 9, pp. 1363–1370, 2007.

[15] P. A. Zandbergen, T. C. Hart, K. E. Lenzer, and M. E. Camponovo, "Error propagation models to examine the effects of geocoding quality on spatial analysis of individual-level datasets," *Spatial and Spatio-Temporal Epidemiology*, vol. 3, no. 1, pp. 69–82, 2012.

[16] M. R. Cayo and T. O. Talbot, "Positional error in automated geocoding of residential addresses," *International Journal of Health Geographics*, vol. 2, article 10, 2003.

[17] B. Jacquemin, J. Lepeule, A. Boudier et al., "Impact of geocoding methods on associations between long-term exposure to urban air pollution and lung function," *Environmental Health Perspectives*, vol. 121, no. 9, pp. 1054–1060, 2013.

[18] G. M. Jacquez, "A research agenda: does geocoding positional error matter in health GIS studies?" *Spatial and Spatio-Temporal Epidemiology*, vol. 3, no. 1, pp. 7–16, 2012.

[19] D. L. Zimmerman and X. Fang, "Estimating spatial variation in disease risk from locations coarsened by incomplete geocoding," *Statistical Methodology*, vol. 9, no. 1-2, pp. 239–250, 2012.

[20] D. T. Duncan, M. C. Castro, J. C. Blossom, G. G. Bennett, and L. G. G. G. Steven, "Evaluation of the positional difference between two common geocoding methods," *Geospatial Health*, vol. 5, no. 2, pp. 265–273, 2011.

[21] P. A. Zandbergen, "A comparison of address point, parcel and street geocoding techniques," *Computers, Environment and Urban Systems*, vol. 32, no. 3, pp. 214–232, 2008.

[22] D. W. Goldberg and M. G. Cockburn, "Improving geocode accuracy with candidate selection criteria," *Transactions in GIS*, vol. 14, no. 1, pp. 149–176, 2010.

[23] P. A. Zandbergen and J. Chakraborty, "Improving environmental exposure analysis using cumulative distribution functions and individual geocoding," *International Journal of Health Geographics*, vol. 5, article 23, 2006.

[24] M. L. Miranda, R. Anthopolos, and D. Hastings, "A geospatial analysis of the effects of aviation gasoline on childhood blood lead levels," *Environmental Health Perspectives*, vol. 119, no. 10, pp. 1513–1516, 2011.

[25] J. Xue, T. McCurdy, J. Burke et al., "Analyses of school commuting data for exposure modeling purposes," *Journal of Exposure Science and Environmental Epidemiology*, vol. 20, no. 1, pp. 69–78, 2010.

[26] M. P. Armstrong, G. Rushton, and D. L. Zimmerman, "Geographically masking health data to preserve confidentiality," *Statistics in Medicine*, vol. 18, no. 5, pp. 497–525, 1999.

[27] K. Sueda, T. Miyaki, and J. Rekimoto, "Social geoscape: visualizing an image of the city for mobile UI using user generated geotagged objects," in *Mobile and Ubiquitous Systems: Computing, Networking, and Services*, pp. 1–12, Springer, 2012.

[28] O. Kounadi, T. J. Lampoltshammer, M. Leitner, and T. Heistracher, "Accuracy and privacy aspects in free online reverse geocoding services," *Cartography and Geographic Information Science*, vol. 40, no. 2, pp. 140–153, 2013.

[29] J. S. Brownstein, C. A. Cassa, and K. D. Mandl, "No place to hide—reverse identification of patients from published maps," *New England Journal of Medicine*, vol. 355, no. 16, pp. 1741–1742, 2006.

[30] J. Krumm, "A survey of computational location privacy," *Personal and Ubiquitous Computing*, vol. 13, no. 6, pp. 391–399, 2009.

[31] J. Rekimoto, T. Miyaki, and T. Ishizawa, "LifeTag: WiFi-based continuous location logging for life pattern analysis," in *Location- and Context-Awareness*, vol. 4718 of *Lecture Notes in Computer Science*, pp. 35–49, 2007.

[32] K. R. Searight, D. J. Logan, J. Bourland II Freddie, C. J. Loher, and B. R. Charlton, "Reverse geocoding system using combined street segment and point datasets," Google Patents, 2010.

[33] R. Marshall, J. Polk, and R. George, "A protocol for location transformations," TCS, 2011.

[34] L.-C. Chen, Y.-C. Lai, Y.-H. Yeh, J.-W. Lin, C.-N. Lai, and H.-C. Weng, "Enhanced mechanisms for navigation and tracking services in smart phones," *Journal of Applied Research and Technology*, vol. 11, pp. 272–282, 2013.

[35] J. S. Brownstein, C. A. Cassa, I. S. Kohane, and K. D. Mandl, "An unsupervised classification method for inferring original case locations from low-resolution disease maps," *International Journal of Health Geographics*, vol. 5, article 56, 2006.

[36] A. J. Curtis, J. W. Mills, and M. Leitner, "Spatial confidentiality and GIS: re-engineering mortality locations from published maps about Hurricane Katrina," *International Journal of Health Geographics*, vol. 5, article 44, 2006.

[37] N. R. Council, *Putting People on the Map: Protecting Confidentiality with Linked Social-Spatial Data*, National Academies Press, 2007.

[38] K. L. Olson, S. J. Grannis, and K. D. Mandl, "Privacy protection versus cluster detection in spatial epidemiology," *American Journal of Public Health*, vol. 96, no. 11, pp. 2002–2008, 2006.

[39] M. N. K. Boulos, A. J. Curtis, and P. Abdelmalik, "Musings on privacy issues in health research involving disaggregate geographic data about individuals," *International Journal of Health Geographics*, vol. 8, p. 46, 2009.

[40] C. Tenopir, S. Allard, K. Douglass et al., "Data sharing by scientists: practices and perceptions," *PLoS ONE*, vol. 6, no. 6, Article ID e21101, 2011.

[41] P. N. Schofield, T. Bubela, T. Weaver et al., "Post-publication sharing of data and tools," *Nature*, vol. 461, no. 7261, pp. 171–173, 2009.

[42] G. T. Duncan and R. W. Pearson, "Enhancing access to microdata while protecting confidentiality: prospects for the future," *Statistical Science*, vol. 6, no. 3, pp. 219–232, 1991.

[43] L. Cox, "Matrix masking methods for disclosure limitation in microdata," *Survey Methodology*, vol. 20, no. 2, pp. 165–169, 1994.

[44] W. B. Allshouse, M. K. Fitch, K. H. Hampton et al., "Geomasking sensitive health data and privacy protection: an evaluation using an E911 database," *Geocarto International*, vol. 25, no. 6, pp. 443–452, 2010.

[45] M. Fitch, "Geomasking algorithms to protect confidentiality of sexually transmitted infections in spatial epidemiology," in *Proceedings of the American Public Health Association Annual Meeting and Exposition*, 2007.

[46] K. H. Hampton, M. K. Fitch, W. B. Allshouse et al., "Mapping health data: improved privacy protection with donut method geomasking," *American Journal of Epidemiology*, vol. 172, no. 9, pp. 1062–1069, 2010.

[47] Y. Lu, C. Yorke, and F. B. Zhan, "Considering risk locations when defining perturbation zones for geomasking," *Cartographica*, vol. 47, no. 3, pp. 168–178, 2012.

[48] J. L. French and M. P. Wand, "Generalized additive models for cancer mapping with incomplete covariates," *Biostatistics*, vol. 5, no. 2, pp. 177–191, 2004.

[49] B. S. Bell, "Spatial analysis of disease-applications," in *Biostatistical Applications in Cancer Research*, pp. 151–182, Springer, 2002.

[50] X. Shi, J. Alford-Teaster, and T. Onega, "Kernel density estimation with geographically masked points," in *Proceedings of the 17th International Conference on Geoinformatics (Geoinformatics '09)*, August 2009.

[51] S. S. Francis, S. Selvin, W. Yang, P. A. Buffler, and J. L. Wiemels, "Unusual space-time patterning of the Fallon, Nevada leukemia cluster: evidence of an infectious etiology," *Chemico-Biological Interactions*, vol. 196, no. 3, pp. 102–109, 2012.

[52] J. Claridge, P. Diggle, C. M. McCann et al., "Fasciola hepatica is associated with the failure to detect bovine tuberculosis in dairy cattle," *Nature Communications*, vol. 3, article 853, 2012.

[53] S. Liang, S. Banerjee, and B. P. Carlin, "Bayesian wombling for spatial point processes," *Biometrics*, vol. 65, no. 4, pp. 1243–1253, 2009.

[54] A. L. Choi, J. I. Levy, D. W. Dockery et al., "Does living near a Superfund site contribute to higher polychlorinated biphenyl (PCB) exposure?" *Environmental Health Perspectives*, vol. 114, no. 7, pp. 1092–1098, 2006.

[55] G. Pereira, A. J. B. M. De Vos, A. Cook, and C. D'Arcy J. Holman, "Vector fields of risk: a new approach to the geographical representation of childhood asthma," *Health and Place*, vol. 16, no. 1, pp. 140–146, 2010.

[56] M.-P. Kwan, I. Casas, and B. C. Schmitz, "Protection of geo-privacy and accuracy of spatial information: how effective are geographical masks?" *Cartographica*, vol. 39, no. 2, pp. 15–28, 2004.

[57] D. L. Zimmerman and C. Pavlik, "Quantifying the effects of mask metadata disclosure and multiple releases on the confidentiality of geographically masked health data," *Geographical Analysis*, vol. 40, no. 1, pp. 52–76, 2008.

[58] C. A. Cassa, S. C. Wieland, and K. D. Mandl, "Re-identification of home addresses from spatial locations anonymized by Gaussian skew," *International Journal of Health Geographics*, vol. 7, article 45, 2008.

[59] D. Stinchcomb, "Procedures for geomasking to protect patient confidentiality," in *Proceedings of the ESRI International Health GIS Conference*, Washington, DC, USA, 2004.

[60] K. J. Clifton and S. R. Gehrke, "Application of geographic perturbation methods to residential locations in the oregon household activity survey: proof of concept," in *Proceedings of the Transportation Research Board 92nd Annual Meeting*, 2013.

[61] C. A. Cassa, S. J. Grannis, J. M. Overhage, and K. D. Mandl, "A context-sensitive approach to anonymizing spatial surveillance data: impact on outbreak detection," *Journal of the American Medical Informatics Association*, vol. 13, no. 2, pp. 160–165, 2006.

[62] M. Leitner and A. Curtis, "Cartographic guidelines for geographically masking the locations of confidential point data," *Cartographic Perspectives*, no. 49, pp. 22–39, 2004.

[63] P. Zandbergen, "Validation of masking techniques for location privacy protection of individual-level health data," in *Proceedings of the American Public Health Association Annual Meeting*, Washington, DC, USA, 2011.

[64] M. Leitner and A. Curtis, "A first step towards a framework for presenting the location of confidential point data on maps-results of an empirical perceptual study," *International Journal of Geographical Information Science*, vol. 20, no. 7, pp. 813–822, 2006.

[65] S. C. Wieland, C. A. Cassa, K. D. Mandl, and B. Berger, "Revealing the spatial distribution of a disease while preserving privacy," *Proceedings of the National Academy of Sciences of the United States of America*, vol. 105, no. 46, pp. 17608–17613, 2008.

[66] L. Sweeney, "k-anonymity: a model for protecting privacy," *International Journal of Uncertainty, Fuzziness and Knowledge-Based Systems*, vol. 10, no. 5, pp. 557–570, 2002.

[67] K. El Emam and F. K. Dankar, "Protecting privacy using k-anonymity," *Journal of the American Medical Informatics Association*, vol. 15, no. 5, pp. 627–637, 2008.

[68] L. Sweeney, "Achieving k-anonymity privacy protection using generalization and suppression," *International Journal of Uncertainty, Fuzziness and Knowledge-Based Systems*, vol. 10, no. 5, pp. 571–588, 2002.

[69] G. Aggarwal, T. Feder, K. Kenthapadi et al., "Approximation algorithms for k-anonymity," *Journal of Privacy Technology (JOPT)*, 2005.

[70] K. El Emam, F. K. Dankar, R. Issa et al., "A globally optimal k-anonymity method for the de-identification of health data," *Journal of the American Medical Informatics Association*, vol. 16, no. 5, pp. 670–682, 2009.

[71] P. Kalnis, G. Ghinita, K. Mouratidis, and D. Papadias, "Preventing location-based identity inference in anonymous spatial queries," *IEEE Transactions on Knowledge and Data Engineering*, vol. 19, no. 12, pp. 1719–1733, 2007.

[72] A. Khoshgozaran, C. Shahabi, and H. Shirani-Mehr, "Location privacy: going beyond K-anonymity, cloaking and anonymizers," *Knowledge and Information Systems*, vol. 26, no. 3, pp. 435–465, 2011.

[73] B. Gedik and L. Liu, "Protecting location privacy with personalized k-anonymity: architecture and algorithms," *IEEE Transactions on Mobile Computing*, vol. 7, no. 1, pp. 1–18, 2008.

[74] G. Ghinita, K. Zhao, D. Papadias, and P. Kalnis, "A reciprocal framework for spatial K-anonymity," *Information Systems*, vol. 35, no. 3, pp. 299–314, 2010.

[75] M. Xue, P. Kalnis, and H. K. Pung, "Location diversity: enhanced privacy protection in location based services," in *Location and Context Awareness*, pp. 70–87, Springer, 2009.

[76] P. A. Zandbergen, "Influence of street reference data on geocoding quality," *Geocarto International*, vol. 26, no. 1, pp. 35–47, 2011.

[77] P. A. Zandbergen and T. C. Hart, "Geocoding accuracy considerations in determining residency restrictions for sex offenders," *Criminal Justice Policy Review*, vol. 20, no. 1, pp. 62–90, 2009.

[78] K. Zinszer, C. Jauvin, A. Verma et al., "Residential address errors in public health surveillance data: a description and analysis of the impact on geocoding," *Spatial and Spatio-Temporal Epidemiology*, vol. 1, no. 2-3, pp. 163–168, 2010.

[79] S. Mazumdar, G. Rushton, B. J. Smith, D. L. Zimmerman, and K. J. Donham, "Geocoding accuracy and the recovery of relationships between environmental exposures and health," *International Journal of Health Geographics*, vol. 7, article 13, 2008.

[80] B. Jacquemin, J. Lepeule, A. Boudier et al., "Impact of geocoding methods on associations between long-term exposure to urban air pollution and lung function," *Environmental Health Perspectives*, 2013.

[81] M. A. Healy and J. A. Gilliland, "Quantifying the magnitude of environmental exposure misclassification when using imprecise address proxies in public health research," *Spatial and Spatio-Temporal Epidemiology*, vol. 3, no. 1, pp. 55–67, 2012.

[82] D. Roongpiboonsopit and H. A. Karimi, "Quality assessment of online street and rooftop geocoding services," *Cartography and Geographic Information Science*, vol. 37, no. 4, pp. 301–318, 2010.

[83] P. A. Zandbergen, "Positional accuracy of spatial data: non-Normal distributions and a critique of the national standard for spatial data accuracy," *Transactions in GIS*, vol. 12, no. 1, pp. 103–130, 2008.

[84] N. Krieger, P. Waterman, K. Lemieux, S. Zierler, and J. W. Hogan, "On the wrong side of the tracts? Evaluating the accuracy of geocoding in public health research," *American Journal of Public Health*, vol. 91, no. 7, pp. 1114–1116, 2001.

[85] Y. Zhou, F. Dominici, and T. A. Louis, "A smoothing approach for masking spatial data," *The Annals of Applied Statistics*, vol. 4, no. 3, pp. 1451–1475, 2010.

[86] H. Wang and J. P. Reiter, "Multiple imputation for sharing precise geographies in public use data," *The Annals of Applied Statistics*, vol. 6, no. 1, pp. 229–252, 2012.

[87] J. C. Huckett, *Synthetic Data Methods for Disclosure Limitation*, ProQuest, 2008.

[88] M. N. Kamel Boulos, Q. Cai, J. A. Padget, and G. Rushton, "Using software agents to preserve individual health data confidentiality in micro-scale geographical analyses," *Journal of Biomedical Informatics*, vol. 39, no. 2, pp. 160–170, 2006.

[89] C. Young, D. Martin, and C. Skinner, "Geographically intelligent disclosure control for flexible aggregation of census data," *International Journal of Geographical Information Science*, vol. 23, no. 4, pp. 457–482, 2009.

15

Prevalence and Correlates of Peripheral Arterial Disease in Nigerians with Type 2 Diabetes

D. O. Soyoye,[1] R. T. Ikem,[1] B. A. Kolawole,[1] K. S. Oluwadiya,[2] R. A. Bolarinwa,[3] and O. J. Adebayo[4]

[1]*Department of Medicine, Obafemi Awolowo University, Ile-Ife, Nigeria*
[2]*Department of Surgery, Ekiti State University, Ado-Ekiti, Nigeria*
[3]*Department of Haematology and Immunology, Obafemi Awolowo University, Ile-Ife, Nigeria*
[4]*Department of Medicine, Federal Medical Centre, Lokoja, Nigeria*

Correspondence should be addressed to D. O. Soyoye; bksoyoye@yahoo.com

Academic Editor: Marianne Brodmann

Background. Peripheral arterial disease (PAD) is a major risk factor for nonhealing foot ulcers in people with diabetes. A number of traditional risk factors have been reported to be associated with PAD; however, there may be a need to consider nontraditional risk factors especially in some vulnerable populations. This study determined the prevalence and risk factors associated with PAD in diabetics. *Methods.* One hundred and fifty type 2 diabetics and an equal number of age- and sex-matched apparently healthy controls were studied. Assessment of PAD was made using history, palpation of lower limb vessels, and measurement of ankle-brachial index (ABI). Statistically significant differences between categorical and continuous variables were determined using Chi square (χ^2) and Student *t*-tests, respectively. Regression analysis was done to determine the associated risk factors for PAD. *Results.* Prevalence of PAD using ABI was 22.0% and 8.0% among diabetic and nondiabetic populations, respectively. Peripheral arterial disease was associated with age, male gender, waist circumference, and high-sensitivity C-reactive protein. *Conclusion.* This study highlights the high prevalence of PAD in people with type 2 diabetes mellitus and in apparently healthy controls; age, male gender, abdominal obesity, and high hs-CRP values were the associated risk factors.

1. Introduction

Peripheral arterial disease (PAD) reflects systemic atherosclerosis and is associated with long-term disability and increased cardiovascular complications [1–3]. Lower extremity PAD is the third leading cause of atherosclerotic cardiovascular morbidity after coronary heart disease and stroke, and it is estimated to affect 200 million people globally [4, 5]. Risk factors for PAD, similar to those of other atherosclerotic vascular diseases, include smoking, obesity, diabetes, hypertension, and dyslipidaemia, with smoking and diabetes having the strongest association with PAD [4–8].

Inflammation is known to play a major role in the initiation and progression of atherosclerosis and its complications, and this discovery explains the adoption of inflammatory biomarkers for cardiovascular risk prediction and monitoring [9, 10]. Since the major risk factors such as diabetes and smoking do not explain the increased occurrence of critical limb ischaemia, there is a need to further investigate the contribution of nontraditional factors such as inflammation to peripheral arterial disease. This study assessed the contribution of inflammatory markers, high-sensitivity C-reactive protein (hs-CRP) and white blood cells, to the occurrence of PAD. These have not been previously studied in relation to PAD among indigenous Nigerians. It is hoped that this study will provoke further study of this previously underreported phenomenon in our environment, thus shedding more light on the exact role of these markers in PAD.

2. Patients and Methods

One hundred and fifty patients with type 2 diabetes attending the outpatient clinic were selected using systematic sampling in which one in four participants were selected as they registered on clinic days. A total of 150 age- and gender-matched apparently healthy, nondiabetic individuals, who were not being managed for any chronic disease, served as controls. People with ankle-brachial index (ABI) > 1.30, those with febrile illness within one month of study, and those with casts, ulcers, and other conditions that may cause an increase in levels of hs-CRP or interfere with examination of posterior tibial and dorsalis pedis arteries were excluded from the study. Type 2 diabetes mellitus was diagnosed among people who satisfy the World Health Organization (WHO) criteria for the diagnosis of DM and were treated and/or controlled initially using oral hypoglycaemic agents and were being treated with oral hypoglycaemic agents and/or insulin [11, 12].

Peripheral arterial disease (PAD) was defined by the presence of intermittent claudication [13], by detection of two or more reduced or absent pulses of the dorsalis pedis and posterior tibial arteries, with at least one of the legs having both the dorsalis pedis and posterior tibial arteries affected [14–16], and also by an ankle-brachial index (ABI) of ≤0.9 in either of the legs [17]. The lower ABI was used in the analysis. PAD was categorized using ABI into normal (ABI = 0.91–1.30), mild (ABI = 0.70–0.90), moderate (ABI = 0.40–0.69), and severe (ABI < 0.40) [13]. ABI was measured using LifeDop handheld Doppler with 8 Hz probe (Model 150R, Madras Engineering, Chennai).

Baseline information regarding the medical and social history of the respondents was obtained. Blood sample was collected for relevant laboratory investigations: fasting lipid profile, fasting plasma glucose, high-sensitivity C-reactive protein, glycated haemoglobin, and white blood cells count (total and differential). High-sensitivity CRP was measured using enzyme linked immunosorbent assay (Diagnostic Automation, Inc., Calabasas, CA, USA). Total and differential white cell count was done using an automated haematology analyzer (Sysmex America Inc., Mundelein, IL, USA). Written informed consent was sought from and granted by the participants. The study was approved by the Ethics and Research Committee of the hospital. Data was analyzed using SPSS 20. Prevalence of PAD was expressed in percentage. Possible association between categorical variables was determined using Chi square test (χ^2), and Student's t-test was used to detect significant differences between continuous variables. Binary logistic regression analysis was done to determine the associated risks for PAD. The outcome variable was presence or absence of PAD as determined by ABI (lower value of the two legs), while the independent variables were known risk factors for PAD (based on literature review), as well as variables found to be significantly different on bivariate analysis between the diabetic and control groups. p value of less than 0.05 was taken as statistically significant.

3. Results

A total of 300 subjects were recruited comprising 150 diabetics (66 males and 84 females) and 150 apparently healthy controls (68 males and 82 females) ($p = 0.908$). During

TABLE 1: Comparison of traditional and nontraditional factors among diabetics and controls.

Parameter	Diabetics $N = 150$	Controls $N = 150$	p value
Smokers (past & present)	22 (14.7%)	9 (6.0%)	0.368
<5 pack-years	16 (10.7%)	9 (6.0%)	0.986
>5 pack-years	6 (4.0%)	0 (0%)	
Alcohol intake (individuals)	38 (25.3%)	19 (12.6%)	0.039
BMI (kg/m^2)	27.8 ± 4.8	25.8 ± 4.7	<0.001
WC (cm)	95.9 ± 11.7	88.8 ± 9.4	<0.001
SBP	132.8 ± 17.6	117.7 ± 11.2	<0.001
FPG (mmol/L)	7.7 ± 3.5	4.4 ± 0.7	<0.001
HbA1c (%)	7.9 ± 2.1	ND	
TC (mmol/L)	4.3 ± 0.9	3.8 ± 0.7	<0.001
HDL (mmol/L)	1.0 ± 0.2	1.1 ± 0.3	0.001
LDL (mmol/L)	2.8 ± 0.8	2.6 ± 0.7	0.009
hs-CRP (mg/L)	1.49 ± 1.64	0.74 ± 0.82	<0.001
Total white cell count (×10^3)	5.90 ± 1.21	4.97 ± 0.99	<0.001
Lymphocyte count (×10^3)	2.68 ± 0.83	2.37 ± 0.65	<0.001
Neutrophil count (×10^3)	3.16 ± 0.87	2.57 ± 0.80	<0.001

BMI: body mass index; WC: waist circumference; WHR: waist-to-hip ratio; SBP: systolic blood pressure; FPG: fasting plasma glucose; HbA1c: glycated haemoglobin; ND: not done; TC: total cholesterol; HDL: high-density lipoprotein; LDL: low-density lipoprotein; hs-CRP: high-sensitivity C-reactive protein.

screening, 32 patients with diabetes and 12 controls with ABI value >1.3 were excluded from the study. Mean ages of diabetics and controls were 56.12 ± 7.65 years and 55.76 ± 7.49 years, respectively ($p = 0.681$). Thirty-one (10.3%) participants were either current or past smokers; two (0.7%) participants (both controls) were current smokers. Table 1 compares some demographic, physical, and biochemical characteristics of the diabetic and the control groups.

3.1. Prevalence of Peripheral Arterial Disease. Intermittent claudication, a historical indicator of PAD, was present in 27 (18.0%) diabetics and 13 (8.7%) controls ($p = 0.026$). 18 (6.0%) male subjects and 22 (7.3%) female subjects, respectively, had intermittent claudication ($p = 0.964$).

The prevalence of PAD based on palpation method was 19.3% among diabetics and 8.0% among controls ($p = 0.007$). 28 (18.7%) diabetics and 12 (8.0%) controls, respectively, had at least one reduced dorsalis pedis artery pulsation ($p = 0.011$). A similar finding was elicited on examination of the posterior tibial artery: 29 (19.3%) diabetics and 13 (8.7%) controls had reduced pulsation ($p = 0.018$). None of the subjects had absent pulsation.

The prevalence of PAD defined by ABI of <0.9 was 22% in the diabetic group and 8.0% in the control group ($p = 0.001$). Mean ABI for diabetic and control groups were 0.99 ± 0.14 and 1.00 ± 0.08, respectively ($p = 0.312$), with mean ABI in males being 1.00 ± 0.10 (diabetics = 0.99 ± 0.13; controls = 1.00 ± 0.07) and in females 0.99 ± 0.12 (diabetics = 0.98 ± 0.16; controls = 1.00 ± 0.08) ($p = 0.813$). Severity of PAD was graded using ABI, which revealed that 26 (17.3%) diabetics

TABLE 2: Association of traditional and nontraditional risk factors and peripheral arterial disease.

Variable	Subjects with PAD (n = 45)	Subjects without PAD (n = 255)	p value
	Mean values ± SD		
Age (years)	58.24 ± 7.73	55.53 ± 7.47	0.033
BMI (kg/m^2)	29.07 ± 5.92	26.39 ± 4.48	0.005
WC (cm)	100 ± 13.09	90.95 ± 10.28	<0.001
SBP (mmHg)	133.16 ± 22.03	123.81 ± 14.97	0.009
FPG (mmol/L)	7.52 ± 4.10	5.74 ± 2.66	0.007
TC (mmol/L)	4.62 ± 1.24	3.98 ± 0.79	0.001
HDL (mmol/L)	1.01 ± 0.21	1.04 ± 0.23	0.429
LDL (mmol/L)	3.09 ± 0.96	2.63 ± 0.71	0.003
TG (mmol/L)	1.01 ± 0.35	0.90 ± 0.33	0.046
Total white cell (×10^3)	6.16 ± 1.53	5.31 ± 1.08	0.001
Neutrophil count	3.00 ± 1.12	2.84 ± 0.84	0.381
Lymphocyte count	3.11 ± 1.15	2.42 ± 0.62	<0.001
hs-CRP (mg/L)	1.83 ± 1.12	0.88 ± 1.08	<0.001

PAD: peripheral arterial disease; BMI: body mass index; WC: waist circumference; SBP: systolic blood pressure; DBP: diastolic blood pressure; FPG: fasting plasma glucose; HDL: high-density lipoprotein; LDL: low-density lipoprotein; hs-CRP: high-sensitivity C-reactive protein.

and 12 (8.0%) controls had mild impairment while 7 (4.7%) diabetics had moderate impairment ($p = 0.001$). None of the participants in the control group had moderate impairment and none of the participants in the two groups had severe PAD. The prevalence of PAD increased with age from 0.3% in subjects aged 31 to 40 years to 2.7% in subjects aged 41 to 50 years, 3.3% in subjects aged 51 to 60 years, and 8.7% in subjects aged more than 60 years.

Using ABI as the reference diagnostic method for PAD, the sensitivity and specificity of the historical method were 45% and 94%, respectively. Similarly, the sensitivity and specificity of the palpation method were 80% and 98%, respectively. Twenty-two (14.7%) diabetics and 7 (4.7%) controls satisfied the criteria for diagnosis of PAD using all the three diagnostic methods ($p = 0.005$).

3.2. Factors Predicting Occurrence of PAD. There was significant association between age, body mass index (BMI), waist circumference, systolic blood pressure, fasting plasma glucose, serum total cholesterol, serum low-density lipoprotein, serum triglycerides, total white blood cell count, lymphocyte count, serum C-reactive protein, and prevalent PAD, but not with high-density lipoprotein or neutrophil count (Table 2).

Mean ± SD glycated haemoglobin in diabetics who had PAD (8.79 ± 2.37%) was significantly higher than in those without PAD (7.66 ± 1.96%) ($p = 0.006$). Correlation analysis showed negative correlation between glycated haemoglobin and ankle-brachial index ($r = -0.191$, $p = 0.019$). Binary logistic regression showed waist circumference (OR = 13.648; 95% CI = 2.046–91.025; $p = 0.007$), hs-CRP (OR = 1.617; 95%

CI = 1.046–2.499; $p = 0.031$), age (OR = 1.110; 95% CI = 1.010–1.221; $p = 0.031$), and male gender (OR = 4.323; 95% CI = 1.153–16.210; $p = 0.030$) as risk factors for PAD in our study population.

4. Discussion

Peripheral arterial disease is a reflection of systemic atherosclerosis and diabetes is a major risk factor for atherosclerosis [7, 18, 19]. Prevalence of PAD may vary with age and method of diagnosis and possibly with the gender of the population studied [13, 14, 20]. In this study, we determined the prevalence of peripheral arterial disease using history, palpation method, and ABI measurement.

The prevalence of PAD elicited by history of intermittent claudication was significantly higher in people with diabetes compared with controls. This is similar to what was reported by Bembi et al. [11], who reported prevalence of 16% and 8% in diabetics and controls, respectively. Intermittent claudication may not be a true indicator of PAD due to the presence of physical impairment and cardiovascular diseases in people with PAD, resulting in their inability to walk far or fast enough to experience muscle ischaemia which brings about intermittent claudication [21, 22]. This may particularly apply among the elderly, where the presence of other conditions such as osteoarthritis may also affect walking [23]. In addition, conditions such as degenerative joint disease, spinal stenosis, and herniated disc may also cause exertional leg pain; hence, intermittent claudication may be nonspecific [20].

The prevalence of PAD using palpation was 19.3% among people with diabetes, which was significantly higher than the 8.0% obtained among controls. More subjects had reduced pulsation of posterior tibial artery compared with dorsalis pedis artery, and none of the subjects had absent pulsation. It is known that dorsalis pedis artery may be absent in a proportion of normal individuals [24, 25]; this was not the case in our study.

Prevalence of PAD (defined by an ABI of <0.9%) was 22.0% and 8% among the diabetics and controls, respectively; none of our participants had severe PAD. The prevalence rates were similar to results obtained by Bembi et al. [11], who obtained prevalence rates of 24% and 8%, respectively, in diabetics and controls. The prevalence rate of PAD in our study is also similar to that reported by Beach et al. [26], who examined people aged 50–70 years using ABI. They found prevalence of 22% among diabetics compared with 3% among controls [26]. We excluded people with leg ulcer; this could inadvertently exclude people with severe arterial disease, and this may explain the absence of people with absent peripheral pulses on palpation and severe PAD on ABI estimation among our study participants.

The prevalence of PAD varied, depending on the method utilized in this study. This is similar to the findings of Ogbera et al. [27] who obtained values of 10.7% for each of intermittent claudication and palpation and 12% for ABI in diabetics with foot at risk. The prevalence in this study was lower than that obtained in our earlier study [16] where we obtained prevalence of PAD of 25.7% and 55.4% on pulse palpation and ABI, respectively [16]. The disparity between this and our earlier study may be explained by the fact that most (62.2%) of the patients reviewed in our earlier study already had foot ulcer, which is one of the major complications of PAD, hence the higher prevalence rates of PAD. Participants with ulcer were excluded from our present study. Palpation may be affected by such factors as ambient temperature, anatomical variations, and interobserver differences. The presence of claudication and an abnormal pulse may therefore underestimate the prevalence of PAD [14, 28].

Inaccurate measurements from ankle-brachial index studies may occur due to the presence of calcified or incompressible vessels (which would produce falsely elevated readings), especially in diabetic and elderly patients, and subclavian-artery stenosis [15]. Despite these limitations, ABI measurement has a sensitivity above 90% in contrast to intermittent claudication with a sensitivity of about 50% [15, 24] and a specificity of 95% for the diagnosis of peripheral arterial disease [15]. It has also been reported to have marginal observer variability [24]. In our study, the sensitivity and specificity of intermittent claudication were 45% and 94%, respectively, and the sensitivity and specificity of the palpation method were 80% and 98%, respectively, with reference to the ankle-brachial index. History of intermittent claudication and detection of reduced peripheral pulses are diagnostic indicators of peripheral arterial disease and are relevant in clinical practice, but the use of ankle-brachial index should be more sensitive in detecting PAD.

Early risk factor identification and treatment may be a cost-effective means of preventing peripheral arterial disease and its complications. Previous studies [17, 24, 29] have suggested the association of PAD with both modifiable and nonmodifiable risk factors. The most common risk factors associated with PAD were advanced age, diabetes, and smoking [24, 26, 30].

As previously reported [31], our study also showed significant association between waist circumference (WC) and PAD, with an almost fourteenfold risk of peripheral arterial disease with increasing waist circumference (OR = 13.648; 95% CI = 2.046–91.025). Also, WC values were significantly higher in diabetics compared with controls. Waist circumference is a measure of central obesity (adiposity), and adipocytes function as an endocrine organ releasing some cytokines and adiponectins such as the tumour necrosis factor (TNF) α, leptin, interleukin-6 (IL-6), prothrombotic agents such as plasminogen activator inhibitor 1 (PAI-1), and angiotensinogen [32, 33]. These factors have their roles in inflammation, coagulation, and atherogenesis [32, 33]. In addition, abdominal obesity is also associated with an atherogenic lipid profile [32].

The level of hs-CRP was higher among diabetics compared with controls. There is about twofold risk of PAD with increasing levels of hs-CRP (OR = 1.617; 95% CI = 1.046–2.499). This finding is consistent with previous reports [17, 34], demonstrating significant association between CRP and PAD. CRP is a marker of inflammation, a characteristic of all phases of atherothrombosis [9, 10, 35]. CRP is also postulated to directly influence vascular vulnerability

and progression of atherosclerosis through several mechanisms, including enhanced expression of local adhesion molecules, increased expression of endothelial plasminogen activator inhibitor 1 (PAI-1), reduced endothelial nitric oxide bioactivity, altered low-density lipoprotein (LDL) uptake by macrophages, and colocalization with complement within atherosclerotic lesions [9, 10, 35].

Advancing age was another associated risk for PAD in this study, which was also reported as a risk in previous studies [11, 17, 36]. Association of PAD with advancing age may be explained by the fact that the incidence of other risk factors associated with atherosclerosis, such as diabetes and hypertension, also increases with age [12, 37]. These risks are further accentuated by physical inactivity which is worsened by degenerative joint disease in the elderly. The favourable lipoprotein pattern and reduced incidence of atherosclerosis in premenopausal women is also lost after menopause [38].

Male sex increased the risk of PAD in this study more than four times (OR = 4.323; 95% CI = 1.153–16.210), a similar finding in other studies [22, 36]. Increased prevalence of PAD in males may be due to the relatively lower levels of high-density lipoprotein (HDL) in men compared with women [38]. The protective role of HDL may be due to its role in augmenting peripheral catabolism of cholesterol via the reverse cholesterol transfer and its carriage of antioxidant enzymes which reduce the level of oxidized phospholipids in atheromatous lesions [35].

There was a significant negative correlation between glycated haemoglobin (a measure of long-term glycaemic control) and ABI ($r = -0.191$, $p = 0.019$). Glycated haemoglobin level was also significantly higher among diabetics who had PAD compared with diabetics without PAD. This association between PAD and hyperglycaemia has been found in several studies [36, 39, 40]. Hyperglycaemia may potentiate atherogenesis by inhibiting arterial endothelial nitric oxide (NO) production, enhancing platelet-derived growth factor- (PGDF-) induced vascular smooth muscle cell proliferation, stimulating PAI-1 production, and accumulating advanced glycation end products [6, 35]. In addition, hyperglycaemia, especially in the setting of insulin resistance, may be associated with atherogenic diabetic dyslipidaemia [38].

Smoking has been reported to be an important risk for PAD [17, 24, 26, 29]; however, smoking was not a significant factor in this study. The reason for this may be that few subjects (10.3%) in both diabetic (less than 15%) and control (6%) groups ever smoked. This smoking rate compares with a rate of 7.0% of adult Nigerians who ever smoked reported in Global Adult Tobacco Survey (GATS) Nigeria [41]. Smoking cessation counseling, which is part of diabetes care, may explain the absence of current smokers among the diabetics. A dose-response relationship exists between pack-year history and PAD risk [26]. None of the subjects actively smoked during the time of the study, and most smoked less than five (5) pack-years. Hence, the smaller number of smokers and the minimal smoking dose in those that smoked may explain the lack of association between smoking and PAD that we observed.

5. Conclusion

The prevalence of peripheral arterial disease is high among diabetic patients and may be a major contributor to lower limb morbidities. Early detection and reliable diagnosis can be made using simple methods such as palpation and measurement of ankle-brachial index. We have shown that peripheral arterial disease is associated with increasing age, male gender, abdominal obesity, and high hs-CRP levels, suggesting that strategies to reduce the occurrence of PAD in people with type 2 diabetes mellitus should not only focus on controlling traditional risk factors, but also consider the effects of inflammation. Future research into strategies aimed at controlling inflammation among people with type 2 diabetes should be considered.

Competing Interests

The authors declare that there are no competing interests regarding the publication of this paper.

Acknowledgments

The authors appreciate Dr. O. O. Ayoola of the Radiology Department and residents of the Endocrinology Unit for their involvement in the recruitment of study participants.

References

[1] N. C. Dolan, K. Liu, M. H. Criqui et al., "Peripheral artery disease, diabetes, and reduced lower extremity functioning," *Diabetes Care*, vol. 25, no. 1, pp. 113–120, 2002.

[2] S. P. Marso and W. R. Hiatt, "Peripheral arterial disease in patients with diabetes," *Journal of the American College of Cardiology*, vol. 47, no. 5, pp. 921–929, 2006.

[3] A. C. Powers, "Diabetes mellitus," in *Harrison's Principles of Internal Medicine*, D. L. Kasper, E. Braunwald, A. S. Fauci, S. L. Hauser, D. L. Longo, and J. L. Jameson, Eds., pp. 2152–2180, McGraw-Hill, New York, NY, USA, 16th edition, 2005.

[4] F. G. R. Fowkes, D. Rudan, I. Rudan et al., "Comparison of global estimates of prevalence and risk factors for peripheral artery disease in 2000 and 2010: a systematic review and analysis," *The Lancet*, vol. 382, no. 9901, pp. 1329–1340, 2013.

[5] I. J. Kullo and T. W. Rooke, "Peripheral artery disease," *The New England Journal of Medicine*, vol. 374, no. 9, pp. 861–871, 2016.

[6] M. Browlee, L. P. Aiello, M. E. Cooper, A. I. Vinik, R. W. Nesto, and A. J. M. Boulton, "Complications of diabetes mellitus," in *William's Textbook of Endocrinology*, H. M. Kronenberg, S. Melmed, K. S. Polonsky, and P. R. Larsen, Eds., pp. 1417–1501, Elsevier, New York, NY, USA, 11th edition, 2008.

[7] W. R. Hiatt, "Medical treatment of peripheral arterial disease and claudication," *The New England Journal of Medicine*, vol. 344, no. 21, pp. 1608–1621, 2001.

[8] V. Fonseca, C. Desouza, S. Asnani, and I. Jialal, "Nontraditional risk factors for cardiovascular disease in diabetes," *Endocrine Reviews*, vol. 25, no. 1, pp. 153–175, 2004.

[9] P. Libby, P. M. Ridker, and A. Maseri, "Inflammation and atherosclerosis," *Circulation*, vol. 105, no. 9, pp. 1135–1143, 2002.

[10] R. R. S. Packard and P. Libby, "Inflammation in atherosclerosis: from vascular biology to biomarker discovery and risk prediction," *Clinical Chemistry*, vol. 54, no. 1, pp. 24–38, 2008.

[11] V. Bembi, S. Singh, P. Singh, G. K. Aneja, T. V. S. Arya, and R. Arora, "Prevalence of peripheral arterial disease in a cohort of diabetic patients," *Southern Medical Journal*, vol. 99, no. 6, pp. 564–569, 2006.

[12] World Health Organisation, "Definition, diagnosis and classification of diabetes mellitus and its complications," Report of WHO Consultation WHO/NCD/NCS/99.2, WHO, 1998.

[13] American Diabetes Association, "Peripheral arterial disease in people with diabetes—a consensus statement," *Diabetes Care*, vol. 26, pp. 3333–3341, 2003.

[14] W. R. Hiatt, S. Hoag, and R. F. Hamman, "Effect of diagnostic criteria on the prevalence of peripheral arterial disease—the San Luis Valley Diabetes Study," *Circulation*, vol. 91, no. 5, pp. 1472–1479, 1995.

[15] R. Ramos, M. Quesada, P. Solanas et al., "Prevalence of symptomatic and asymptomatic peripheral arterial disease and the value of the ankle-brachial index to stratify cardiovascular risk," *European Journal of Vascular and Endovascular Surgery*, vol. 38, no. 3, pp. 305–311, 2009.

[16] R. Ikem, I. Ikem, O. Adebayo, and D. Soyoye, "An assessment of peripheral vascular disease in patients with diabetic foot ulcer," *Foot*, vol. 20, no. 4, pp. 114–117, 2010.

[17] E. Selvin and T. P. Erlinger, "Prevalence of and risk factors for peripheral arterial disease in the United States: results from the National Health and Nutrition Examination Survey, 1999–2000," *Circulation*, vol. 110, no. 6, pp. 738–743, 2004.

[18] J. Belch, A. MacCuish, I. Campbell et al., "The Prevention of Progression of Arterial Disease and Diabetes (POPADAD) trial: factorial randomised placebo controlled trial of aspirin and antioxidants in patients with diabetes and asymptomatic peripheral arterial disease," *British Medical Journal*, vol. 337, article a1840, 10 pages, 2008.

[19] C. White, "Intermittent claudication," *The New England Journal of Medicine*, vol. 356, no. 12, pp. 1241–1250, 2007.

[20] M. A. Creager and P. Libby, "Peripheral arterial disease," in *Braunwald's Heart Disease. A Textbook of Cardiovascular Medicine*, P. Libby, R. O. Bonow, D. L. Mann, D. P. Zipes, and E. Braunwald, Eds., pp. 1491–1513, Saunders, Philadelphia, Pa, USA, 8th edition, 2008.

[21] J. M. Murabito, R. B. D'Agostino, H. Silbershatz, and P. W. F. Wilson, "Intermittent claudication: a risk profile from the Framingham Heart Study," *Circulation*, vol. 96, no. 1, pp. 44–49, 1997.

[22] W. S. Aronow, "Peripheral arterial disease in the elderly," *Clinical Interventions in Aging*, vol. 2, no. 4, pp. 645–654, 2007.

[23] W. T. Meijer, A. W. Hoes, D. Rutgers, M. L. Bots, A. Hofman, and D. E. Grobbee, "Peripheral arterial disease in the elderly: the rotterdam study," *Arteriosclerosis, Thrombosis, and Vascular Biology*, vol. 18, no. 2, pp. 185–192, 1998.

[24] F. G. R. Fowkes, "The measurement of atherosclerotic peripheral arterial disease in epidemiological surveys," *International Journal of Epidemiology*, vol. 17, no. 2, pp. 248–254, 1988.

[25] J. W. Olin and B. A. Sealove, "Peripheral artery disease: current insight into the disease and its diagnosis and management," *Mayo Clinic Proceedings*, vol. 85, no. 7, pp. 678–692, 2010.

[26] K. W. Beach, G. R. Bedford, R. O. Bergelin et al., "Progression of lower-extremity arterial occlusive disease in type II diabetes mellitus," *Diabetes Care*, vol. 11, no. 6, pp. 464–472, 1988.

[27] A. O. Ogbera, A. Adedokun, O. A. Fasanmade, A. E. Ohwovoriole, and M. Ajani, "The foot at risk in nigerians with diabetes mellitus—the Nigerian scenario," *International Journal of Endocrinology and Metabolism*, vol. 4, pp. 165–173, 2005.

[28] M. H. Criqui, A. Fronek, M. R. Klauber, E. Barrett-Connor, and S. Gabriel, "The sensitivity, specificity, and predictive value of traditional clinical evaluation of peripheral arterial disease: results from noninvasive testing in a defined population," *Circulation*, vol. 71, no. 3, pp. 516–522, 1985.

[29] A. T. Hirsch, M. H. Criqui, D. Treat-Jacobson et al., "Peripheral arterial disease detection, awareness, and treatment in primary care," *The Journal of the American Medical Association*, vol. 286, no. 11, pp. 1317–1324, 2001.

[30] L. Norgren, W. R. Hiatt, J. A. Dormandy et al., "Inter-society consensus for the management of peripheral arterial disease (TASC II)," *Journal of Vascular Surgery*, vol. 45, no. 1, pp. S5–S67, 2007.

[31] J. Golledge, A. Leicht, R. G. Crowther, P. Clancy, W. L. Spinks, and F. Quigley, "Association of obesity and metabolic syndrome with the severity and outcome of intermittent claudication," *Journal of Vascular Surgery*, vol. 45, no. 1, pp. 40–46, 2007.

[32] E. T. Fung, A. M. Wilson, F. Zhang et al., "A biomarker panel for peripheral arterial disease," *Vascular Medicine*, vol. 13, no. 3, pp. 217–224, 2008.

[33] "Obesity," in *Harrison's Principles of Internal Medicine*, J. S. Flier, E. Maratos-Flier, E. Braunwald et al., Eds., pp. 422–429, McGraw-Hill, New York, NY, USA, 16th edition, 2005.

[34] P. Poirier, T. D. Giles, G. A. Bray et al., "Obesity and cardiovascular disease: pathophysiology, evaluation, and effect of weight loss: an update of the 1997 American Heart Association Scientific Statement on obesity and heart disease from the Obesity Committee of the Council on Nutrition, Physical Activity, and Metabolism," *Circulation*, vol. 113, no. 6, pp. 898–918, 2006.

[35] P. M. Ridker and P. Libby, "Risk Factors for atherothrombotic disease," in *Braunwald's Heart Disease. A textbook of Cardiovascular Medicine*, P. Libby, R. O. Bonow, D. L. Mann, D. P. Zipes, and E. Braunwald, Eds., pp. 1491–1513, Elsevier, 8th edition, 2008.

[36] M. T. Alzamora, R. Forés, J. M. Baena-Díez et al., "The Peripheral Arterial disease study (PERART/ARTPER): prevalence and risk factors in the general population," *BMC Public Health*, vol. 10, article 38, 11 pages, 2010.

[37] A. V. Chobanian, G. L. Bakris, H. R. Black et al., "The seventh report of the Joint National Committee on prevention, detection, evaluation, and treatment of high blood pressure," *Journal of the American Medical Association*, vol. 289, no. 19, pp. 2560–2571, 2003.

[38] P. Libby, "Prevention and treatment of atherosclerosis," in *Harrison's Principles of Internal Medicine*, D. L. Kasper, E. Braunwald, A. S. Fauci, S. L. Hauser, D. L. Longo, and J. L. Jameson, Eds., pp. 2152–2180, McGraw-Hill, 16th edition, 2005.

[39] A. I. Adler, R. J. Stevens, A. Neil, I. M. Stratton, A. J. M. Boulton, and R. R. Holman, "UKPDS 59: hyperglycemia and other potentially modifiable risk factors for peripheral vascular disease in type 2 diabetes," *Diabetes Care*, vol. 25, no. 5, pp. 894–899, 2002.

[40] V. Aboyans, M. H. Criqui, J. O. Denenberg, J. D. Knoke, P. M. Ridker, and A. Fronek, "Risk factors for progression of peripheral arterial disease in large and small vessels," *Circulation*, vol. 113, no. 22, pp. 2623–2629, 2006.

[41] Federal Ministry of Health Nigeria, Global Adult Tobacco Survey (GATS) Nigeria: Country Report 2012, Nigeria, http://www.who.int/tobacco/surveillance/survey/gats/nigeria_country_report.pdf.

16

Current Options for Determining Fracture Union

Saam Morshed

Department of Orthopaedic Surgery, University of San Francisco School of Medicine, San Francisco, CA 94143-0410, USA

Correspondence should be addressed to Saam Morshed; morsheds@orthosurg.ucsf.edu

Academic Editor: Patrizia D'Amelio

Determining whether a bone fracture is healed is one of the most important and fundamental clinical determinations made in orthopaedics. However, there are currently no standardized methods of assessing fracture union, which in turn has created significant disagreement among orthopaedic surgeons in both clinical and research settings. An extensive amount of research has been dedicated to finding novel and reliable ways of determining healing with some promising results. Recent advancements in imaging techniques and introduction of new radiographic scores have helped decrease the amount of disagreement on this topic among physicians. The knowledge gained from biomechanical studies of bone healing has helped us refine our tools and create more efficient and practical research instruments. Additionally, a deeper understanding of the molecular pathways involved in the bone healing process has led to emergence of serologic markers as possible candidates in assessment of fracture union. In addition to our current physician centered methods, patient-centered approaches assessing quality of life and function are gaining popularity in assessment of fracture union. Despite these advances, assessment of union remains an imperfect practice in the clinical setting. Therefore, clinicians need to draw on multiple modalities that directly and indirectly measure or correlate with bone healing when counseling patients.

1. Introduction

There are about 6 million fractures in the United States annually and 5–10% of these fractures proceed to nonunion [1]. The risk of nonunion is increased based on certain patient factors such as smoking habit or diabetes and varies by location of fracture with those of the scaphoid waist, neck of femur, and open fractures of the tibia being especially susceptible [2–6]. Nonunions are associated with significantly higher rate of healthcare resource use, drastically higher per patient cost, and use of stronger opioid medications [7–10]. Infection can present as a delay or failure of fracture repair, and the clinician should always consider this in the differential diagnosis. Determining when a fracture is healed is a routine part of orthopaedic clinical care. It is crucial to making the right clinical decision for patients including determining their weight-bearing status, appropriate time for hardware removal, and diagnosis and treatment of nonunions. It is also tremendously important in interpreting research studies on treatment and therapeutics of fracture repair. Therefore, a valid and standard definition of fracture union should be an essential and fundamental goal in orthopaedics. Lack

of such standardized and unified definition can lead to questionable and controversial results or more importantly expose the patients to additional and avoidable risks. The recent controversies surrounding the use of recombinant human bone morphogenetic protein-2 are an example of how assessment of fracture union is crucial to generating valid inferences in pivotal studies leading to approval of novel therapeutic modalities [11–13].

There has been considerable clinical and basic science research dedicated to better defining fracture healing and developing more efficient diagnostic tools for earlier and more accurate diagnosis of nonunions. However, it still largely remains a subjective topic and there is a significant amount of disagreement among physicians in regard to when a fracture is healed. A survey of 444 orthopaedic surgeons a decade ago identified that there is a lack of consensus in defining delayed union and nonunion in tibial fractures among orthopaedic surgeons. There was considerable disagreement in both clinical and radiographic criteria to define fracture union as well as the average time required for diagnosis of delayed or failed union [14]. The same level of disagreement and variability seems to exist among researchers in regard to clinical and radiographic definitions of fracture healing. A systematic review of 92 studies published between year 2000 and 2006 showed similar trends of a lack of objective tools to radiographically or clinically assess fracture healing [15].

This subjectivity and lack of agreement among clinicians and researchers in definition of fracture union are a major obstacle in conducting clinical trials in this field. Recently, there has been some effort to create standardized fracture union checklists. Though not completely validated, the initial assessments of these diagnostic tools are promising. The goal of this paper is to review the current options for determining fracture union and to explore recent advancements made in the field. The target audience of this review is the clinician who takes care of patients with bone fracture, be they a primary care physician or orthopaedic surgeon, as the diagnosis of fracture healing is fundamental to caring for these patients at any level of specialization.

2. Biology of Fracture Healing

To fully grasp the reason behind the lack of a gold standard in determining union, it is important to understand the complex molecular pathways and mechanical factors involved in bone healing. A detailed discussion of the molecules and cytokines involved in bone healing is beyond the scope of our review; however, a large number of these factors have been identified and extensively studied in both animal and human models [17–19]. Skeletal tissue has a great regenerative ability and it is now known that bone is one of the few tissues that can heal without forming fibrous scar tissue and regain its prefracture mechanical properties. A significant number of factors work in a highly coordinated and complex fashion at the molecular level to achieve this goal.

It is helpful to think of the bone healing process in a stepwise fashion, even though in reality there is a great overlap among these different stages. In general, it is possible to divide this process into an initial hematoma formation step, followed by inflammation, proliferation and differentiation, and eventually ossification and remodeling [20]. Shortly after a fracture ocurrs, the vascular injury to periosteum, endosteum, and the surrounding soft tissue causes hypoperfusion in the adjacent area. The coagulation cascade is activated which leads to the formation of a hematoma rich in platelets and macrophages. Cytokines from these macrophages initiate an inflammatory response, including increased blood flow and vascular permeability at the fracture site. Mechanical and molecular signals dictate what happens subsequently. Fracture healing can occur either through direct intramembranous healing or more commonly through indirect or secondary healing. The major difference between these two pathways is that direct healing requires absolute stability and lack of interfragmentary motion, whereas, in secondary healing, presence of interfragmentary motion at the site of fracture creates relative stability. In secondary healing, this mechanical stimulation in addition to the activity of the inflammatory molecules leads to formation of fracture callus followed by woven bone which is eventually remodeled to lamellar bone.

At a molecular level secretion of numerous cytokines and proinflammatory factors coordinate these complex pathways. Tumor necrosis factor-α (TNF-α), interleukin-1 (IL-1), IL-6, IL-11, and IL-18 are responsible for the initial inflammatory response [21]. Mesenchymal stem cells are recruited from the surrounding soft tissue and differentiate into osteogenic cells which are involved in generation of cartilaginous and periosteal bony callus [22]. Revascularization, an essential component of bone healing, is achieved through different molecular pathways requiring either angiopoietin or vascular endothelial growth factors (VEGF) [23]. VEGF's importance in the process of bone repair has been shown in a number of studies involving animal models [24, 25]. As the collagen matrix is invaded by blood vessels, the mineralization of the soft callus occurs through the activity of osteoblasts resulting in hard callus, which is remodeled into lamellar bone. Inhibition of angiogenesis in rats with closed femoral fractures completely prevented healing and resulted in atrophic nonunions [26]. On the other hand, inadequate fixation in presence of good vascularity has been shown to lead to hypertrophic nonunion [22, 27]. Therefore, successful fracture healing requires a balanced interaction between biological and biomechanical forces.

As evident, fracture healing is a continuous and complex biological and molecular process. However, in the clinical setting, physicians often dichotomize healing to aid in clinical decision-making and draw conclusions about efficacy of treatment. This oversimplification can lead to loss of valuable information along the spectrum of healing and more importantly misdiagnosis and misguided treatment decisions.

3. Nonunion

There is currently no accepted standardized definition of fracture nonunion among orthopaedic surgeons. According to the definition provided by the American Food and Drug Administration (FDA) a minimum of at least nine months has to elapse since the initial injury and there should be no signs of healing for the final three months for diagnosis of fracture nonunion [28]. There are a few different classification systems of nonunions, but nonunions are most commonly divided into two categories of hypervascular nonunion and avascular nonunion [29, 30]. In hypervascular nonunions, also known as hypertrophic nonunion, fracture ends are vascular and are capable of biological activity. There is evidence of callus formation around the fracture site (Figure 1) and it is thought to be in response to excessive micromotion at the fracture site [31]. Avascular nonunions, also known as atrophic nonunion, are caused by avascularity or poor blood supply of the fracture ends [32, 33]. There is no or minimal callus formation and fracture line remains visible (Figure 2). This type of nonunion requires biological enhancement in addition to adequate immobilization to heal [29].

4. Measures of Healing

Our current available tools in assessment of fracture healing can be broadly divided into four categories: (1) imaging studies, (2) mechanical assessment, (3) serologic markers,

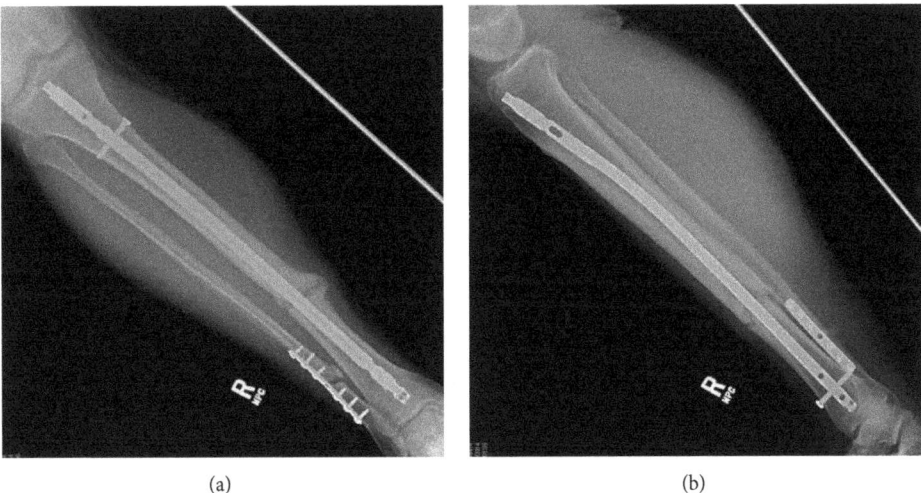

FIGURE 1: ((a) and (b)) Radiographs of a hypertrophic tibial nonunion in a 35-year-old man ten months status after medullary fixation of an open tibial shaft fracture with persistent pain and inability to weight bare. Note abundant callus formation but persistent fracture line.

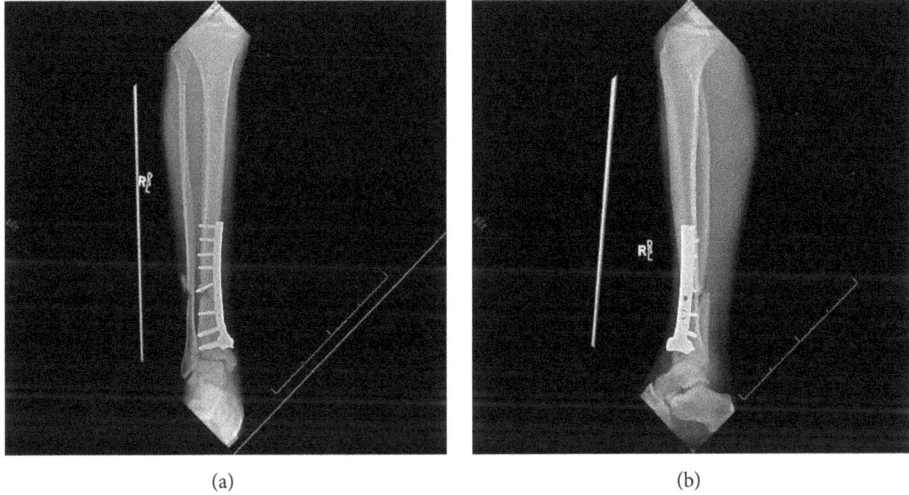

FIGURE 2: ((a) and (b)) Radiographs of an atrophic nonunion of the tibia with hardware failure one year after motorcycle collision resulting in an open tibial fracture. In this patient, little or no callus is evident.

and (4) clinical examination. We will explore each of these categories and their current use in clinical or research settings in detail.

4.1. Imaging Measures. Despite their limitations, radiographic assessment has remained a crucial tool in determining fracture healing. This stems from clinicians' familiarity with plain radiography and their widespread availability and accessibility. Bhandari et al. showed in an international survey of 444 orthopaedic surgeons in 2002 that 39.7% to 45.8% of surgeons always used radiographic data, including callus size, cortical continuity, and progressive loss of fracture line in assessment of tibial fracture healing [14]. Despite developments of advanced imaging techniques to quantitatively and qualitatively assess bone health and fracture healing, plain radiography remains the most commonly used radiographic tool for this purpose. This is due to lower cost, wider availability, and lower radiation exposure of plain radiography compared to other available modalities. However, the few studies that looked at reliability of plain radiography in detecting fracture healing concluded that radiographs do not define union with enough accuracy and are generally inconclusive in determining the stage of union [34–36]. Research into validation and standardization of these radiographic tools is surprisingly sparse. There have been a few recent studies that attempted to standardize radiographic healing criteria for tibia and femur fractures with promising initial results [16, 37–39]. We review these studies along with a few other imaging modalities used in determination of union, including computed tomography and ultrasound.

4.1.1. Radiographic Union Scores. The teams at the University of Toronto and McMaster University have recently developed

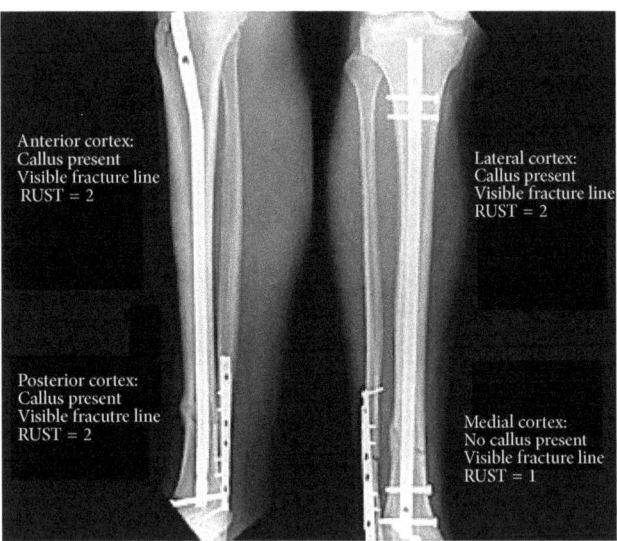

FIGURE 3: Assignment of the RUST in a patient with distal tibial shaft fracture at 3 months postoperatively. Overall RUST = 7.

TABLE 1: Individual cortex score based on radiographic findings. These scores are added to calculate the RUST [16].

Score per cortex	Callus	Fracture line
1	Absent	Visible
2	Present	Visible
3	Present	Invisible

two radiographic scoring systems, radiographic union score for hip (RUSH) and radiographic union score for tibia (RUST), that have been shown to increase agreement among surgeons and radiologists in assessing fracture repair [16, 38–40]. After pointing out the limitations of older radiographic scoring systems, they showed that assessment of the number of cortices bridged by callus had higher reliability in determining healing [41]. Based on this finding they attempted to improve accuracy of radiographic fracture union assessment by developing scaling systems that were mainly based on the appearance of the cortex on plain films.

The RUST is based on callus formation and visibility of fracture line at 4 cortices observed on AP and lateral radiographs (Figure 3). Minimum score of 4 indicates no healing and maximum of 12 indicates a healed fracture. Score for each cortex is assigned according to the criteria shown in Table 1. Whelan et al. looked at 45 sets of anteroposterior and lateral radiographs of tibial shaft fractures treated with intramedullary nails [39]. Seven reviewers, including orthopaedic residents, orthopaedic surgeons, and orthopaedic traumatologists independently evaluated the images for fracture healing using the RUST score. Agreement was measured using intraclass correlation coefficients (ICC) with 95% confidence intervals (CI). They found that overall interobserver agreement was substantial at both the initial assessment (ICC = 0.86, 95% CI 0.79–0.91) and 9 weeks after (ICC = 0.88, 95% CI 0.80–0.96). However, since there is

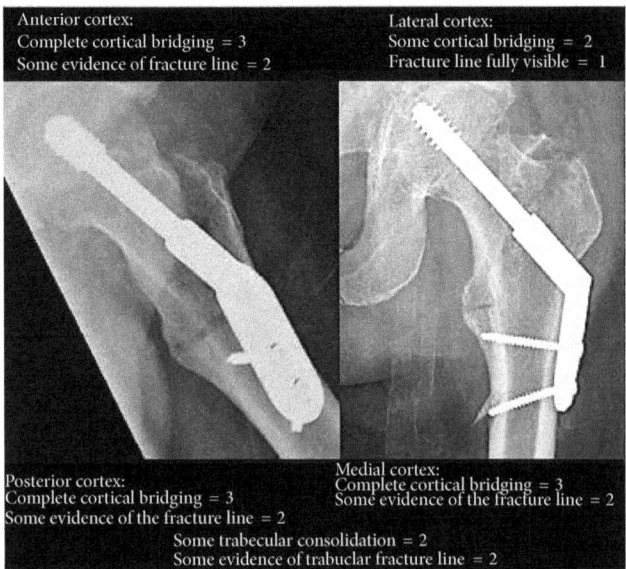

FIGURE 4: Assignment of the RUSH in a patient with an acute intertrochanteric fracture at 6 weeks postoperatively. The overall score in this patient is 22. As evident, the RUSH checklist incorporates cortical and trabecular bridging and fracture line disappearance in its scoring system.

currently no gold standard to compare the RUST to, they concluded that further research is required to fully validate this scoring system as a clinical tool.

Similarly, the RUSH provides a standardized radiographic assessment of hip fracture healing based on absence or presence of bridging and appearance of the fracture line. Figure 4 provides an example of using the RUSH in assessment of fracture union.

Bhandari et al. reviewed 150 cases of femoral neck fractures at two time points by a panel of three radiologists and three orthopaedic surgeons [37]. Reviewers were blinded to the time that the images were taken postoperatively. They reviewed each image to subjectively determine healing using anteroposterior and lateral images followed by assessment of the same images using the RUSH. They found higher agreement of fracture healing with use of the RUSH (ICC = 0.53, 95% CI: 0.30–0.69) compared to subjective assessment (ICC = 0.22, CI: 0.01–0.41). The same group conducted another similar study in which the six reviewers (three orthopaedic surgeons and three radiologists) had access to the time the images were taken after injury [38]. They assessed fracture healing using sequential radiographs in 100 patients with femoral neck fractures and 100 patients with intertrochanteric fractures. Agreement was almost perfect for both femoral neck and intertrochanteric fractures using RUSH score (ICC = 0.85, 95% CI: 0.82–0.87, and ICC = 0.88, 95% CI: 0.86–0.90, resp.) The RUSH score could potentially be used as a clinical tool given the evidence of increased reliability and agreement among clinicians. However, both the RUST and RUSH currently remain to be validated in terms of prediction of fracture union. This requires larger clinical studies to compare data from the RUST and RUSH with other

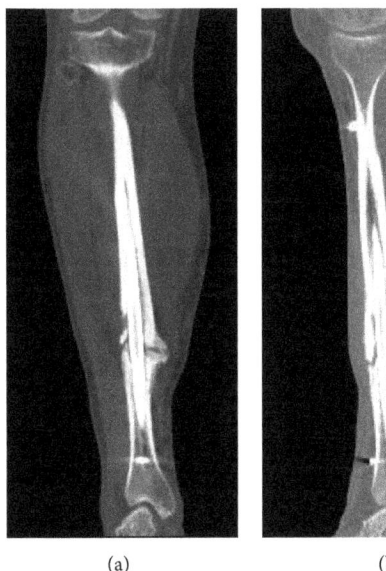
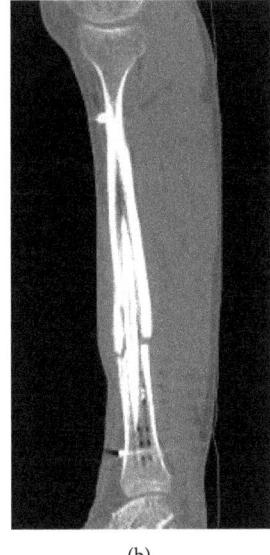

(a)   (b)

FIGURE 5

available outcome measures of healing including physical exam findings, other imaging modalities, and biomechanical data.

4.1.2. Computed Tomography. Computed tomography (CT) is superior to plain radiography in assessment of union and visualizing of fracture in presence of abundant callus or overlaying cast (Figure 5) [42]. There have been studies to test accuracy and efficacy of computed tomography in assessment of fracture union in clinical settings. Bhattacharyya et al. showed that computed tomography has 100% sensitivity for detecting nonunion; however, it is limited by a low specificity of 62% [43]. Three of the 35 patients in the study were misdiagnosed as tibial nonunion based on CT scan findings but were actually healed when fracture was visualized during surgical intervention. In a study of 18 patients with complex fractures of tibia shaft stabilized initially with external fixator, it was shown that an increase of more than 50% callus formation after 12 weeks on CT was an indicator of stability with sensitivity of 100% and specificity of 83% [44]. These findings correlated well with the data obtained from refractometry, a noninvasive method of measuring stability in fractures treated with external fixators. In another study investigators compared quantitative and qualitative changes of fracture healing in 39 patients with closed fractures of distal radius, tibia and/or fibular malleoli, or tibial shaft using both computed tomography and conventional radiography [45]. They found that early manifestations of healing, including blurring of fracture margins and formation of external callus, were observed earlier with CT scan. Most of the discrepancies between X-ray and CT scan findings were in periarticular and metaphyseal injuries. Overall, the findings of both modalities matched in 64% of cases. Overall the investigators concluded that CT scans have some advantages over radiographs in early detection of fracture healing in radius fractures. A limitation of CT is beam-hardening artifact from internal and external fixation. Despite reductions in image degradation from these artifacts using modern software, resolution is still affected when the region of interest is adjacent to metal implants. Currently, cost and radiation dose of CT scans limit their widespread use as the main clinical assessment tool for assessment of fracture healing despite evidence of their good diagnostic accuracy and correlation with other clinical markers of healing.

A new technology called virtual stress testing (VST) draws on improving resolution provided by CT-based finite element analysis. Finite element analysis (FE) is a mathematical tool initially designed for structural and stress analysis of buildings, bridges, and other architectural structures. Its use in orthopaedics involves simulation of either static problems, such as weight bearing capacity of implants and prosthetics or dynamic problems, such as fall analysis [46]. Finite element analysis uses information from CT images to provide quantitative assessment of bone strength [47]. Orwoll and his colleagues recently showed that biomechanical data obtained from finite element analysis correlate well with risk of hip fractures in men above the age of 65 [47]. This correlation remained statistically significant after adjusting for age and BMI.

Recently this technology was expanded from prediction of fracture risk to evaluation of fracture repair. In a pilot study Petfield used VST in complex tibia fractures treated with ring fixators to identify patients who would have a clinical event including refracture, malunion, or need for surgical revision if their hardware was removed. They retrospectively included 66 patients with CT scans of their fracture 2–4 weeks prior to removal of their ring fixators. With virtual stress testing they were able to use the information obtained from CT images and simulate multiple loading conditions after subtracting the mechanical contribution of the external fixator and therefore predict outcomes like axial compression, bending, and area of tissue failure. Eleven patients eventually had one of the above clinical events. Using quantitative data on failed tissue percentage and bone strength to body weight ratio, they were able to predict 9 of these 11 events [48]. More prospective studies with large sample sizes are required at this point to validate this technology and expand its use to other forms of internal fixations.

4.1.3. Ultrasound.

Ultrasound is unable to penetrate cortical bone, but there is evidence that it is able to detect callus formation before radiographic changes are visible [49, 50]. Following the promising results of their pilot study in which ultrasound was able to correctly predict union at a much shorter period of time compared to X-ray [51], Moed conducted a larger prospective study which showed that ultrasound findings at 6 and 9 weeks have a 97% positive predictive value (95% CI: 0.9-1) and 100% sensitivity in determining fracture healing in patients with acute tibial fractures treated with locked intramedullary nailing [52]. Time to determination of healing was also shorter using ultrasound (6.5 weeks) compared to nineteen-week average of radiographic data ($P < 0.001$). Ultrasound has additional advantages over other imaging modalities including lower cost, no ionizing radiation exposure, and being noninvasive. However its use and interpretation of findings are thought to be highly dependent on operator's expertise. Furthermore, thick layers of soft tissue can obscure adequate view of bones with ultrasound. As ultrasound technology advances, many of these limitations will likely be addressed. As with other imaging modalities, further prospective validation is required.

4.1.4. Positron Emission Tomography.

Positron emission tomography (PET) imaging generates imaging based on metabolic activity of different tissues. It has been historically used in detection of highly metabolic active tumors. A study in 2007 used PET scan with ^{18}F-fluoride ion in assessment of bone healing in rats with femur fractures [53]. ^{18}F-fluoride ion deposits in regions of the bone with high osteoblastic activity and high rate of turnover, such as endosteal and periosteal surfaces [54, 55]. In this study, one group of rats received intramedullary fixation for their femur fractures while in the second group investigators placed spacers at fracture sites to interfere with the healing process throughout the study. They evaluated the bone healing of both groups by weekly PET scans and plain radiographs. In treatment group uptake of ^{18}F-fluoride ion increased consistently between 1-3 weeks and remained elevated at 4 weeks after treatment. Radiographic and histologic analysis of femurs in this group also showed clear signs of healing. In contrast, ^{18}F-fluoride ion uptake in the group of rats with spacers was significantly lower at all time points throughout the study compared to the treatment group ($P < 0.005$). They concluded that ^{18}F-fluoride ion PET could potentially play an important part in assessment of fracture healing given its ability to quantitatively monitor metabolic activity and provide objective evaluation of fracture repair.

4.2. Mechanical Property Testing.

Mechanical testing measures fracture stiffness and stability. Modulating stability is a concept that orthopaedic surgeons think about and deal with on a daily basis. Increase in fracture stiffness is an indication of healing and it also correlates well with strength in the early phases of callus formation after injury [56, 57]. Biomechanical testing and vibrational analysis both utilize this concept in assessment of fracture healing. While the majority of these modalities cannot assist in assessment of fractures treated with internal fixation, many are still in use as research tools and may have some clinical role when external fixation is used.

4.2.1. Biomechanical Testing.

Biomechanical testing methods can be divided into direct and indirect measurement of stiffness. In direct measurement displacement angle across the fracture is measured by radiograph or surface measurements using four-point bending in the setting of applied load [58, 59]. The degree of deflection by the bending moment was assumed to be inversely proportional to the stability of the fracture union. The authors referred to this technique as "shift comparison" and introduced it as a quantitative method of measuring stability. This technique requires that no cast or hardware be present. Marsh defined nonunion in the study of 43 isolated closed tibial shaft fractures as failure to reach a stiffness of 7 Nm per degree by 20 weeks after injury since none of the fractures that reached this value failed to heal [60]. There was also high degree of correlation between stiffness measurements with injury severity and functional outcomes (SF-36) at 6 months. He explained delayed union as the cessation of periosteal activity before the completion of fracture bridging and nonunion as the cessation of both periosteal and endosteal responses with no bridging in the case of conservatively managed fractures.

In indirect testing fracture stiffness is measured by using strain-gauge units attached to external fixators to measure the strain in the fixator column [57]. Jorgensen measured fracture bending at a known amount of load in tibial fractures [61]. Richardson et al. noted that this method provides only indirect measurement of changes in stress in the fixator as the fracture heals; however, there are currently methods available to measure absolute values of stiffness using the same system [57, 62, 63]. Using this technique, Richardson et al. showed that most patients were able to weight-bear without support when their fracture stiffness reached 15 Nm per degree and that use of this threshold as compared to clinical and radiographic assessment was a better predictor of likelihood of refracture ($P = 0.02$) and also decreased the time to independent weight-bearing ($P = 0.02$) [57, 64].

4.2.2. Vibrational Analysis.

Vibrational testing uses either resonant frequency or computerized sonometry to assess mechanical properties of healing bones. The advantage of these methods compared to biomechanical testing is that they are noninvasive and painless. Resonant frequency analysis (RFA) is based on the principle that there is a direct correlation between the natural frequency of a beam and its stiffness. Long bones act as beams and therefore the same principle can be applied to long bones [65]. Early studies were done by Jurist who proposed that estimation of

Young's modulus of bones *in vivo* could be used to assess bone quality [66]. His lab measured resonant frequency by detecting bones' response to vibratory changes. Biological and physical changes in bone throughout the healing process change this resonant frequency [65–68]. Benirschke et al. showed that resonant frequency correlated well with both bending rigidity ($r^2 = 0.815$) of tibia and time to fracture healing [67]. Lowet used finite element modeling to show that there is a linear correlation between resonant frequencies and torsional stiffness of the healing tibia once callus stiffness reached 5% or higher of the stiffness of the intact bone [69]. Despite all these evidences for resonant frequency analysis as a quantitative tool for assessment of fracture healing, there are shortcomings associated with this method that limit its use. In a study of 74 tibial fractures it was shown that resonant frequency analysis was significantly inaccurate in assessment of healing in fractures of the proximal fourth of the tibia and fractures treated with interlocking nails [65]. They detected similar errors in a few patients treated with external fixators. Many of these fractures were falsely identified as healed by resonant frequency analysis. Authors explained this by proposing that RFA was most probably measuring the stiffness of the fixation instead of the healing fracture. Also quantity and quality of the overlaying soft tissue have a significant impact on the measurements of vibrational testing [70].

Quantitative ultrasonometry has also been studied for assessment of its efficacy in measurement of bone healing. Early studies in animal models demonstrated that ultrasound propagation velocity (USPV) across fractures approaches values of normal bone throughout the healing process [71]. Fellinger et al. used a system consisting of two sound transducers on two ends of tibial fractures with external fixators to evaluate the healing process by detecting sound transmission across these fractures [72]. Using computerized analysis of vibration reaction and sound propagation along fractures they were able to detect early signs of delayed union before radiographic signs were evident. Since then more precise devices have been developed and tested *in vitro* with similar results, showing high accuracy in predicting simulated fracture gap using ultrasound propagation velocity ($r^2 = 0.994$) [73]. Investigators used a tibia phantom with simulated transverse fractures for this study, which as they acknowledged is a simplification of actual clinical fractures with various anatomical characteristics and amount of soft tissue damage. Overlaying soft tissues limit *in vivo* studies of computerized sonometry to subcutaneous bones. Lack of large-scale reports of diagnostic accuracy and reliability of this modality in assessment of healing of various types of fractures in humans is the major barrier to its transition into the clinical and research practice.

5. Serologic Markers

As discussed above, prediction and early detection of nonunions could lead to lower medical costs and better clinical outcomes for patients. Given what we know about the early local and systemic molecular changes following a fracture, serologic biomarkers are gaining popularity as possible early predictors of fracture healing [74–77]. While C-reactive protein (CRP) and erythrocyte sedimentation rate (ESR) are commonly used in the evaluation of nonunion, particularly those where infection is suspected, much research has recently been focused on the identification of more sensitive and specific markers of delayed or failed fracture repair. Studies in human and animal models have identified many candidate biomarkers and potential limitations associated with their use as clinical diagnostic tools.

Moghaddam et al. conducted a prospective cohort study to assess changes in serum concentrations of a few serologic markers in normal and delayed fracture healing [78]. He was able to show significantly lower levels of tartrate-resistant acid phosphatase 5b (TRACP 5b) and C-terminal cross-linking telopeptide of type I collagen (CTX) in patients who developed nonunions compared to patients with normal healing. TRACP 5b is a direct marker of osteoclastic activity and bone resorption, while CTX is an indirect measure of osteoclastic activity by reflecting collagen degradation. Following a bone fracture, increased bone metabolism is observed in patients with normal healing. This is reflected by a sudden increase in osteoclastic markers, namely, CTX and TRACP 5b, during the first few weeks [79]. However, this increase was not observed in the delayed healing group, indicating a lower initial bone turnover following their injury. On the other hand, osteoblastic markers, total N-terminal propeptide of type I collagen (PINP), and bone specific alkaline phosphatase (BAP) initially decrease followed by an increase in both treatment and control groups without any significant difference between the two groups.

Another serologic marker of healing that has been extensively studied within the past decade is transforming growth factor-beta 1 (TGF-β1) [80–84]. It is a member of the TGF-β family and has been shown to be an essential regulatory molecule in fracture healing. It has been detected in callus of human and animal fracture models [74, 85] and its systemic and local administration enhanced bone remodeling and fracture healing in animal models [82, 86]. Zimmermann et al. prospectively assessed systemic changes of TGF-β1 levels in patients with delayed healing and nonunion of long bone fractures [87]. He found that in both normal and nonhealing groups serum level of TGF-β1 increased within the first 2 weeks after fracture. However, the delayed healing group had a faster decline of serum concentration between 2 and 4 weeks after trauma and its level was significantly lower in the delayed fracture-healing group at 4 weeks. However, a more recent study by Sarahrudi found no significant differences in the TGF-β1 concentrations of delayed and normal fracture healing groups [88].

Collagen III amino-terminal propeptide (PIIINP) is the N-terminal peptide cleaved from type-III procollagen during the process of type-III collagen synthesis [75]. Stoffel et al. [89] showed PIIINP becomes elevated during fracture healing and reaches its maximum at two weeks in malleolar fractures and 12 weeks in tibial fractures. Its level decreases afterwards and normalizes, which preceded radiographic and clinical evidence of healing. Kurdy [90] showed in 20 patients with isolated tibial shaft fractures that serum PIIINP levels were significantly higher in the nonhealing group at 10 weeks. This difference in PIIINP levels between healing and nonhealing groups was evident within the first 10 weeks after the initial injury.

Despite these encouraging findings there are a few issues that make the use of these biomarkers as diagnostic tools problematic. Secretion of many of the cytokines and biologic markers is also influenced by other factors. For example, systemic levels of TGF-β were found to vary based on smoking status, age, gender, diabetes mellitus, and chronic alcohol abuse at different time points [91]. The same factors, excluding alcohol abuse, have been shown to affect expression of macrophage colony stimulating factor (M-CSF) and vascular endothelial growth factors (VEGF) [92]. A recent systematic review concluded after thorough analysis of data presented in 44 studies that no recommendations in terms of clinical use of these serologic biomarkers can be made at this point [93]. Some of the limitations they identified include the small number of patients recruited in these studies, genetic heterogeneity among individuals, variation of the populations used in studies, and lack of large randomized trials in assessment of nonunion biomarkers.

6. Clinical Assessment of Healing

Despite all the advancements in developing fracture assessment instruments reviewed above, physical exam remains one of the mainstays of determining fracture union in the clinical setting. Patients with suspected nonunion should always be inspected for local signs of infection such as erythema, drainage, and wound problems. In a recent international survey of 335 orthopaedic surgeons, 88% of the participants agreed that radiographic and clinical data are required for adequate definition of union [94]. For delayed union and nonunion a majority of the respondents (83% and 84%, resp.) indicated that lack of weight-bearing ability was the most important clinical criterion for diagnosis, followed by fracture pain (78% and 74%, resp.) and weight-bearing status (48% and 51%, resp.). In a systematic review in 2008, out of fifty nine studies that used clinical criteria in defining union, absence of pain or tenderness at the fracture site on weight-bearing (31/59), absence of pain on palpation at the site of fracture (23/59), and the ability to weight-bear (12/59) were the most commonly used criteria to define fracture healing [15]. Lack of a standardized clinical definition of union contributes to this observed variability among clinicians and researchers in defining union.

Weight-bearing status has been shown to correlate relatively well with fracture stiffness in tibial fractures treated with external fixation [95]; however, physicians' ability to judge stiffness and weight-bearing ability based on physical exam alone is not very reliable. Webb et al. showed that manual assessment of stiffness by orthopaedic surgeons was not superior to that of medical students [96]. Additionally, it was shown that physicians, regardless of number of years of experience, are not reliable in judging stability with increasing stiffness of fractures [97]. As discussed above,

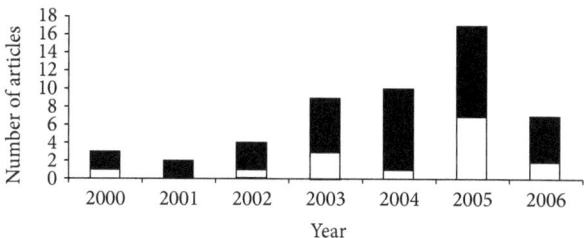

FIGURE 6: Distribution of general and region-specific instrument usage over time from 2000 to 2006 showing an increase in use of regional questionnaires between 2000 and 2005.

other more reliable biomechanical modalities of assessment of stiffness are not currently used as clinical tools. Pain on palpation at the site of injury is also currently widely used among physicians to judge union; however, it is a highly subjective outcome given individual and cultural differences in perception and tolerance level of pain among the population.

It is important to consider that patients might think very differently about the process of healing compared to physicians and other healthcare professionals. None of the tools we described so far assesses patients' goals and expectations in terms of their daily physical and mental health during the healing period. Therefore, use of tools to evaluate patient-reported outcome measures should be an important part of both research and clinical assessment of fracture healing. The increase in number of clinical studies between 2000 and 2005 that used patient-reported health-related questionnaires in assessment of fracture healing could indicate a shift towards a more patient-centered approach in dealing with this topic (Figure 6) [15].

The currently available patient-reported functional outcome assessment tools either measure general physical and psychological health, as in the Short Form-36 (SF-36) [98, 99], or are disease-specific, as in disability of the arm, shoulder, and hand (DASH) [100] or Western Ontario McMaster Arthritis Index (WOMAC) [101]. Disease-specific or region-specific questionnaires generally provide information on pain, physical status, and functional assessment of a specific body region, whereas general health questionnaires like SF-36 are generic measures of functional wellbeing and mental health [102]. Another class of questionnaires is health related quality of life (HRQoL) that measures patients' quality of life and how it is affected by a disease, disability, or treatment. Health Utility Index [103] and EuroQol-5D [104] are examples of the health related quality of life questionnaires. In the future, computer-assisted testing implementing item response theory is likely to streamline the process of gathering patient reported outcomes as evidenced by the National Institutes of Health PROMISE initiative [105]. These more efficient instruments are currently being validated in a number of different orthopaedic clinical settings including orthopaedic trauma.

7. Conclusion

As evident by now, fracture healing requires a complex interplay of biological pathways and mechanical forces. This process occurs in a continuum that varies dramatically based on fracture location, type, choice of treatment, and other host and injury related factors. Therefore, dichotomization of this complicated phenomenon is a clear oversimplification with subsequent loss of valuable information. This lack of standardized definition of fracture healing impairs our ability to compare findings from various studies on this topic. Recent developments of the RUSH and RUST score aim to improve reliability among assessors. Serologic markers also show promising results in more accurately predicting rate and quality of fracture healing; however, genetic and environmental variations among individuals limit their current clinical utility.

The future direction of fracture healing assessment should focus on further validation of the current available tools and development of better physician-assessed and patient-assessed instruments in measurement of union. The quality of these tools should be determined by evaluating their measurement properties, including reliability, validity, and reproducibility of results [106]. Defining a gold standard that incorporates all the different clinical, radiographic, biological, and biomechanical factors of healing has proven to be a difficult task. An endpoint Adjudication Committee can and should help increase agreement in assessment of fracture healing in clinical trials [107], as long as it is recognized that this may incompletely measure the impact of a treatment on overall injury recovery and health-related quality of life. Measurement of patient-reported outcomes can enhance our understanding of what radiographs and physical examination tell us about the degree of bone healing, though they may also enlighten clinicians and researchers as to how little an intervention meant to affect fracture repair impacts general health.

Conflict of Interests

The author declares that there is no conflict of interests regarding the publication of this paper.

Acknowledgment

This review article could not have been completed without the dedication of Pouriya Ghayoumi, BS, whose hard work and systematic research were vital to summarizing this vast body of knowledge.

References

[1] T. A. Einhorn, "Enhancement of fracture-healing," *Journal of Bone and Joint Surgery*, vol. 77, no. 6, pp. 940–956, 1995.

[2] R. C. Castillo, M. J. Bosse, E. J. MacKenzie, and B. M. Patterson, "Impact of smoking on fracture healing and risk of complications in limb-threatening open tibia fractures," *Journal of Orthopaedic Trauma*, vol. 19, no. 3, pp. 151–157, 2005.

[3] C. Tzioupis and P. V. Giannoudis, "Prevalence of long-bone non-unions," *Injury*, vol. 38, no. 2, pp. S3–S9, 2007.

[4] N. Osman, C. Touam, E. Masmejean, H. Asfazadourian, and J. Y. Alnot, "Results of non-operative and operative treatment of humeral shaft fractures. A series of 104 cases," *Annales de Chirurgie de la Main et du Membre Supérieur*, vol. 17, no. 3, pp. 195–206, 1998.

[5] P. R. Wolinsky, E. McCarty, Y. Shyr, and K. Johnson, "Reamed intramedullary nailing of the femur: 551 cases," *The Journal of Trauma*, vol. 46, no. 3, pp. 392–399, 1999.

[6] R. A. Winquist, S. T. Hansen Jr., and D. K. Clawson, "Closed intramedullary nailing of femoral fractures. A report of five hundred and twenty cases," *Journal of Bone and Joint Surgery*, vol. 66, no. 4, pp. 529–539, 1984.

[7] E. Antonova, T. K. Le, R. Burge, and J. Mershon, "Tibia shaft fractures: costly burden of nonunions," *BMC Musculoskeletal Disorders*, vol. 14, article 42, 2013.

[8] Z. Dahabreh, G. M. Calori, N. K. Kanakaris, V. S. Nikolaou, and P. V. Giannoudis, "A cost analysis of treatment of tibial fracture nonunion by bone grafting or bone morphogenetic protein-7," *International Orthopaedics*, vol. 33, no. 5, pp. 1407–1414, 2009.

[9] R. Beaver, M. R. Brinker, and R. L. Barrack, "An analysis of the actual cost of tibial nonunions," *The Journal of the Louisiana State Medical Society*, vol. 149, no. 6, pp. 200–206, 1997.

[10] N. K. Kanakaris and P. V. Giannoudis, "The health economics of the treatment of long-bone non-unions," *Injury*, vol. 38, supplement 2, pp. S77–S84, 2007.

[11] S. Govender, C. Csimma, H. K. Genant et al., "Recombinant human bone morphogenetic protein-2 for treatment of open tibial fractures a prospective, controlled, randomized study of four hundred and fifty patients," *The Journal of Bone & Joint Surgery A*, vol. 84, no. 12, pp. 2123–2134, 2002.

[12] E. J. Carragee, G. Chu, R. Rohatgi et al., "Cancer risk after use of recombinant bone morphogenetic protein-2 for spinal arthrodesis," *Journal of Bone and Joint Surgery A*, vol. 95, no. 17, pp. 1537–1545, 2013.

[13] H. T. Aro, S. Govender, A. D. Patel et al., "Recombinant human bone morphogenetic protein-2: a randomized trial in open tibial fractures treated with reamed nail fixation," *Journal of Bone and Joint Surgery—Series A*, vol. 93, no. 9, pp. 801–808, 2011.

[14] M. Bhandari, G. H. Guyatt, M. F. Swiontkowski, P. Tornetta III, S. Srpague, and E. H. Schemitsch, "A lack of consensus in the assessment of fracture healing among orthopaedic surgeons," *Journal of Orthopaedic Trauma*, vol. 16, no. 8, pp. 562–566, 2002.

[15] S. Morshed, L. Corrales, H. Genant, and T. Miclau III, "Outcome assessment in clinical trials of fracture-healing," *The Journal of Bone and Joint Surgery American*, vol. 90, supplement 1, pp. 62–67, 2008.

[16] B. W. Kooistra, B. G. Dijkman, J. W. Busse, S. Sprague, E. H. Schemitsch, and M. Bhandari, "The radiographic union scale in tibial fractures: reliability and validity," *Journal of Orthopaedic Trauma*, vol. 24, supplement 1, pp. S81–S86, 2010.

[17] T. A. Einhorn, "The science of fracture healing," *Journal of Orthopaedic Trauma*, vol. 19, supplement 10, pp. S4–S6, 2006.

[18] P. V. Giannoudis, T. A. Einhorn, and D. Marsh, "Fracture healing: the diamond concept," *Injury*, vol. 38, no. 4, pp. S3–S6, 2007.

[19] B. McKibbin, "The biology of fracture healing in long bones," *Journal of Bone and Joint Surgery B*, vol. 60, no. 2, pp. 150–162, 1978.

[20] P. J. Harwood, J. B. Newman, and A. L. R. Michael, "An update on fracture healing and non-union," *Orthopaedics and Trauma*, vol. 24, no. 1, pp. 9–23, 2010.

[21] L. C. Gerstenfeld, D. M. Cullinane, G. L. Barnes, D. T. Graves, and T. A. Einhorn, "Fracture healing as a post-natal developmental process: molecular, spatial, and temporal aspects of its regulation," *Journal of Cellular Biochemistry*, vol. 88, no. 5, pp. 873–884, 2003.

[22] R. Marsell and T. A. Einhorn, "The biology of fracture healing," *Injury*, vol. 42, no. 6, pp. 551–555, 2011.

[23] E. Tsiridis, N. Upadhyay, and P. Giannoudis, "Molecular aspects of fracture healing: which are the important molecules?" *Injury*, vol. 38, no. 1, pp. S11–S25, 2007.

[24] T.-W. Chu, Z.-G. Wang, P.-F. Zhu, W.-C. Jiao, J.-L. Wen, and S.-G. Gong, "Effect of vascular endothelial growth factor in fracture healing," *Chinese Journal of Reparative and Reconstructive Surgery*, vol. 16, no. 2, pp. 75–78, 2002.

[25] J. Street, M. Bao, L. DeGuzman et al., "Vascular endothelial growth factor stimulates bone repair by promoting angiogenesis and bone turnover," *Proceedings of the National Academy of Sciences of the United States of America*, vol. 99, no. 15, pp. 9656–9661, 2002.

[26] M. R. Hausman, M. B. Schaffler, and R. J. Majeska, "Prevention of fracture healing in rats by an inhibitor of angiogenesis," *Bone*, vol. 29, no. 6, pp. 560–564, 2001.

[27] E. Green, J. D. Lubahn, and J. Evans, "Risk factors, treatment, and outcomes associated with nonunion of the midshaft humerus fracture," *Journal of Surgical Orthopaedic Advances*, vol. 14, no. 2, pp. 64–72, 2005.

[28] United States Food and Drug Administration (USFDA), Office of Device Evaluation, Guidance Document for Industry and CDRH Staff for the Preparation of Investigational Device Exemptions and Premarket Approval Application for Bone Growth Stimulator Devices, 1988.

[29] J. P. M. Frölke and P. Patka, "Definition and classification of fracture non-unions," *Injury*, vol. 38, supplement 2, pp. S19–S22, 2007.

[30] A. Naimark, K. Miller, D. Segal, and J. Kossoff, "Nonunion," *Skeletal Radiology*, vol. 6, no. 1, pp. 21–25, 1981.

[31] B. G. Weber and O. Cech, *Pseudoarthrosis: Pathology, Biomechanics, Therapy, Results*, Hans Huber Medical Publisher, Berne, Switzerland, 1976.

[32] V. Perumal and C. S. Roberts, "(ii) Factors contributing to nonunion of fractures," *Current Orthopaedics*, vol. 21, no. 4, pp. 258–261, 2007.

[33] A. A. C. Reed, C. J. Joyner, S. Isefuku, H. C. Brownlow, and A. H. R. W. Simpson, "Vascularity in a new model of atrophic nonunion," *The Journal of Bone and Joint Surgery B*, vol. 85, no. 4, pp. 604–610, 2003.

[34] R. R. R. Hammer, S. Hammerby, and B. Lindholm, "Accuracy of radiologic assessment of tibial shaft fracture union in humans," *Clinical Orthopaedics and Related Research*, vol. 199, pp. 233–238, 1985.

[35] T. J. Blokhuis, J. H. D. De Bruine, J. A. M. Bramer et al., "The reliability of plain radiography in experimental fracture healing," *Skeletal Radiology*, vol. 30, no. 3, pp. 151–156, 2001.

[36] B. J. Davis, P. J. Roberts, C. I. Moorcroft, M. F. Brown, P. B. M. Thomas, and R. H. Wade, "Reliability of radiographs in defining union of internally fixed fractures," *Injury*, vol. 35, no. 6, pp. 557–561, 2004.

[37] M. Bhandari, M. Chiavaras, O. Ayeni et al., "Assessment of radiographic fracture healing in patients with operatively treated femoral neck fractures," *Journal of Orthopaedic Trauma*, vol. 27, no. 9, pp. e213–e219, 2013.

[38] M. Bhandari, M. M. Chiavaras, N. Parasu et al., "Radiographic union score for hip substantially improves agreement between surgeons and radiologists," *BMC Musculoskeletal Disorders*, vol. 14, article 70, 2013.

[39] D. B. Whelan, M. Bhandari, D. Stephen et al., "Development of the radiographic union score for tibial fractures for the assessment of tibial fracture healing after intramedullary fixation," *The Journal of Trauma*, vol. 68, no. 3, pp. 629–632, 2010.

[40] M. M. Chiavaras, S. Bains, H. Choudur et al., "The Radiographic Union Score for Hip (RUSH): the use of a checklist to evaluate hip fracture healing improves agreement between radiologists and orthopedic surgeons," *Skeletal Radiology*, vol. 42, no. 8, pp. 1079–1088, 2013.

[41] D. B. Whelan, M. Bhandari, M. D. McKee et al., "Interobserver and intraobserver variation in the assessment of the healing of tibial fractures after intramedullary fixation," *Journal of Bone and Joint Surgery B*, vol. 84, no. 1, pp. 15–18, 2002.

[42] E. M. Braunstein, S. A. Goldstein, J. Ku, P. Smith, and L. S. Matthews, "Computed tomography and plain radiography in experimental fracture healing," *Skeletal Radiology*, vol. 15, no. 1, pp. 27–31, 1986.

[43] T. Bhattacharyya, K. A. Bouchard, A. Phadke, J. B. Meigs, A. Kassarjian, and H. Salamipour, "The accuracy of computed tomography for the diagnosis of tibial nonunion," *Journal of Bone and Joint Surgery—Series A*, vol. 88, no. 4, pp. 692–697, 2006.

[44] P. Schnarkowski, J. Redei, C. G. Peterfly et al., "Tibial shaft fractures: assessment of fracture healing with computed tomography," *Journal of Computer Assisted Tomography*, vol. 19, no. 5, pp. 777–781, 1995.

[45] M. Grigoryan, J. A. Lynch, A. L. Fierlinger et al., "Quantitative and qualitative assessment of closed fracture healing using computed tomography and conventional radiography," *Academic Radiology*, vol. 10, no. 11, pp. 1267–1273, 2003.

[46] G. L. Roberts and I. Pallister, "Finite element analysis in trauma and orthopaedics—an introduction to clinically relevant simulation and its limitations," *Orthopaedics and Trauma*, vol. 26, no. 6, pp. 410–416, 2012.

[47] E. S. Orwoll, L. M. Marshall, C. M. Nielson et al., "Finite element analysis of the proximal femur and hip fracture risk in older men," *Journal of Bone and Mineral Research*, vol. 24, no. 3, pp. 475–483, 2009.

[48] J. L. Petfield, M. Kluk, E. Shin et al., "Virtual stress testing of regenerating bone in Tibia fractures," in *Proceedings of the 23rd Annual Scientific Meeting of Limb Lengthening and Reconstruction Society*, New York, NY, USA, July 2013, http://www.llrs.org/PDFs/Annual%20Meeting%20Presentations/Saturday%20Meeting/16.Petfield.pdf.

[49] J. G. Craig, J. A. Jacobson, and B. R. Moed, "Ultrasound of fracture and bone healing," *Radiologic Clinics of North America*, vol. 37, no. 4, pp. 737–751, 1999.

[50] B. R. Moed, E. C. Kim, M. van Holsbeeck et al., "Ultrasound for the early diagnosis of tibial fracture healing after static interlocked nailing without reaming: histologic correlation using a canine model," *Journal of Orthopaedic Trauma*, vol. 12, no. 3, pp. 200–205, 1998.

[51] B. R. Moed, J. T. Watson, P. Goldschmidt, and M. van Holsbeeck, "Ultrasound for the early diagnosis of fracture healing after

interlocking nailing of the tibia without reaming," *Clinical Orthopaedics and Related Research*, no. 310, pp. 137–144, 1995.

[52] B. R. Moed, S. Subramanian, M. van Holsbeeck et al., "Ultrasound for the early diagnosis of tibial fracture healing after static interlocked nailing without reaming: clinical results," *Journal of Orthopaedic Trauma*, vol. 12, no. 3, pp. 206–213, 1998.

[53] W. K. Hsu, B. T. Feeley, L. Krenek, D. B. Stout, A. F. Chatzi-ioannou, and J. R. Lieberman, "The use of 18F-fluoride and 18F-FDG PET scans to assess fracture healing in a rat femur model," *European Journal of Nuclear Medicine and Molecular Imaging*, vol. 34, no. 8, pp. 1291–1301, 2007.

[54] N. Narita, K. Kato, H. Nakagaki, N. Ohno, Y. Kameyama, and J. A. Weatherell, "Distribution of fluoride concentration in the rat's bone," *Calcified Tissue International*, vol. 46, no. 3, pp. 200–204, 1990.

[55] N. Narita, K. Kato, and H. Nakagaki, "Distribution pattern of fluoride concentration in the bones of the rabbit and the rat," *Aichi Gakuin Daigaku Shigakkai Shi*, vol. 27, no. 1, pp. 317–321, 1989.

[56] M. J. Chehade, A. P. Pohl, M. J. Pearcy, and N. Nawana, "Clinical implications of stiffness and strength changes in fracture healing," *Journal of Bone and Joint Surgery*, vol. 79, no. 1, pp. 9–12, 1997.

[57] J. B. Richardson, J. L. Cunningham, A. E. Goodship, B. T. O'Connor, and J. Kenwright, "Measuring stiffness can define healing of tibial fractures," *Journal of Bone and Joint Surgery B*, vol. 76, no. 3, pp. 389–394, 1994.

[58] P. Edholm, R. Hammer, S. Hammerby, and B. Lindholm, "The stability of union in tibial shaft fractures: its measurement by a non-invasive method," *Archives of Orthopaedic and Traumatic Surgery*, vol. 102, no. 4, pp. 242–247, 1984.

[59] P. Edholm, R. Hammer, S. Hammerby, and B. Lindholm, "Comparison of radiographic images. A new method for analysis of very small movements," *Acta Radiologica—Diagnosis*, vol. 24, no. 3, pp. 267–272, 1983.

[60] D. Marsh, "Concepts of fracture union, delayed union, and nonunion," *Clinical Orthopaedics and Related Research*, no. 355 supplement, pp. S22–S30, 1998.

[61] T. E. Jorgensen, "Measurements of stability of crural fractures treated with Hoffmann osteotaxis. 2. Measurements on crural fractures," *Acta Orthopaedica Scandinavica*, vol. 43, no. 3, pp. 207–218, 1972.

[62] A. E. Churches, K. E. Tanner, and J. D. Harris, "The Oxford External Fixator: fixator stiffness and the effects of bone pin loosening," *Engineering in Medicine*, vol. 14, no. 1, pp. 3–11, 1985.

[63] F. Burny, R. Bourgeois, M. Donkerwolcke, and F. Moulart, "Clinical use of external fixation. Current situation and future prospects," *Acta Orthopaedica Belgica*, vol. 44, no. 6, pp. 895–920, 1978.

[64] J. B. Richardson, J. Kenwright, and J. L. Cunningham, "Fracture stiffness measurement in the assessment and management of tibial fractures," *Clinical Biomechanics*, vol. 7, no. 2, pp. 75–79, 1992.

[65] S. S. Tower, R. K. Beals, and P. J. Duwelius, "Resonant frequency analysis of the tibia as a measure of fracture healing," *Journal of Orthopaedic Trauma*, vol. 7, no. 6, pp. 552–557, 1993.

[66] J. M. Jurist, "In vivo determination of the elastic response of bone. I. Method of ulnar resonant frequency determination," *Physics in Medicine and Biology*, vol. 15, no. 3, pp. 417–426, 1970.

[67] S. K. Benirschke, H. Mirels, D. Jones, and A. F. Tencer, "The use of resonant frequency measurements for the noninvasive

assessment of mechanical stiffness of the healing tibia," *Journal of Orthopaedic Trauma*, vol. 7, no. 1, pp. 64–71, 1993.

[68] A. Alizad, M. Walch, J. F. Greenleaf, and M. Fatemi, "Vibrational characteristics of bone fracture and fracture repair: application to excised rat femur," *Journal of Biomechanical Engineering*, vol. 128, no. 3, pp. 300–308, 2006.

[69] G. Lowet, X. Dayuan, and G. van der Perre, "Study of the vibrational behaviour of a healing tibia using finite element modelling," *Journal of Biomechanics*, vol. 29, no. 8, pp. 1003–1010, 1996.

[70] S. Saha and R. S. Lakes, "The effect of soft tissue on wave propagation and vibration tests for determining the in vivo properties of bone," *Journal of Biomechanics*, vol. 10, no. 7, pp. 393–401, 1977.

[71] I. M. Siegel, G. T. Anast, and T. Fields, "The determination of fracture healing by measurement of sound velocity across the fracture site," *Surgery, Gynecology & Obstetrics*, vol. 107, no. 3, pp. 327–332, 1958.

[72] M. Fellinger, N. Leitgeb, R. Szyszkowitz et al., "Early detection of delayed union in lower leg fractures using a computerised analysis of mechanical vibration reactions of bone for assessing the state of fracture healing," *Archives of Orthopaedic and Trauma Surgery*, vol. 113, no. 2, pp. 93–96, 1994.

[73] C. F. Njeh, J. R. Kearton, D. Hans, and C. M. Boivin, "The use of quantitative ultrasound to monitor fracture healing: a feasibility study using phantoms," *Medical Engineering & Physics*, vol. 20, no. 10, pp. 781–786, 1999.

[74] M. P. Bostrom, "Expression of bone morphogenetic proteins in fracture healing," *Clinical Orthopaedics and Related Research*, vol. 355, supplement, pp. S116–S123, 1998.

[75] G. Cox, T. A. Einhorn, C. Tzioupis, and P. V. Giannoudis, "Bone-turnover markers in fracture healing," *The Bone & Joint Journal*, vol. 92, no. 3, pp. 329–334, 2010.

[76] T. A. Einhorn, "The cell and molecular biology of fracture healing," *Clinical Orthopaedics and Related Research*, supplement 355, pp. S7–S21, 1999.

[77] L. M. Hoesel, U. Wehr, W. A. Rambeck, R. Schnettler, and C. Heiss, "Biochemical bone markers are useful to monitor fracture repair," *Clinical Orthopaedics and Related Research*, no. 440, pp. 226–232, 2005.

[78] A. Moghaddam, U. Müller, H. J. Roth, A. Wentzensen, P. A. Grützner, and G. Zimmermann, "TRACP 5b and CTX as osteological markers of delayed fracture healing," *Injury*, vol. 42, no. 8, pp. 758–764, 2011.

[79] S. W. Veitch, S. C. Findlay, A. J. Hamer, A. Blumsohn, R. Eastell, and B. M. Ingle, "Changes in bone mass and bone turnover following tibial shaft fracture," *Osteoporosis International*, vol. 17, no. 3, pp. 364–372, 2006.

[80] M. E. Joyce, S. Jingushi, and M. E. Bolander, "Transforming growth factor-β in the regulation of fracture repair," *The Orthopedic Clinics of North America*, vol. 21, no. 1, pp. 199–209, 1990.

[81] G. L. Barnes, P. J. Kostenuik, L. C. Gerstenfeld, and T. A. Einhorn, "Growth factor regulation of fracture repair," *Journal of Bone and Mineral Research*, vol. 14, no. 11, pp. 1805–1815, 1999.

[82] M. Lind, B. Schumacker, K. Soballe, J. Keller, F. Melsen, and C. Bunger, "Transforming growth factor-β enhances fracture healing in rabbit tibiae," *Acta Orthopaedica Scandinavica*, vol. 64, no. 5, pp. 553–556, 1993.

[83] B. Wildemann, G. Schmidmaier, S. Ordel, R. Stange, N. P. Haas, and M. Raschke, "Cell proliferation and differentiation during

fracture healing are influenced by locally applied IGF-I and TGF-betal: comparison of two proliferation markers, PCNA and BrdU," *Journal of Biomedical Materials Research B: Applied Biomaterials*, vol. 65, no. 1, pp. 150–156, 2003.

[84] M. E. Joyce, A. B. Roberts, M. B. Sporn, and M. E. Bolander, "Transforming growth factor-beta and the initiation of chondrogenesis and osteogenesis in the rat femur," *The Journal of Cell Biology*, vol. 110, no. 6, pp. 2195–2207, 1990.

[85] X. Si, Y. Jin, L. Yang, G. L. Tipoe, and F. H. White, "Expression of BMP-2 and TGF-β1 mRNA during healing of the rabbit mandible," *European Journal of Oral Sciences*, vol. 105, no. 4, pp. 325–330, 1997.

[86] G. Schmidmaier, B. Wildemann, J. Heeger et al., "Improvement of fracture healing by systemic administration of growth hormone and local application of insulin-like growth factor-1 and transforming growth factor-β1," *Bone*, vol. 31, no. 1, pp. 165–172, 2002.

[87] G. Zimmermann, P. Henle, M. Küsswetter et al., "TGF-β1 as a marker of delayed fracture healing," *Bone*, vol. 36, no. 5, pp. 779–785, 2005.

[88] K. Sarahrudi, A. Thomas, M. Mousavi et al., "Elevated transforming growth factor-beta 1 (TGF-β1) levels in human fracture healing," *Injury*, vol. 42, no. 8, pp. 833–837, 2011.

[89] K. Stoffel, H. Engler, M. Kuster, and W. Riesen, "Changes in biochemical markers after lower limb fractures," *Clinical Chemistry*, vol. 53, no. 1, pp. 131–134, 2007.

[90] N. M. G. Kurdy, "Serology of abnormal fracture healing: the role of PIIINP, PICP, and BsALP," *Journal of Orthopaedic Trauma*, vol. 14, no. 1, pp. 48–53, 2000.

[91] G. Kaiser, A. Thomas, J. Kottstorfer, M. Kecht, and K. Sarahrudi, "Is the expression of transforming growth factor-Betal after fracture of long bones solely influenced by the healing process?" *International Orthopaedics*, vol. 36, no. 10, pp. 2173–2179, 2012.

[92] J. Köttstorfer, G. Kaiser, A. Thomas et al., "The influence of non-osteogenic factors on the expression of M-CSF and VEGF during fracture healing," *Injury*, vol. 44, no. 7, pp. 930–934, 2013.

[93] I. Pountos, T. Georgouli, S. Pneumaticos, and P. V. Giannoudis, "Fracture non-union: can biomarkers predict outcome?" *Injury*, vol. 44, no. 12, pp. 1725–1732, 2013.

[94] M. Bhandari, K. Fong, S. Sprague, D. Williams, and B. Petrisor, "Variability in the definition and perceived causes of delayed unions and nonunions: a cross-sectional, multinational survey of orthopaedic surgeons," *The Journal of Bone and Joint Surgery (American Volume)*, vol. 94, no. 15, pp. e1091–e1096, 2012.

[95] C. C. Joslin, S. J. Eastaugh-Waring, J. R. W. Hardy, and J. L. Cunningham, "Weight bearing after tibial fracture as a guide to healing," *Clinical Biomechanics*, vol. 23, no. 3, pp. 329–333, 2008.

[96] J. Webb, G. Herling, T. Gardner, J. Kenwright, and A. H. R. W. Simpson, "Manual assessment of fracture stiffness," *Injury*, vol. 27, no. 5, pp. 319–320, 1996.

[97] R. Hammer and H. Norrbom, "Evaluation of fracture stability: a mechanical simulator for assessment of clinical judgement," *Acta Orthopaedica Scandinavica*, vol. 55, no. 3, pp. 330–333, 1984.

[98] J. C. Theis, "Clinical priority criteria in orthopaedics: a validation study using the SF36 quality of life questionnaire," *Health Services Management Research*, vol. 17, no. 1, pp. 59–61, 2004.

[99] C. A. McHorney, J. E. Ware Jr., and A. E. Raczek, "The MOS 36-Item Short-Form Health Survey (SF-36): II. Psychometric and clinical tests of validity in measuring physical and mental health constructs.," *Medical Care*, vol. 31, no. 3, pp. 247–263, 1993.

[100] P. L. Hudak, P. C. Amadio, and C. Bombardier, "Development of an upper extremity outcome measure: the DASH (disabilities of the arm, shoulder and hand) [corrected]. The Upper Extremity Collaborative Group (UECG)," *American Journal of Industrial Medicine*, vol. 29, no. 6, pp. 602–608, 1996.

[101] N. Bellamy, "WOMAC: a 20-year experiential review of a patient-centered self-reported health status questionnaire," *Journal of Rheumatology*, vol. 29, no. 12, pp. 2473–2476, 2002.

[102] J. Ware, sf-36.org: SF-36 Health Survey Update, 2013, http://www.sf-36.org/tools/sf36.shtml.

[103] Health Utilities Group/Health Utilities Index and Quality of Life, 2013, http://www.fhs.mcmaster.ca/hug.

[104] What is EQ-5D, 2013, http://www.euroqol.org.

[105] "PROMIS: Dynamic Tools to Measure Health Outcomes from the Patient Perspective," 2013, http://www.nihpromis.org/?AspxAutoDetectCookieSupport=1.

[106] V. A. Scholtes, C. B. Terwee, and R. W. Poolman, "What makes a measurement instrument valid and reliable?" *Injury*, vol. 42, no. 3, pp. 236–240, 2011.

[107] C. Vannabouathong, S. Sprague, and M. Bhandari, "Guidelines for fracture healing assessments in clinical trials. Part I: definitions and endpoint committees," *Injury*, vol. 42, no. 3, pp. 314–316, 2011.

17

The Protocol of Choice for Treatment of Snake Bite

Afshin Mohammad Alizadeh,[1] Hossein Hassanian-Moghaddam,[2,3] Nasim Zamani,[2,3] Mitra Rahimi,[2,3] Mohammad Mashayekhian,[2] Behrooz Hashemi Domeneh,[2] Peyman Erfantalab,[2,4] and Ali Ostadi[2,5]

[1]Department of Bone Marrow Transplantation, Taleghani Hospital, Shahid Beheshti University of Medical Sciences, Tehran, Iran
[2]Toxicological Research Center, Department of Clinical Toxicology, Loghman-Hakim Hospital, School of Medicine, Shahid Beheshti University of Medical Sciences, Tehran, Iran
[3]Excellence Center of Clinical Toxicology, Iranian Ministry of Health, Tehran, Iran
[4]Department of Emergency Medicine, School of Medicine, Iran University of Medical Sciences, Tehran, Iran
[5]Department of Internal Medicine, School of Medicine, Tabriz University of Medical Sciences, Tabriz, Iran

Correspondence should be addressed to Hossein Hassanian-Moghaddam; hassanian@sbmu.ac.ir

Academic Editor: Giovanni Storto

The aim of the current study is to compare three different methods of treatment of snake bite to determine the most efficient one. To unify the protocol of snake bite treatment in our center, we retrospectively reviewed files of the snake-bitten patients who had been referred to us between 2010 and 2014. They were contacted for follow-up using phone calls. Demographic and on-arrival characteristics, protocol used for treatment (WHO/Haddad/GF), and outcome/complications were evaluated. Patients were entered into one of the protocol groups and compared. Of a total of 63 patients, 56 (89%) were males. Five, 19, and 28 patients were managed by Haddad, WHO, or GF protocols, respectively. Eleven patients had fallen into both GF and WHO protocols and were excluded. Serum sickness was significantly more common when WHO protocol was used while 100% of the compartment syndromes and 71% of deformities had been reported after GF protocol. The most important complications were considered to be deformity, compartment syndrome, and amputation and were more frequent after the use of WHO and GF protocols (23.1% versus 76.9%; none in Haddad; P = NS). Haddad protocol seems to be the best for treatment of snake-bitten patients in our region. However, this cannot be strictly concluded because of the limited sample size and nonsignificant P values.

1. Introduction

Snake bite is a common and very important health problem in many parts of the world including our country [1, 2]. Apart from the production of antivenom, snake envenomation shares all characteristics of a neglected tropical disease in Asia [3]. Snake bite has caused almost from 4.5 to 9.1 effect rate in each 100000 Iranian population and 67 deaths (0.1% mortality rate) during 2002 to 2011 [2]. Although mortality rate of snake bite is fairly low, the complications due to it or its treatment (including coagulopathies, renal and/or pulmonary failure, disseminated intravascular coagulopathy, hemorrhages, deformities, compartment syndrome, limb amputation, and serum sickness syndrome) are rather frequent [1, 4].

Different protocols exist to manage snake bite, some of the very commonly used ones of which are the protocols suggested by the World Health Organization (WHO), *Goldfrank's Toxicologic Emergencies* (GF) textbook (Figure 1), and *Haddad and Winchester's (Haddad) Clinical Management of Poisoning and Drug Overdose* textbook (Figure 2) [5–7].

Interestingly, these protocols are far different from each other regarding management of the patients and even in the determination of the severity of poisoning (Table 1) [6, 7]. They all have their own fans. No study has compared the efficacy of these protocols to determine the most efficient one with the least complications.

In Iran, of three types of antivenom, only polyvalent one is produced by the Razi Vaccine and Serum Research

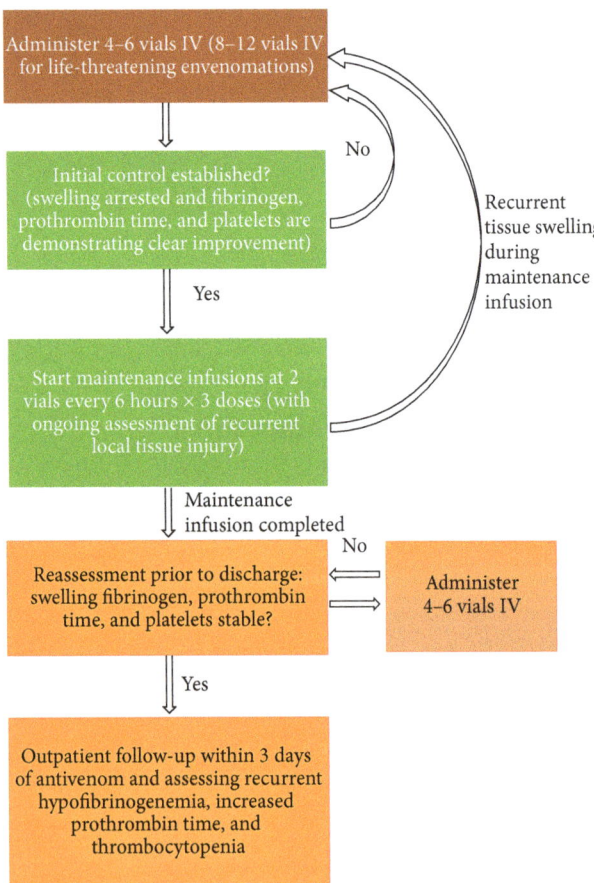

FIGURE 1: Flowchart of treatment of snake bite by *Goldfrank's Toxicologic Emergencies* textbook [6].

TABLE 1: Iranian-modified WHO diagram for management of snake bite.

Severity of envenomation	Signs/symptoms	Number of the vials that should be given
Mild	Local swelling without systemic signs/symptoms	3–5
Moderate	Extension of swelling with systemic signs/symptoms (paresthesia, nausea and vomiting, diarrhea, fatigue, lightheadedness, sweating, and chills) ± lab test abnormalities	6–10
Severe	Extension of swelling to all affected limb with systemic signs/symptoms (respiratory failure, shock, bleeding, loss of consciousness, fasciculation, and seizure) and severe lab test abnormalities	11–20

Institute. The polyvalent product can neutralize the venom of six different venomous snake species including *Naja naja oxiana*, *Pseudocerastes persicus fieldi*, *Echis carinatus*, *Vipera albicornuta*, *Vipera lebetina obtusa*, and *Agkistrodon halys* [2]. They are produced by plasma condensation and purification of immunized horses and contain 10 mLs of effective substance which can intravenously or intramuscularly be administered. Our center is a tertiary clinical toxicology center with an annual admission rate of about 30 to 40 snake-bitten patients. In a previous study from our center, two deaths were reported following venomous animals envenomation [8]. Five attending physicians of this center use different protocols of snake bite treatment (mostly GF and WHO) based on their personal favorite but not on the patients' clinical condition. In a try to unify the protocol of snake bite treatment in our center, we reviewed the files of the snake-bitten patients and compared the outcome and frequency of complications between them to determine which protocol was probably the best for the management of these patients.

2. Methods

Files of all patients who had been bitten by snakes and referred to a single tertiary toxicology center within five years (April 2010 to April 2014) were retrospectively evaluated.

Data was extracted by a single abstractor. The data extracted included patients' demographics (age and sex), the site of snake bite, time elapsed between bite and hospital presentation, on-arrival signs and symptoms, treatment protocol used for the treatment of the patient (WHO versus Haddad versus GF), numbers of the vials given to each patient, complications during the hospital stay (development of cellulitis, compartment syndrome, fasciotomy, and limb amputation), complications developed after hospital discharge (fever, swelling, and redness for determination of cellulitis; fever, rash, and arthritis/arthralgia for serum sickness syndrome; and limb deformities), hospital stay, and final outcome of the patients (complete recovery, recovery with sequelae, or death). However, since WHO has no suggested specific protocol for our region, a modified WHO protocol focused on specific snakes of Iran (developed by Iranian Ministry of Health) is used in our country [5]. Compartment syndrome was confirmed by doppler ultrasonography in each case.

Two fellows reviewed all charts and determined if the patient had been managed by WHO, GF, or Haddad protocols. The criteria for assessing compliance to the treatment protocol were based on severity of envenomation defined in each protocol, number of used vials, and repetition of it during hospitalization course. In case they disagreed on one decision, a third expert (an attending physician) entered their decision making process and convinced them to reach the same decision. Finally, the experts agreed on all charts and their protocol. For their follow-up, the patients were contacted using phone calls.

Their main postdischarge complications were evaluated using a self-made questionnaire evaluating the development of serum sickness, cellulitis, and permanent complications such as deformity of the bitten limb. The patients were then

5 general questions	Answers for crotaline antivenoms	
Indications	Mild crotaline envenomations with progression	
	Moderate and severe crotalid envenomations	
Contraindications	Relative contraindications	
	Horse product allergy (Wyeth-Ayerst)	
	Sheep product allergy (CroFab)	
	Papaya or papain allergy (CroFab)	
	Inability to manage anaphylactic and anaphylactoid reactions with life-threatening envenomations	
	Absolute contraindications	
	Refusal after informed consent	
	Inability to manage anaphylactic and anaphylactoid reactions with non-life-threatening envenomations	
Complications	Immediate	
	Anaphylactoid reactions	
	Anaphylactic reactions (type I hypersensitivity, IgE mediated)	
	More common with Wyeth-Ayers	
	Less common with CroFab	
	Delayed	
	Serum sickness (type III hypersensitivity; antigen-antibody, immune complex mediated)	
	Virtually inevitable with Wyeth-Ayerst	
	Uncommon with CroFab	
	Recurrent coagulopathy	
	Less common with Wyeth-Ayers	
	More common with CroFab	

Dosage		Initial number of vials	
	Degree of envenomations	Wyeth-Ayerst	CroFab
	Dry bite (no envenomations)	0	0
	Mild with progression	10	4–6
	Moderate	10–20	6
	Severe	20	6–12
Route	Intravenous in an intensive care setting in the emergency department or intensive care unit		

FIGURE 2: Flowchart of treatment of snake bite by *Haddad and Winchester's (Haddad) Clinical Management of Poisoning and Drug Overdose* textbook [7].

entered into one of the protocol groups and compared regarding the treatment performed, complications developed, and final outcome.

The data was entered into statistical package for social sciences (SPSS) version 17 and analyzed using Student's t-test (mean difference) and Kruskal-Wallis H test (median difference) for continuous data and chi-square test (for categorical data). A P value less than 0.05 was considered to be statistically significant. The study was approved by the Local Ethics Committee of Shahid Beheshti University of Medical Sciences.

3. Results

A total of 147 viper-bitten patients had been referred to us during the study period. Of them, only 63 could be followed up by phone calls and 56 (89%) were males. Five, 19, and 28 patients were managed by Haddad, WHO, or GF protocols, respectively, while 11 had fallen into both GF and WHO protocols and were therefore excluded. In fact, due to the similarity of these two protocols in mild cases, we could not determine which protocol the treating physician had chosen and thus we excluded the patients. In the remaining 52 patients, 46 (88%) were males. The most common site of snake bite was fingers (24 patients; 46%)

followed by feet (12 patients; 23%) and calves (5 patients; 10%). None of the patients were bitten in the head and neck. The most common signs/symptoms on presentation were swelling (51 patients; 98%) and pain (44 patients; 85%). The patients were considered to have mild, moderate, or severe envenomations according to the protocol applied for their treatment as this classification may significantly differ in different treatment protocols. Complications including serum sickness, deformity, compartment syndrome needing fasciotomy, amputation, necrosis, and neuropathy were detected in 10 (19.2%), 7 (13.5%), 4 (7.7%), 2 (3.8%), 2 (3.85), and 1 (1.9%) patients, respectively. Serum sickness was significantly ($P = 0.04$) more common when WHO protocol was applied (70% of all cases of serum sickness), while 100% of the compartment syndromes and 71% of all deformities had been reported after treatment with GF protocol. The most important complications were considered to be deformity, compartment syndrome, and amputation and were more frequent after use of WHO and GF protocols (23.1% versus 76.9%; none in Haddad; $P = $ NS; Table 2).

4. Discussion

According to our results, although the sample size is limited, Haddad protocol seems to be the best method of snake bite

TABLE 2: Follow-up data on three common snakebite protocols ($n = 52$).

Variable	WHO $n = 19$	GF $n = 28$	Haddad $n = 5$	Sig.	Posttest
Antivenom used vials (min, max)	5 [2, 6] (2, 18)	5 [5, 8] (0, 30)	10 [10, 12] (10, 12)	.016	$P = 0.013$, Haddad-WHO* $P = 0.021$, GF-Haddad*
Deformity n (%)	2 (10.5)	5 (17.9)	0	NS	—
Amputation n (%)	1 (5.3)	1 (3.6)	0	NS	—
Fasciotomy n (%)	0	4 (14.3)	0	NS	—
Necrosis n (%)	1 (5.3)	0	1 (20)	NS	—
Neuropathy n (%)	0	1 (3.6)	0	NS	—
Serum sickness n (%)	7 (36.8)	2 (7.1)	1 (20)	.04	$P = 021$, GF-WHO**
Hospital stay (day) (min, max)	2 [1, 2] (1, 12)	3 [2, 4] (1, 9)	3 [1.5, 4.5] (1, 5)	.035	$P = 0.035$, WHO-GF*

*Using post hoc adjusted test. **Using Pearson chi-square.

treatment. It causes least important complications (deformity, compartment syndrome needing fasciotomy, and amputation) and even less serum sickness in comparison with the other two protocols. However, based on the number of the vials advised by each protocol, Haddad suggests the most invasive treatment. As shown in Table 2, the amount of recommended antivenom is significantly more in Haddad protocol.

Increasing amount of administrated antivenom usually increases the risk of serum sickness [9]. Haddad generally advises 10, 10–20, and more than 20 vials for mild, moderate, and severe envenomations, which is far beyond the vials recommended by GF (4–6 in each step before reconsideration) while having 3 to maximum 20 vials by WHO [5–7]. We think this is mainly due to the fact that the earlier the patients receive their antivenom, the faster they improve. Previous authors have also emphasized the protective role of early antivenom administration on the snake-bitten patients and its fair effects on their final outcome [10].

We believe that although administration of 4–6 vials and reconsideration of the patients according to the GF protocol (and somehow WHO protocol) prevent administration of excessive antivenom vials, it predisposes the patient to higher risk of insufficient vial administration in the early hours after bite which are the critical hours in patient management since the best results are withdrawn when the antivenom is initiated within 24 hours [11]. On the other hand, it seems that early administration of high numbers of vials—as suggested by Haddad—should predispose the patient to higher risk of later serum sickness syndrome; this was not supported by our study, a result that we could not explain.

5. Limitations of This Study

The retrospective nature of the study was definitely a limitation of the current study. Also, difference between the common snakes at the home of the textbooks and ours, difference in the antivenoms available in our country and theirs, and very few numbers of the studied patients who were even needed to be reduced to only 52 cases are possibly other limitations that should be considered in future studies. In fact most of our patients were shepherds and could not be followed up through phone calls. However, it should be mentioned that a possible strength of our study is that we used the same polyvalent antivenoms manufactured by a single factory for all patients and in all episodes.

Also, the occurrence of serum sickness might relate to the dose of antivenoms and their quality and it was unreasonable to find serum sickness more common in group of WHO protocol. This was however a finding of the current study that should be further investigated in the future studies. In conclusion, although Haddad's protocol seems to be the best for treatment of snake-bitten patients in our region, this cannot be strictly concluded because of the limited sample size. Further prospective studies on more sample sizes are warranted to determine the best protocol for snake-bitten patients in different regions.

Competing Interests

The authors declare that they have no competing interests.

Authors' Contributions

Hossein Hassanian-Moghaddam and Nasim Zamani made contribution to conception and design. Mitra Rahimi, Mohammad Mashayekhian, Peyman Erfantalab, Ali Ostadi, and Behrooz Hashemi Domeneh contributed to the study implementation. Afshin Mohammad Alizadeh, Hossein Hassanian-Moghaddam, and Nasim Zamani analyzed and interpreted the data. Hossein Hassanian-Moghaddam and

Nasim Zamani drafted the article or revised it critically for important intellectual content. Afshin Mohammad Alizadeh, Hossein Hassanian-Moghaddam, Nasim Zamani, Mitra Rahimi, Mohammad Mashayekhian, Behrooz Hashemi Domeneh, Peyman Erfantalab, and Ali Ostadi participated in the final approval of the version to be published.

References

[1] R. Dehghani, B. Fathi, M. P. Shahi, and M. Jazayeri, "Ten years of snakebites in Iran," *Toxicon*, vol. 90, pp. 291–298, 2014.

[2] R. Dehghani, O. Mehrpour, M. P. Shahi et al., "Epidemiology of venomous and semi-venomous snakebites (Ophidia: Viperidae, Colubridae) in the Kashan city of the Isfahan province in Central Iran," *Journal of Research in Medical Sciences*, vol. 19, no. 1, pp. 33–40, 2014.

[3] E. Alirol, S. K. Sharma, H. S. Bawaskar, U. Kuch, and F. Chappuis, "Snake bite in south asia: a review," *PLoS Neglected Tropical Diseases*, vol. 4, no. 1, article e603, 2010.

[4] G. Bhalla, D. Mhaskar, and A. Agarwal, "A study of clinical profile of snake bite at a tertiary care centre," *Toxicology International*, vol. 21, no. 2, pp. 203–208, 2014.

[5] S. Shadnia, K. Soltaninejad, and A. Moghisi, *Country-Wide Guide to Treat Snake Bite in Iran*, Markaze-Nashre-Seda Publication, Tehran, Iran, 2009 (Persian).

[6] A. F. Pizon and A. M. Ruha, "Antivenom: snakes," in *Goldfrank's Toxicologic Emergencies*, R. S. Hoffman, M. A. Howland, N. A. Lewin, L. S. Nelson, and L. R. Goldfrank, Eds., pp. 1547–1551, McGraw Hill, New York, NY, USA, 2015.

[7] F. G. Walter, P. B. Chase, M. C. Fernandez, and J. McNally, "Venomous snakes," in *Haddad and Winchester's Clinical Management of Poisoning and Drug Overdose*, M. W. Shannon, S. W. Borron, and M. J. Burns, Eds., pp. 399–432, Elsevier, New York, NY, USA, 1998.

[8] H. Hassanian-Moghaddam, N. Zamani, M. Rahimi, S. Shadnia, A. Pajoumand, and S. Sarjami, "Acute adult and adolescent poisoning in Tehran, Iran; the epidemiologic trend between 2006 and 2011," *Archives of Iranian Medicine*, vol. 17, no. 8, pp. 534–538, 2014.

[9] C.-Y. Huang, D.-Z. Hung, and W.-K. Chen, "Antivenin-related Serum Sickness," *Journal of the Chinese Medical Association*, vol. 73, no. 10, pp. 540–542, 2010.

[10] K. S. Girish and K. Kemparaju, "Overlooked issues of snakebite management: time for strategic approach," *Current Topics in Medicinal Chemistry*, vol. 11, no. 20, pp. 2494–2508, 2011.

[11] J. Ashurst and R. Cannon, "Approach and management of venomous snake bites: a guide for the primary care physician," *Osteopathic Family Physician*, vol. 4, no. 5, pp. 155–159, 2012.

18

Surgical Management of Massive Pericardial Effusion and Predictors for Development of Constrictive Pericarditis in a Resource Limited Setting

Emeka B. Kesieme,[1] **Peter O. Okokhere,**[2] **Christopher Ojemiega Iruolagbe,**[2] **Angela Odike,**[3] **Clifford Owobu,**[4] **and Theophilus Akhigbe**[5]

[1]*Department of Surgery, Irrua Specialist Teaching Hospital, PMB 8, Irrua, Edo State, Nigeria*
[2]*Department of Medicine, Irrua Specialist Teaching Hospital, PMB 8, Irrua, Edo State, Nigeria*
[3]*Department of Paediatrics, Irrua Specialist Teaching Hospital, PMB 8, Irrua, Edo State, Nigeria*
[4]*Department of Pathology, Irrua Specialist Teaching Hospital, PMB 8, Irrua, Edo State, Nigeria*
[5]*Department of Radiology, Irrua Specialist Teaching Hospital, PMB 8, Irrua, Edo State, Nigeria*

Correspondence should be addressed to Emeka B. Kesieme; ekesieme@gmail.com

Academic Editor: Ville Kyto

Background. The diagnosis and treatment of massive pericardial effusion and cardiac tamponade have evolved over the years with a tendency towards a more comprehensive diagnostic workup and less traumatic intervention. *Method.* We reviewed and analysed the data of 32 consecutive patients who underwent surgery on account of massive pericardial effusion and cardiac tamponade in a semiurban university hospital in Nigeria from February 2010 to February 2016. *Results.* The majority of patients (34.4%) were between 31 and 40 years. Fourteen patients (43.8%) presented with clinical and echocardiographic feature of cardiac tamponade. The majority of patients (59.4%) presented with haemorrhagic pericardial effusion and the average volume of fluid drained intraoperatively was 846 mL ± 67 mL. Pericardium was thickened in 50% of cases. Subxiphoid pericardiostomy was performed under local anaesthesia in 28 cases. No postoperative recurrence was observed; however 5 patients developed features of constrictive pericarditis. The relationship between pericardial thickness and development of pericardial constriction was statistically significant ($p = 0.004$). *Conclusion.* Subxiphoid pericardiostomy is a very effective way of treating massive pericardial effusion. Removing tube after adequate drainage (50 mL/day) and treatment of primary pathology are key to preventing recurrence. There is also a need to follow up patients to detect pericardial constriction especially those with thickened pericardium.

1. Introduction

Massive pericardial effusion and cardiac tamponade are life-threatening cardiac pathologies that require urgent intervention.

The challenges in managing these conditions are not just only in treatment, but also in identifying the aetiological agent. In developing countries, the dominant cause of massive pericardial effusion is tuberculosis whereas in developed countries it is more likely to be caused by cancer, infectious, iatrogenic, connective tissue diseases and perhaps, in a good number of patients, the cause remains idiopathic [1, 2].

The nature of effusion drained from the pericardial space may be serous, haemorrhagic, or purulent. It may be massive, usually caused by malignancy followed by uraemia in the developed world [3]. A large effusion becomes a powerful predictor for development of cardiac tamponade when it has a circumferential echo space of more than 1 cm anteriorly and posteriorly [4].

Cardiac tamponade is a clinical emergency. Patients with cardiac tamponade present with features of elevated systemic venous pressure and the diagnosis is confirmed echocardiographically by right atrial or right ventricular diastolic collapse.

Patients that present with this condition should ideally be well investigated to diagnose the cause. Where facilities are available, pericardial fluid analysis for tumour markers (carcinoembryonic antigen, carbohydrate antigen CA-125, 19-9) is important in patients with suspected malignant effusion. In those with suspected tuberculous pericardial effusion, adenosine deaminase (ADA), interferon-gamma, PCR analysis for tuberculosis, and pericardial lysozymes should be done in addition to the routine pericardial fluid acid-fast bacilli staining and mycobacterium culture. High ADA level may predict the evolution towards constriction [5]. GeneXpert-MTB/RIF assay has been highly recommended as an initial diagnostic platform for early and quick detection of TB cases and hence can be very useful in diagnosing TB pericardial effusion [6]. Pericardioscopy can be useful in obtaining pericardial biopsy [5]. However in the setting of a developing country, there is significant challenge acquiring and performing the entire investigative armamentarium required for diagnosing the cause of massive pericardial effusion.

Pericardiocentesis which can be percutaneous or guided by echocardiography and subxiphoid pericardiostomy are effective ways of drainage in patients presenting with massive pericardial effusion and cardiac tamponade. Successful drainage has been achieved by use of percutaneous pigtail pericardial catheter [7]. Other methods of drainage include the transthoracic approach and video-assisted thoracoscopy.

We herein present our unit experience with surgical management of this condition to highlight challenges faced managing this condition with limited diagnostic facilities in the developing world. We surveyed factors that might suggest the possibility of future development of pericardial constriction.

2. Materials/Methods

We reviewed all cases of massive pericardial effusion and cardiac tamponade that presented to Irrua Specialist Teaching Hospital, Irrua, between February 2010 and February 2016. Irrua Specialist Teaching Hospital is a 375-bedded hospital located in a rural community and serving primarily the central, northern, and southern senatorial districts of Edo State, Nigeria.

Information was obtained from case notes, operating register, and surgeon's note. The following were documented: age, sex, clinical features suggestive of massive pericardial effusion and cardiac tamponade, investigative modalities, operative findings (thickness of pericardium, volume, and colour of fluid drained), subsequent development of recurrence, and constrictive pericarditis.

A 2D echocardiography was used to confirm the diagnosis of pericardial effusion by the presence of an echo-free space surrounding the heart. The diagnosis of cardiac tamponade was made based on the echocardiographic findings of right atrial or ventricular collapse during diastole. Chest radiograph and ECG were done in all cases.

Inclusion criteria include all patients who had moderate (10–20 mm), large (20 mm or more), and very large effusion (20 mm or more with evidence of compression of the heart).

We excluded patients with small effusion, patients with effusive-constrictive pericarditis, and two patients with cardiac tamponade who died shortly after pericardiocentesis.

Most patients had subxiphoid pericardiostomy under local anaesthesia which was augmented by conscious sedation in a handful of patients. A few patients with loculated pericardial effusion with background extensive adhesion had a limited lateral thoracostomy with creation of pericardial window.

Fluid was sent for cytology, Ziehl-Neelsen staining, and Gram staining if effluent was purulent. Pericardial biopsy was done in all cases and sent for histology.

Seventeen cases were followed up for evidence of recurrence and for development of constrictive pericarditis for a period of one to four years.

Data was entered into SPSS Version 16, statistical software package (SPSS Inc; Chicago, IL). Categorical data was calculated in frequencies and percentages. Chi-square was used for categorical variable and p value < 0.05 was considered statistically significant.

3. Result

The majority of patients (34.4%, $n = 11$) were between 31 and 40 years, followed by those between 41 and 50 years, who accounted for 18.8% of cases (Table 1). Eighteen respondents (56.2%) were males while 14 (43.8%) were females. Most of them presented with varying degrees of dyspnoea (87.5%), orthopnea (40.6%), cough (34.4%), and chest pain (28.1%). One of the patients presented with high grade fever (40–41°C) and widespread petechial haemorrhage.

Criteria for probable and definitive diagnosis of TB pericardial effusion were met in 14 patients, which accounted for the majority of cases (43.8%). This was followed by idiopathic causes, responsible for pericardial effusion in 18.7% of cases (Table 1). Out of the 32 patients studied, fourteen patients (43.8%) presented with clinical and echocardiographic features in keeping with cardiac tamponade. Electrocardiogram (ECG) showed mainly low QRS voltages.

The mean volume of fluid drained was 846 mL ± 67 mL. The majority of respondents (53.1%) drained between 500 mL and 1,000 mL. Macroscopic appearance revealed that most of the effusions (59.4%) were haemorrhagic (Table 1). The majority of haemorrhagic effusion was probably secondary to tuberculosis (68.4%), idiopathic cause (15.8%), and uraemia (10.5%) and a case, which was suspected to be due to viral haemorrhagic fever. The patient with suspected viral haemorrhagic fever presented with high grade pyrexia (41°C) and petechial haemorrhage in addition to the haemorrhagic pericardial effusion and cardiac tamponade. Lassa polymerase chain reaction (PCR) was negative but the fever underwent resolution by lysis after initial doses of ribavirin. The patient resided in a community that is endemic for Lassa fever. Purulent pericardial effusion was observed in the 3 paediatric patients aged between 1 and 10 years. The culture grew colonies of *Staph. aureus* in 2 patients. Malignant pleural effusion was seen in 4 patients. All of the malignant effusions were secondary to metastatic carcinoma of the breast. Sixteen patients (50%) had evidence of thickened

TABLE 1: Demographic characteristics of respondents.

Demographic variables	Number	%
Age		
0–10	3	9.4
11–20	2	6.2
21–30	5	15.6
31–40	11	34.4
41–50	6	18.8
51–60	3	9.4
>60	2	6.2
Sex		
Male	18	56.2
Female	14	43.8
Causes		
Bacterial infection	3	9.4
Idiopathic	6	18.7
Malignant	4	12.5
Tuberculosis	14	43.8
Steroid-resistant nephritic syndrome	1	3.1
Suspected haemorrhagic fever	1	3.1
Uraemia	3	9.4
Volume of fluid drained intraoperatively		
<500	5	15.6
500–1000	17	53.1
>1000	10	31.3
Nature of fluid		
Serous	10	31.3
Haemorrhagic	19	59.4
Purulent	3	9.3

TABLE 2: Effect of age, pericardial thickness, and nature of effusion on development of pericardial constriction.

Variables		Development of constrictive pericarditis (CP)		p value
		Developed CP	Has not developed CP	
Age				0.409
0–10		—	3	
11–20		—	2	
21–30		1	3	
31–40		1	9	
41–50		2	2	
51–60		1	1	
>60		—	2	
Thickened pericardium	No			0.004
Present	12	5	7	
Absent	15	0	15	
Nature of effusion	No			0.296
Haemorrhagic	16	4	12	
Nonhaemorrhagic	11	1	10	

the development of pericardial constriction is statistically significant ($p < 0.004$) (Table 2).

4. Discussion

To make a definitive diagnosis of TB pericardial effusion involves demonstrating tubercle bacilli in pericardial fluid or on histologic section of the pericardium. A probable or presumed diagnosis of TB pericardial effusion involves the proof of TB elsewhere in a patient with otherwise unexplained pericarditis, a lymphocytic pericardial exudate with elevated biomarkers of TB infection, and/or appropriate response to a trial of antituberculous chemotherapy [8].

All the cases of TB pericarditis presented with infiltration of lymphocytes; however the yield of AFB on pericardial fluid and pericardial tissue was considerably low. This was obvious in the positive histology result of 3 out of 14 cases. Pericardial biopsy is positive in 10–64% of cases [9]. This was not surprising because conventional diagnostic methods used for detection of tuberculous pericarditis have been shown to be usually insensitive and require long culture periods. This may be due to the paucibacillary nature of disease and nonuniform distribution of microorganisms, coupled with the fact that precise and accurate diagnosis of pericardial effusion requires good laboratory equipment with highly trained personnel, which seems to be lacking in resource challenged settings [10]. There is therefore a need to incorporate other tests that are very sensitive for detecting TB pericardial effusion.

Tuberculosis is the most likely common cause of massive pleural effusion and cardiac tamponade and it is responsible for 43.8% of cases. Our finding is in keeping with findings

pericardium. Pericardium was considered thickened if it is ≥4 mm.

The histology revealed mainly chronic pericarditis with chronic inflammatory cells and they were either specific or nonspecific. Three out of 14 patients had histological evidence of tuberculosis. Malignant cells were seen in 1 out of all the 4 patients who presented with suspected malignant pericardial effusion.

Subxiphoid pericardiostomy was performed in 28 patients while 3 patients had limited lateral thoracotomy. Limited lateral thoracotomy was used in localized pericardial effusion, one purulent and two haemorrhagic effusions with extensive adhesions to the anterior fibrous pericardium.

There was one operative death in a patient with cardiac tamponade. Postoperative mortality from pulmonary embolism was recorded in a patient who had previous venous thromboembolism and another who died from severe renal impairment.

Seventeen cases were followed up for one to four years. No postoperative recurrence was observed. Five patients developed features of pericardial constriction. Out of these, 3 had pericardial stripping. The relationship between age at the onset of disease and nature of effusion and the development of pericardial constriction is not statistically significant; however the relationship between thickened pericardium and of Agner and Gallis, who observed that tuberculosis and malignant effusion were more likely to cause large pericardial effusion, effusion causing haemodynamic compromise compared to those secondary to idiopathic pericarditis [11]. Other studies done in regions with high endemicity for TB also revealed TB as the most common cause of pericardial effusion [12, 13]. All our patients suspected to have TB pericardial effusion received an initial 4-drug therapy for 2 months (isoniazid, rifampicin, pyrazinamide, and ethambutol) followed by isoniazid and rifampicin for the remaining 4 months. The findings of TB as the most common cause of pericardial effusion contrasts the findings in developed countries. In a study by Colombo et al., the most frequent causes of pericardial effusion were neoplastic (36%), idiopathic (32%), and uraemic (20%) whereas in the series of 57 patients investigated by Corey et al. the most common diagnoses were malignancy (23%), viral infection (14%), radiation induced inflammation (14%), collagen-vascular disease (12%), and uraemia (12%) [3, 14]. Sagristà-Sauleda et al. documented acute idiopathic pericarditis as the most common cause of massive pericardial effusion and this accounted for 20% of cases. This was followed by iatrogenic effusion (16%), neoplastic effusion (13%), and chronic idiopathic pericarditis (9%) [15]. A more recent study by Abdallah and Atar revealed that the most frequent aetiology of large symptomatic pericardial effusion was idiopathic [36% (77% with a clinical diagnosis of pericarditis)], followed by malignancy (31.4%), ischemic heart disease (16.3%), renal failure (4.6%), trauma (4.6%), and autoimmune disease (4.6%) [16].

In our study, TB pericardial effusion was the most likely cause of haemorrhagic pericardial effusion. In a study, haemorrhagic pericardial effusion was secondary to TB in 80% of patients [17]. Haemorrhagic pericardial effusion has been associated with neoplasia and poor survival in some studies, whereas others have implicated iatrogenic disease, malignancy, atherosclerotic heart disease, and idiopathic diseases as the major causes of haemorrhagic pericardial effusion [14, 18].

Purulent pericardial effusion was observed only in 3 paediatric patients. 1.2 L of pus was drained from the pericardium of one of these patients. Purulent pericarditis is a suppurative complication of bacterial infection of the pericardial space that can arise as a result of direct extension from an adjacent infection. This is supported by one of the patients who presented with extensive pyomyositis. *Staphylococcus aureus* is the most commonly identified pathogen as in our study, though other organisms as nontypeable *H. influenzae* (NTHi) and *Streptococcus pneumoniae* have been isolated [19–21].

The most common symptom was dyspnoea. Orthopnea was particularly observed in patients who presented with cardiac tamponade. Other studies have reported dyspnoea as the most common symptoms [11, 12]. Many patients (43.8%) presented with history and echocardiographic features in keeping with cardiac tamponade because generally in the developing world most of our patients present late.

The majority of pericardial effusion was drained by subxiphoid pericardiostomy; hence we strongly advocate this technique. Other researchers have also advocated this route [22–24]. We performed 28 out of 32 cases under local anaesthesia. Palatianos et al. used general anaesthesia in 35 out of 42 cases that they performed on [22]. Subxiphoid pericardiostomy offers rapid access to the pericardium and has low morbidity and excellent long term results as noted in other studies [23]. It is also performed under local anaesthesia and contamination of pleural space especially in cases of purulent pericarditis is avoided. It is also easy to obtain satisfactory pleural biopsy.

We used limited lateral thoracostomy on few occasions, when there is extensive adhesion anteriorly. This is to avoid inadvertent entry to the heart. Thoracotomy has been shown to result in a higher incidence of respiratory complications, as defined by the presence of pneumonia, pleural effusion, prolonged ventilation, and need for reintubation. Thoracotomy also has a longer mean hospital stay [25]. We have never considered video-assisted thoracoscopy because we do not have the facilities. We did not perform initial pericardiocentesis on most cases of cardiac tamponade because we have no delay operating on them. Most of our effusions are haemorrhagic and it may be difficult to differentiate a haemorrhagic pericardial effusion ab initio and one secondary to myocardial puncture especially when the procedure is performed without echocardiographic guidance. Pericardiocentesis is also not without risk of atrial and ventricular arrhythmias, vasovagal episodes, and pneumothorax.

We did not record any case of recurrence following drainage. This contrasts the findings of Sarigül et al., who recorded recurrence of 10.2%, and recurrence was most commonly observed in uraemic patients [13]. Our zero recurrence may be related to our protocol for management of these patients, as we ensure drainage less than 50 mL before removal of tubes. The normal pericardial sac contains 10–50 mL of pericardial fluid, which acts as a lubricant between the pericardial layers. We also ensured that patient adhered strictly to the management of the primary pathology. Shahbaz Sarwar and Fatimi recorded recurrence in 32 out of 99 patients treated for pericardial effusion. TB was the most common cause of recurrent effusion in their study [26]. In a study by Mueller et al., 18% had recurrent pericardial effusion [24].

A constrictive physiology can develop within months and years after pericardiostomy. Five patients developed constrictive pericarditis. Out of this, 3 had pericardiectomy. They were more likely to present with echocardiographic findings of thickened pericardium. Studies have also that a high risk of constriction has been observed in cases of purulent pericarditis, tubercular pericarditis, and radiation pericarditis [21, 27, 28]. Late pericardial constriction has also been noted in a patient with idiopathic pericardial effusion [24]. We followed up our cases of purulent pericarditis and we did not encounter features of constriction.

Our study is limited by the number of cases seen over the 6-year period. A result from a sizeable study population may be more relevant.

5. Conclusion

Massive pericardial effusion and cardiac tamponade are largely secondary to tuberculosis in the developing world.

Subxiphoid pericardiostomy is a satisfactory method of drainage of pericardial effusion and postoperatively those with thickened pericardium need to be closely monitored.

Competing Interests

The authors declare that there are no competing interests regarding the publication of this paper.

References

[1] M. Imazio and Y. Adler, "Management of pericardial effusion," *European Heart Journal*, vol. 34, no. 16, pp. 1186–1197, 2013.

[2] F. F. Syed, M. Ntsekhe, and B. M. Mayosi, "Tailoring diagnosis and management of pericardial disease to the epidemiological setting," *Mayo Clinic Proceedings*, vol. 85, no. 9, p. 866, 2010.

[3] G. R. Corey, P. T. Campbell, P. Van Trigt et al., "Etiology of large pericardial effusions," *The American Journal of Medicine*, vol. 95, no. 2, pp. 209–213, 1993.

[4] M. J. Eisenberg, M. M. Dunn, N. Kanth et al., "Prognostic value of echocardiography in hospitalised patients with pericardial effusion," *Journal of the American College of Cardiology*, vol. 22, no. 2, pp. 588–592, 1993.

[5] L. J. Burgess, H. Reuter, M. E. Carstens, J. J. F. Taljaard, and A. F. Doubell, "The use of adenosine deaminase and interferon-γ as diagnostic tools for tuberculous pericarditis," *Chest*, vol. 122, no. 3, pp. 900–905, 2002.

[6] N. Negi and B. K. Das, "Genexpert technology: a new ray of hope for the diagnosis of tuberculour pericardial effusion," *Journal of the Practice of Cardiovascular Sciences*, vol. 1, no. 3, pp. 233–240, 2015.

[7] T. Yousuf, J. Kramer, A. Kopiec, Z. Bulwa, S. Sanyal, and J. Ziffra, "A rare case of cardiac tamponade induced by chronic rheumatoid arthritis," *Journal of Clinical Medicine Research*, vol. 7, no. 9, pp. 720–723, 2015.

[8] B. Maisch, P. M. Seferović, A. D. Ristić et al., "The Task Force on the Diagnosis and Management of Pericardial Diseases of the European Society of Cardiology. Guidelines on the diagnosis and management of pericardial diseases executive summary," *European Heart Journal*, vol. 25, no. 7, pp. 587–610, 2004.

[9] P. Ong, S. Greulich, J. Schumm et al., "Favorable course of pericardial angiosarcoma under paclitaxel followed by pazopanib treatment documented by cardiovascular magnetic resonance imaging," *Circulation*, vol. 126, no. 18, pp. e279–e281, 2012.

[10] M. Purohit and T. Mustafa, "Laboratory diagnosis of extrapulmonary tuberculosis (EPTB) in resource-constrained setting: state of the art, challenges and the need," *Journal of Clinical and Diagnostic Research*, vol. 9, no. 4, pp. EE01–EE06, 2015.

[11] R. C. Agner and H. A. Gallis, "Pericarditis: differential diagnostic considerations," *Archives of Internal Medicine*, vol. 139, no. 4, pp. 407–412, 1979.

[12] R. Hoque, M. Nuruzzaman, S. S. Husain, and Z. Rahman, "Subxiphoid window drainage of pericardial effusion—study of 35 cases," *University Heart Journal*, vol. 5, no. 2, pp. 71–74, 2010.

[13] A. Sarigül, B. Farsak, M. S. Ateş, M. Demircin, and I. Paşaoğlu, "Subxiphoid approach for treatment of pericardial effusion," *Asian Cardiovascular and Thoracic Annals*, vol. 7, no. 4, pp. 297–300, 1999.

[14] A. Colombo, H. G. Olson, J. Egan, and J. M. Gardin, "Etiology and prognostic implications of a large pericardial effusion in men," *Clinical Cardiology*, vol. 11, no. 6, pp. 389–394, 1988.

[15] J. Sagristà-Sauleda, J. Mercé, G. Permanyer-Miralda, and J. Soler-Soler, "Clinical clues to the causes of large pericardial effusions," *American Journal of Medicine*, vol. 109, no. 2, pp. 95–101, 2000.

[16] R. Abdallah and S. Atar, "Etiology and characteristics of large symptomatic pericardial effusion in a community hospital in the contemporary era," *QJM*, vol. 107, no. 5, Article ID hct255, pp. 363–368, 2014.

[17] C. R. Gibbs, R. D. S. Watson, S. P. Singh, and G. Y. H. Lip, "Management of pericardial effusion by drainage: a survey of 10 years' experience in a city centre general hospital serving a multiracial population," *Postgraduate Medical Journal*, vol. 76, no. 902, pp. 809–813, 2000.

[18] S. Atar, J. Chiu, J. S. Forrester, and R. J. Siegel, "Bloody pericardial effusion in patients with cardiac tamponade. Is the cause cancerous, tuberculous, or latrogenic in the 1990s?" *Chest*, vol. 116, no. 6, pp. 1564–1569, 1999.

[19] K. J. Downes, K. Abulebda, C. Siracusa, R. Moore, M. A. Staat, and S. E. Poynter, "Non-typeable *Haemophilus influenzae* purulent pericarditis in a child with cystic fibrosis," *Pediatrics International*, 2016.

[20] K. J. Downes, K. Abulebda, C. Siracusa, R. Moore, M. A. Staat, and S. E. Poynter, "Non-typeable *Haemophilus influenzae* purulent pericarditis in a child with cystic fibrosis," *Pediatrics International*, 2016.

[21] R. J. Morgan, L. W. Stephenson, P. K. Woolf, R. N. Edie, and L. H. Edmunds Jr., "Surgical treatment of purulent pericarditis in children," *Journal of Thoracic and Cardiovascular Surgery*, vol. 85, no. 4, pp. 527–531, 1983.

[22] G. M. Palatianos, R. J. Thurer, M. Q. Pompeo, and G. A. Kaiser, "Clinical experience with subxiphoid drainage of pericardial effusions," *Annals of Thoracic Surgery*, vol. 48, no. 3, pp. 381–385, 1989.

[23] D. W. O. Moores and S. W. Dziuban Jr., "Pericardial drainage procedures," *Chest Surgery Clinics of North America*, vol. 5, no. 2, pp. 359–373, 1995.

[24] X. M. Mueller, H. T. Tevaearai, M. Hurni et al., "Long-term results of surgical subxiphoid pericardial drainage," *Thoracic and Cardiovascular Surgeon*, vol. 45, no. 2, pp. 65–69, 1997.

[25] K. S. Naunheim, K. A. Kesler, A. C. Fiore et al., "Pericardial drainage: subxiphoid vs. transthoracic approach," *European Journal of Cardio-Thoracic Surgery*, vol. 5, no. 2, pp. 99–104, 1991.

[26] C. M. Shahbaz Sarwar and S. Fatimi, "Characteristics of recurrent pericardial effusions," *Singapore Medical Journal*, vol. 48, no. 8, pp. 725–728, 2007.

[27] R. Long, M. Younes, N. Patton, and E. Hershfield, "Tuberculous pericarditis: long-term outcome in patients who received medical therapy alone," *American Heart Journal*, vol. 117, no. 5, pp. 1133–1139, 1989.

[28] R. G. Martin, J. C. Ruckdeschel, P. Chang, R. Byhardt, R. J. Bouchard, and P. H. Wiernik, "Radiation-related pericarditis," *The American Journal of Cardiology*, vol. 35, no. 2, pp. 216–220, 1975.

19

Lipopolysaccharide-Induced Spatial Memory and Synaptic Plasticity Impairment Is Preventable by Captopril

Azam Abareshi,[1] **Akbar Anaeigoudari,**[2] **Fatemeh Norouzi,**[3] **Mohammad Naser Shafei,**[1] **Mohammad Hossein Boskabady,**[4] **Majid Khazaei,**[4] **and Mahmoud Hosseini**[1]

[1]*Neurocognitive Research Center, Faculty of Medicine, Mashhad University of Medical Sciences, Mashhad, Iran*
[2]*Department of Physiology, School of Medicine, Jiroft University of Medical Sciences, Jiroft, Iran*
[3]*Department of Physiology, Esfarayen Faculty of Medical Sciences, Esfarayen, Iran*
[4]*Neurogenic Inflammation Research Center, Faculty of Medicine, Mashhad University of Medical Sciences, Mashhad, Iran*

Correspondence should be addressed to Mahmoud Hosseini; hosseinim@mums.ac.ir

Academic Editor: João Quevedo

Introduction. Renin-angiotensin system has a role in inflammation and also is involved in many brain functions such as learning, memory, and emotion. Neuroimmune factors have been proposed as the contributors to the pathogenesis of memory impairments. In the present study, the effect of captopril on spatial memory and synaptic plasticity impairments induced by lipopolysaccharide (LPS) was investigated. *Methods.* The rats were divided and treated into control (saline), LPS (1 mg/kg), LPS-captopril (LPS-Capto; 50 mg/kg captopril before LPS), and captopril groups (50 mg/kg) before saline. Morris water maze was done. Long-term potentiation (LTP) from CA1 area of hippocampus was assessed by 100 Hz stimulation in the ipsilateral Schaffer collateral pathway. *Results.* In the LPS group, the spent time and traveled path to reach the platform were longer than those in the control, while, in the LPS-Capto group, they were shorter than those in the LPS group. Moreover, the slope and amplitude of field excitatory postsynaptic potential (fEPSP) decreased in the LPS group, as compared to the control group, whereas, in the LPS-Capto group, they increased compared to the LPS group. *Conclusion.* The results of the present study showed that captopril improved the LPS-induced memory and LTP impairments induced by LPS in rats. Further investigations are required in order to better understand the exact responsible mechanism(s).

1. Introduction

Renin-angiotensin system (RAS) is one of the neuropeptide systems in the brain. The substrate of RAS, angiotensinogen, is cleaved by the renin enzyme to form the decapeptide angiotensin (Ang I) in the brain [1]. Ang I is then converted to an octapeptide, Ang II, by angiotensin converting enzyme (ACE) [2] which is extensively located within various areas of central nervous system (CNS) [3]. Ang II is cleaved by glutamyl aminopeptidase A (AP-A) to form heptapeptide, Ang III. Ang II can also be cleaved to Ang (1-7) by carboxypeptidase P [2]. In addition, ACE2 acts on Ang I and Ang II to form Ang 1-9 and Ang 1-7, respectively. ACE2 has been shown to have a higher efficiency for conversion of Ang II to Ang 1-7 than for conversion of Ang I to Ang 1-9. This enzyme has been expressed in a low concentration in the CNS [4]. The

main effector of RAS, Ang II, binds to specific receptors in the brain to induce multiple actions [5]. It also regulates blood pressure, sodium and water balance, and sexual behaviors [2, 6]. The brain RAS has been shown to be involved in memory loss associated diseases such as Alzheimer's disease (AD) [1, 7] and cognitive dysfunctions which are preventable by angiotensin converting enzymes (ACE) inhibitors including captopril [1, 8]. Long-term potentiation (LTP), one of the major forms of activity dependent synaptic plasticity, is the primary experimental model for evaluating the synaptic basis of learning and memory in the hippocampus of vertebrates [9, 10]. An enhanced level of Ang II has been reported to be able to inhibit LTP induction in hippocampus [8].

In addition, RAS has been proposed to have a role in inflammatory responses and lipopolysaccharide- (LPS-) mediated microglial activation [11]. On the other hand, ACE inhibitors such as captopril have also been reported to have anti-inflammatory effects both in vitro and in vivo through reducing inflammatory cytokines such as tumor necrosis factor α (TNFα) and interleukin 1 (IL-1) [12, 13].

LPS, a potent inflammation-inducing agent in experimental studies, mimics the role of live bacteria and affects cognition and induces sickness behaviors when administered systemically or centrally [14]. These effects are attributed to overproduction of cytokines including interleukin-1β (IL-1β) and TNFα from immune cells [15]. Additionally, brain tissues oxidative damage has been reported to have an important role in learning and memory impairments induced by LPS [16]. Interestingly, an increased level of malondialdehyde (MDA) as an index of oxidative stress and a reduced level of total thiol content had been accompanied with increase in IL-1β, cognitive dysfunction, spatial learning deficits in Morris water maze (MWM), and synaptic plasticity impairment followed by LPS administration [14, 16]. It has also been reported that captopril is able to increase blood brain barrier permeability in rats [17]. Captopril also affects generation of proinflammatory and anti-inflammatory cytokines induced by LPS [18, 19]. We, therefore, decided to test whether captopril can prevent LPS-induced spatial memory and synaptic plasticity impairments.

2. Materials and Methods

2.1. Animals and Drugs. Male Wistar rats, 12 weeks old (240 ± 10 g), were purchased from the animal house of Mashhad University of Medical Sciences, Mashhad, Iran. The animals were housed in standard conditions (temperature 22 ± 2°C and 12 h light/dark cycle). The rats had free access to food and water. The animals were treated in accordance with approved procedures by the Committee on Animal Research of Mashhad University of Medical Sciences. Forty of the animals were divided into four groups (n = 10 in each group) and used for behavioral studies: (1) control, (2) LPS, (3) LPS-captopril (LPS-Capto), and (4) Capto groups. The animals in the LPS and LPS-Capto groups were treated by LPS (1 mg/kg; i.p.) [20], which began one week prior to the behavioral tests and continued to be injected 2 h before each trial of MWM test (Figure 1). The animals in the control and Capto groups received 1 mL/kg of saline instead of LPS. In the LPS-Capto and Capto groups, 50 mg/kg of captopril (i.p.) [21–23] was daily injected one week prior to start of the experiments and also was injected 30 min before LPS or saline. It has also been reported that captopril is bale to increase blood brain barrier permeability in rats [17]. The rest of the animals [23] were grouped into (1) control, (2) LPS, and (3) LPS-Capto (n = 8 in each group) and used for electrophysiological experiments after receiving a single dose of drugs or vehicle. LPS was purchased from Sigma (Sigma Chemical Co.). Captopril was provided by Daroupakhsh Company, Iran.

2.2. Morris Water Maze (MWM) Test. MWM apparatus was made of a circular black pool (136 cm diameter, 60 cm high, and 30 cm deep) with boundaries of the four quadrants including Q1 (northwest), Q2 (northeast), Q3 (southwest), and Q4 (southeast) that was filled with water (23–25°C).

A circular platform (10 cm diameter and 28 cm high) was hidden within the pool approximately 2 cm below the surface of the water in the center of the northwest quadrant. To determine the path, visual cues were fixed at several locations around the room outside the maze. The path, time, and speed of the animals to find the platform were traced by a camera. Before each experiment, the rats were familiarized with the water maze without a platform for 30 seconds. The animals performed four trials each day for five consecutive days and, in each trial, they were released randomly at one of the four positions. In each trial, the rat was allowed to swim until it found and remained on the platform for 20 seconds. If the animal was not able to find the platform within 60 seconds, it was guided to the platform by the experimenter and allowed to stay on it for 20 seconds. After removing from the pool, it was dried and placed in the cage for another 20 seconds. The time spent and distance traveled to reach the platform were recorded by a video tracking system. On the sixth day, the platform was removed, and the animals were allowed to swim for 60 seconds. The time spent and path traveled in the target quadrant (Q1) were compared between the groups.

2.3. Electrophysiological Study. For electrophysiological experiments, 24 of the animals were divided into three groups: (1) control, (2) LPS, and LPS-Capto (n = 8 in each group). The animals were anesthetized with urethane (1.6 g/kg) and their heads were then fixed in a stereotaxic apparatus. After exposing the skull, two small holes were drilled, under sterile conditions, to place stimulating and recording electrodes. Field potential was recorded from CA1 area of hippocampus. For this purpose, a bipolar stimulating electrode (stainless steel, 0.125 mm diameter, AM system) was infixed in the ipsilateral Schaffer collateral pathway (AP = 3 mm; ML = 3.5 mm; DV = 2.8–3 mm) and a unipolar recording electrode was lowered into the stratum radiatum of right CA1 area of hippocampus (AP = 4.1 mm; ML = 3 mm; DV = 2.5 mm). To ensure proper placement of the electrodes, physiological and stereotaxic indicators were used. Paired pulse facilitation (PPF) was considered as physiological indicator, and coordinates obtained from atlas of Paxinos and Watson were considered as stereotaxic indicators. PPF was measured by delivering ten consecutive evoked responses of paired pulses at 50 ms interpulse interval to the Schaffer collateral pathway at frequency 0.1 Hz (10 s interval). The stimulating electrode was connected to a stimulator and recording electrode was connected to an amplifier. Obtained extracellular field potential from CA1 area of hippocampus following stimulation of the Schaffer collateral pathway was amplified (100x) and filtered (1 Hz to 3 kHz band pass) using differential amplifier. A maximum field excitatory postsynaptic potential (fEPSP) was obtained by stimulating the Schaffer collateral pathway and recording in CA1 area. After a 30 min stabilization period, in order to evaluate synaptic potency before induction of LTP, an input-output (I/O) function was exerted by gradually increasing the stimulus intensities with constant current (input) and recording fEPSP (output). A baseline recording was then taken at 30 min before induction of LTP. After ensuring a steady state baseline response, in order for LTP induction, a high frequency stimulus (HFS) protocol of

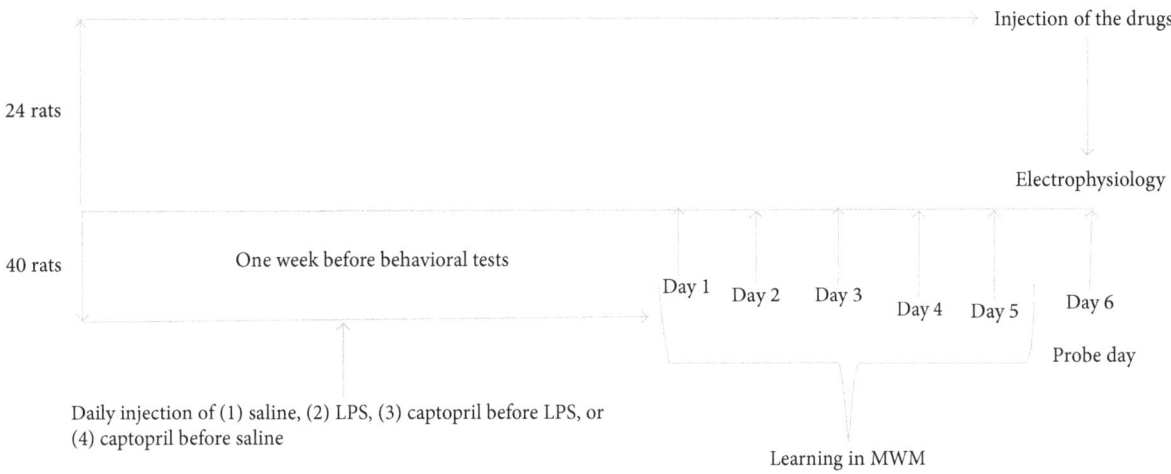

FIGURE 1: The protocol for the experiments.

100 Hz was applied. The stimuli with the intensities which produced 50% of the maximum response were applied to induce LTP.

The fEPSP was then recorded for 90 min after high frequency stimuli. Computer-based stimulation and recording were performed using Neurotrace software version 9 and Eletromodule 12 (Science Beam Institute, Tehran, Iran), respectively. The values of the slope and amplitude of the fEPSP were averaged of the 10 consecutive traces. Reponses were analyzed using custom software from the same institute.

2.4. Statistical Analysis. All data were expressed as means ± SEM and analyzed using two-way ANOVA followed by Tukey's post hoc test. Differences were considered statistically significant when $P < 0.05$.

3. Results

3.1. MWM Results. Using two-way ANOVA, the results showed that the treatment significantly affected the escape latency to reach the platform ($f_{(3,767)} = 23.28$; $P < 0.001$). There were also significant effects for days on the escape latency to reach the platform ($f_{(4,767)} = 64.04$; $P < 0.001$). There was a significant interaction between the treatment and days on the escape latency to reach the platform ($f_{(12,767)} = 2.50$; $P < 0.01$). The results also showed that the escape latency to reach the platform in the LPS group was significantly higher than that in the control group at days 3 ($P < 0.05$), 4 ($P < 0.001$), and 5 ($P < 0.001$). The animals in the LPS-Capto group had a significantly shorter time latency to reach the platform in comparison to those of the LPS group at days 3 ($P < 0.01$), 4 ($P < 0.01$), and 5 ($P < 0.001$). There was no significant difference in the time spent to reach the platform between the control and LPS-Capto groups. There was also no significant difference between the Capto and control groups (Figure 2).

Using two-way ANOVA, the results showed that the treatment significantly affected the distance traveled to reach the platform ($f_{(3,767)} = 23.56$; $P < 0.001$). There were also

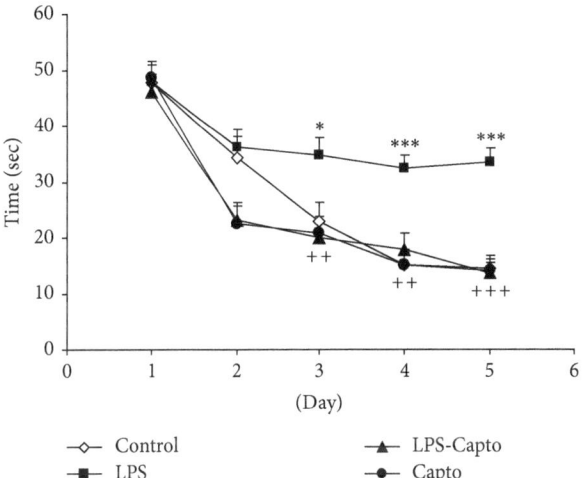

FIGURE 2: Comparison of time latency to reach the platform in the Morris water maze test between the four groups. Data are presented as mean ± SEM ($n = 10$ in each group). $^{*}P < 0.05$ and $^{***}P < 0.001$ compared with the control group and $^{++}P < 0.01$ and $^{+++}P < 0.001$ compared with the LPS group.

significant effects for days on the distance traveled to reach the platform ($f_{(4,767)} = 34.20$; $P < 0.001$). There was a significant interaction between the treatment and days on the distance traveled to reach the platform ($f_{(12,767)} = 2.45$; $P < 0.01$). The results also showed that the distance traveled to reach the platform in the LPS group was significantly higher than that in the control group at days 3 ($P < 0.01$), 4 ($P < 0.01$), and 5 ($P < 0.001$). The animals had a significantly shorter traveled distance to reach the platform in the LPS-Capto group in comparison to the LPS group at days 3 ($P < 0.01$), 4 ($P < 0.01$), and 5 ($P < 0.001$). There was no significant difference in the length of the swimming path between the control and LPS-Capto groups. There was also no significant difference between the Capto and control groups (Figure 3).

In the probe day, the animals of the LPS group spent lower time ($P < 0.001$) and traveled shorter distance ($P < 0.001$)

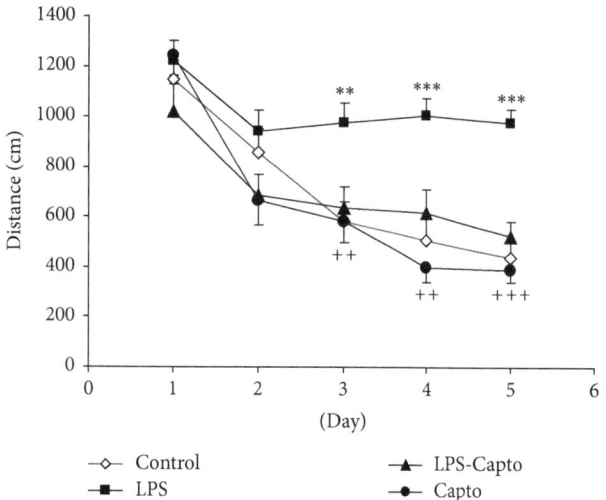

FIGURE 3: Comparison of the distance traveled to reach the platform in the Morris water maze test between the four groups. Data are presented as mean ± SEM (n = 10 in each group). $^{**}P < 0.01$ and $^{***}P < 0.001$ compared with the control group and $^{++}P < 0.01$ and $^{+++}P < 0.001$ compared with the LPS group.

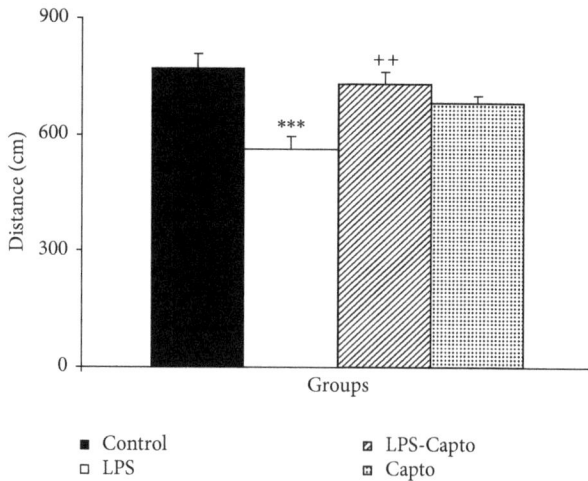

FIGURE 5: The results of the distance traveled in the target quadrant (Q1) in probe day, 24 hours after the last learning session. The platform was removed and the distance traveled in the target quadrant was compared between the groups. Data are shown as mean ± SEM (n = 10 in each group). $^{***}P < 0.001$ compared with the control group and $^{++}P < 0.01$ compared with the LPS group.

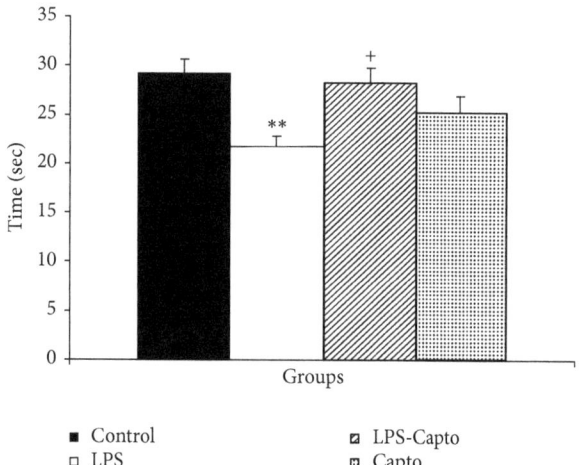

FIGURE 4: The results of the time spent in the target quadrant (Q1) in probe day, 24 hours after the last learning session. The platform was removed and the time spent in the target quadrant was compared between the groups. Data are shown as mean ± SEM (n = 10 in each group). $^{**}P < 0.01$ compared with the control group and $^{+}P < 0.01$ compared with the LPS group.

in the target quadrant (Q1) than those of the control group. The animals in the LPS-Capto group spent greater time and traveled longer distance in the Q1 compared to those in the LPS group ($P < 0.05$ and $P < 0.01$, resp.). There was no significant difference in the time spent and distance traveled in the Q1 between the control and LPS-Capto groups. The results also showed that there was no significant difference in the time spent and distance traveled in the target quadrant between the Capto and control groups (Figures 4 and 5).

3.2. Electrophysiological Results. After inducing HFS, the mean fEPSP amplitude in the LPS group decreased

significantly with respect to the control group ($P < 0.01$). The mean fEPSP amplitude in the LPS-Capto group was significantly higher than that in the LPS group ($P < 0.05$). There was no significant difference in fEPSP amplitude between the control and LPS-Capto groups (Figure 6(a)). In addition, after applying HFS, the fEPSP slope in the LPS group was significantly lower than that in the control group ($P < 0.01$). Injection of captopril increased the mean fEPSP slope in the LPS-Capto group in comparison to the LPS group ($P < 0.05$); however, there was no significant difference in fEPSP slope between the control and LPS-Capto groups (Figure 6(b)).

4. Discussion

Previous studies have demonstrated that LPS impairs learning and memory [14, 24]. In parallel with such reports, in the current study, intraperitoneal injection of LPS also impaired spatial learning and memory in the Morris water maze [25]. The results showed that the animals of the LPS group had more time latency (Figure 2) and longer traveled distance (Figure 3) to find the escape platform compared with those of the control group. The results of probe trial also showed that the animals of the LPS group did not well look for the location of the escape platform and spent less time (Figure 4) and traveled shorter distance (Figure 5) in the target quadrant (Q1) with respect to those of the control group.

LTP is a form of activity dependent synaptic plasticity which is suggested to be a predominant mechanism of learning and memory processes [9]. In hippocampus, LTP induction has been well known as a principle experimental model for studying synaptic basis of learning and memory in vertebrates [26]. In previous studies, LPS administration has resulted in suppression of LTP induction in rat dentate gyrus in vitro [27] and subiculum in vivo [28]. In the current study,

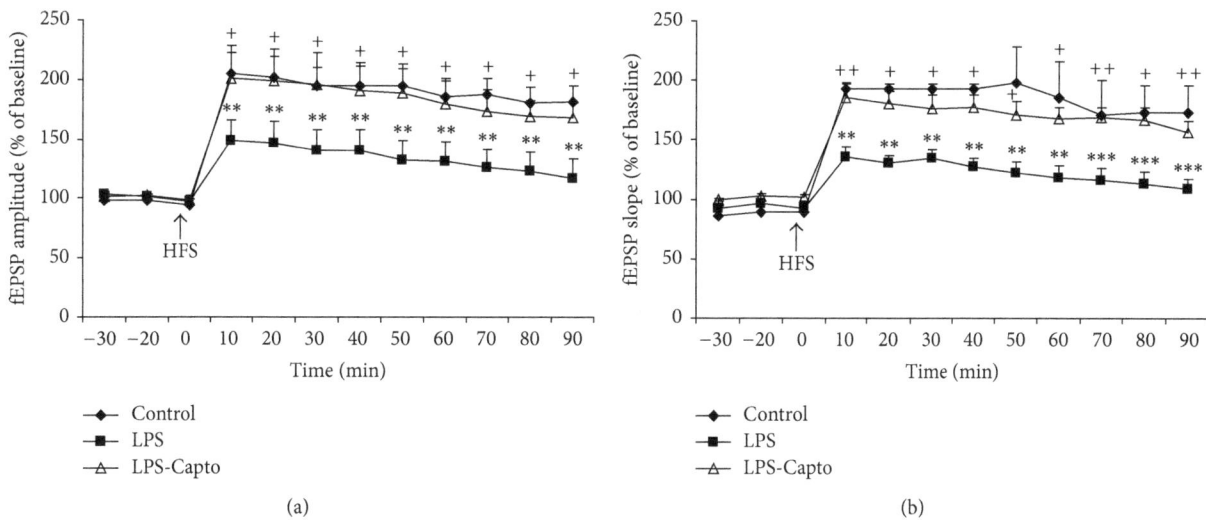

FIGURE 6: The results of LTP induction in CA1 area of the hippocampus using 100 Hz tetanic stimulation at (a) the fEPSP amplitude and (b) the fEPSP slope. Data are presented as the average percentage changes from baseline responses. Each point shows mean ± SEM ($n = 8$ in each group). The amplitude and slope of fEPSP in the LPS group were lower than those in the control group ($^{**}P < 0.01$ and $^{***}P < 0.001$) and in the LPS-Capto group they were higher with respect to the LPS group ($^{+}P < 0.05$ and $^{++}P < 0.01$).

LPS administration also impaired LTP induction in rats' hippocampus which was reflected by decreasing of amplitude (Figure 6(a)) and slope (Figure 6(b)) of fEPSP in the LPS group compared to the control group.

Deleterious effects of LPS on neuronal function such as synaptic plasticity, learning, and memory have been attributed to inflammatory responses and overproduction of proinflammatory cytokines including TNFα and IL-1β [29]. Experimental findings have indicated that serum level of TNFα, IL-1β, and IL-6 increases after LPS administration [14]. In addition, it has been reported that detrimental effects of LPS, IL-1β, and IL-6 on spatial learning and memory are probably mediated by inhibiting LTP induction in the hippocampus [14, 30]. Considering these facts, it seems that an excessive production of proinflammatory cytokines followed by injection of LPS plays an important role in spatial memory and synaptic plasticity deficits caused by LPS in the present study. Supporting this idea, we have previously shown that administration of LPS (1 mg/kg) increases serum TNFα levels [10, 16, 31].

In addition, the results of our study also indicated that intraperitoneal administration of captopril 30 min before LPS diminished harmful effects of LPS on spatial learning and memory and synaptic plasticity. In the current study, behavioral results revealed that the animals of the LPS-Capto group not only had a lower latency (Figure 2) and shorter traveled distance (Figure 3) to find the escape platform in comparison with those of the LPS group but also spent more time (Figure 4) and traveled longer distance (Figure 5) to look for the location of the platform in the target quadrant in probe day. In electrophysiological experiments, administration of captopril also enhanced both the amplitude (Figure 6(a)) and the slope (Figure 6(b)) of fEPSP.

RAS system is one of the neuropeptide systems in the brain that is considered to have some effects on neuronal functions [32]. RAS of the brain has been proposed to be involved in processing of sensory information, learning and memory, and regulation of emotional behaviors [7, 33]. Researches have suggested that an increased level of RAS activity is accompanied with cognitive functions impairments. It has also been reported that injection of Ang II or renin into the CNS disturbs retention of passive avoidance tasks [34]. In addition, Ang II and its specific analogues inhibited LTP induction and spatial learning when administered into the hippocampus [4]. On the other hand, ACE inhibitors such as captopril and perindopril were able to increase conditioned avoidance and habituation memory [1]. It has been demonstrated that intraperitoneal and intracerebroventricular injection of captopril improved cognitive processes in radial 8 arm maze and Y maze paradigms [35]. Sepehri et al. also confirmed that captopril improved spatial memory of aged rats [36]. Captopril was also reported to be able to block trimethyltin-induced spatial memory deficits in rats [37]. According to these facts, an increased level of RAS activity followed by LPS injection which was restored by captopril might be suggested in development of the results of the current study. However, more researches are needed to be done to elucidate this subject. Ability of captopril to pass from brain barrier may elucidate central acting effects of the drug which was seen in the present study [38, 39].

In recent studies, activation of RAS has been exhibited to have a significant proinflammatory action. It has been indicated that locally produced Ang II by inflamed vessels promotes synthesis and secretion of inflammatory cytokines such as IL-6 [40]. The results of previous studies have confirmed that administration of LPS increases RAS activity which is reflected by an enhanced level of Ang II in the plasma of rats [41]. On the other hand, anti-inflammatory effects of certain ACE inhibitors have been reported in both in vivo and in vitro studies [42]. Captopril, as a well-known

ACE inhibitor, has been demonstrated to inhibit LPS-induced inflammatory responses [18]. It has also been reported that pretreatment with captopril suppresses expression of inflammatory cytokines such as TNFα in rabbits [43]. Captopril has also been shown to increase concentration of anti-inflammatory cytokines such as IL-10 [37]. Considering this scientific evidence, improving effects of captopril on spatial memory and synaptic plasticity observed in the present study may be, at least in part, due to inhibition of production of proinflammatory cytokines, which needs, however, to be more evaluated.

Additionally, the reactive oxygen species (ROS) and brain tissues oxidative damage play an important role in learning and memory impairment [44]. The RAS is also proposed to have a crucial implication in induction of ROS [45]. Previous studies indicated that produced Ang II by vascular tissues enhances the production of ROS via activating AT_1 receptors [46]. It has been reported that chronic activation of the brain RAS with sustained generation of Ang II causes cardiovascular remodeling, inflammation responses, and oxidative stress leading to endothelial dysfunction and, finally, disrupts regulation of cerebral blood flow [4]. It has also been documented that age-related cognition deficits are associated with the stimulation of AT_1, reduction of cerebral blood flow, and enhancement of oxidative stress [47]. Previously, we also suggested a role for the brain tissues oxidative damage in memory impairment following peripheral LPS administration [16]. On the other hand, treatment with ACE inhibitors such as captopril has been proposed to enhance the activities of antioxidant enzymes as well as nonenzymatic antioxidant defense [48, 49]. Captopril is able to scavenge free radicals and also is able to inhibit reactive oxygen and nitrogen species production [50]. It has also been reported that captopril pulls up GSH depletion and GSSG formation caused by doxorubicin [51]. Given these facts, it seems that oxidative stress following administration of LPS along with excessive activation of RAS accounted for the development of the results of the present study. It also seems that inhibition of LPS-induced spatial memory and synaptic plasticity impairments by captopril is in part by preventing the brain tissues oxidative damage. However, these mechanisms should be clarified in the future.

In summary, it seems that administration of LPS enhances RAS activity which impairs spatial memory and synaptic plasticity. The results of the present study showed that pretreatment with captopril prevented LPS-induced spatial learning and memory and synaptic plasticity impairments, confirming a relationship between RAS and LPS-induced brain dysfunctions.

Disclosure

The project reported in this paper was part of M.S. thesis.

Competing Interests

The authors have no conflict of interests to declare.

Acknowledgments

The authors would like to thank the Vice Presidency of Research of Mashhad University of Medical Sciences for their financial support.

References

[1] A. Ciobica, W. Bild, L. Hritcu, and I. Haulica, "Brain renin-angiotensin system in cognitive function: pre-clinical findings and implications for prevention and treatment of dementia," *Acta Neurologica Belgica*, vol. 109, no. 3, pp. 171–180, 2009.

[2] J. W. Wright and J. W. Harding, "The brain angiotensin system and extracellular matrix molecules in neural plasticity, learning, and memory," *Progress in Neurobiology*, vol. 72, no. 4, pp. 263–293, 2004.

[3] M. J. McKinley, A. L. Albiston, A. M. Allen et al., "The brain renin-angiotensin system: location and physiological roles," *International Journal of Biochemistry and Cell Biology*, vol. 35, no. 6, pp. 901–918, 2003.

[4] V. L. Bodiga and S. Bodiga, "Renin angiotensin system in cognitive function and dementia," *Asian Journal of Neuroscience*, vol. 2013, Article ID 102602, 18 pages, 2013.

[5] Z. Lenkei, M. Palkovits, P. Corvol, and C. Llorens-Cortès, "Expression of angiotensin type-1 (AT1) and type-2 (AT2) receptor mRNAs in the adult rat brain: a functional neuroanatomical review," *Frontiers in Neuroendocrinology*, vol. 18, no. 4, pp. 383–439, 1997.

[6] P. R. Gard, "The role of angiotensin II in cognition and behaviour," *European Journal of Pharmacology*, vol. 438, no. 1-2, pp. 1–14, 2002.

[7] C. Llorens-Cortes and F. A. O. Mendelsohn, "Organisation and functional role of the brain angiotensin system," *Journal of the Renin-Angiotensin-Aldosterone System*, vol. 3, supplement 1, pp. S39–S48, 2002.

[8] N. Hirawa, Y. Uehara, Y. Kawabata et al., "Long-term inhibition of renin-angiotensin system sustains memory function in aged Dahl rats," *Hypertension*, vol. 34, no. 3, pp. 496–502, 1999.

[9] V. Paul and P. Ekambaram, "Involvement of nitric oxide in learning & memory processes," *Indian Journal of Medical Research*, vol. 133, no. 5, pp. 471–478, 2011.

[10] A. Anaeigoudari, M. Soukhtanloo, M. N. Shafei et al., "Neuronal nitric oxide synthase has a role in the detrimental effects of lipopolysaccharide on spatial memory and synaptic plasticity in rats," *Pharmacological Reports*, vol. 68, no. 2, pp. 243–249, 2016.

[11] H. Shimizu, M. Miyoshi, K. Matsumoto, O. Goto, T. Imoto, and T. Watanabe, "The effect of central injection of angiotensin-converting enzyme inhibitor and the angiotensin type 1 receptor antagonist on the induction by lipopolysaccharide of fever and brain interleukin-1β response in rats," *Journal of Pharmacology and Experimental Therapeutics*, vol. 308, no. 3, pp. 865–873, 2004.

[12] A. Tarkowski, H. Carlsten, H. Herlitz, and G. Westberg, "Differential effects of captopril and enalapril, two angiotensin converting enzyme inhibitors, on immune reactivity in experimental lupus disease," *Agents and Actions*, vol. 31, no. 1-2, pp. 96–101, 1990.

[13] A. C. T. M. Peeters, M. G. Netea, B. J. Kullberg, T. Thien, and J. W. M. Van Der Meer, "The effect of renin-angiotensin system inhibitors on pro- and anti- inflammatory cytokine production," *Immunology*, vol. 94, no. 3, pp. 376–379, 1998.

[14] K. M. Sell, S. F. Crowe, and S. Kent, "Lipopolysaccharide induces memory-processing deficits in day-old chicks," *Pharmacology Biochemistry and Behavior*, vol. 68, no. 3, pp. 497–502, 2001.

[15] E. Tyagi, R. Agrawal, C. Nath, and R. Shukla, "Influence of LPS-induced neuroinflammation on acetylcholinesterase activity in rat brain," *Journal of Neuroimmunology*, vol. 205, no. 1-2, pp. 51–56, 2008.

[16] A. Anaeigoudari, M. N. Shafei, M. Soukhtanloo et al., "Lipopolysaccharide-induced memory impairment in rats is preventable using 7-nitroindazole," *Arquivos de Neuro-Psiquiatria*, vol. 73, no. 9, pp. 784–790, 2015.

[17] H. S. Sharma, "Effect of captopril (a converting enzyme inhibitor) on blood-brain barrier permeability and cerebral blood flow in normotensive rats," *Neuropharmacology*, vol. 26, no. 1, pp. 85–92, 1987.

[18] R. Schindler, C. A. Dinarello, and K.-M. Koch, "Angiotensin-converting-enzyme inhibitors suppress synthesis of tumour necrosis factor and interleukin 1 by human peripheral blood mononuclear cells," *Cytokine*, vol. 7, no. 6, pp. 526–533, 1995.

[19] K. Amirshahrokhi, M. Ghazi-Khansari, A. Mohammadi-Farani, and G. Karimian, "Effect of captopril on TNF-α and IL-10 in the livers of bile duct ligated rats," *Iranian Journal of Immunology*, vol. 7, no. 4, pp. 247–251, 2010.

[20] N. Terrando, A. Rei Fidalgo, M. Vizcaychipi et al., "The impact of IL-1 modulation on the development of lipopolysaccharide-induced cognitive dysfunction," *Critical Care*, vol. 14, no. 3, article R88, 2010.

[21] C. C. Barney, M. J. Katovich, and M. J. Fregly, "The effect of acute administration of an angiotensin converting enzyme inhibitor, captopril (SQ 14,225), on experimentally induced thirsts in rats," *Journal of Pharmacology and Experimental Therapeutics*, vol. 212, no. 1, pp. 53–57, 1980.

[22] D. Kumaran, M. Udayabanu, M. Kumar, R. Aneja, and A. Katyal, "Involvement of angiotensin converting enzyme in cerebral hypoperfusion induced anterograde memory impairment and cholinergic dysfunction in rats," *Neuroscience*, vol. 155, no. 3, pp. 626–639, 2008.

[23] K. Łukawski, T. Jakubus, G. Raszewski, and S. J. Czuczwar, "Captopril potentiates the anticonvulsant activity of carbamazepine and lamotrigine in the mouse maximal electroshock seizure model," *Journal of Neural Transmission*, vol. 117, no. 10, pp. 1161–1166, 2010.

[24] A. H. Swiergiel and A. J. Dunn, "Effects of interleukin-1β and lipopolysaccharide on behavior of mice in the elevated plus-maze and open field tests," *Pharmacology Biochemistry and Behavior*, vol. 86, no. 4, pp. 651–659, 2007.

[25] N. L. Sparkman, L. A. Martin, W. S. Calvert, and G. W. Boehm, "Effects of intraperitoneal lipopolysaccharide on Morris maze performance in year-old and 2-month-old female C57BL/6J mice," *Behavioural Brain Research*, vol. 159, no. 1, pp. 145–151, 2005.

[26] T. V. P. Bliss and G. L. Collingridge, "A synaptic model of memory: long-term potentiation in the hippocampus," *Nature*, vol. 361, no. 6407, pp. 31–39, 1993.

[27] A. J. Cunningham, C. A. Murray, L. A. J. O'Neill, M. A. Lynch, and J. J. O'Connor, "Interleukin-1β (IL-1β) and tumour necrosis factor (TNF) inhibit long-term potentiation in the rat dentate gyrus in vitro," *Neuroscience Letters*, vol. 203, no. 1, pp. 17–20, 1996.

[28] S. Commins, L. A. J. O'Neill, and S. M. O'Mara, "The effects of the bacterial endotoxin lipopolysaccharide on synaptic transmission and plasticity in the CA1-subiculum pathway in vivo," *Neuroscience*, vol. 102, no. 2, pp. 273–280, 2001.

[29] L. M. Thomson and R. J. Sutherland, "Systemic administration of lipopolysaccharide and interleukin-1β have different effects on memory consolidation," *Brain Research Bulletin*, vol. 67, no. 1-2, pp. 24–29, 2005.

[30] W. P. Luk, Y. Zhang, T. D. White et al., "Adenosine: a mediator of interleukin-1β-induced hippocampal synaptic inhibition," *Journal of Neuroscience*, vol. 19, no. 11, pp. 4238–4244, 1999.

[31] A. Anaeigoudari, M. Soukhtanloo, P. Reisi, F. Beheshti, and M. Hosseini, "Inducible nitric oxide inhibitor aminoguanidine, ameliorates deleterious effects of lipopolysaccharide on memory and long term potentiation in rat," *Life Sciences*, vol. 158, pp. 22–30, 2016.

[32] O. von Bohlen und Halbach and D. Albrecht, "The CNS renin-angiotensin system," *Cell and Tissue Research*, vol. 326, no. 2, pp. 599–616, 2006.

[33] I. Haulică, W. Bild, and D. Boişteanu, "Biosynthesis and physio-pharmacological actions of angiotensin peptides: 2. Physio-pharmacological properties," *Revista Medico-Chiruricala A Societatii de Medici si Naturalisti Din Iasi*, vol. 110, no. 2, pp. 384–390, 2006.

[34] S. Inaba, M. Iwai, M. Furuno et al., "Continuous activation of renin-angiotensin system impairs cognitive function in renin/angiotensinogen transgenic mice," *Hypertension*, vol. 53, no. 2, pp. 356–362, 2009.

[35] W. Bild, L. Hritcu, A. Ciobica, V. Artenie, and I. Haulica, "P02-170 Comparative effects of captopril, losartan and PD123319 on the memory processes in rats," *European Psychiatry*, vol. 24, p. S860, 2009.

[36] H. Sepehri, F. Ganji, and F. Bakhshandeh, "Effect of short time captopril administration on spatial memory in aging rats," *Physiology and Pharmacology*, vol. 19, no. 1, pp. 68–75, 2015.

[37] M. H. Skinner, D.-X. Tan, M. Grossmann, M. T. Pyne, and R. K. Mahurin, "Effects of captopril and propranolol on cognitive function and cerebral blood flow in aged hypertensive rats," *Journals of Gerontology, Series A: Biological Sciences and Medical Sciences*, vol. 51, no. 6, pp. B454–B460, 1996.

[38] O. Marson, A. B. Ribeiro, S. Tufik, O. Kohlmann Jr., and O. L. Ramos, "Inhibition of central angiotensin I conversion by oral captopril," *Brazilian Journal of Medical and Biological Research*, vol. 14, no. 1, pp. 73–76, 1981.

[39] S. Kato, K. Itoh, T. Yaoi et al., "Organ distribution of quantum dots after intraperitoneal administration, with special reference to area-specific distribution in the brain," *Nanotechnology*, vol. 21, no. 33, Article ID 335103, 2010.

[40] A. R. Brasier, A. Recinos, and M. S. Eledrisi, "Vascular inflammation and the renin-angiotensin system," *Arteriosclerosis, Thrombosis, and Vascular Biology*, vol. 22, no. 8, pp. 1257–1266, 2002.

[41] R. J. Bolterman, M. C. Manriquez, M. C. Ortiz Ruiz, L. A. Juncos, and J. C. Romero, "Effects of captopril on the renin angiotensin system, oxidative stress, and endothelin in normal and hypertensive rats," *Hypertension*, vol. 46, no. 4, pp. 943–947, 2005.

[42] K. Amirshahrokhi, M. Ghazi-Khansari, A. Mohammadi-Farani, and G. Karimian, "Effect of captopril on TNF-α and IL-10 in the livers of bile duct ligated rats," *Iranian Journal of Immunology*, vol. 7, no. 4, pp. 247–251, 2010.

[43] A. Zagariya, R. Bhat, S. Navale, G. Chari, and D. Vidyasagar, "Inhibition of meconium-induced cytokine expression and cell apoptosis by pretreatment with captopril," *Pediatrics*, vol. 117, no. 5, pp. 1722–1727, 2006.

[44] F. Beheshti, M. Hosseini, M. N. Shafei et al., "The effects of *Nigella sativa* extract on hypothyroidism-associated learning and memory impairment during neonatal and juvenile growth in rats," *Nutritional Neuroscience*, 2016.

[45] K. Husain, W. Hernandez, R. A. Ansari, and L. Ferder, "Inflammation, oxidative stress and renin angiotensin system in atherosclerosis," *World Journal of Biological Chemistry*, vol. 6, no. 3, pp. 209–217, 2015.

[46] M. Pacurari, R. Kafoury, P. B. Tchounwou, and K. Ndebele, "The renin-angiotensin-aldosterone system in vascular inflammation and remodeling," *International Journal of Inflammation*, vol. 2014, Article ID 689360, 13 pages, 2014.

[47] N.-C. Li, A. Lee, R. A. Whitmer et al., "Use of angiotensin receptor blockers and risk of dementia in a predominantly male population: prospective cohort analysis," *British Medical Journal*, vol. 340, Article ID b5465, 2010.

[48] E. M. V. de Cavanagh, F. Inserra, L. Ferder, and C. G. Fraga, "Enalapril and captopril enhance glutathione-dependent antioxidant defenses in mouse tissues," *American Journal of Physiology—Regulatory Integrative and Comparative Physiology*, vol. 278, no. 3, pp. R572–R577, 2000.

[49] A. Abareshi, M. Hosseini, M. N. Shafei, M. H. Boskabady, and H. R. Sadeghnia, *The effects of captopril on behavioral dysfunctions induced by lipopolysaccharide in male rats [M.S. of Physiology]*, School of Medicine, Mashhad University of Medical Sciences, Mashhad, Iran, 2016.

[50] M. Tamba and A. Torreggiani, "Free radical scavenging and copper chelation: a potentially beneficial action of captopril," *Free Radical Research*, vol. 32, no. 3, pp. 199–211, 2000.

[51] H. Niknahad, A. Taghdiri, A. Mohammadi-Bardbori, and A. Rezaeian Mehrabadi, "Protective effect of captopril against doxorubicin-induced oxidative stress in isolated rat liver mitochondria," *Iranian Journal of Pharmaceutical Sciences*, vol. 6, no. 2, pp. 91–98, 2010.

20

Molecular Analysis of Vancomycin-Resistant Enterococci Isolated from Regional Hospitals in Trinidad and Tobago

Patrick E. Akpaka,[1] Shivnarine Kissoon,[1] and Padman Jayaratne[2]

[1]Department of Paraclinical Sciences, Faculty of Medical Sciences, The University of the West Indies, St. Augustine Campus, St. Augustine, Trinidad and Tobago
[2]Department of Pathology and Molecular Medicine, McMaster University, 1280 Main Street W., Hamilton, ON, Canada L8S 4L8

Correspondence should be addressed to Patrick E. Akpaka; peakpaka@yahoo.co.uk

Academic Editor: Gabriel Dimitriou

Geographic spread of vancomycin-resistant enterococci (VRE) clones in cities, countries, or even continents has been identified by molecular techniques. This study aimed at characterizing virulent genes and determining genetic relatedness of 45 VRE isolates from Trinidad and Tobago using molecular tools, including polymerase chain reaction, pulsed-field gel electrophoresis (PFGE), and Random Amplification Polymorphic DNA (RAPD). The majority (84%) of the isolates were *Enterococcus faecium* possessing *van*A gene while the rest (16%) were *Enterococcus faecalis* possessing *van*B. The *esp* gene was found in all 45 VRE isolates while *hyl* genes were found only in *E. faecium* species. The *E. faecium* species expressed five distinct PFGE patterns. The predominant clones with similar or common patterns belonged to clones one and three, and each had 11 (29%) of the VRE isolates. Plasmid content was identified in representative isolates from each clonal group. By contrast, the *E. faecalis* species had one PFGE pattern suggesting the presence of an occult and limited clonal spread. The emergence of VRE in the country seems to be related to intra/interhospital dissemination of an epidemic clone carrying the *van*A element. Therefore, infection control measures will be warranted to prevent any potential outbreak and spread of VRE in the country.

1. Introduction

Vancomycin-resistant enterococci (VRE) were first described in Great Britain in 1988 and shortly afterwards were reported in other European countries and the USA [1, 2]. In Latin America, VRE have been reported in Brazil, Colombia, and Argentina [3]. Several reports of outbreaks and spread in hospitals, communities, nursing homes, and long term care institutions have been documented [3]. Epidemiologic links of VRE clones occurring in different hospitals, countries, and regions have been demonstrated in several places [3]. Understanding disease mechanisms, organism's virulence, and host predisposition must be considered. Enterococcal surface protein encoded by the *esp* gene is a virulence factor found in both *Enterococcus faecalis* and *Enterococcus faecium*. In addition, the presence of the variant *esp* gene in *E. faecium* was reported to be associated with in-hospital spread whereas the hyaluronidase (*hyl*) gene was also regarded as a potential virulence gene associated with invasive disease

[4, 5]. Although the prevalence rate of VRE in Trinidad and Tobago is low, 3.9% [6], there are no molecular analysis or epidemiologic reports of VRE isolates available in the country.

Understanding the molecular epidemiology of VRE is crucial for assessing and implementing infection control measures in any healthcare institution or country [7]. The aim of this study was to detect the phenotypes and genotypes of vancomycin resistance, their plasmid contents, virulence factors, analysis of the *esp* repeat profile, and molecular relatedness among enterococci isolated from hospitals in Trinidad and Tobago. This information may provide the background level of VRE in Trinidad and Tobago and be of help in controlling nosocomial spread if a VRE outbreak occurs.

2. Materials and Methods

The 45 VRE bacterial isolates used for this analysis were those identified among 1,141 enterococcal isolates from previously reported study [6]. These isolates were from five regional hospitals (tagged as A–E) in the country and were identified phenotypically by standard microbiologic laboratory procedures [8]. No duplicate isolates from a single patient were included and there was no history of VRE outbreak during the study period.

The antimicrobial susceptibility tests were performed by the standard disk diffusion method and minimum inhibitory concentration (MIC) determined using the Microscan WalkAway 96 SI (Siemens, USA). *Staphylococcus aureus* ATCC 25923 and *E. faecalis* ATCC 29212 strains were used as controls. The antibiotics ampicillin, ciprofloxacin, levofloxacin, linezolid, nitrofurantoin, penicillin, quinupristin/dalfopristin, rifampicin, tetracycline, and vancomycin included in the Gram-positive panel 20 of the Microscan were tested. The MIC values were interpreted according to approved CLSI breakpoints [9] as previously reported [6]. The MIC values of the enterococcal isolates were as follows for the antibiotics: AMP $\leq 8\,\mu$g/mL; CIP $\leq 1\,\mu$g/mL; LEV $\leq 2\,\mu$g/mL; LZD $\leq 2\,\mu$g/mL; PEN $\leq 8\,\mu$g/mL; Q-D ≤ 1; RIF $\leq 1\,\mu$g/mL; TET $\leq 4\,\mu$g/mL; VAN $\leq 8\,\mu$g/mL.

2.1. Multiplex Polymerase Chain Reaction (PCR).

Determination of glycopeptide resistance genotypes and confirmation of species identification were performed by multiplex polymerase chain reaction (PCR), as previously described by Jayaratne and Rutherford [10]. Briefly, prepared bacteria cells in normal saline mixed in lysis buffer were subjected to PCR amplification in $50\,\mu$L reaction mixtures containing deoxynucleoside triphosphate, two primers (*van*A: forward, 175-GGGAAAACGACAATTGC-191; reverse, 907-GTACAATGCGCCGTTA-891; *van*B: forward, 173-ATG-GGAAGCCGATAGTC-189; reverse, 807-GATTTCGTT-CCTCGACC-791), Taq polymerase, MgCl$_2$, buffer, and H$_2$O.

The samples were subjected to 30 PCR cycles, each consisting of one minute of denaturation at 94°C, one minute of annealing at 58°C, and one minute of elongation at 72°C. PCR products were analyzed by electrophoresis on 1% agarose gels and were stained with ethidium bromide.

A *van*A strain (*E. faecium* ATCC 700221), a *van*B strain (*E. faecalis* ATCC 51299), and a vancomycin susceptible *E. faecalis* (ATCC 29212), 16S rDNA Internal Amplification Control, were run with each set of reactions as quality positive and negative controls (Figure 1).

2.1.1. Pulsed-Field Gel Electrophoresis (PFGE).

Genomic DNA was prepared in agarose plugs as described by Murray et al. and Turabelidze et al. with some modifications [11, 12]. After cell lysis by mutanolysin in lysoenzyme and incubation with proteinase, the DNA was digested with *Sma*I. The PFGE was performed using a contour-clamped homogenous electric field apparatus (CHEF DRIII, Bio-Rad Laboratories, Hercules, CA, USA). Gel images were captured on the Gel Doc imaging system using Quality One Software version 4.4.1 (Bio-Rad Laboratories, Hercules, CA, USA). The resulting banding patterns were analyzed by visual inspection according to previously established criteria [13, 14]. Gel analysis was performed using Bionumerics version 3.5 (Applied Maths, Austin, TX, USA) and cluster analysis was achieved using Dice coefficient and UPGMA.

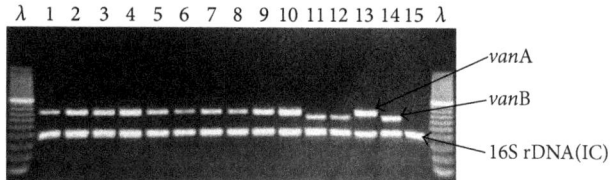

FIGURE 1: Agarose gel electrophoresis of PCR amplified products of vancomycin-resistant enterococci (VRE) isolates obtained from Trinidad and Tobago in 2008 to 2012. Lane λ is the markers. Lanes one–ten represent *van*A positive *E. faecium* and lanes 11 and 12 represent *van*B positive *E. faecalis* from Trinidad and Tobago. Lanes 13–15 represent control strains of *van*A (*E. faecium* ATCC 700221), with *van*B (*E. faecalis* ATCC 51299) and *Enterococcus* vancomycin-sensitive (*E. faecalis* ATCC 29212), and 16S rDNA is the Internal Amplification Control (IC), respectively.

2.1.2. Random Amplified Polymorphic DNA (RAPD)/PCR Amplification.

PCR assays were routinely performed in a $25\,\mu$L reaction mixture containing 20–30 g of genomic DNA, $2.5\,\mu$L 10x buffer, one-unit Taq DNA polymerase, two μmol primer, one mmol each of dCTP, dGTP, dATP, and dTT, and 2.5 mmol MgCl$_2$. AP4 ($5'$ TCA CGC TGC A-$3'$) random primer was used for RAPD. PCR reactions were performed on Perkin Elmer 9600 under the following conditions: 30 cycles of 94°C for one minute, 36°C for one minute, and 72°C for two minutes, with a final extension of 72°C for five minutes. PCR products were run on 1.5% agarose gels and stained with ethidium bromide. DNA ladder (Promega, USA) was used as DNA size markers. AP4 ($5'$ TCA CGC TGC A-$3'$) primers were chosen for RAPD analysis because on PCR they yielded clear patterns [15].

2.1.3. Repetitive-Sequence-Based-PCR (Rep-PCR).

Repetitive-sequence-based-PCR (Rep-PCR) methods are rapid typing procedures that amplify the regions between the noncoding repetitive sequences in bacterial genomes [16]. The ERICIR ($5'$ ATG TAA GCT CCT GGG GAT TCA C-$3'$) was used for Rep-PCR. The genetic relatedness of VRE isolates was determined by Rep-PCR typing as previously described in Healy et al. [17]. DNA was extracted using a one μL loop of plated culture or one mL of broth culture and the Ultraclean Microbial DNA Isolation Kit (Mo Bio Laboratories, Solana Beach, Calif.) following the manufacturer's instructions. The extracted DNA was amplified using the DiversiLab *Enterococcus* fingerprinting (Spectral Genomics, Inc., Houston, TX) according to the manufacturer's instructions. Genomic DNA, the Rep-PCR primer (*Enterococcus*) Ampli*Taq*, and PCR buffer (Applied Biosystems) were all mixed together and subjected to thermal cycling. Amplicons were separated by 1.5% agarose gel electrophoresis (gels, 25 by 25 cm^2) containing ethidium bromide ($3\,\mu$g/mL in gel and in 1x tris-acetate-EDTA running buffer) for six hours at 120 V in a recirculating electrophoresis unit. DNA ladder (Promega, USA) was used as DNA size markers. Gel images were captured on the Gel Doc imaging system using Quality One Software version 4.4.1 (Bio-Rad Laboratories, Hercules, CA, USA).

2.2. Detection of esp and hyl Genes by PCR. The presence of *esp* and *hyl* genes was determined for all 45 VRE isolates by PCR as described by Vankerckhoven et al. [18, 19]. Bacteria cultures grown on Columbia agar (Becton Dickinson, MD) supplemented with 5% sheep blood were incubated at 37°C. Bacterial DNA suspension, 0.1 μm of primer *hyl* and 0.2 μm of *esp* primer including HotStar Taq Master Mixture (Qiagen, Hilden, Germany), Taq DNA polymerase, and deoxynucleoside triphosphates were all subjected to 30 PCR cycles. The PCR products were analyzed by electrophoresis on 1.5% pronarose gel for one hour at 150 V and were stained with ethidium bromide. *E. faecium* strain C68 (hyl_{Efm} and esp_{Efm}) was used as the positive control. A 100 bp DNA ladder (Bio-Rad) was used as a molecular size marker.

2.2.1. Determination of Variation in the esp A and C Repeats. For determining repeat number variations of *esp* A and C repeats, two different primer combinations were used: esp_{fs} 7F-esp_{fm} 5R and esp_{fs} 5F-esp_{fm} 3R, respectively [17]. Briefly, chromosomal DNA was purified as described elsewhere [11]. PCR conditions for all amplification reactions were performed in 25 μL volumes with HotStar Taq Polymerase and HotStar Master Mix buffers (Qiagen Inc., Valencia, CA). Subsequently, the amplicons were subjected to agarose gel electrophoresis (1%) in order to determine their sizes. From the sizes of the amplicons the numbers of repeats were deduced. Amplicon size differences corresponded to multiples of either 252 bp (A repeats) or 246 bp (C repeats).

2.2.2. Determination of Plasmid Content. A subset of isolates representing at least one isolate indicative of each major PFGE pattern was assessed for the presence of the plasmids by the SI nuclease method as described by Barton et al. [20].

3. Results

All 45 VRE isolates used for this analysis and their hospital and facility distribution were from work previously reported [6]. More than half (54%, 24/45) of the VRE isolates were recovered from urogenital tract system infections, and 42.2% (19/45) were from skin and soft tissue infections (Table 1). One isolate each was recovered from blood and gastrointestinal tract, respectively. The GIT isolate was from peritoneal fluid of a patient who had peritonitis. All isolates (100%) were from hospitalized patients and thus represented healthcare-associated isolates and infections. Most (84%, 38/45) of the isolates were *E. faecium* and the rest (16%, 7/45) are *E. faecalis*. All enterococcal isolates had an MIC value for vancomycin $\geq$ 32 μg/mL; they all were 100% susceptible to linezolid. Although only 18% of the *E. faecium* were resistant to quinupristin-dalfopristin but 100% resistant to ciprofloxacin, erythromycin, and levofloxacin, all *E. faecalis* were 100% resistant to ciprofloxacin, erythromycin, levofloxacin, and quinupristin-dalfopristin.

All the *E. faecium* isolates possessed the *van*A genes while all *E. faecalis* possessed the *van*B genes. Overall, the *esp* gene was detected in all (100%) VRE isolates. None of the isolates had *hyl* genes. Analysis of the *esp* repeat profiles produced similar results. The numbers of A and C repeats of the *esp*

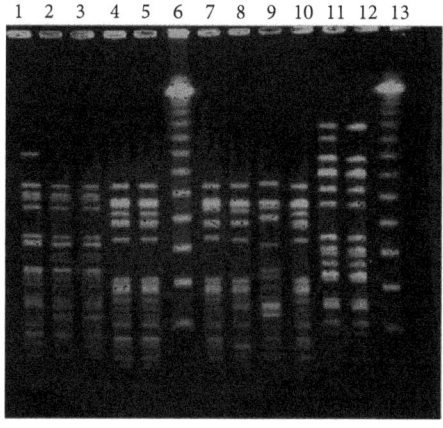

FIGURE 2: *Sma*I PFGE profiles of vancomycin-resistant *E. faecium* from major regional hospitals in Trinidad and Tobago, 2008–2012. Lanes one to five and seven to 12 are representative of vancomycin-resistant *E. faecium* isolates from Trinidad and Tobago regional hospitals. Lambda (λ) DNA PFGE molecular size marker is indicated in marker lanes 6 and 13. Lane one = PFGE-1 or clone one; lanes two and three = PFGE-2 or clone two; lanes four, five, seven, eight, and ten = PFGE-3 or clone three; lane nine = PFGE-4 or clone four; lanes 11 and 12 = PFGE-5 or clone five.

gene seen in the *E. faecium* isolates varied from three to seven and from three to eight, respectively. Based on the *esp* A and C repeat profile, these *E. faecium* isolates belonged to five different groups. The most prevalent *esp* profile was A6-C5 (28.9%, 11/38 isolates), followed by A5-C6 (23.9%, 9/38 isolates), A6-C3 (15.8%, 6/38 isolates), A4-C5 (13.2%, 5/38 isolates), and A5-C7 (10.5%, 4/38 isolates).

3.1. PFGE Typing. The analysis of molecular typing demonstrated five PFGE patterns (Figure 2) among the 38 vancomycin-resistant *E. faecium* isolates. The predominant clones were one and three (PFGE-1 and PFGE-3), and each clone occurred in 11 (29%) isolates, respectively. Clone one was present in two hospitals: "D" and "C" hospitals located in the southern and northern geographic areas of Trinidad. Clone three was present in four of five hospitals, "A," "C," "D," and "E," in the country. Clones two and five (PFGE-2 and PFGE-5) were represented by six (16%) and eight (21%) isolates, respectively, from the two hospitals "C" and "D." Clone four (PFGE-4) had two isolates, one from "C" and the other from "A" hospitals and both from the urogenital tract (UGT). All the seven vancomycin-resistant *E. faecalis* had an identical PFGE pattern indicating they belong to the same clone (PFGE result not shown). The cluster analysis was achieved by the Bionumerics software (Applied Maths, Austin, TX, USA). Percentages of similarity were determined using the Dice correlation coefficient and a dendrogram (Figure 3) was produced via the unweighted pair group method with arithmetic mean clustering (UPGMA).

RAPD produced concordant patterns to PFGE. Five different RAPD and Rep-PCR types were obtained for the 38 *E. faecium* strains. Seven *E. faecalis* isolates showed one Rep-PCR type. The five Rep-PCR types were as follows: type one (29%, 11 isolates), type two (15.8%, 6 isolates), type three

TABLE 1: Showing various pulsed-field gel electrophoresis (PFGE) groups of 45 vancomycin-resistant enterococcal isolates from regional hospitals in Trinidad and Tobago (%).

Source	N	E. faecium					E. faecalis
		PFGE-1	PFGE-2	PFGE-3	PFGE-4	PFGE-5	PFGE
UGT	17 (38)	4	1	6	2	4	7
SSTI	19 (42)	6	4	5	0	4	0
Blood	1	0	1	0	0	0	0
GIT*	1	1	0	0	0	0	0
Total	38	11 (29)	6 (16)	11 (29)	2 (5)	8 (21)	7

N = number of isolates distribution; PFGE = pulsed-field gel electrophoresis pattern signifying the same clone; UGT = urogenital tract; SSTI = skin and soft tissue infections; GIT* = gastrointestinal tract, and this sole isolate was from the peritoneal fluid of a patient who had peritonitis. All seven vancomycin-resistant E. faecalis had an identical PFGE pattern indicating they belong to the same clone.

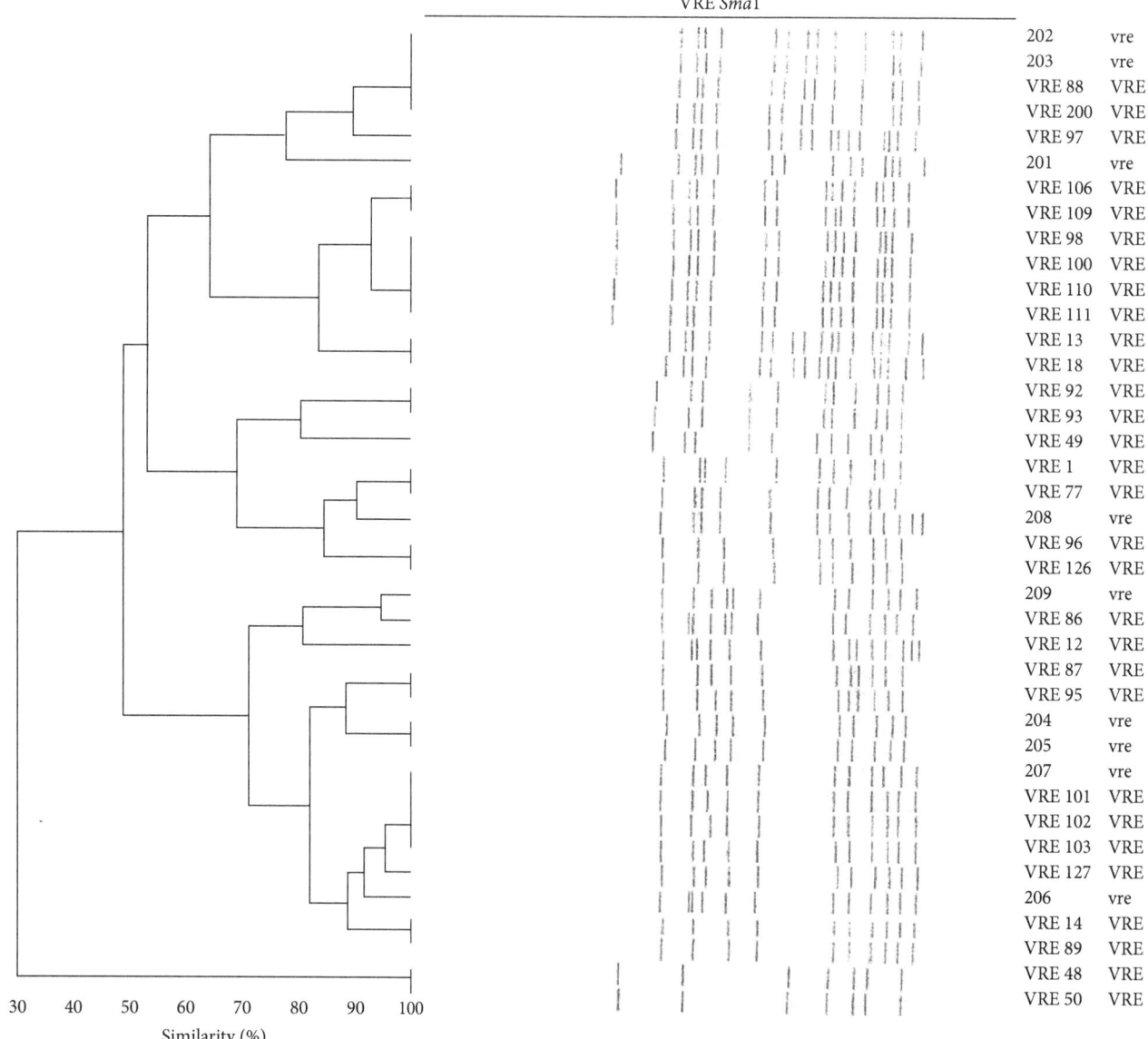

FIGURE 3: Dendrogram of PFGE vancomycin-resistant E. faecium. Molecular typing of vancomycin-resistant E. faecium from regional hospitals in Trinidad and Tobago. The phylogenetic tree was constructed by use of the Dice coefficient and UPGMA clustering; the band tolerance was set at 1.5%, and the threshold cut-off value was set at 85%.

(29%, 11 isolates), type four (5.2%, 2 isolates), and type five (21%, 8 isolates). The vancomycin-resistant *E. faecalis* had one RAPD and Rep-PCR type and all had similar banding patterns. These results were concordant with PFGE types which were visually inspected according to Tenover et al. criteria [13].

3.2. Plasmid Results. Seven VRE isolates representing the various clones and from different hospitals were randomly chosen for plasmid determination. All the isolates examined had at least one plasmid ranging in size from 48.5 kbp to 200 kbp. One isolate from hospital "C" had multiple plasmids.

4. Discussions

In the current study, the genetic characteristics of all vancomycin-resistant enterococci were investigated by PFGE, RAPD, Rep-PCR, and *esp* repeat profiles. Each method had a different ability to analyze the genotypes of VRE isolates.

E. faecium remained as in many countries the most prevalent species among VRE (86% of the isolates) which is similar to reports from North America, Australia, and Italy, where prevalence ranged from 79.5% to 99% [21–23]. The majority of vancomycin-resistant *E. faecium* from this current study were multiply resistant to antibiotics such as ciprofloxacin, erythromycin, levofloxacin, rifampicin, and tetracycline, similar to results from other places [22, 23]. In contrast, vancomycin-resistant *E. faecalis* showed high (100%) resistance to erythromycin, vancomycin, and quinupristin/dalfopristin. Similar results were observed by Corso et al. [3]. This high resistance observed was probably due to prior exposure and high consumption and usage of antibiotics as previously reported [6].

All vancomycin-resistant *E. faecium* isolates in this study were of the *van*A genotype which showed a high vancomycin MIC of ≥32 μg/mL. A similar high vancomycin MIC has been reported in the United States and Europe [24]. The predominance also of *van*A *E. faecium* in our study is similar to findings in Northern Asia, Europe, and the United States [24, 25]. The predominance of *van*B *E. faecalis* in our study is also similar to findings from Australia and Taiwan where *van*B gene is more common [24].

This present study found the *esp* gene to be present in all the 45 VRE isolates. Although reports of *esp* prevalence vary according to region and population, our results are consistent with those of Shankar et al., who found the prevalence of *esp* to be 77% in a sample of *E. faecium* (predominantly *van*A) from eight European countries [5, 26]. Also in the USA, UK, and Spain there have been various prevalence reports ranging from 61% to 70% [26]. The *esp* gene is part of a putative pathogenicity island considered to be a marker for epidemicity and could putatively contribute to the spread of vancomycin-resistant *E. faecium* isolates in hospitals [27–29]. The presence of *esp* genes was not associated with the invasiveness or outbreak potential of VRE. Shankar et al. reported that *esp* genes can be deleted from the pathogenicity island of vancomycin-resistant *E. faecalis* at a high frequency [30]. Oancea et al. also demonstrated that the *esp* gene is transferable by conjugation among enterococcal isolates [31].

The *esp* repeat profiles used to analyze the VRE isolates revealed that the *E. faecium* strains in the different groups had identical *esp* repeat profiles which were relatively stable and this was similar to other studies by Leavis et al. [19]. The *esp* repeat profiles could be utilized to investigate the outbreaks of resistant clones in combination with other genotyping methods [19].

In this study, the PFGE and the *esp* gene repeat profiles showed multiple genotypes of *E. faecium* isolates which were consistent with the result of RAPD and Rep-PCR. The presence of a dominant vancomycin-resistant *E. faecium* clone (clones 1 and 3) in several major hospitals shows that their spread has occurred not only within individual hospitals but also between hospitals of various geographic locations in the country. Other studies have documented the spread of vancomycin-resistant *E. faecium* and *E. faecalis* clones among hospitals [32, 33]. The spread of clones in different institutions in the country may suggest that some strains contain bacterial factors that enhance their spread within hospitals. Some other researchers [5, 28] have identified the *esp* gene encoding a surface protein associated with virulence for *E. faecalis* and *E. faecium* residing on a pathogenicity island. Studies by Harrington et al. support the hypothesis that a combination of vancomycin resistance and the *esp* gene could lead to dissemination of particular clones [34]. The finding of no *hyl* gene in clinical VRE isolates in this current study suggests a low prevalence or nonexistence of this gene in Trinidad and Tobago. This will definitely be a sharp contrast to the prevalence of *hyl* gene that varies from 3% to 71% among European VRE [4, 18].

In our study, molecular typing results indicate the dominant dissemination of vancomycin-resistant *E. faecium* clones one and three in different wards of the same hospital, in different hospitals, and in different cities. The reason for this may be due to the absence of an alert system for patients infected or colonized with vancomycin-resistant enterococci in the hospitals. There are equally no consistent effective screening mechanisms or policies in place for VRE infections or colonization, and all these could contribute to this dissemination. The isolates in this study were polyclonal with two major clones, suggesting a highly diverse population of hospital acquired *E. faecium* strains. This picture can possibly be explained by exchange of a mobile resistance determinant between various enterococci as reported in other places [35–37].

Five different RAPD types were obtained for the 38 vancomycin-resistant *E. faecium* isolates. This demonstrates that *E. faecium* strains could be easily differentiated by RAPD fingerprinting, thus supporting the validity of this fast and accurate technique in studying diversity of *E. faecium* population [38]. This result is in agreement with findings by Quednau et al. (1999) who reported genetic variability within *E. faecium* [39]. During an outbreak, the identity of isolates should ideally be confirmed by two different methods. Although RAPD requires testing of the reproducibility of the patterns, this technique is easier to perform and less time-consuming than other phenotyping or genotyping techniques proposed for enterococci [38, 39]. Therefore, the RAPD method with AP4 plus ERICIR primers is a powerful tool for microbiologists to investigate VRE isolates in cases of nosocomial infection [15].

The Rep-PCR has been reported to have good typeability and reproducibility [17] and has been used to investigate several nosocomial outbreaks [40]. Comparable findings have been reported for Rep-PCR and PFGE for *Acinetobacter baumannii*, *Streptococcus pneumoniae*, and methicillin-resistant *Staphylococcus aureus* (MRSA) [41]. Rep-PCR may be more suitable as a rapid screening method to exclude the possibility of clonal spread and to facilitate prompt intervention for outbreaks, whereas PFGE could be reserved for confirmation. Using both methods simultaneously could be costly. In areas where there is low VRE prevalence and low clonal spread as in this present study, Rep-PCR may be used as an ideal quick screening tool [42]. The isolates analyzed in this study by Rep-PCR and PFGE showed good reproducibility; the Rep-PCR was highly correlated with PFGE typing to evaluate the clonal spread of VRE in this study.

Plasmid analysis has been used for epidemiologic studies of several outbreaks involving aminoglycosides-resistant and β-lactamase producing enterococci [43, 44]. Studies by Dutka-Malen et al. [45] of glycopeptide-resistant enterococci isolates in hospitals in Europe and the United States concluded that the spread of high level resistance (*van*A phenotype) is due to dissemination of a gene rather than a bacterial clone or a single plasmid. Many attempts have been made to show the ability of enterococci to transfer genes encoding for antibiotic resistance with the same or different enterococci species, as well as to other members of other bacteria genera [36]. The plasmid carriage by *E. faecium* identified in this present study appears to be low, limiting the usefulness of plasmid typing of these isolates.

The significantly higher prevalence of VRE in the two regional hospitals, "C" and "D" hospitals, suggests that these hospitals may be at a greater risk of VRE dissemination as there was evidence of high consumption and usage of antibiotics in these institutions [6].

5. Conclusion

This analysis indicates that the prevalence of VRE is low among clinical isolates in the country. Our findings confirm the potential for interhospital spread of VRE and highlight the importance of strengthening the practice of appropriate infection control protocols or early implementation in hospitals in Trinidad and Tobago.

The PFGE, RAPD, and Rep-PCR proved useful in typing vancomycin-resistant enterococci isolates from Trinidad and Tobago. A high prevalence of the *esp* gene was seen among the polyclonal VRE infection isolates and molecular analysis suggests that intra- and interhospital spread of vancomycin-resistant enterococci clone carrying *van*A elements seem to be the main mechanism of vancomycin-resistance dissemination in Trinidad and Tobago.

Continued surveillance activities for VRE are needed to detect early occurrence, dissemination, and corresponding increase in VRE prevalence locally. Further studies such as determination of sequence typing (ST) by multilocus sequence typing (MLST) or multiple-locus variable number tandem repeat analysis (MLVA) are warranted, and carriage rate of VRE among individuals in the country should be investigated.

Ethical Approval

Approval for this study was given by the Institutional Review Ethics Committee of the University of the West Indies, St. Augustine, Trinidad and Tobago. Permission to conduct this study at the various hospital institutions was also obtained.

Consent

No consent was obtained from any patients since data were only extracted from their case notes using codes and there was no way any information obtained would have been related to the patient in this study.

Competing Interests

The authors declare that there is no conflict of interests regarding the publication of this paper.

Acknowledgments

The authors are indebted to the staff at the different laboratory and health facilities where this study was carried out for their support.

References

[1] A. C. Uttley, C. H. Collins, J. Naidoo, and R. C. George, "Vancomycin-resistant enterococci," *The Lancet*, vol. 331, no. 8575-8576, pp. 57–58, 1988.

[2] R. LeClercq, E. Derlot, J. Duval, and P. Courvalin, "Plasmid-mediated resistance to vancomycin and teicoplanin in *Enterococcus faecium*," *The New England Journal of Medicine*, vol. 319, no. 3, pp. 157–161, 1988.

[3] A. C. Corso, P. S. Gagetti, M. M. Rodríguez et al., "Molecular epidemiology of vancomycin-resistant *Enterococcus faecium* in Argentina," *International Journal of Infectious Diseases*, vol. 11, no. 1, pp. 69–75, 2007.

[4] L. B. Rice, L. Carias, S. Rudin et al., "A potential virulence gene, hyl_{Efm}, predominates in *Enterococcus faecium* of clinical origin," *The Journal of Infectious Diseases*, vol. 187, no. 3, pp. 508–512, 2003.

[5] V. Shankar, A. S. Baghdayan, M. M. Huycke, G. Lindahl, and M. S. Gilmore, "Infection-derived *Enterococcus faecalis* strains are enriched in *esp*, a gene encoding a novel surface protein," *Infection and Immunity*, vol. 67, no. 1, pp. 193–200, 1999.

[6] S. Kissoon, P. E. Akpaka, and W. H. Swanston, "Vancomycin resistant enterococci infections in Trinidad and Tobago," *British Microbiology Research Journal*, vol. 9, no. 3, pp. 20–28, 2015.

[7] S. F. Oprea, N. Zaidi, S. M. Donabedian, M. Balasubramaniam, E. Hershberger, and M. J. Zervos, "Molecular and clinical epidemiology of vancomycin-resistant *Enterococcus faecalis*," *Journal of Antimicrobial Chemotherapy*, vol. 53, no. 4, pp. 626–630, 2004.

[8] K. Becker and C. von Eiff, "Staphylococcus, micrococcus, and other catalase-positive cocci," in *MCM*, K. C. Carroll, G. Funke, J. H. Jorgenson, M. L. Landry, and D. W. Warnock, Eds., ASM Press, Washington, DC, USA, 10th edition, 2011.

[9] Clinical and Laboratory Standards Institute, "Performance standards for antimicrobial susceptibility testing," Twenty-Third Informational Supplement M100-S23, Clinical and Laboratory Standards Institute (CLSI), Wayne, Pa, USA, 2013.

[10] P. Jayaratne and C. Rutherford, "Detection of clinically relevant genotypes of vancomycin-resistant enterococci in nosocomial surveillance specimens by PCR," *Journal of Clinical Microbiology*, vol. 37, no. 6, pp. 2090–2092, 1999.

[11] B. E. Murray, K. V. Singh, J. D. Heath, B. R. Sharma, and G. M. Weinstock, "Comparison of genomic DNAs of different enterococcal isolates using restriction endonucleases with infrequent recognition sites," *Journal of Clinical Microbiology*, vol. 28, no. 9, pp. 2059–2063, 1990, Erratum: *Journal of Clinical Microbiology*, vol. 29, pp. 418, 1991.

[12] D. Turabelidze, M. Kotetishvili, A. Kreger, J. G. Morris Jr., and A. Sulakvelidze, "Improved pulsed-field gel electrophoresis for typing vancomycin-resistant enterococci," *Journal of Clinical Microbiology*, vol. 38, no. 11, pp. 4242–4245, 2000.

[13] F. C. Tenover, R. D. Arbeit, R. V. Goering et al., "Interpreting chromosomal DNA restriction patterns produced by pulsed-field gel electrophoresis: criteria for bacterial strain typing," *Journal of Clinical Microbiology*, vol. 33, no. 9, pp. 2233–2239, 1995.

[14] T. L. Bannerman, G. A. Hancock, F. C. Tenover, and J. M. Miller, "Pulsed-field gel electrophoresis as a replacement for bacteriophage typing of *Staphylococcus aureus*," *Journal of Clinical Microbiology*, vol. 33, no. 3, pp. 551–555, 1995.

[15] N. Barbier, P. Saulnier, E. Chachaty, S. Dumontier, and A. Andremont, "Random amplified polymorphic DNA typing versus pulsed-field gel electrophoresis for epidemiological typing of vancomycin-resistant enterococci," *Journal of Clinical Microbiology*, vol. 34, no. 5, pp. 1096–1099, 1996.

[16] Y.-C. Chuang, J.-T. Wang, M.-L. Chen, and Y.-C. Chen, "Comparison of an automated repetitive-sequence-based PCR microbial typing system with pulsed-field gel electrophoresis for molecular typing of vancomycin-resistant *Enterococcus faecium*," *Journal of Clinical Microbiology*, vol. 48, no. 8, pp. 2897–2901, 2010.

[17] M. Healy, J. Huong, T. Bittner et al., "Microbial DNA typing by automated repetitive-sequence-based PCR," *Journal of Clinical Microbiology*, vol. 43, no. 1, pp. 199–207, 2005.

[18] V. Vankerckhoven, T. Van Autgaerden, C. Vael et al., "Development of a multiplex PCR for the detection of asa1, gelE, cylA, esp, and hyl genes in enterococci and survey for virulence determinants among european hospital isolates of *Enterococcus faecium*," *Journal of Clinical Microbiology*, vol. 42, no. 10, pp. 4473–4479, 2004.

[19] H. Leavis, J. Top, N. Shankar et al., "A novel putative Enterococcal pathogenicity island linked to the esp virulence gene of *Enterococcus faecium* and associated with epidemicity," *Journal of Bacteriology*, vol. 186, no. 3, pp. 672–682, 2004.

[20] B. M. Barton, G. P. Harding, and A. J. Zuccarelli, "A general method for detecting and sizing large plasmids," *Analytical Biochemistry*, vol. 226, no. 2, pp. 235–240, 1995.

[21] R. R. S. Nelson, K. F. McGregor, A. R. Brown, S. G. B. Amyes, and H.-K. Young, "Isolation and characterization of glycopeptide-resistant enterococci from hospitalized patients over a 30-month period," *Journal of Clinical Microbiology*, vol. 38, no. 6, pp. 2112–2116, 2000.

[22] G. G. Zhanel, N. M. Laing, K. A. Nichol et al., "Antibiotic activity against urinary tract infection (UTI) isolates of vancomycin-resistant enterococci (VRE): results from the 2002 North

American vancomycin resistant enterococci susceptibility study (NAVRESS)," *Journal of Antimicrobial Chemotherapy*, vol. 52, no. 3, pp. 382–388, 2003.

[23] W. M. Dunne Jr. and W. Wang, "Clonal dissemination and colony morphotype variation of vancomycin-resistant *Enterococcus faecium* isolates in metropolitan Detroit, Michigan," *Journal of Clinical Microbiology*, vol. 35, no. 2, pp. 388–392, 1997.

[24] L. J. Worth, M. A. Slavin, V. Vankerckhoven, H. Goossens, E. A. Grabsch, and K. A. Thursky, "Virulence determinants in vancomycin-resistant *Enterococcus faecium vanB*: clonal distribution, prevalence and significance of esp and hyl in Australian patients with haematological disorders," *Journal of Hospital Infection*, vol. 68, no. 2, pp. 137–144, 2008.

[25] T. M. Coque, R. J. L. Willems, J. Fortún et al., "Population structure of *Enterococcus faecium* causing bacteremia in a Spanish University Hospital: setting the scene for a future increase in vancomycin resistance?" *Antimicrobial Agents and Chemotherapy*, vol. 49, no. 7, pp. 2693–2700, 2005.

[26] X. Zhu, B. Zheng, S. Wang et al., "Molecular characterisation of outbreak-related strains of vancomycin-resistant *Enterococcus faecium* from an intensive care unit in Beijing, China," *Journal of Hospital Infection*, vol. 72, no. 2, pp. 147–154, 2009.

[27] R. J. L. Willems, W. Homan, J. Top et al., "Variant esp gene as a marker of a distinct genetic lineage of vancomycin-resistant *Enterococcus faecium* spreading in hospitals," *The Lancet*, vol. 357, no. 9259, pp. 853–855, 2001.

[28] R. J. L. Willems, J. Top, M. van Santen et al., "Global spread of vancomycin-resistant *Enterococcus faecium* from distinct nosocomial genetic complex," *Emerging Infectious Diseases*, vol. 11, no. 6, pp. 821–828, 2005.

[29] R. J. L. Willems and M. J. M. Bonten, "Glycopeptide-resistant enterococci: deciphering virulence, resistance and epidemicity," *Current Opinion in Infectious Diseases*, vol. 20, no. 4, pp. 384–390, 2007.

[30] N. Shankar, A. S. Baghdayan, and M. S. Gilmore, "Modulation of virulence within a pathogenicity island in vancomycin-resistant *Enterococcus faecalis*," *Nature*, vol. 417, no. 6890, pp. 746–750, 2002.

[31] C. Oancea, I. Klare, W. Witte, and G. Werner, "Conjugative transfer of the virulence gene, esp, among isolates of *Enterococcus faecium* and *Enterococcus faecalis*," *Journal of Antimicrobial Chemotherapy*, vol. 54, no. 1, pp. 232–235, 2004.

[32] H. S. Sader, M. A. Pfaller, F. C. Tenover, R. J. Hollis, and R. N. Jones, "Evaluation and characterization of multiresistant *Enterococcus faecium* from 12 U.S. medical centers," *Journal of Clinical Microbiology*, vol. 32, no. 11, pp. 2840–2842, 1994.

[33] R. Del Campo, C. Tenorio, M. Zarazaga, R. Gomez-Lus, F. Baquero, and C. Torres, "Detection of a single vanA-containing *Enterococcus faecalis* clone in hospitals in different regions in Spain," *Journal of Antimicrobial Chemotherapy*, vol. 48, no. 5, pp. 746–747, 2001.

[34] S. M. Harrington, T. L. Ross, K. A. Gebo, and W. G. Merz, "Vancomycin resistance, esp, and strain relatedness: a 1-year study of enterococcal bacteremia," *Journal of Clinical Microbiology*, vol. 42, no. 12, pp. 5895–5898, 2004.

[35] S. Handwerger and J. Skoble, "Identification of chromosomal mobile element conferring high-level vancomycin resistance in *Enterococcus faecium*," *Antimicrobial Agents and Chemotherapy*, vol. 39, no. 11, pp. 2446–2453, 1995.

[36] R. Son, F. Nimita, G. Rusul, E. Nasreldin, L. Samuel, and M. Nishibuchi, "Isolation and molecular characterization of

vancomycin-resistant *Enterococcus faecium* in Malaysia," *Letters in Applied Microbiology*, vol. 29, no. 2, pp. 118–122, 1999.

[37] M. Quednau, S. Ahrné, and G. Molin, "Genomic relationships between *Enterococcus faecium* strains from different sources and with different antibiotic resistance profiles evaluated by restriction endonuclease analysis of total chromosomal DNA using *Eco*RI and *Pvu*II," *Applied and Environmental Microbiology*, vol. 65, no. 4, pp. 1777–1780, 1999.

[38] J. F. Tomayko and B. E. Murray, "Analysis of *Enterococcus faecalis* isolates from intercontinental sources by multilocus enzyme electrophoresis and pulsed-field gel electrophoresis," *Journal of Clinical Microbiology*, vol. 33, no. 11, pp. 2903–2907, 1995.

[39] N. Woodford, D. Morrison, A. P. Johnson, V. Briant, R. C. George, and B. Cookson, "Application of DNA probes for rRNA and *van*A genes to investigation of a nosocomial cluster of vancomycin-resistant enterococci," *Journal of Clinical Microbiology*, vol. 31, no. 3, pp. 653–658, 1993.

[40] M. L. Bertin, J. Vinski, S. Schmitt et al., "Outbreak of methicillin-resistant *Staphylococcus aureus* colonization and infection in a neonatal intensive care unit epidemiologically linked to a healthcare worker with chronic otitis," *Infection Control and Hospital Epidemiology*, vol. 27, no. 6, pp. 581–585, 2006.

[41] S. Saeed, M. G. Fakih, K. Riederer, A. R. Shah, and R. Khatib, "Interinstitutional and intrainstitutional transmission of a strain of *Acinetobacter baumannii* detected by molecular analysis: comparison of pulsed-field gel electrophoresis and repetitive sequence-based polymerase chain reaction," *Infection Control and Hospital Epidemiology*, vol. 27, no. 9, pp. 981–983, 2006.

[42] C. R. Sherer, B. M. Sprague, J. M. Campos et al., "Characterizing vancomycin-resistant enterococci in neonatal intensive care," *Emerging Infectious Diseases*, vol. 11, no. 9, pp. 1470–1472, 2005.

[43] J. E. Patterson, B. L. Masecar, C. A. Kauffman, D. R. Schaberg, W. J. Hierholzer Jr., and M. J. Zervos, "Gentamicin resistance plasmids of enterococci from diverse geographic areas are heterogeneous," *The Journal of Infectious Diseases*, vol. 158, no. 1, pp. 212–216, 1988.

[44] N. C. Clark, R. C. Cooksey, B. C. Hill, J. M. Swenson, and F. C. Tenover, "Characterization of glycopeptide-resistant enterococci from U.S. hospitals," *Antimicrobial Agents and Chemotherapy*, vol. 37, no. 11, pp. 2311–2317, 1993.

[45] S. Dutka-Malen, S. Evers, and P. Courvalin, "Detection of glycopeptide resistance genotypes and identification to the species level of clinically relevant enterococci by PCR," *Journal of Clinical Microbiology*, vol. 33, no. 1, pp. 24–27, 1995.

Permissions

List of Contributors

Mathias Zink
Central Institute of Mental Health, Department of Psychiatry and Psychotherapy, Medical Faculty Mannheim, HeidelbergUniversity, P.O. Box 12 21 20, 68072Mannheim, Germany

Ruta Sakiene
Lithuanian University of Health Sciences, Medical Academy, Eiveniu 2, LT-50009 Kaunas, Lithuania

Alvita Vilkeviciute
Neuroscience Institute, Lithuanian University of Health Sciences, Medical Academy, Eiveniu 2, LT-50009 Kaunas, Lithuania

Loresa Kriauciuniene and Rasa Liutkeviciene
Neuroscience Institute, Lithuanian University of Health Sciences, Medical Academy, Eiveniu 2, LT-50009 Kaunas, Lithuania
Department of Ophthalmology, Lithuanian University of Health Sciences, Medical Academy, Eiveniu 2, LT-50009 Kaunas, Lithuania

VilmaJurate Balciuniene, Dovile Buteikiene and Goda Miniauskiene
Department of Ophthalmology, Lithuanian University of Health Sciences, Medical Academy, Eiveniu 2, LT-50009 Kaunas, Lithuania

Douglas M. Durrant, Jessica L. Williams and Brian P. Daniels
Department of Internal Medicine, Washington University School of Medicine, Campus Box 8051,660 S. Euclid Avenue, St. Louis, MO 63110, USA

Robyn S. Klein
Department of Internal Medicine, Washington University School of Medicine, Campus Box 8051,660 S. Euclid Avenue, St. Louis, MO 63110, USA
Department of Anatomy and Neurobiology, Washington University School of Medicine, Campus Box 8051, 660 S. Euclid Avenue, St. Louis, MO 63110, USA
Department of Pathology and Immunology, Washington University School of Medicine, Campus Box 8051, 660 S. Euclid Avenue, St. Louis, MO 63110, USA

MeikeVogler
Department of Biochemistry, University of Leicester, Henry-Wellcome Building, Lancaster Road, Leicester LE19HN, UK

Manijeh Kahbazi,Marzieh Ebrahimi, Nader Zarinfar, Mohammad Arjomandzadegan, Taha Fereydouni, Fatemeh Karimiand Amir Reza Najmi
Infectious Diseases Research Centre (IDRC), Arak University of Medical Sciences, Arak, Iran

Manuel López-Cabrera
Centro de Bioloáia Molecular-Severo Ochoa, CSIC, UAM, Cantoblanco, C/Nicolás Cabrera 1, 28049 Madrid, Spain

Zainab Khan, Karim Rahim, Jaspreet S. Rayat, Lin Xing, MunirIqbal, Karim Mohamed and Sanjay Sharma
Department of Ophthalmology, Hotel Dieu Hospital, Queen's University, 166 Brock Street, Kingston, ON, Canada K7L 5G2

Puneet S. Braich
Department of Ophthalmology, Virginia Commonwealth University School of Medicine,401 N. 11th Street, Suite 439, Richmond, VA 23219, USA

David Almeida
Vitreo Retinal Surgery, PA, 7760 France Avenue S., Minneapolis, MN 55435, USA

Dong Joon Lee
Oral and Craniofacial Health Sciences Research, School of Dentistry, University of North Carolina, Chapel Hill, NC 27599-7455, USA

Yonsil Park Wei-Shou Hu
Department of Chemical Engineering and Materials Science, University of Minnesota, Minneapolis, MN 55455-0132, USA

Ching-Chang Ko
Oral and Craniofacial Health Sciences Research, School of Dentistry, University of North Carolina, Chapel Hill, NC 27599-7455, USA
Department of Orthodontics, School of Dentistry, University of North Carolina, Chapel Hill, NC 27599-7454, USA

Loubna Shamseddine
Department of Prosthodontics, Lebanese University, School of Dentistry, P.O. Box 6573/14, Beirut, Lebanon

Farid Chaaban
Faculty of Engineering and Architecture, American University of Beirut, Mazraa-Daybess Street, Ferdawss Building, First Floor, P.O. Box 11-0236, Beirut 1107 2020, Lebanon

Rodney R. Dietert
Department of Microbiology and Immunology, College of Veterinary Medicine, Cornell University, North Tower Road, Ithaca, NY 14853, USA

Meirigeng Qi
Division of Transplantation/Department of Surgery, University of Illinois at Chicago, IL 60612, USA
Department of Diabetes and Metabolic Diseases Research, Beckman Research Institute of the City of Hope, 1500 E. Duarte Road, Duarte, CA 91010, USA

Khalid Abusaada, Fnu Asad-ur-Rahman, Vladimir Pech, Umair Majeed, Shengchuan Dai, Xiang Zhu and Sally A. Litherland
Florida Hospital Internal Medicine Program, Florida Hospital, 601 Rollins Street, Orlando, FL 32803, USA

Alice Zwerling, Sourya Shresthaand DavidW. Dowdy
Johns Hopkins Bloomberg School of Public Health, Baltimore, MD 21205, USA

Paul A. Zandbergen
Department of Geography, University of New Mexico, Albuquerque, NM 87131, USA

D. O. Soyoye, R. T. Ikem and B. A. Kolawole
Department of Medicine, ObafemiAwolowo University, Ile-Ife, Nigeria

K. S. Oluwadiya
Department of Surgery, Ekiti State University, Ado-Ekiti, Nigeria

R. A. Bolarinwa
Department of Haematology and Immunology, ObafemiAwolowo University, Ile-Ife, Nigeria

O. J. Adebayo
Department of Medicine, Federal Medical Centre, Lokoja, Nigeria

SaamMorshed
Department of Orthopaedic Surgery, University of San Francisco School of Medicine, San Francisco, CA 94143-0410, USA

Afshin Mohammad Alizadeh
Department of Bone Marrow Transplantation, Taleghani Hospital, ShahidBeheshtiUniversity of Medical Sciences, Tehran, Iran

Hossein Hassanian-Moghaddam, Nasim Zamani and Mitra Rahimi
Toxicological Research Center, Department of Clinical Toxicology, Loghman-Hakim Hospital, School of Medicine, ShahidBeheshti University of Medical Sciences, Tehran, Iran

Excellence Center of Clinical Toxicology, Iranian Ministry of Health, Tehran, Iran

Mohammad Mashayekhian and Behrooz Hashemi Domeneh
Toxicological Research Center, Department of Clinical Toxicology, Loghman-Hakim Hospital, School of Medicine, ShahidBeheshti University of Medical Sciences, Tehran, Iran

Peyman Erfantalab
Toxicological Research Center, Department of Clinical Toxicology, Loghman-Hakim Hospital, School of Medicine, ShahidBeheshti University of Medical Sciences, Tehran, Iran
Department of Emergency Medicine, School of Medicine, Iran University of Medical Sciences, Tehran, Iran

Ali Ostadi
Toxicological Research Center, Department of Clinical Toxicology, Loghman-Hakim Hospital, School of Medicine, ShahidBeheshti University of Medical Sciences, Tehran, Iran
Department of Internal Medicine, School of Medicine, Tabriz University of Medical Sciences, Tabriz, Iran

Emeka B. Kesieme
Department of Surgery, Irrua Specialist Teaching Hospital, PMB 8, Irrua, Edo State, Nigeria

Peter O. Okokhere and Christopher OjemiegaIruolagbe
Department of Medicine, Irrua Specialist Teaching Hospital, PMB 8, Irrua, Edo State, Nigeria

Angela Odike
Department of Paediatrics, Irrua Specialist Teaching Hospital, PMB 8, Irrua, Edo State, Nigeria

Clifford Owobu
Department of Pathology, Irrua Specialist Teaching Hospital, PMB 8, Irrua, Edo State, Nigeria

TheophilusAkhigbe
Department of Radiology, Irrua Specialist Teaching Hospital, PMB 8, Irrua, Edo State, Nigeria

Azam Abareshi, Mohammad NaserShafei and Mahmoud Hosseini
Neurocognitive Research Center, Faculty of Medicine, Mashhad University of Medical Sciences, Mashhad, Iran

Akbar Anaeigoudari
Department of Physiology, School of Medicine, Jiroft University of Medical Sciences, Jiroft, Iran

Fatemeh Norouzi
Department of Physiology, Esfarayen Faculty of Medical Sciences, Esfarayen, Iran

Mohammad Hossein Boskabady and MajidKhazaei
Neurogenic Inflammation Research Center, Faculty of Medicine, Mashhad University of Medical Sciences, Mashhad, Iran

Patrick E. Akpaka and Shivnarine Kissoon
Department of Paraclinical Sciences, Faculty of Medical Sciences, The University of theWest Indies, St. Augustine Campus, St. Augustine, Trinidad and Tobago

Padman Jayaratne
Department of Pathology and Molecular Medicine, McMaster University, 1280 Main Street W.,Hamilton, ON, Canada L8S 4L8

Index

Lightning Source UK Ltd.
Milton Keynes UK
UKHW05n0847250518
323150UK00002B/147/P